Preface to the Third Edition

In the nine years since the Second Edition of this book was published, a number of changes have occurred. Almost imperceptibly new information on fluorides in caries prevention has built up consistently over the past 11 years, to such an extent that there was a chance that if we didn't try to update our knowledge now, the opportunity would be lost.

New information on the metabolism of fluoride has become available. Rather than try to update this part of the book ourselves, we decided to ask Professor-Emeritus G. N. Jenkins to join us to improve the chapters on physiology, toxicity and mode of action of fluoride. We were delighted when he agreed to help us with the present edition.

There have been changes too in the publishing world. John Wright became Wright PSG and then in 1986 came under the umbrella of Butterworths. It was decided that the Third Edition should be developed as a book in its own right rather than continue as one of the Dental Practitioner Series. We are most grateful to Ms Lucy Sayer of Butterworths for encouraging us to embark on this edition.

Newcastle upon Tyne, 1991

J.J.M.
A.J.R.-G.
G.N.J.

Preface to the Second Edition

In an age when so many dental textbooks have a multiplicity of authors, I was pleased to have the opportunity, in 1976, to draw together my own thoughts on fluorides in caries prevention. One reviewer wrote that he hoped the book would be kept up to date, but added that it would be 'a labour of Hercules'. I was delighted when Andrew Rugg-Gunn agreed to join me in attempting the Second Edition, and hope that our efforts have produced a more comprehensive summary of the effects of fluoride on dental caries.

One of the major developments in fluoride therapy since the publication of the First Edition has been the increasing use of combinations of types of fluoride used to prevent caries, either as part of the care of the individual patient or in community preventive schemes. This aspect has been expanded in this edition and examples given of fluoride-based schemes which have been implemented at the community level in some areas of the world. The number of countries operating water fluoridation schemes has expanded and these are now brought together in a new chapter.

Newcastle upon Tyne, 1982

J.J.M.
A.J.R.-G.

Fluorides in caries prevention

Third Edition

J. J. Murray PhD, MChD, FDS RCS (Eng.), MCCD RCS (Eng.)
Professor and Head, Department of Child Dental Health, Dental School, University of Newcastle upon Tyne
Formerly Reader and Honorary Consultant, Department of Children's Dentistry, Institute of Dental Surgery, Eastman Dental Hospital

A. J. Rugg-Gunn *RD*, PhD, DSc, BDS, FDS RCS (Edin.)
Professor of Preventive Dentistry, Departments of Child Dental Health and Oral Biology, Dental School, University of Newcastle upon Tyne

G. N. Jenkins PhD, DSc, DOdont, FDS RCS (Eng.)
Emeritus Professor, Oral Physiology, University of Newcastle upon Tyne

Wright

Wright
An imprint of Butterworth-Heinemann Ltd
Linacre House, Jordan Hill, Oxford OX2 8DP

 PART OF REED INTERNATIONAL BOOKS

OXFORD LONDON BOSTON
MUNICH NEW DELHI SINGAPORE SYDNEY
TOKYO TORONTO WELLINGTON

First published by John Wright & Sons Ltd 1976
Second edition 1982
Third edition published by Butterworth-Heinemann Ltd 1991

British Library Cataloguing in Publication Data
Murray, John J.
Fluorides in caries prevention. – 3rd ed.
I. Title II. Rugg-Gunn, A.J.
III. Jenkins, G.N.
617.6

ISBN 0 7236 2363 5

Library of Congress Cataloguing in Publication Data
Murray, John J.
Fluorides in caries prevention. – 3rd ed./J.J. Murray, A.J.
Rugg-Gunn, G.N. Jenkins.
p. cm.
Includes index.
ISBN 0 7236 2363 5:£25.00
1. Dental caries–Prevention. 2. Fluorides–Therapeutic use.
3. Fluorides–Physiological effect. I. Rugg-Gunn, A. J.
II. Jenkins, G. Neil (George Neil) III. Title.
[DNLM: 1. Dental Caries–prevention & control. 2. Fluoridation.
3. Fluorides, Topical–therapeutic use. WU 270 M982f]
RK331.M85 1991
617.6′7052–dc20
DNLM/DLC
for Library of Congress 91-13785
CIP

Composition by Genesis Typesetting, Laser Quay, Rochester, Kent
Printed and bound in Great Britain by The University Press, Cambridge

Preface to the First Edition

Any clinical therapy must have a firm rational basis for its application. If a supposed caries-inhibitory agent is to be used clinically, its effectiveness must be confirmed by carefully controlled clinical trials, the results of which have been confirmed by several independent investigators. In addition, dentists, although being predominantly concerned with the effects of treatment at the individual dentist–patient level, also have the responsibility of appreciating the effectiveness of measures designed to reduce the prevalence of dental caries within the community.

The main aim of this book is to present the evidence concerning the clinical effectiveness of fluoride, in its various forms, as a caries-inhibitory agent. The first four chapters of the book are concerned with the systemic administration of fluoride; the next five chapters consider the effect of fluoride applied topically in toothpaste, prophylactic paste, solutions, gels, varnishes and mouth rinses. The final three chapters are concerned with the physiology and toxicity of fluoride and with the possible mechanisms by which fluoride exerts its caries-preventive effect.

London, 1975 J.J.M.

Acknowledgements

The changes and additions incorporated in this edition could not have been achieved without help and encouragement from a number of people. The enthusiasm of Mr P. D. Stocker and his perseverance in tracing the early history of fluoridation provided the stimulus to the information included in Chapter 1. Information on fluoride levels in water supplies in England and Wales was collated by Miss S. R. Bickley and Professor Lennon in 1988 and first published in *Community Dental Health* in 1989. We are indebted to the Editor, Professor P. M. C. James, for granting us permission to reproduce this information.

The update on fluoride dentrifrices was made possible by contact with Mr S. Hartley (Procter and Gamble), Mr T. G. H. Davies (Colgate-Palmolive), Dr R. Chesters (Unilever) and Mr A. G. McGree (Beecham Products). Their help is greatly appreciated.

Most of the references concerning the effectiveness of Duraphat Fluoride Varnish were provided by Mr D. Glover for a lecture given by one of the authors in 1986, which forms the basis of the information included in Chapter 11.

Permission to reproduce the Water (Fluoridation) Act 1985 was granted by HMSO. Our thanks go also to the Editors of *Acta Odontologica Scandinavica, Archives of Oral Biology, British Dental Journal, Caries Research, Community Dentistry and Oral Epidemiology, Community Health, Fluoride Drinking Water, Helvetica Odontologica Acta, Journal of the American Dental Association, Journal of Dental Research, Journal of Pathology and Bacteriology*, and *Scandinavian Journal of Dental Research*, and to Blackwell Scientific Publications, Professor I. J. Moller, Charles C. Thomas, Publishers, University of Chicago Press, and the World Health Organisation, for permission to reproduce illustrations. We are especially grateful to Dr W. Driscoll and the Editor of the *Journal of the American Dental Association* for the provision of Plates 1–6, and to Professor O. Fejerskov and Munksgaard Publishers, Copenhagen, for providing Plates 7–12. Appropriate acknowledgement is made in the text.

We are indebted to Miss Louise Carter and Mrs Karen Khan, who have been responsible for the secretarial work involved in compiling the current edition, and to Mr Bob Pearson for his meticulous checking of our manuscript.

Finally, we dedicate this book to Valerie, Diane and Olive.

Contents

Chapter 1

Fluoride and dental health in the nineteenth century

According to Arnold (1957) the early interest in fluoride appeared to be concerned with the content of fluoride in bones. In 1802, Morozzo described a fossilized elephant; a couple of years later the fluoride content of this animal's tooth was determined. In 1805, Morichini found fluoride in human enamel, although for many years there was much controversy as to the presence or absence of fluoride in bones and teeth, depending on the chemical methods used. Fluorine is said to have been discovered by the chemist Scheele in 1771, but not isolated until 1886 by Moissan (West, Selby and Hodgman, 1964). Ficinus reported his belief in the presence of fluoride in enamel and dentine in 1847 and Fremy found fluoride in fresh bones, bone powders and bone ash in 1855.

Arnold (1957) cites a reference to Berzelius, who in 1822 suspected that fluoride was present in water. Probably the first reference to the presence of fluoride in water in Britain was made by Wilson (1846), who reported the presence of calcium fluoride in one of the wells of Edinburgh (supplying the brewery of Mr Campbell in the Cowgate, behind Minto House). He believed he was the first to detect fluoride in sea water, where, by using the bittern or mother liquor of the salt pans in which water from the Firth of Forth is evaporated, he found calcium fluoride present 'in most notable quantity'. In 1849, Wilson reported an experiment on the hard crust which collects at the bottom and sides of the boilers used in the evaporation of sea water from the Firths of Forth and Clyde. The crust or deposit consisted mainly of 'sulphate of lime, and carbonate of lime and magnesia, as well as sodium chloride'. However, when sulphuric acid was poured on the specimens it gave off hydrochloric, carbonic and hydrofluoric acid which caused glass to corrode. He concluded that 'From what is known of the comparative uniformity in composition of sea water, it may safely be inferred, that if fluorine be present in the waters of the Firths of Forth and Clyde, and in the German Ocean, it will be found universally present in the sea' (Wilson, 1849). By the latter part of the nineteenth century the presence of fluoride and its possible role in tissue physiology was vaguely evident to some investigators. Probably the first report of fluoride concentration in drinking water quoted in parts per million was given by Hillebrand (1893) (Table 1.1). He reported a value of 5.2 ppm F (10.7% as calcium fluoride) in water from a thermal spring in New Mexico.

It is difficult to determine when the first association between fluoride and teeth was made. Desirabode in 1847 referred to fluates (which is presumed to mean fluoride); he mixed 'equal parts of siliciate or fluate of lime and alumine, dried and pulverized, with a sufficient quantity of water to form it into a homogeneous paste;

Table 1.1 Water from Ojo Caliente, New Mexico – A Thermal Spring near Taos (Analysis by W. F. Hillebrand, 1893. In parts per million)

Found		*Hypothetical combination*		*Per cent total solids*
SiO_2	60.2	LiCl	20.9	0.62
SO_2	151.0	KCl	59.9	1.76
PO_4	0.2	NaCl	305.5	9.01
CO_3	2153.5	$Na_2B_4O_7$	5.4	0.16
B_4O_7	4.2	Na_2SO_4	233.3	6.59
Cl	231.4	Na_2CO_3	1846.9	54.49
F	5.2	$Ca_3P_2O_8$	0.3	0.01
Fe_2O_3*	1.6	CaF_2	10.7	0.32
Al_2O_3	0.5	$CaCO_3$	43.0	1.27
Ca	22.8	$SrCO_3$	2.4	0.07
Sr	1.4	$MgCO_3$	33.2	0.98
Mg	9.5	SIO_2	60.2	1.78
K	31.4	Fe_2O_3	1.6	0.05
Na	995.1	Al_2O_3	0.5	0.01
Li	3.4	CO_2 bicarb.	775.6	22.88
	3671.4		3399.4	100.00

* State of oxidation unknown. Fe_2O_3 all sediment.

The water also contains traces of arsenic, nitrates, iodine (?), barium, and ammonium. No organic matter. Titanium, bromine, manganese, and sulphides were looked for but not found.

this is introduced into the cavity and its desiccation favored by the approach of a heated instrument'.

The first reference to a prophylactic role for fluoride may well have been made by Erhadt in 1874. In a contribution to *Memorabilia* – a monthly publication in German for 'rational physicians' – he reported:

> As, for a long time, Iron was given for the blood, Calcium and Phosphorus for the bones, so has it been successful to add Fluoride to the tooth enamel in a soluble and absorbable form. It is Fluoride that gives hardness and durability to the tooth enamel and protects against caries.
>
> Fluoride pills were recommended in England, in the form of Potassium Fluoride, an easily soluble salt which in small doses does not disturb the gastro-intestinal tract. Potassium Fluoride must be given for months, and it comes in a pleasant tasting form as 'Hunter's Pills', of which one is taken daily. These pills have special application during 'change of teeth' in children and in women during pregnancy, when teeth frequently suffer.

Another German, Dr A. Denninger gave a lecture entitled 'Fluoride: an agent to combat dental disease and perhaps also appendicitis' to the Rhenish Natural Science Society in Mainz in 1896. He summarized existing knowledge in the following way:

> Fluorine is an element which is close to chlorine, bromine and iodine and, most frequently bound to calcium, occurs as calcium fluoride in minerals. Absorbed by the roots of plants, it reaches fruits, tubers and foliage and through these the bodies of animals. The bones and particularly the enamel of teeth contain demonstrable quantities of fluorine, which of course can also occur by direct

uptake of fluorine-containing particles of earth and dust, as contaminations of food. The tooth enamel protects the softer dentine from small organisms, bacteria etc. which cause diseases in the dentine when the enamel is injured. The stronger the enamel layer, the better protected the tooth. The tiny quantities of fluorine which are available for uptake in vegetables, do not seem to be sufficient to form a powerful enamel layer. The administration of calcium fluoride is simple and cheap; it is sufficient if one takes a few specks of finely powdered calcium fluoride daily with meals; for more idle persons a chemist's shop in Mainz keeps dosed pills.

The lack of fluorine in foodstuffs still seems to be a very important factor in the cause of dental diseases. To prove this, of course, is not easy. To make a large number of analyses of soil and foodstuffs, to start investigations into the teeth of people in separate districts as well, would be a very difficult job that could not be carried out by an individual. However, experiment offers better prospects. Eighteen years ago the author took a fairly large quantity of calcium fluoride daily to determine whether this powder had harmful effects or not. After a year's use, however, the harmlessness of calcium fluoride having been established, it was possible to bring others into the experiment. Children in particular were able to provide the best information and suitable and willing subjects were found. Although improvement in the teeth of elderly people could hardly be expected, it was still possible to ascertain a good result in this respect as well. The teeth were significantly stronger, and in addition to greater hardness the teeth show a greater capacity for resistance. More important, however, were trials in children. During pregnancy several women ingested calcium fluoride daily. The teeth of the children born to these women were good without exception, and the mothers retained all their teeth in full health. A mother's body did not need to supply fluorine since enough was present in the food. But in case of older children who received fluorine too, the dental formation was really good, in some it was even magnificent. Now many years have gone by, and a large number of persons, particularly children receive calcium fluoride on medical and dental prescription with great benefit for their teeth.

Let us briefly summarize the main points of this presentation. In our foodstuffs there is usually not enough fluorine for strong tooth enamel. Therefore diseases of the teeth occur. To nourish the teeth correctly, finely powdered calcium fluoride, fluorspar, should be taken. Buy 100 g of finely powdered fluorspar (price 10 to 30 pfennigs) in a suitable shop (drug, materials supply stores etc.) and take some, first daily, then after about two weeks only every two to four days, later on a small quantity at even longer intervals.

Pindborg (1965) and Hunsfadbraten (1982) both refer to a pamphlet published in 1902 by Cross and Co. in Copenhagen, Denmark, entitled 'Fluoridens. How to Remedy the Decay of our Teeth'. The Danish Apothecary Society analysed the tablets and found they contained 83.7% calcium fluoride.

The text of the brochure (Figures 1.1 and 1.2) stated that various substances were essential for the health of the teeth, above all fluorine. In England this preparation was mixed with table salt in the proportion of 1 teaspoon of Fluoridens to 2 tablespoons of table salt. In this way all members of the family had their daily doses of fluorine without any special effort. It was felt it was never too late to combat the decay of the teeth, even though it was understood that the best results were achieved when fluorine was given regularly to children. The author of the Danish

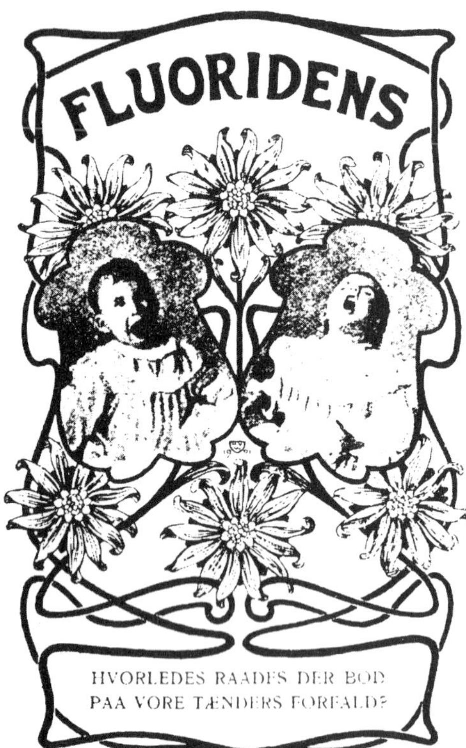

Figure 1.1 Front cover of a leaflet, 'Fluoridens: How to Remedy the Decay of Our Teeth', c.1902 (Pindborg, 1965)

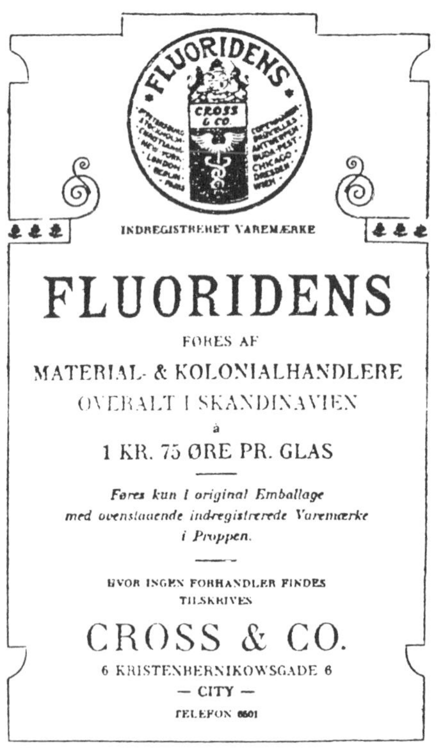

Figure 1.2 Back cover of a brochure from Cross and Co., advertising Fluoridens, c.1902 (Hunsfadbraten, 1982)

brochure recommended that mothers sprinkle Fluoridens on the popular open sandwiches which children took to school. Pregnant and nursing women were also urged to take their daily doses. The author of the pamphlet maintained that 'the decay of the teeth was due mainly to the refined foodstuffs which do not contain a sufficient quantity of fluorine. However, no dentist is in doubt that the teeth should contain fluorine and that this element is of great importance to the enamel, which is the shield and protector of the teeth against all pernicious influences'.

The importance of fluorine was emphasized by Sir James Crichton Browne in an address to the Eastern Counties Branch of the British Dental Association in 1892:

> I would name to you, as a specific cause of the increase of dental caries, a change that has taken place in a food stuff of a particular kind, and of primary importance. I mean bread, the staff of life, from which, in the progress of civilisation, the coarse elements – and the coarse elements consist of the outer husks of the grains of which it is composed – have been eliminated. In as far as our own country, at any rate, is concerned, this is essentially an age of white bread and fine flour, and it is an age therefore in which we are no longer partaking to anything like the same amount that our ancestors did of the bran or husky parts of wheat, and so are deprived to a large degree of a chemical element which they received in abundance, namely, fluorine. The late Dr George Wilson

showed that fluorine is more widely distributed in nature than was before his time supposed; but still, as he pointed out, it is but sparingly present where it does occur, and the only channels by which it can apparently find its way into the animal economy is through the siliceous stems of grasses and the outer husks of grain in which it exists in comparative abundance. But analysis has proved that the enamel of the teeth contains more fluorine in the form of fluoride of calcium than any other part of the body, and fluorine might, indeed, be regarded as the characteristic chemical constituent of this structure – the hardest of all animal tissue, and containing 95.5 per cent of salts against 72 per cent in the dentine. I think it well worthy of consideration whether the re-introduction into our diet, and especially into the diet of child-bearing women and of children, of a supply of fluorine in some suitable natural form – and what can be more suitable than that in which it exists in the pellicles of our grain stuffs? – might not do something to fortify the teeth of the next generation.

In 1908 the *British Dental Journal*, under the heading 'Calcium fluoride in therapeutics' gave over half a page to an abstract from a French pharmaceutical journal on fluoride dosages. The article referred to the beneficial effect of fluoride in the healing of bone fractures and stated that it was 'generally recognized' that fluoride is necessary for the health of teeth. A powder prescribed by A. Robin included magnesium and calcium carbonate, calcium triphosphate, calcium fluoride and one gram of white sugar(!) Brissemort (1908) reported that the administration of 5 mg of calcium fluoride, 15 days a month, had a marked influence in arresting dental caries.

Thus it can be seen that the use of fluorides for dental purposes began in the nineteenth century. The first entirely speculative ideas led to the development of fluoride-containing pills in the 1890s. This aspect of fluoride and dental health then lay dormant for over 40 years.

References

Arnold, F. A. Jr (1957) *A Brief History of the Research on the Role of Fluorides to Dental Health*, Publication No. WHO/DH/7, Expert Committee on the Public Health Aspects of Water Fluoridation, World Health Organisation, Geneva

Brissemort (1908) *L'Union Pharm.*, **49**, 352 (cited in Miscellanea: calcium fluoride in therapeutics. *Br. Dent. J.* (1909), **29**, 1155–1156)

British Dental Association (1908) *Lindsay Club Newsl.*, no. 14

Crichton Browne, Sir J. (1892) An address on tooth culture. *Lancet* **2**, 6–10

Denninger, A. (1896) Fluoride: an agent to combat dental disease and perhaps also appendicitis. *Rundsch. Prometheus,* **50**, 795–796

Desirabode, M. (1847) *Complete Elements of the Science and Art of the Dentist*, 2nd edn, American Society of Dental Surgeons, Baltimore, p. 285

Erharde, A. (1874) Kali Fluoratum zur Erhaltung der Zahne. *Memorabilien ans der Praxis,* **19**, 359–360

Ficinus, R. (1847) Ueber das Ausfallen der Zähne und das Wesen der Zahnkaries. *J. Chirurg. Augenheilk* [ns], 6.1

Fremy, E. (1855) Recherches chimiques sur les os. *Ann. Chim. Phys.*, **43**, 47

Hillebrand, W. F. (1893) Water from Ojo Caliente, New Mexico. *Bull. U.S. Geol. Surv.,* **113**, 114

Hunsfadbraten, K. (1982) Fluoride in caries prophylaxis at the turn of the century. *Bull. Hist. Dentist.*, **30**, 117–120

Morichini, D. (1805) Analisi dello smalto di un dente fossile di elefante e dei denti umani. *Mem. Mat. Fis. Soc. Italiana Sci.,* **12**, pt 2, 73

Morozzo, C. L. (1802) Notice sur un squelette d'un gros animal trouvé aux environs de Rome par le comte Morozzo. *J. Phys.,* **54**, 441

Pindborg, J. J. (1965) En Dansk Fluorideringspjece Fra 1902. *Tandlaegebladet,* **69**, 557–561

West, R. C., Selby, S. M. and Hodgman, C. D. (1964) *Handbook of Chemistry and Physics*, 45th edn, Chemical Rubber Co., Cleveland, Ohio

Wilson, G. (1846) On the solubility of fluoride of calcium in water and the relation of this property to the occurrence of that substance in minerals and in recent and fossil plants and animals. *Proc. Roy. Soc. Edinb.,* **2**, 91

Wilson, G. (1849) On the presence of fluorine in the waters of the Firth of Forth, the Firth of Clyde and the German Ocean. *Chem. Gax.,* **7**, 404

Further reading

Berzelius, J. (1807) Analyse der Knochen. *J. Chem. U. Phys.,* **3**, 1

Berzelius, J. (1822) Estrait d'une lettre de M. Berzelius à M. Berthollet. *Ann. Chim. Phys.,* **21**, 246

Berzelius, J. (1823) *Untersuchung der Mineral-Wässer von Karlsbad, von Teplitz und Konigswart*, Leipzig, 126 pp.

Cawson, R. A. and Stocker, I. P. D. (1984) The early history of fluorides as anticaries-agents. *Br. Dent. J.,* **157**, 403–404

Churchill, H. V. (1931) Occurrence of fluorides in some water of the United States. *Ind. Eng. Chem.,* **23**, 996–998

Middleton, J. (1844) On fluorine in recent and fossil bones and the sources from which it is derived. *Mem. Proc. Chem. Soc.,* **2**, 134

Middleton, J. (1845) On fluorine in bones, its source and its application to the determination of the geological age of fossil bones. *Q. J. Geol. Soc. Lond.,* **1**, 214

Murray, M. M. and Wilson, D. C. (1942) Distribution of fluorosis in India and in England. *Nature,* **144**, 155

Nicklès, M. J. (1857) Recherches sur la diffusion du fluor. *Compt. Send.,* **45**, 331

Silliman, B., Jr (1846) On the chemical composition of the calcareous corals. *Am. J. Sci. Arts*, 2nd ser., **1**, 189

Smith, H. V. and Smith, M. C. (1931) Mottled enamel in Arizona and its correlation with the concentration of fluorides in water supplies. *Bull. Ariz. Agric. Exp. Stn*, no. 32

Stocker, I. D. P. (transl.) (1988) *Deutsche Zahnarzliche Wochenschrift* (1907), **10**, 196–198

Wilson, D. C. (1939) Distribution of fluorosis in India and in England. *Nature,* **144**, 155

Wilson, D. C. (1941) Fluorine and dental caries. *Lancet,* **1**, 375

Wilson, G. (1850) On the presence of fluorine in blood and milk. *Edinb. New Phil. J.,* **49**, 227

Wilson, G. (1857) On M. J. Nicklès claim to be the discoverer of fluorine in the blood. *Proc. Roy. Soc. Edinb.,* **3**, 463

Chapter 2

A history of water fluoridation

Colorado Stain

The history of fluoridation is more than 80 years old. It started with the arrival of Dr Frederick McKay in Colorado Springs, Colorado, USA, in 1901, the year following his graduation from the University of Pennsylvania Dental School. He soon noticed that many of his patients, particularly those who had lived in the area all their lives, had an apparently permanent stain on their teeth, which was known to the local inhabitants as 'Colorado Stain'. McKay checked the lecture notes he had saved from dental school but found nothing to describe such markings, nor could he find any reference to them in any of the available scientific literature. He called the stain 'mottled enamel' and said that it was characterized by:

> Minute white flecks, or yellow or brown spots or areas, scattered irregularly or streaked over the surface of a tooth, or it may be a condition where the entire tooth surface is of a dead paper-white, like the colour of a china dish. (McKay, 1916a.)

The first systematic endeavour to investigate this lesion was made by the Colorado Springs Dental Society in 1902.

> At that time it was generally supposed that a limited area of territory, measured by a comparatively short radius of miles, was the only area affected, and as a first step toward defining its limits, a series of letters were addressed to dentists practising in various portions of the Rocky Mountain region. The answers received brought very little information of value and the matter of further investigation was allowed to rest for the next six years. (McKay, 1916a.)

In 1905, McKay moved to St Louis to practise orthodontics. He stayed there for three years, during which time he never saw a case of mottled enamel, whereas in Colorado Springs he saw cases every day. He returned to Colorado in 1908 and the stain problem struck him with more force than ever. At the May 1908 meeting of the El Paso County Odontological Society, McKay revived the question. After hearing his talk, the society sent him, together with a patient whose teeth bore the markings of the stain, to the annual meeting in June of the State Dental Association in Boulder. McKay exhibited the patient and, though dentists showed a passing interest in the problem, he learned of similar conditions in several other towns. The dentists in these towns, unimpressed by an almost universal condition, had not bothered to report the stain (Minutes of Colorado Springs Dental Society, 1908).

By showing an actual case of Colorado Stain to dentists from all over the State, McKay scattered the seeds of interest beyond the borders of his recently adopted home. As a result of the meeting in Boulder, McKay decided that, first, he needed help from a recognized dental research worker and, secondly, he needed to define the exact geographical area of the stain – the endemic area. To attain his first objective he approached one of America's foremost authorities on dental enamel, Dr Greene Vardiman Black, Dean of the Northwestern University Dental School in Chicago. At first Black thought that McKay was mistaking the stain for something else. He could scarcely believe there could be a dental lesion affecting so many people which still remained unmentioned in the dental literature. Black asked that some of the mottled teeth be sent to him for examination (Black, 1916). He agreed to attend the Colorado State Dental Association meeting in July 1909, and promised to spend some weeks in Colorado Springs before the annual meeting.

In preparation for this visit, and as a first step in mapping out the entire endemic area, McKay and a fellow townsman, Dr Isaac Binton, examined the children in the public schools of Colorado Springs. In all they inspected 2945 children and discovered to their complete astonishment that 87.5 per cent of the children native to the area had mottled teeth (McKay, 1916a). For the first time investigators had statistical data detailing the prevalence of the lesion in the community. This new information was given to Black when he arrived in Denver, in June 1909, to tour the Colorado Springs area. Black addressed the State Dental Association meeting: he described the histological examination of the lesion and recounted his personal observations noted during the several weeks he had been touring the Rocky Mountain area. His interest, together with his authority and prestige, raised the study of the problem from the status of a local curiosity to that of an investigation meriting the earnest concern of all dental research workers. Black's histological findings were published in a paper entitled: 'An endemic imperfection of the enamel of the teeth heretofore unknown in the literature of dentistry' (Black, 1916).

The endemic area

Despite Black's involvement other dentists were unimpressed and showed little enthusiasm for carrying on the investigation. It was left to McKay to sustain the study by his persistent interest. His Colorado Springs survey had shown that almost nine out of ten of the native children had mottled teeth: he began searching for other endemic areas. His travels took him up and down the creek valleys of the mountainous region and out onto the nearby plains. He examined children living in Pueblo, Maniton, La Junta, Cripple Creek, Woodland Park and Great Mountain Falls. A few trips convinced McKay that the phenomenon called 'mottling' was much more widespread than he had thought. Slowly, too, McKay began to get help from other dentists in the country. As a result of a short article by Dr Black in the newspaper *Dental Brief*, a Dr W. H. Arthur wrote a letter to the newspaper describing the condition in a town in one of the Southern States on the Atlantic seaboard. The letter was brought to the notice of McKay by a dental nurse, Mrs Mayhall, and he immediately wrote to Dr Arthur requesting information. The reply, dated 18 April 1912, described the classic picture of mottled enamel: the condition was confined to a 'small circumscribed geographical area, it was confined exclusively to children and young people born in the territory, but not to any set or class of people'. (McKay, 1916b.)

Another dentist, Dr Rice, reported the stain at Smavillo, Texas, and donated two incisor teeth from that district which exactly corresponded in appearance with those from previously studied districts (McKay, 1916c). McKay was greatly helped by Dr Joseph Murphy, medical supervisor of the US Indian Service, who instructed his field dentists to examine and report on the prevalence of mottling among the Indians in all schools under his jurisdiction. From as far away as Tacoma, Washington, Rapid City, South Dakota and Mojave City, Arizona, McKay received reports which broadened the boundaries of the endemic areas (McKay, 1916d).

The horizons were broadened still further when, in 1912, McKay discovered that people from parts of Naples in Italy also had stained teeth. He came across an article written in 1902 by Dr J. M. Eager, a United States Marine Hospital Service surgeon stationed in Italy, who reported that a high proportion of certain Italian emigrants embarking at Naples had a dental peculiarity known locally as *denti di Chiaie* (Eager, 1902). Some of these Italians had ugly brown stains on their teeth; others had a fine horizontal black line crossing the incisor teeth. McKay heard that a young doctor, Dr J. F. McConnell from Colorado Springs, was planning a holiday in Italy, and asked him to examine some Naples children and report back. The doctor was familiar with the stain in Colorado Springs and wrote back from Naples that there was no doubt that the mottled teeth in Naples were the same as those being investigated by McKay (McKay, 1916c).

Mottled enamel and dental caries

Throughout this period the energy and enthusiasm which kept McKay going was generated by a desire to find out the cause of mottling so that some means might be found of preventing the unsightly stains on people's teeth. The histological investigations by Black (1916) showed that in mottled teeth there was a failure of the cementing substance of the enamel. One would have expected that imperfect, hypocalcified enamel would have decalcified more readily than normal enamel. However, throughout his investigations, McKay was struck by the fact that caries experience was no higher in mottled teeth. In 1916 he wrote:

> This mottled condition, in itself, does not seem to increase the susceptibility of the teeth to decay, which is perhaps contrary to what might be expected, because the enamel surface is much more corrugated and rougher than normal enamel. (McKay, 1916a.)

This contradiction must have been in the back of McKay's mind throughout the whole period of his research. He expressed it more forcibly in a paper to the Chicago Society on 17 April 1928:

> Mottled enamel is a condition in which the enamel is most obviously and unmistakably defective. In fact it is the most poorly calcified enamel of which there is any record in dental literature. If the chief determining factor governing the susceptibility to decay is the integrity or perfection of the calcification of enamel, then by all the laws of logic this enamel is deprived of the one essential element for its protection. . . . In spite of this the outstanding fact is that mottled enamel shows no greater susceptibility to the onset of caries than does enamel that may be considered to have been normally or perfectly calcified. This statement is made as a result of extensive observations and examinations of

> several thousand cases during the past years. . . . My testimony has been supplemented by that of others, who report that these mottled enamel cases, in the various districts, are singularly free from caries. One of the first things noted by Dr Black during his first contact with an endemic locality was the singular absence of decay, and it can hardly be said that his faculty for observations was superficial. (McKay, 1928.)

Mottled enamel: aetiological factors

Yet in the forefront of McKay's mind all the time was the desire to determine the cause of mottled enamel. He established that the occurrence of mottled enamel was localized in definite geographical areas. Within these endemic areas a very high proportion of children were affected; only children who had been born and lived all their lives in an endemic area had mottled enamel; children who had been born elsewhere and brought to the district when 2 to 3 years of age were not affected. The condition was not affected by home or environment factors; families whether rich or poor were affected. This factor tended to eliminate diet as an aetiological factor. McKay observed that three cities in Arkansas, where mottling occurred, although separated from each other by some miles, all received their water supply from one source, Fountain Creek. This, together with many other reports, led him to believe that something in the water supply was responsible for mottled enamel.

> Even from the very beginning of the notice taken of this lesion and before any definite steps were taken to study it, the sentiment of both the profession and the laity in the areas of susceptibility was that the water was in some way responsible. Indeed it was hardly possible to mention this condition without at once encountering a question, and often a dogmatic assertion, indicating the water as the cause. (McKay, 1916b.)

Further evidence supporting the water-supply hypothesis came from a dentist, Dr O. E. Martin, practising in Britton, South Dakota. On reading McKay's 1916 article in the *Dental Cosmos*, he felt that McKay's description of mottling sounded suspiciously like the blemishes he had seen on certain local children and asked for McKay's advice. McKay visited Britton in October 1916. He discovered that in 1898 Britton had changed its water supply from individual shallow wells to a deep-drilled artesian well. Without exception, McKay found that all those who had passed through childhood prior to the changing of the water supply had normal teeth, while natives who had grown up in Britton since 1898 had mottling. He concluded that some mysterious element in the water supply was responsible (McKay, 1918).

So convinced was he that something in the water supply was reponsible for causing mottling, that McKay persuaded a community to change its water supply solely because of the existence of a dental abnormality. The town was Oakley, Idaho, a tiny frontier village 75 miles north-west of Great Salt Lake. In 1908 the community had constructed a pipeline from a warm spring 5 miles out of town. A few years after they began using the water from this source, people began to notice that their children's teeth had a peculiar brownish discoloration. In contrast, children in neighbouring communities seemed to have normal teeth. By 1923, the mothers of the town were so concerned that, with the help of the local dentist, they initiated a survey of children attending the local schools. They found that every child who had been born and lived in the town since 1908 had mottled teeth (McKay, 1925). The mothers of the town demanded action. They appointed a committee and appealed to Dr McKay to visit the town to support them in their efforts to raise a $35 000 bond issue to change the water supply. Several influential townspeople thought the water theory was absurd. They asked the proponents that if they were so certain the present water supply was the cause of the mottling, how could they predict that a different supply would not do the same thing? McKay gave a lecture on his findings in other areas to a mass meeting in the community. Recalling the incident some years later he wrote:

> It was a source of regret to be unable to give any definite answer to the most important question; of a proper substitute for the then existing water supply at Oakley, but I did state that the most valuable and conclusive evidence that could be obtained would be to locate individuals who had spent the years of enamel development in contact with a contemporary source of a new supply. The condition of their enamel would determine the question more definitely than any other means at our disposal. (McKay, 1933.)

Located near Oakley was Carpenter Spring, which had a different water supply; 4 children raised on this water had normal teeth free from brown stain. This meagre information was sufficient to sway the officials of Oakley and they voted to lay a new pipeline to bring water from Carpenter Spring, which was opened on 1 July 1925. The climax came 7½ years later in February 1933 when McKay again examined the teeth of Oakley children. Of 24 children born in Oakley following the change in water supply, none had any brown stain in those permanent teeth which had erupted (McKay, 1933).

A similar occurrence was reported in the town of Bauxite, a community formed in 1901 to provide homes for employees of the Republic Mining and Manufacturing Company, a subsidiary of the Aluminium Company of America (ALCOA). The first domestic water supply to Bauxite came from shallow wells and springs, but in 1909 a new source of water was obtained from a 297 ft (90 m) well. A practising dentist, Dr F. L. Robertson, of nearby Benton, reported to the State Board of Health that the younger citizens of Bauxite seemed to have badly stained teeth, whereas children living in Benton had normal teeth. The State health officer made a formal request to the US Public Health Service in Washington to examine the children living in Bauxite and Benton. In 1928 the US Public Health Service asked Dr McKay to accompany Dr Gromer Kempf, one of their medical officers, to carry out the examinations. They found that no mottling occurred in people who grew up on Bauxite water prior to 1909, but all native Bauxite children who used the deep-well water after that date had mottled teeth. No individual whose enamel developed during residence in Benton had mottled teeth. They reported that the standard water analysis of Bauxite water 'throws little light whatever on the probable causal agent' (Kempf and McKay, 1930). Another piece of evidence had been gathered, but McKay seemed no closer to the solution.

Mottled enamel and fluoride concentration in the drinking water

The answer was now close at hand. In New Kensington, Pennsylvania, the chief chemist of ALCOA, Mr H. V. Churchill, read Kempf and McKay's paper and was greatly disturbed. Certain people in the USA were condemning the use of aluminium-ware for cooking. ALCOA mined most of its aluminium supply from Bauxite: if the story of the stain in Bauxite got into the hands of those who claimed that aluminium cooking utensils caused poisoning, ALCOA would have to reply to the charge. When Churchill received a sample of Bauxite water he instructed Mr A. W. Petrey, head of the testing division of the ALCOA laboratory, to look for traces of rare elements – those not usually tested for. Petrey ran a spectrographic analysis and noted that fluoride was present in Bauxite water at a level of 13.7 parts per million (ppm). Churchill wrote to McKay on 20 January 1931:

> We have discovered the presence of hitherto unsuspected constituents in this water. The high fluorine content was so unexpected that a new sample was taken with extreme precautions and again the test showed fluorine in the water. (Churchill, 1931a.)

He also asked McKay to send samples of water from other endemic areas with a 'minimum of publicity'. McKay quickly arranged for dentists in Britton, South Dakota, Oakley, Idaho and Colorado Springs to send samples of the water in their areas. The results of these analyses were published in 1931:

Location of sample	*Fluorine as fluoride* (ppm)
Deep Well, Bauxite, Ark.	13.7
Colorado Springs, Colo.	2.0
Well near Kidder, S. Dak.	12.0
Well near Lidgerwood, N. Dak.	11.0
Oakley, Idaho	6.0

Churchill emphasized the fact that no precise correlation between the fluoride content of these waters and the mottled enamel had been established. All that was shown was the presence of a hitherto unsuspected common constituent of the waters from the endemic areas (Churchill, 1931b).

Confirmation of Churchill's findings came from a husband and wife team, working at the Arizona Agricultural Experiment Station, Dr Margaret Cammack Smith, head of the nutrition department, and Howard V. Smith, agricultural chemist. They observed that mottled enamel occurred in residents of St David and decided to try to produce mottled enamel experimentally in rats. Their first experiment, with ordinary diet and water taken from St David, was a failure. In their next experiment they concentrated St David water to one-tenth of its original volume by boiling and within a week a difference was noted – the rats' incisor teeth lost translucency. Within a month the enamel was 'strikingly dull, white in appearance and pitted' (Smith, 1931). A review of the literature revealed that a report had been written in 1925 on the effect of additions of fluorine to the diet of rats on the quality of their teeth (McCollum *et al.*, 1925). The Arizona workers then carried out further experiments, feeding sodium fluoride to rats in amounts equalling 0.025%, 0.1% and 0.5% of the diet. The characteristic enamel defects which developed in the rats were so strikingly similar to those produced by the feeding of the residue from St David water that no one could fail to associate the two (Smith, 1931). An analysis of St David water supply was carried out and showed that the fluoride concentration was 3.8–7.2 ppm. Further analyses of 185 public and private water supplies in Arizona were carried out – the fluoride concentration varied from 0.0 to 12.6 ppm fluoride (Smith and Smith, 1931).

An abstract of Churchill's work appeared on 10 April 1931 in the *Industrial and Engineering Chemistry, News Edition*. His complete report was published in the September issue of the journal. Only three weeks after Churchill's preliminary report had been published, Margaret Cammack Smith presented her findings to the Tucson Dental Association at a dinner on 2 May 1931. After nearly 30 years, the solution to McKay's problem had been obtained by two independent workers, reaching the same conclusion within a few days of one another.

Mottled enamel in the United Kingdom

McKay's work had not gone unnoticed in the UK. Reference to McKay's and Black's articles in *Dental Cosmos* of 1916 had been made in the fifth edition of Colyer's *Dental Surgery and Pathology* (London, Longmans) which was required reading for all dental students of that time. One such dental student was Norman Ainsworth.

> Having read this [account of mottled teeth] as a dental student I regret to say that I forgot it, together with a great many other paragraphs in that volume, immediately after qualifying. When I was a student in Middlesex Hospital in 1921, I chanced to be given charge of a girl patient, aged 15, in one of the surgical wards and noticed that her teeth showed a very unusual appearance. They were curiously opaque and flecked with brownish black spots. It appeared that many other people in her home town, Maldon, Essex, were affected in the same way, and it was generally supposed that the drinking water was responsible. I fear that I had already forgotten Rocky Mountain mottled teeth, but the condition was so unusual that I made a mental note that I would look for a chance to verify the girl's statements. A year later I undertook a tour of council schools in various parts of England and Wales for the Dental Diseases Committee of the Medical Research Council, and remembering the incident I arranged that Maldon should be included. (Ainsworth, 1933.)

The MRC report was published in 1925 (*Special Report Series*, no. 97). Ainsworth examined 4258 children aged 2–15 years attending 36 schools in England and Wales. He visited two schools in Maldon, examining 202 children aged 5–15 years. His results showed that, taking all children, the percentage of permanent teeth with dental caries was 13.1%. Considering Maldon children only, the percentage was 7.9%. Ainsworth was particularly interested in the prevalence of mottling in Maldon children. He recorded that of 134 children who were lifelong residents of Maldon, 125 showed mottling. He concluded:

> The distribution of the stain . . . points to an outside origin for the stain, either atmospheric or in the water, since these are precisely the surfaces most exposed to air and fluid in the acts of speaking and drinking respectively. My own view, and it is little more than a guess, is that the cause of both mottling and stain will be found in some quality or impurity of the drinking water not ascertainable by ordinary analytical methods. (Ainsworth, 1928.)

At this time Ainsworth had not read Black's and McKay's (1916) accounts of mottled teeth in America. When he did so he knew that 'the similarity between my own description and theirs is so striking in every detail as to leave no reasonable doubt that the conditions are identical' (Ainsworth, 1933). Ainsworth read the reports by Churchill showing that water from endemic areas contains fluorides in quantities varying from 2 to 13 ppm and wanted to test the Maldon water fluoride concentration.

> I will not weary you with the last stage. Public authorities are slow-moving bodies, and in the end I paid a surprise visit to Maldon with a car and a crate of Winchester quart bottles. They were filled at the various pumping stations in the district and, as a control, one from the drinking water of Witham, a town a few miles distant, which I had already found to be immune, though the water supply was declared exactly similar by the county analyst. The National Physical Laboratory, at my request, had already worked out a method of measuring minute quantities of fluorine in water, and they found that they could be reasonably sure by using de Boer's colorimetric method of attaining an accuracy of 0.1 part per million. Using this method, they tested the five samples and reported that, whereas Witham water contained 0.5 parts of fluorine per million, the water from the four endemic areas contained 4.5–5.5 parts per million. (Ainsworth, 1933.)

The significance of Ainsworth's contribution was that he gave statistical data showing that caries experience in a fluoride area was lower than average. McKay had stressed that mottled teeth had a caries rate no higher than normal teeth.

'Shoe leather survey'

The study of the relationship between fluoride concentration in drinking water, mottled enamel and dental caries was given an impetus by the decision of Dr Clinton T. Messner, Head of the US Public Health Service, in 1931, to assign a young dental officer, Dr H. Trendley Dean, to pursue full-time research on mottled enamel. Dean was responsible for the research unit within the US Public Health Service and was the first dental officer of the service to be given a non-clinical assignment. His first task was to continue McKay's work and to find the extent and geographical distribution of mottled enamel in the USA. He sent a questionnaire to the secretary of every local and state dental society in the country asking if mottled enamel existed in their areas and if so how extensive was it and from what source was the drinking water obtained. Out of 415 questionnaires distributed, 207 replied. In cases where Polk's Dental Register (1928) failed to show a dentist practising in a county, the questionnaire was sent to the county health officer, and in a few cases to local physicians. In all, 1197 of these individual questionnaires were sent and 632 replies were received. As a result of this investigation Dean reported that there were 97 localities in the country where mottled enamel was said to occur and this claim had been confirmed by a dental survey. There were a further 28 areas referred to in the literature where mottled enamel was said to be endemic, but no confirmatory dental surveys had yet been carried out, and there were 70 areas which had been reported by questionnaires but which had not yet been confirmed by extensive surveys (Dean, 1933).

Many of these confirmatory surveys were carried out by Dean himself. He started in Courtland, Virginia, and then followed with examinations in North Carolina, Tennessee and Illinois. Dean and his colleagues referred to the investigations as 'shoe leather epidemiology'. His travels gave Dean a very clear

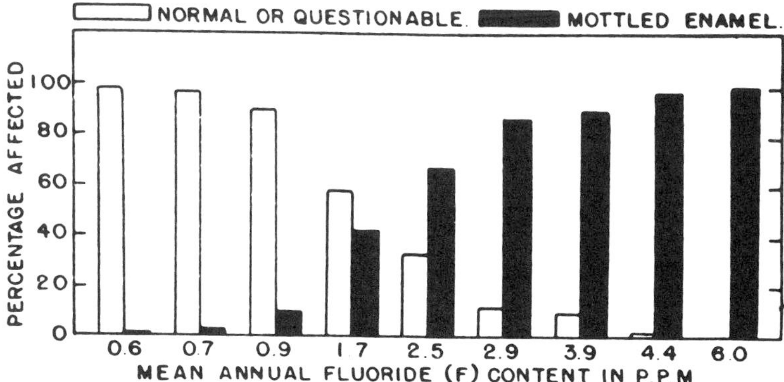

Figure 2.1 Prevalence of mottled enamel in areas with differing concentrations of fluoride in the water supply (From Dean, 1936; reproduced from *Fluoride Drinking Waters*, edited by McClure, F. J., by kind permission of the US Department of Health, Education and Welfare, 1962)

picture of the variations in mottling which could occur. He developed a standard of classification of mottling in order to record quantitatively the severity of mottling within a community (Dean, 1934) so that he could relate the fluoride concentration in the drinking water to the severity of mottling in a given area. His aim was to find out the 'minimal threshold' of fluorine – the level at which fluorine began to blemish the teeth. He showed conclusively that the severity of mottling increased with increasing fluoride concentration in the drinking water (Dean and Elvove, 1936; Dean, 1936). His results are expressed diagrammatically in Figure 2.1. He concluded that:

> From the continuous use of water containing about one part per million, it is possible that the very mildest form of mottled enamel may develop in about 10 per cent of the group. In waters containing 1.7 or 1.8 parts per million the incidence may be expected to rise to 40 or 50 per cent, although the percentage distribution of severity would be largely of the 'very mild' and 'mild' types. (Dean, 1936.)

Dean continued his studies into the relationship between the severity of mottled enamel and the fluoride concentration in the water supply. He presented additional evidence to show that amounts of fluoride not exceeding 1 ppm were of no public health significance (Dean and Elvove, 1936). On 25 October 1938, in conjunction with Frederick McKay, he summarized the knowledge of mottled enamel in a paper to the Epidemiology Section of the American Public Health Association. He reported that in the USA there were now 375 known areas, in 26 states, where mottled enamel of varying degrees of severity was found. He also stated that the production of mottled enamel had been halted at Oakley, Idaho, Bauxite, Arkansas, and Andover, South Dakota, simply by changing the water supply, which contained high concentrations of fluoride, to one whose fluoride concentration did not exceed 1 ppm. This information was 'the most conclusive and direct proof that fluoride in the domestic water is the primary cause of human mottled enamel' (Dean and McKay, 1939). The publication of this information brought to a successful conclusion McKay's search for the cause of mottled enamel which began in Colorado Springs in 1902 and lasted for almost 40 years.

Dental caries prevalence in natural fluoride areas

The story of fluoridation now entered a new and, from a public health point of view, a most important phase. Dean was aware of the reports from the literature that there may be an inverse relationship between the level of mottling and the prevalence of caries in a community. He knew of McKay's observations, first made in 1916, that mottled enamel was no more susceptible to decay than normal enamel. He had read Ainsworth's report in 1933 that caries experience in the high fluoride area was markedly lower than caries experience in all other districts examined. During his study to determine the minimum threshold of mottling, Dean had, in some cities, also examined the children for dental caries. Taking a selected sample of 9-year-old children, he found that of 114 children who had continuously used a domestic water supply comparatively low in fluoride (0.6–1.5 ppm) only 5, or 4%, were caries-free. On the other hand, of the 122 children who had continuously used domestic water containing 1.7–2.5 ppm F, 27 (22%) were caries-free. He concluded: 'Inasmuch as it appears that the mineral composition of the drinking water may have an important bearing on the incidence of dental caries in a community, the possibility of partially controlling dental caries through the domestic water supply warrants thorough epidemiological-chemical study'. (Dean, 1938.)

To test further the hypothesis that an inverse relationship existed between endemic dental fluorosis and dental caries, a survey of four Illinois cities was planned. The cities were Galesburg and Monmouth (water supply contained 1.8 and 1.7 ppm F, respectively), and the nearby cities of Macomb and Quincy (water supply contained 0.2 ppm F). Altogether 885 children, aged 12–14 years, were examined. The results were clear: caries experience in Macomb and Quincy was more than twice as high as that in Galesburg and Monmouth (Dean *et al.*, 1939).

This study paved the way for a much larger investigation of caries experience of 7257 12–14-year-old children from 21 cities in four States. The results are shown diagrammatically in Figure 2.2 and depict with startling clarity the association between increasing fluoride concentration in the drinking water and decreasing caries experience in the population. Furthermore this study showed that near maximal reduction in caries experience occurred with a concentration of 1 ppm F in the drinking water. At this concentration, fluoride caused only 'sporadic instances of the mildest forms of dental fluorosis of no practical aesthetic significance' (Dean, Arnold and Elvove, 1942).

In the UK, a natural fluoride area was discovered as a result of children being evacuated from an industrial area because of World War II. In 1941, Robert Weaver was told by Mr Irvine, Senior School Dentist for Westmorland, that children evacuated to the Lake District from South Shields, on the mouth of the River Tyne, 'had remarkably good teeth – much better than those of the local children'. Weaver, who was a dentist in the Ministry of Education, visited Westmorland, examined 117 evacuees (average age 11 years) and found the mean for decayed, missing or filled (DMF) teeth was 1.7. Weaver (1944) reported:

> Bearing in mind the work which had been done in America, I got in touch with Dr Campbell Lyons, Medical Officer of Health for South Shields, and asked him if he would have the town's water analysed for fluorine. He did so, and a preliminary analysis suggested that the fluorine content might be as much as two parts per million. It was obvious that the conditions were such as to make possible a perfectly controlled investigation since North Shields, on the opposite

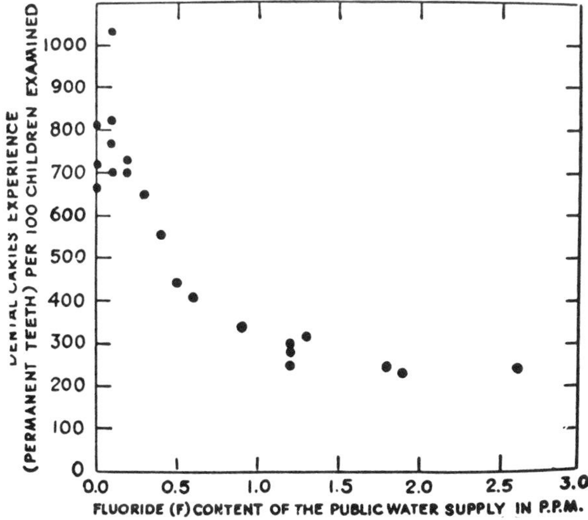

Figure 2.2 Relation between caries experience of 7257 12–14-year-old white schoolchildren of 21 cities in the USA and the fluoride content of the water supply (From Dean, Arnold and Elvove, 1942; reproduced from *Fluoride Drinking Waters*, edited by McClure, F. J., by kind permission of the US Department of Health, Education and Welfare, 1962)

bank of the River Tyne has an entirely different water supply. [The River Tyne at this part varies in width from 350 to 500 yd (320 to 457 m) and the two communities are linked by a ferry.]

At Weaver's request Dr Dawson, the Medical Officer of Health for the North Shields area, arranged for the water to be analysed and this showed a fluorine content of less than 0.25 ppm. Subsequently Weaver (1944) examined 1000 children on each side of the River Tyne. He reported that the mean dmft in 5-year-old children was 6.6 in North Shields and 3.9 in South Shields; the comparable figures for 12-year-old children were 4.3 and 2.4 DMF teeth. Weaver's observations were extremely important because he focused attention on the deciduous dentition as well as the permanent dentition.

Dental caries prevalence in artificially fluoridated areas

Grand Rapids–Muskegon study

The fluoridation story now entered the final phase. The crucial step was to see if dental caries could be reduced in a community by adding fluoride at 1 ppm to a fluoride-deficient water supply. The US Public Health Service was ready to embark on such an experiment. In December 1942 the service began talks with city officials of two cities in the Lake Michigan area, Grand Rapids and Muskegon. Extensive field and laboratory studies were carried out on the physiological effects of fluoride ingestion and it was concluded that not only was a fluoride concentration of 1 ppm the best for caries control, but also it was well within the limits of safety (Moulton, 1942).

In view of this information both city councils agreed in August 1944 to conduct the experiment, which would be carried out by Dr Dean, in conjunction with the Michigan State Health Department and the University of Michigan Dental School. It was decided that Grand Rapids would be the experimental town and that Muskegon would be the control town. In September 1944, Dean and his co-workers – Francis Arnold, Philip Jay and John Knutson – began the dental examinations of 19 680 Grand Rapids children and 4291 Muskegon children aged 4–16 years. All were continuous residents of the two cities. These baseline studies showed that caries experience in the deciduous and permanent dentitions in Grand Rapids was similar to that of Muskegon (Dean *et al.*, 1950). The method used to measure caries experience was to count the number of decayed, missing the filled teeth for each child – the DMF index (Klein, Palmer and Knutson, 1938). In addition, 5116 children continuously resident in the natural fluoride area of Aurora, Illinois (F = 1.4 ppm), were examined to provide further baseline information. On 25 January 1945 sodium fluoride was added to the Grand Rapids water supply. This was an historic occasion, because for the first time a permissible quantity of a beneficial dietary nutrient was added to the communal drinking water.

The effects of 6½ years of fluoridation in Grand Rapids were reported by Arnold, Dean and Knutson (1953). The results were clear: caries experience of 6-year-old Grand Rapids children was almost half that of 6-year-old Muskegon children (Table 2.1). The city officials of Muskegon, convinced of the efficacy of fluoridation, decided to fluoridate their own water supply in July 1951, so from this date Muskegon could no longer be used as a control town.

Table 2.1 Mean def in Grand Rapids and Muskegon, 1951

Age	*Grand Rapids*		*Muskegon*	
	No. children	*Mean def*	*No. children*	*Mean def*
4	168	2.13	63	4.46
5	853	2.27	351	5.25
6	750	2.98	294	5.67

The only control left for Grand Rapids was a retrospective comparison with baseline data. Results after 10 years of fluoridation (Arnold *et al.*, 1956) and 15 years of fluoridation (Arnold *et al.*, 1962) are recorded in Figure 2.3. They indicate that caries experience in 15-year-old Grand Rapids children had fallen from 12.48 DMF teeth per mouth in 1944 to 6.22 DMF teeth per mouth in 1959, a reduction of approximately 50%. Furthermore, caries experience in the fluoridated community of Grand Rapids was very similar to that occurring in the natural fluoride area of Aurora. This was the experimental proof that the previously observed inverse relationship between fluoride in drinking water and dental caries experience was a cause and effect relationship.

The feelings that Trendley Dean and his co-workers had when they started the Grand Rapids experiment were recalled in an article by John Knutson (1970):

> It is now 25 years ago that the late Trendley Dean and I journeyed by train from Washington, D.C., to Grand Rapids, Michigan, to be joined by Philip Jay for a

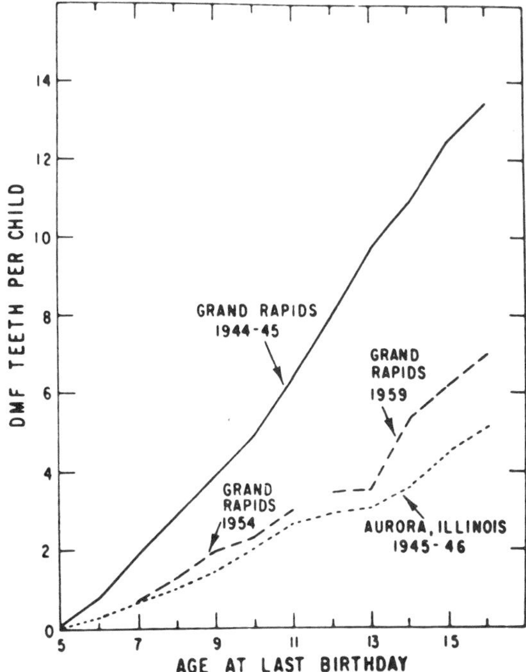

Figure 2.3 Dental caries in Grand Rapids children after 10 and 15 years of fluoridation (From Arnold *et al.*, 1962; copyright by the American Dental Association. Reprinted by permission.)

meeting with the mayor to gain his approval for a water fluoridation experiment. . . . There were no signs of apprehension or daring or of pioneering. There were no implications or inferences that we were being foolhardy in subjecting a population of 160,000 people to a procedure which might have either short or long-range hazards. We were merely replicating nature's best, based on an extensive background of study data in nature's laboratory, a laboratory which was extremely large. In the United States alone, some seven million people in 1,900 communities had throughout life used drinking water which was naturally fluoridated with a fluoride concentration of 0.7 ppm or greater. We knew what too much did, we knew what too little did, we knew what the optimum amount was and we had assurance that one part per million fluoride in the drinking water had the same biological effect whether it got there from flowing over rocks or from a feeding machine.

Newburgh–Kingston study

In addition to the Grand Rapids–Muskegon study, two other fluoridation studies were carried out in the USA. On 2 May 1945, sodium fluoride was added to the drinking water of Newburgh, on the Hudson river. The town of Kingston, situated 35 miles away from Newburgh, was chosen as a control town. This study was directed by David B. Ast, Chief of the Dental Bureau, State of New York Department of Health. Baseline studies were carried out in the two communities in

1944–46 (Ast, Finn and McCafferty, 1950). Clinical examinations after 10 years of fluoridation were carried out in 1954–55 (Ast *et al.*, 1956). They reported that while caries experience in 10–12-year-old Kingston children had changed little from 1945 (23.1% of teeth were carious) to 1955 (26.3%), in contrast in similarly aged Newburgh children over the 10-year period, the DMF rate had fallen from 23.5% to 13.9%, thus confirming the caries-inhibitory property of fluoride drinking water.

Evanston–Oak Park study

A third American fluoridation experiment began in January 1946 in Evanston, Illinois; the nearby community of Oak Park acted as the control town. Drs J. R. Blayney, I. N. Hill and S. O. Zimmerman of the University of Chicago Memorial Dental Clinic conducted the study and their findings after 14 years of fluoridation in Evanston were published in 1967 (Blayney and Hill, 1967). Whereas the DMF values of 14-year-old Evanston children fell from 11.66 to 5.95 between 1946 and 1960 (a reduction of 49%), no change was observed in the DMF values of 14-year-old Oak Park children over the intervening years. Here again was experimental proof of the caries-inhibitory property of fluoride in drinking water at a concentration of 1 ppm. The Evanston–Oak Park study presented the most detailed data of all the fluoridation studies. In an introduction to the report, Dr F. A. Arnold, Jr., Chief Dental Officer, United States Public Health Service, wrote:

> Here in a single report are data on the effect of water fluoridation on dental caries so completely documented that the article is virtually a textbook for use in further research. It is an important scientific contribution towards betterment of the dental health of our nation. It is a classic in this field. (Arnold, 1967.)

Yet the strength of the experimental proof of the caries-inhibitory property of fluoride drinking water lies not only in the conclusion of one study, but also in the fact that the three American studies, carried out by different investigators in different parts of the country, reached similar conclusions: addition of 1 ppm fluoride in the drinking water reduced caries experience by approximately 50%.

Canadian study (Brantford, Sarnia and Stratford)

In Canada, a project was undertaken in Brantford, Ontario, where fluoride was added to the water supply in June 1945. The community of Sarnia was established as the control town; in addition, the community of Stratford, where fluoride was naturally present in the drinking water at a level of 1.3 ppm, was used as an auxiliary control. After 17 years of fluoridation in Brantford, caries experience was similar to that occurring in the natural fluoride area of Stratford and was 55% lower than in the control town of Sarnia (Hutton, Linscott and Williams, 1951; Brown and Poplove, 1965).

Dutch study (Tiel–Culemborg)

The caries-inhibitory action of fluoride in drinking water is not uniform: fluoride inhibits smooth-surface caries much more than pit and fissure caries. Investigation of this selective property of fluoride was an important component of the Dutch study, instituted in 1953 in Tiel and Culemborg.

This study was designed to assess the preventive effect of fluoride drinking water on the anatomical siting of caries attack: approximal surfaces, free smooth surfaces (buccal and lingual) and pit and fissure sites. In March 1953 the drinking water in Tiel was fluoridated at a level of 1.1 ppm. Culemborg, with a fluoride concentration of 0.1 ppm, was to serve as a control. Baseline examinations of 11–15-year-old children were carried out in 1952. There were no significant differences between Tiel and Culemborg data at the beginning of the investigation (Backer Dirks, Houwink and Kwant, 1961).

The examinations in 1969 provided data on 15-year-old children who had been born within the first year after the introduction of fluoridation 16 years previously (Kwant *et al.*, 1973). Approximal cavities were established from radiographs only; caries in pits and fissures and on free smooth surfaces was determined clinically. The 135 Culemborg 15-year-olds had a mean of 25.8 carious sites or surfaces compared with 11.3 carious sites or surfaces in the 147 Tiel 15-year-olds. Over all the sites there was, therefore, 56% less caries in Tiel (Table 2.2). The percentage reduction was highest (86%) in the free smooth surfaces (buccal and lingual) and least (31%) in the pit and fissure sites. A 75% reduction was observed for approximal surfaces, which amounted to a difference of 7.6 approximal surfaces per child between Tiel and Culemborg. The number of teeth which had been extracted due to caries was 85% less in Tiel 15-year-olds (1.55 extractions per child) compared with Culemborg 15-year-olds (0.23 extractions per child).

Table 2.2 Mean number of pit and fissure, approximal and smooth-surface cavities in 15-year-old children, born in 1954 and examined in 1969, in Tiel and Culemborg (from Kwant *et al.*, 1973)

	No. children	*Pit and fissure*	*Approximal*	*Free smooth surface*	*Total*
Culemborg	135	12.0	10.1	3.6	25.8
Tiel	147	8.3	2.5	0.5	11.3
Difference		3.7	7.6	3.1	14.5
% Difference		31	75	86	56

Kwant *et al.* (1974) reported on the effect of lifelong water fluoridation in 17- and 18-year-olds. The authors pointed out that direct comparisons between the inhabitants of the two towns were becoming more difficult in the older age groups, since the number of extractions had a considerable bearing on the results. In Culemborg, 17- and 18-year-olds had had six times as many teeth extracted as in Tiel. The difference in the number of cavities between the 17-year-olds born in 1954 and examined in 1971 in Tiel and Culemborg was 19 cavities per person, or 53% fewer cavities in Tiel. For the 18-year-olds, born in 1953, the difference was 17 cavities per person or 48% fewer cavities in Tiel.

The epidemiological evidence from this well-conducted Dutch study indicates that adequate ingestion of fluoride at an early stage of enamel formation is important in preventing pit and fissure caries, but is of less importance as far as smooth-surface caries is concerned.

New Zealand study (Hastings)

The effectiveness of fluoridation was also demonstrated in a study carried out in Hastings, New Zealand. This was a retrospective study: baseline examinations were carried out in 1954; further examinations were carried out in 1964 after 10 years of fluoridation (Ludwig, 1965) and in 1970 after 16 years' fluoridation (Ludwig, 1971). The mean DMFT of 15-year-old children fell from 16.8 in 1954 to 8.5 in 1970, a reduction of 8.3 teeth or 49%. This study, like the Dutch study, also demonstrated the selective caries-inhibitory action of fluoride on different tooth surfaces. In these 15-year-old children, free smooth-surface caries was reduced by 87% (a difference of 3.3 surfaces between 1954 and 1970), approximal caries by 73% (a difference of 14.7 surfaces) and occlusal-surface caries by 39% (a difference of 7.2 surfaces).

The effect of fluoridation in Hastings on the cost of a dental public health programme has been reported by Denby and Hollis (1966). There was a 45% increase in the number of children that could be treated by a dental nurse and a decrease in the cost of the General Dental Benefits programme.

British studies

In the UK, the studies by Weaver (1944) had shown that caries experience in South Shields (natural fluoride content 1.4 ppm) was approximately 50% lower than in North Shields (fluoride content 0.25 ppm), thus confirming Dean's findings in Galesburg and Monmouth, Macomb and Quincy (Dean *et al.*, 1939).

In addition, Weaver (1950) carried out a second investigation in 1949, in the North-East of England, including a survey of West Hartlepool children, where fluoride content of the water supply was 2 ppm. He examined 500 5-year-old children and reported that the mean dmft was 1.76 and that 53.6% of the children were caries-free. A similar number of 12-year-old children were examined: the mean DMF was 0.96 and 59.8% were caries-free. He commented: 'There can be few, if any, other areas in this country where the average DMF figure for unselected 12-year-old children is less than 1, as it was found to be in West Hartlepool.

Forrest (1956) studied 324 12–14-year-old children in other parts of Britain with concentrations of fluoride in the drinking water varying from 0.9 to 5.8 ppm. She compared the caries prevalence with 259 children of the same age in non-fluoride areas. Caries was markedly lower in the high-fluoride regions.

A further study of areas with varying concentrations of fluoride in drinking water was carried out by James (1961), who examined 1027 children aged 11–13 years from three areas in East Anglia: Norwich and Yarmouth (Norfolk) (F = 0.17–0.2 ppm), Chelmsford (intermittent fluoride content) and Colchester (F = 1.2–2 ppm). Children from Colchester were further divided into 'continuous' and 'non-continuous' residents. This study showed that the DMF of those children continuously resident in the high-fluoride area was less than half that of corresponding children in the low-fluoride area. Children aged 11–13 years who were continuous residents of Colchester had nearly double the proportion of sound first permanent molars found in the non-continuous residents.

In 1952, the British Government sent a mission to the USA and Canada to study fluoridation in operation. The mission concluded that fluoridation of water supplies was a valuable health measure, but recommended that in this country fluoride should be added to the water supplies of some selected communities before its general adoption was considered (Report of the United Kingdom Mission, 1953). The selected communities chosen were Watford, Kilmarnock and part of Anglesey. Fluoride was added to these drinking waters in 1955–1956. Sutton, Ayr and the remaining part of Anglesey acted as the control towns. The results after 5 years of fluoridation (Department of Public Health and Social Security, 1962) showed that caries experience in 5-year-old children was 50% lower in the fluoride areas than the non-fluoride areas (Table 2.3). In spite of this, fluoridation was discontinued in Kilmarnock in 1962, on the instructions of the local council. However, dental examinations continued to be carried out in all areas and the findings after 11 years' fluoridation were reported in 1969 (Table 2.4). The report confirmed the main findings of 1962, that fluoridation of water supplies is a highly effective method of reducing dental decay.

In addition to demonstrating the beneficial effects of fluoridation, the report also confirmed its complete safety. 'During the eleven years under review, medical practitioners reported only two patients with symptoms which they felt might have been associated with fluoridation. Careful investigation in both instances failed to attribute the symptoms to the drinking of fluoridated water.' (Department of Public Health and Social Security, 1969.) The Government is so confident of the safety of water fluoridation that it is prepared to give unlimited indemnity to any local authority in respect of actions for damages based on alleged harm to health resulting from fluoridation. In the Republic of Ireland, where fluoridation of community water supplies has been mandatory since 1964, legal action has already been taken. After a lengthy case lasting 65 days before Mr Justice Kenny in the Irish High Court, the judge held that the amount of fluoride ingested at a

Table 2.3 Number of children examined and mean dmft in 1956 and 1961 for each year age group in study areas and control areas (From Department of Public Health and Social Security, 1962)

Age	*Study areas*				*Control areas*			
	1956		*1961*		*1956*		*1961*	
	No. children	*Mean dmf*	*No. children*	*Mean dmf*	*No. children*	*Mean dmf*	*No. children*	*Mean dmf*
3*	450	3.80	388	1.29	297	3.53	329	3.32
4*	591	5.39	468	2.31	334	5.18	295	4.83
5†	785	5.81	531	2.91	461	5.66	374	5.39
6†	883	6.49	615	4.81	566	6.32	432	6.22
7†	952	7.06	593	6.05	577	7.08	446	6.89

* Full dentition. † Canines and molars only.

Table 2.4 Number of children examined and mean DMF in study and control areas (From Department of Public Health and Social Security, 1969)

Age	*Study areas*					*Control areas*				
	1956		*1967*			*1956*		*1967*		
	No. children	*Mean DMF*	*No. children*	*Mean DMF*	*Per cent difference*	*No. children*	*Mean DMF*	*No. children*	*Mean DMF*	*Per cent difference*
8	806	2.1	378	1.2	43	499	2.2	204	2.0	8
9	780	2.8	395	1.8	36	491	2.8	229	2.7	3
10	636	3.4	356	2.4	31	460	3.5	213	3.3	5
8–10	2222	2.8	1129	1.8	36	1450	2.8	646	2.7	5

concentration of 1 ppm in the drinking water did not involve any risk to health and concluded that the fluoridation of the public water supplies was not a violation of constitutional rights. His judgement was subsequently upheld in the Supreme Court of the Republic of Ireland. In the UK, the decision to fluoridate the public water supplies is taken by individual local authorities. In 1971, approximately 5% of the total population in this country had the benefit of fluoridated drinking water (Parliamentary News, 1971) and, by 1980, approximately 10% of the population were drinking fluoridated drinking water.

In 1977, Strathclyde Regional Health Authority voted to introduce water fluoridation into the West of Scotland. Strathclyde Regional Council agreed to the proposal, but were taken to court by a Mrs McColl. After a long court case in the Court of Session in Edinburgh, Judge Lord Jauncey ruled that water fluoridation in Scotland was *ultra vires*. The details of his judgement are considered more fully in Chapter 18. The law was changed in the UK in 1985 by means of the Water Fluoridation Bill to ensure that water fluoridation schemes could continue. However, as a result of the 1983 judgement, water fluoridation schemes in Scotland had to stop and none has been restarted, even though the law has been changed.

The number of fluoridation plants, and the population served, in each region in England and Wales, have been updated recently by Bickley and Lennon (1989) and are reproduced in Tables 2.5 and 2.6. Approximately 6.5 million people in England and Wales consume water containing 0.7 ppm or more fluoride. Surveys of the effect of natural and artificially fluoridated water on dental caries have been carried out in various parts of Great Britain (Figure 2.4).

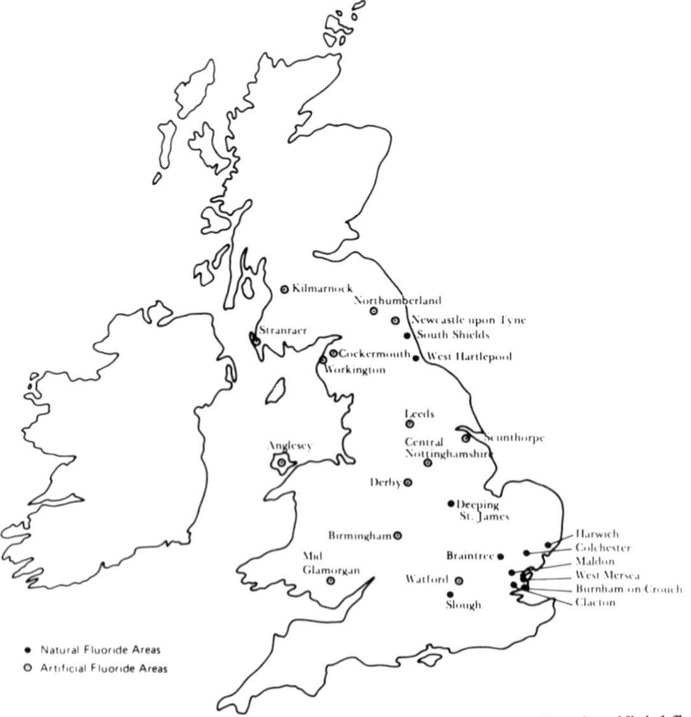

Figure 2.4 Areas of Great Britain in which surveys of natural and artificial fluoridation have been carried out

Table 2.5 Health districts in the 14 English regions, and in Wales, showing the percentages of the populations consuming water containing different concentrations of fluoride. ^{N} denotes natural, ^{A} artificial fluoride. In the latter case, the dates of water fluoridation are given (From Bickley and Lennon, 1989)

NORTHERN REGIONAL HEALTH AUTHORITY

The Districts of North Tees, South Tees and Darlington all receive only water which has a natural fluoride content of less than 0.3 ppm. Districts which have levels greater than 0.3 ppm are shown below.

District	*Population*	*Less than 0.3 ppm*	*% Pop.*	*0.3+ but less than 0.7 ppm*	*% Pop.*	*0.7+ but less than 0.9 ppm*	*% Pop.*	*0.9 ppm and over*	*% Pop.*	*F schemes implemented*
Hartlepool	90 700							90 700^{N}	100	
S. Cumbria	172 600	164 000^{N}	95*							
E. Cumbria	177 400	168 530^{N}	95	887^{N}	0.5			7 983^{A}	4.5	1969/77
W. Cumbria	136 600	17 758^{N}	13					118 842^{A}	87	1969/71
Durham	235 900	99 078^{N}	42	77 847^{N}	33			58 975^{A}	25	1968/89
S. W. Durham	153 600	53 760^{N}	35	89 088^{N}	58			10 752^{A}	7	1984
N. W. Durham	86 100							86 100^{A}	100	1968
Northumberland	301 000	195 650^{N}	65					105 350^{A}	35	1968/82/83
Gateshead	207 300							207 300^{A}	100	1968
Newcastle	281 400							281 400^{A}	100	1968
N. Tyneside	192 300	96 150^{N}	50					96 150^{A}	50	1968
S. Tyneside	156 900			156 900^{N}	100					
Sunderland	297 700	56 563^{N}	19	241 137^{N}	81					
Total				565 859				1 063 552		

* 8 600 (5%) of South Cumbria population on private water supplies, F levels not known.
Regional population 3 080 300

Table 2.5 continued

YORKSHIRE REGIONAL HEALTH AUTHORITY

The Districts of Hull, York, Scarborough, Bradford, Calderdale, Leeds East, Leeds West, Wakefield, Pontefract and East Yorkshire all receive only water which has a natural fluoride content of less than 0.3 ppm. Districts which have levels greater than 0.3 ppm are shown below.

District	*Population*	*Less than 0.3 ppm*	*% Pop.*	*0.3+ but less than 0.7 ppm*	*% Pop.*	*0.7+ but less than 0.9 ppm*	*% Pop.*	*0.9 ppm and over*	*% Pop.*	*F schemes implemented*
Grimsby	159 000	146 280[N]	92					12 720[A]	8	1971
Scunthorpe	193 900	62 048[N]	32					131 852[A]	68	1968/69
Northallerton	113 200	113 000[N]	99.82					200[N]	0.18	
Harrogate	134 600	125 178[N]	93					9 422[N]	7	
Airedale	173 000	172 705[N]	99.83			295[N]	0.17			
Huddersfield	212 500	127 500[N]	60					85 000[A]	40	1970/79
Dewsbury	164 100	150 972[N]	92			13 128[A]	8			1970/86
Total						13 423		239 194		

Regional population 3 601 400

MERSEY REGIONAL HEALTH AUTHORITY

The Districts of Macclesfield, Halton, Warrington, Wirral, St Helens and Knowsley, North Sefton, South Sefton and Liverpool all receive only water which has a natural fluoride content of less than 0.3 ppm. Districts which have levels greater than 0.3 ppm are shown below.

District	*Population*	*Less than 0.3 ppm*	*% Pop.*	*0.3+ but less than 0.7 ppm*	*% Pop.*	*0.7+ but less than 0.9 ppm*	*% Pop.*	*0.9 ppm and over*	*% Pop.*	*F schemes implemented*
Chester	177 700	172 369[N]	97					5 331[A]	3	1975
Crewe	246 700	115 949[N]	47			76 477[A]	31	54 274[A]	22	1975
Total						76 477		59 605		

Regional population 2 414 100

TRENT REGIONAL HEALTH AUTHORITY

The Districts of Leicestershire, Nottingham, Barnsley and Rotherham all receive only water which has a natural fluoride content of less than 0.3 ppm. Districts which have levels greater than 0.3 ppm are shown below.

District	*Population*	*Less than 0.3 ppm*	*% Pop.*	*0.3+ but less than 0.7 ppm*	*% Pop.*	*0.7+ but less than 0.9 ppm*	*% Pop.*	*0.9 ppm and over*	*% Pop.*	*F schemes implemented*
N. Derbyshire	361 600	162 829[N]	45	55 324[N]	15.3	56 936[N]	15.8	86 511[N + A]	23.9	pre-1974
S. Derbyshire	525 600	183 960[N]	35	331 129[N]	63	525[N]	0.1	2 102[N]	0.4	
								7 884[A]	1.5	1987
N. Lincolnshire	267 700	(– varying levels 96 372[N] (36%) of nat. fluoride –)						171 328[A]	64	1970/80
S. Lincolnshire	299 600	176 813[N]	59	42 050[N]	14			80 737[A]	27	1987
Bassetlaw	104 900							104 900[A]	100	1985
Central Notts.	285 100	30 220[N]	10.6					254 880[A]	89.4	1976/84
Doncaster	289 300	287 854[N]	99.5					1 446[A]	0.5	1987
Sheffield	534 300	502 242[N]	94	32 058[N]	6					
Total				566 933		57 461		709 788		

Regional population 4 633 800

NORTH WESTERN REGIONAL HEALTH AUTHORITY

All Districts within the North Western Regional Health Authority receive only water which has a natural fluoride content of less than 0.3 ppm (Stockport, Bolton, Wigan, Oldham, Tameside and Glossop, Rochdale, Blackburn Hyndburn and Ribble, Salford, Trafford, Bury, Burnley Pendel and Rossendal, Blackpool Wyre and Fylde, Lancaster, West Lancashire Chorley and South Ribble, Preston, North Manchester, Central Manchester, South Manchester).

Regional population 3 990 000

Table 2.5 continued

WEST MIDLANDS REGIONAL HEALTH AUTHORITY

The Districts of Shropshire, Hereford, Kidderminster and North Staffs all receive only water which has a natural fluoride content of less than 0.3 ppm. Districts which have levels greater than 0.3 ppm are shown below.

District	*Population*	*Less than 0.3 ppm*	*% Pop.*	*0.3+ but less than 0.7 ppm*	*% Pop.*	*0.7+ but less than 0.9 ppm*	*% Pop.*	*0.9 ppm and over*	*% Pop.*	*F schemes implemented*
Dudley	300 900	54 162^{N}	18					246 728^{A}	82	1986/88
Sandwell	301 100							301 100^{A}	100	1964/86
Walsall	261 800							261 800^{A}	100	1985/87
Wolverhampton	251 900	60 456^{N}	24					191 444^{A}	76	1986
Worcester	236 300	184 314^{N}	78					51 986^{A}	22	1979
Bromsgrove and Redditch	164 000	6 500^{N}	4					157 500^{A}	96	1970/71
N. Warwicks	172 800	864^{N}	0.5					171 936^{A}	99.5	1964/81/87
S. Warwicks	223 000			2 000^{N}	0.9			221 000^{A}	99.1	1970/81
Rugby	84 900			400^{N}	0.4			84 500^{A}	99.6	1969
Coventry	310 400			20 176^{N}	6.5			290 224^{A}	93.5	1981/89
Mid. Staffs	308 100	154 050^{N}	50					154 050^{A}	50	1987/88
S. E. Staffs	252 300							16 652^{N}	6.6	
								235 648^{A}	93.4	1986/87
Solihull	202 200							202 200^{A}	100	1964/81
N. Birmingham	163 900							163 900^{A}	100	1964/86
E. Birmingham	199 900							199 900^{A}	100	1964
C. Birmingham	180 700							180 700^{A}	100	1964
W. Birmingham	211 500							211 500^{A}	100	1964
S. Birmingham	248 100							248 100^{A}	100	1964
Total				22 576				3 590 878		

Regional population 5 181 400

OXFORD REGIONAL HEALTH AUTHORITY

The Districts of Kettering, Northampton, Milton Keynes and Aylesbury Vale all receive only water which has a natural fluoride content of less than 0.3 ppm. Districts which have levels greater than 0.3 ppm are shown below.

District	*Population*	*Less than 0.3 ppm*	*% Pop.*	*0.3+ but less than 0.7 ppm*	*% Pop.*	*0.7+ but less than 0.9 ppm*	*% Pop.*	*0.9 ppm and over*	*% Pop.*	*F schemes implemented*
Oxford	539 600	498 590^{N}	92.4	1 221^{N}	0.2			39 798^{A}	7.4	1972
Wycombe	271 600	260 736^{N}	96					10 864^{A}	4	1973/77
W. Berkshire	445 000	434 765^{N}	97.7					10 235^{N}	2.3	
E. Berkshire	361 300	350 461^{N}	97	10 839^{N}	3					
Total				12 060				60 888		

Regional population 2 476 300

EAST ANGLIAN REGIONAL HEALTH AUTHORITY

The Districts of Cambridge, Peterborough, West Norfolk and Wisbech all receive only water which has a natural fluoride content of less than 0.3 ppm. Districts which have levels greater than 0.3 ppm are shown below.

District	*Population*	*Less than 0.3 ppm*	*% Pop.*	*0.3+ but less than 0.7 ppm*	*% Pop.*	*0.7+ but less than 0.9 ppm*	*% Pop.*	*0.9 ppm and over*	*% Pop.*	*F schemes implemented*
Huntingdon	129 800	42 834^{N}	33	86 966^{N}	67					
Norwich	465 600	339 888^{N}	73	125 712^{N}	27					
Great Yarmouth and Waveney	194 900	160 987^{N}	82.6	17 736^{N}	9.1	16 177^{N}	8.3			
E. Suffolk	318 400		– varying levels-	318 400^{N}	-of nat.	fluoride –				
W. Suffolk	224 500		– varying levels-	224 500^{N}	-of nat.	fluoride –				
Total				773 314		16 177				

Regional population 1 991 700

Table 2.5 continued

NORTH EAST THAMES REGIONAL HEALTH AUTHORITY

The Districts of Basildon and Thurrock, Southend, Barking Havering and Brentford, Waltham Forest, Enfield, Haringey, Newham, Tower Hamlets, City and Hackney, Islington, Bloomsbury and Hampstead all receive only water which has a natural fluoride content of less than 0.3 ppm. Districts which have levels greater than 0.3 ppm are shown below.

District	*Population*	*Less than 0.3 ppm*	*% Pop.*	*0.3+ but less than 0.7 ppm*	*% Pop.*	*0.7+ but less than 0.9 ppm*	*% Pop.*	*0.9 ppm and over*	*% Pop.*	*F schemes implemented*
Mid. Essex	287 100	57 420^{N}	20	175 131^{N}	61	11 484^{N}	4	43 065^{N}	15	
N. E. Essex	298 700			50 779^{N}	17	247 921^{N}	83			
W. Essex	253 800	159 894^{N}	63	93 906^{N}	37					
Redbridge	228 000	120 000^{N}	52.6	107 500^{N}	47.1			500^{N}	0.3	
Total				427 316		259 405		43 565		

Regional population 3 773 100

NORTH WEST THAMES REGIONAL HEALTH AUTHORITY

The Districts of North Hertfordshire, North West Hertfordshire, Barnet, Harrow, Parkside Hillingdon, Hounslow and Spelthorne, Ealing, Riverside and Paddington all receive only water which has a natural fluoride content of less than 0.3 ppm. Districts which have levels greater than 0.3 ppm are shown below.

District	*Population*	*Less than 0.3 ppm*	*% Pop.*	*0.3+ but less than 0.7 ppm*	*% Pop.*	*0.7+ but less than 0.9 ppm*	*% Pop.*	*0.9 ppm and over*	*% Pop.*	*F schemes implemented*
N. Bedfordshire	245 600	58 944^{N}	24					186 656^{A}	76	1972
S. Bedfordshire	275 300	269 794^{N}	98					5 506^{A}	2	1972
E. Herts.	293 800	285 200^{N}	97	8 600						
S. W. Herts.	244 700	171 290^{N}	70					73 410^{A}	30	1955/56
Total				8 600				265 572		

Regional population 3 488 100

SOUTH EAST THAMES REGIONAL HEALTH AUTHORITY

All Districts in the South East Thames Regional Health Authority receive only water which has a natural fluoride content of less than 0.3 ppm (Brighton, Eastbourne, Hastings, South East Kent, Canterbury and Thanet, Maidstone, Tunbridge Wells, Medway, Dartford and Gravesham, Bromley, Greenwich, Bexley, West Lambeth, Camberwell, Lewisham and Southwark).

Regional population 3 618 200

SOUTH WEST THAMES REGIONAL HEALTH AUTHORITY

All Districts in the South West Thames Regional Health Authority receive only water which has a natural fluoride content of less than 0.3 ppm (North West Surrey, Mid Surrey, Kingston and Esher, Merton and Sutton, Richmond Twickenham and Roehampton, Wandsworth, Chichester, Mid Downs, Worthing, Croydon, West Surrey and North East Hampshire, South West Surrey, East Surrey).

Regional population 2 964 500

WESSEX REGIONAL HEALTH AUTHORITY

The Districts of West Dorset, East Dorset, Southampton and South West Hampshire, Winchester, Isle of Wight and Salisbury all receive only water which has a natural fluoride content of less than 0.3 ppm. Districts which have levels greater than 0.3 ppm are shown below.

District	*Population*	*Less than 0.3 ppm*	*% Pop.*	*0.3+ but less than 0.7 ppm*	*% Pop.*	*0.7+ but less than 0.9 ppm*	*% Pop.*	*0.9 ppm and over*	*% Pop.*	*F schemes implemented*
Basingstoke and N. Hampshire	215 000	210 700[N]	98					4 300[N]	2	
Portsmouth and S. E. Hampshire	525 900	475 414[N]	90.4	50 486[N]	9.5					
Swindon	227 700	38 709[N]	17	161 667[N]	71	27 324[N]	12			
Bath	396 400	271 534[N]	68.5	97 118[N]	24.5	27 748[N]	7			
Total				309 271		55 072		4 300		

Regional population 2 876 500

Table 2.5 continued

SOUTH WESTERN REGIONAL HEALTH AUTHORITY

All but one District in the South Western Regional Health Authority receive only water which has a natural fluoride content of less than 0.3 ppm (North Devon, Exeter, Plymouth, Torbay, Cornwall, Cheltenham, Gloucester, Bristol and Weston, Frenchay, Southmead). A small percentage of the population in Somerset District receive supplies with levels greater than 0.3 ppm (shown below).

District	*Population*	*Less than 0.3 ppm*	*% Pop.*	*0.3+ but less than 0.7 ppm*	*% Pop.*	*0.7+ but less than 0.9 ppm*	*% Pop.*	*0.9 ppm and over*	*% Pop.*	*F schemes implemented*
Somerset	396 400	373 806[N]	94.3	22 594[N]	5.7					
Total				22 594						
Regional population 3 177 500										

WALES

The Districts of East Dyfed, Clwyd, Gwent, Mid Glamorgan, South Glamorgan, West Glamorgan and Pembrokeshire all receive only water which has a natural fluoride content of less than 0.3 ppm. Districts which have levels greater than 0.3 ppm are shown below.

District	*Population*	*Less than 0.3 ppm*	*% Pop.*	*0.3+ but less than 0.7 ppm*	*% Pop.*	*0.7+ but less than 0.9 ppm*	*% Pop.*	*0.9 ppm and over*	*% Pop.*	*F schemes implemented*
Gwynedd	234 600	164 924[N]	70.3					69 676[A]	29.7	1955
Powys	112 300	106 236[N]	94.6					6 064[A]	5.4	1971
Total								75 740		
Principality population 2 820 900										

Table 2.6 Regional totals, showing the percentages of populations consuming water containing different concentrations of fluoride in England and Wales (From Bickley and Lennon, 1989)

Region	Population	Less than 0.3 ppm	% Pop.	0.3+ but less than 0.7 ppm	% Pop.	0.7+ but less than 0.9 ppm	% Pop.	0.9 ppm and over	% Pop.
Northern	3 080 300*	1 442 289	47	565 859	18.3			1 063 552	34.5
Yorkshire	3 601 400	3 348 783	93			13 423	0.4	239 194	6.6
Mersey	2 414 100	2 278 018	94			76 477	3	59 605	3
Trent	4 633 800	3 309 618	71.5	556 933	12	57 461	1.2	709 788	15.3
N. Western	3 990 000	3 990 000	100						
W. Midlands	5 181 400	1 567 946	30.2	22 567	0.4			3 590 878	69.4
Oxford	2 476 300	2 403 352	97	12 060	0.5			60 888	2.5
E. Anglian	1 991 700	1 202 209	60.4	773 314	38.8	16 177	0.8		
N. E. Thames	3 773 100	3 042 814	80.6	427 316	11.3	259 405	7	43 565	1.1
N. W. Thames	3 488 100	3 213 928	92	8 600	0.3			265 572	7.7
S. E. Thames	3 618 200	3 618 200	100						
S. W. Thames	2 964 500	2 964 500	100						
Wessex	2 876 500	2 507 857	87	309 271	11	55 072	19	4 300	0.1
S. Western	3 177 500	3 154 906	99.3	22 594	0.7				
Wales	2 820 900	2 745 160	97					75 740	3
Total	50 085 800	40 798 580		2 698 523		478 015 (388 410^{N}) (89 605^{A})		6 113 082 (177 176^{N}) (5 935 906^{A})	

* 8 600 of S. Cumbria pop. on private water supplies. F levels not known (represents 0.2% of Northern Regional population).

^{N}denotes natural, ^{A}artificial fluoride.

The World Health Organisation

Looking further afield, the World Health Organisation has always taken a keen interest in the effect of fluoridation on dental health. In 1958 they produced a first report by an expert committee on water fluoridation and concluded that drinking water containing about 1 ppm fluoride had a marked caries-preventive action and that controlled fluoridation of drinking water was a practicable and effective public health measure (WHO, 1958). In a later article, 'Fluoridation and dental health' (WHO, 1969), it was stated that as a result of the initial controlled fluoridation studies in America and Canada, further programmes were under way in more than 30 countries and territories serving over 120 million people.

In 1962, the World Health Organisation invited 29 experts to collaborate in the preparation of a monograph relating to the effects of fluoride on human health. The object of the monograph was to provide an impartial review of the scientific literature on the varied aspects of fluoridation and the many complex questions relating to the metabolism of fluorides and their use in medicine and public health (WHO, 1970). In a summary of the section on fluorides and general health, A. E. Martin (1970) stated that:

> By their wide distribution in nature, their inevitable presence in man's food and drink and their consequent presence in the tissues of the human body, fluorides form a natural part of man's environment, yet when present in excess they are known to be harmful. Studies of the geographical distribution of dental mottling in the U.S.A. were begun during the early decades of the century and the identification of fluorides in water supplies in 1931 led to a comprehensive survey designed, in the first place, to find the threshold limit for the avoidance of dental fluorosis and, later, to ascertain the concentration in a water supply necessary for optimal dental protection. When the artificial fluoridation of water was first considered, this survey provided a useful starting point for a programme of specific epidemiological and experimental studies which, over the past three decades, has yielded a mass of data confirming the safety of fluoridation. This has been supplemented by independent studies from other countries which have provided further supplementary material for use in defining the upper limits of a safe fluoride intake. The results have shown that for the climatic, nutritional and environmental conditions under which the surveys have been carried out, a level of approximately 1 ppm fluoride in temperate climates has no harmful effects on the community. The margin of safety is such that it will cover any individual variation of intake to be found in such areas.

A report on fluoridation was submitted by the Director of WHO to the 22nd World Health Assembly, as a result of which the following resolution was adopted by the Assembly on 22 July 1969:

> The World Health Organisation recommended member states to examine the possibility of introducing and where practicable to introduce fluoridation of those community water supplies where the fluoride intake from water and other sources for the given population is below optimal levels, as a proven public health measure, and where fluoridation of community water supplies is not practicable to study other methods of using fluorides for the protection of dental health. (WHO, 1969.)

This resolution was reaffirmed in the Report of the WHO Director General in

1975: 'Fluoridation of communal water supplies, where feasible, should be the cornerstone of any national programme of dental caries prevention'.

McKay would have been well pleased. His observations in Colorado Springs over 80 years ago, followed by his persistence in determining the cause of mottled enamel, had transcended national boundaries and resulted in the discovery of a public health measure, which would markedly reduce the prevalence of dental caries, being recommended to all member states of the World Health Organisation. The history of fluoridation must surely rank as one of the classic epidemiological studies of chronic disease in the history of medicine.

References

Ainsworth, N. J. (1928) Mottled teeth. *R. Dent. Hosp. Mag.*, Feb

Ainsworth, N. J. (1933) Mottled teeth. *Br. Dent. J.*, **60**, 233–250

Arnold, F. A. Jun. (1967) Foreword to fluorine and dental caries. *J. Am. Dent. Assoc.*, **74**, 230

Arnold, F. A. Jun., Dean, H. T., Jay, P. and Knutson, J. W. (1956) Effect of fluoridated public water supplies on dental caries prevalence. 10th year of the Grand Rapids–Muskegon Study. *Public Health Rep.*, **71**, 652–658

Arnold, F. A. Jun., Dean, H. T. and Knutson, J. W. (1953) Effect of fluoridated public water supplies on dental caries prevalence. Results of the seventh year of study at Grand Rapids and Muskegon, Mich. *Public Health Rep.*, **68**, 141–148

Arnold, F. A., Likens, R. C., Russell, A. L. and Scott, D. B. (1962) Fifteenth year of the Grand Rapids fluoridation study. *J. Am. Dent. Assoc.*, **65**, 780–785

Ast, D. B., Finn, S. B. and McCafferty, I. (1950) The Newburgh–Kingston caries fluorine study. I, Dental findings after three years of water fluoridation. *Am. J. Public Health*, **40**, 116–124

Ast, D. B., Smith, D. J., Wacks, B. and Cantwell, K. T. (1956) Newburgh–Kingston caries-fluorine study XIV. Combined clinical and roentgenographic dental findings after ten years of fluoride experience. *J. Am. Dent. Assoc.*, **52**, 314–325

Backer Dirks, O., Houwink, B. and Kwant, G. W. (1961) The results of 6½ years of artificial fluoridation of drinking water in the Netherlands. The Tiel–Culemborg experiment. *Arch. Oral Biol.*, **5**, 284–300

Bickley, S. R. and Lennon, M. A. (1989) Fluoride levels in water supplies in health districts in England and Wales. A survey conducted by the British Fluoridation Society in 1988. *Commun. Dental Health*, **6**, 403–414

Black, G. V. (1916) Mottled teeth. *Dent. Cosmos*, **58**, 129–156

Blayney, J. R. and Hill, I. N. (1967) Fluorine and dental caries. *J. Am. Dent. Assoc.*, **74**, 233–302

Brown, H. K. and Poplove, M. (1965) Brantford–Sarnia–Stratford fluoridation caries study: final survey 1963. *J. Can. Dent. Assoc.*, **31**, 505–511

Churchill, H. V. (1931a) Letter to F. S. McKay in the McKay papers. Cited by McNeil (1957), p. 26

Churchill, H. V. (1931b) Occurrence of fluorides in some waters of the United States. *Ind. Eng. Chem.*, **23**, 996–998

Dean, H. T. (1933) Distribution of mottled enamel in the United States. *Public Health Rep.*, **48**, 704–734

Dean, H. T. (1934) Classification of mottled enamel diagnosis. *J. Am. Dent. Assoc.*, **21**, 1421–1426

Dean, H. T. (1936) Chronic endemic dental fluorosis (mottled enamel). *J. Am. Med. Assoc.*, **107**, 1269–1272

Dean, H. T. (1938) Endemic fluorosis and its relation to dental caries. *Public Health Rep.*, **53**, 1443–1452

Dean, H. T., Arnold, F. A. Jun. and Elvove, E. (1942) Domestic water and dental caries, V, additional studies of the relation of fluoride domestic waters to dental caries experience in 4,425 white children aged 12–14 years, of 13 cities in 4 states. *Public Health Rep.*, **57**, 1155–1179

Dean, H. T., Arnold, F. A. Jun., Jay, P. and Knutson, J. W. (1950) Studies on mass control of dental caries through fluoridation of public water supply. *Public Health Rep.*, **65**, 1403–1408

Dean, H. T. and Elvove, E. (1936) Some epidemiological aspects of chronic endemic dental fluorosis. *Am. J. Public Health,* **26**, 567–575

Dean, H. T., Jay, P., Arnold, F. A. Jun. and Elvove, E. (1939) Domestic water and the dental caries including certain epidemiological aspects of oral *L. acidophilus. Public Health Rep.,* **54**, 862–888

Dean, H. T. and McKay, F. S. (1939) Production of mottled enamel halted by a change in common water supply. *Am. J. Public Health,* **29**, 590–596

Denby, G. C. and Hollis, M. J. (1966) The effect of fluoridation on a dental public health programme. *N. Z. Dent. J.,* **62**, 32–36

Department of Public Health and Social Security (1962) The results of fluoridation studies in the United States and the results achieved after five years. *Rep. Public Health Med. Subj.* (*Lond.*), no. 105

Department of Public Health and Social Security (1969) Report of the Committee on Research into Fluoridation. The fluoridation studies in the United Kingdom and the results achieved after eleven years. *Rep. Public Health Med. Subj.* (*Lond.*), no. 122

Eager, J. M. (1902) Abstract: chiaie teeth. *Dent. Cosmos,* **44**, 300–301

Forrest, J. R. (1956) Caries incidence and enamel defects in areas with different levels of fluoride in the drinking water. *Br. Dent. J.,* **100,** 195–200

Hutton, W. L., Linscott, B. W. and Williams, D. B. (1951) Brantford fluorine experiment. *Can. J. Public Health,* **42**, 81

James, P. M. C. (1961) Dental caries prevalence in high and low fluoride areas of East Anglia. *Br. Dent. J.,* **110**, 165–169

Kempf, G. A. and McKay, F. S. (1930) Mottled enamel in a segregated population. *Public Health Rep.,* **45**, 2923–2940

Klein, H., Palmer, G. E. and Knutson, J. W. (1938) Studies on dental caries: (1) Dental status and dental needs of elementary schoolchildren. *Public Health Rep.,* **53**, 751–765

Knutson, J. W. (1970) Water fluoridation after 25 years. *Br. Dent. J.,* **129**, 297–300

Kwant, G. W., Groeneveld, A., Pot, T. J. and Purdell Lewis, D. (1974) Fluoridetoevoeging aan het drinkwater V. *Nederl. Tijds. Tandheelk.,* **81**, 251–261

Kwant, G. W., Houwink, B., Backer Dirks, O., Groeneveld, A. and Pot, T. J. (1973) Artificial fluoridation of drinking water in the Netherlands; results of the Tiel–Culemborg experiment after 16½ years. *Netherl. Dent. J.,* **80**, suppl. 9, 6–27

Ludwig, T. G. (1965) The Hastings Fluoridation Project V – Dental effects between 1954 and 1964. *N.Z. Dent. J.,* **61**, 175–179

Ludwig, T. G. (1971) Hastings fluoridation project VI. *N.Z. Dent. J.,* **67**, 155–160

McCollum, E. V., Simmonds, N., Becker, J. E. and Bunting, R. W. (1925) The effect of additions of fluoride to the diet of rats on the quality of their teeth. *J. Biol. Chem.,* **63**, 553

McKay, F. S. (1916a) An investigation of mottled teeth (I). *Dent. Cosmos,* **58**, 477–484

McKay, F. S. (1916b) An investigation of mottled teeth (II). *Dent. Cosmos,* **58**, 627–644

McKay, F. S. (1916c) An investigation of mottled teeth (III). *Dent. Cosmos,* **58**, 781–792

McKay, F. S. (1916d) An investigation of mottled teeth (IV). *Dent. Cosmos,* **58**, 894–904

McKay, F. S. (1918) Progress of the year in the investigation of mottled enamel with special reference to its association with artesian water. *J. Natl Dent. Assoc.,* **5**, 721–750

McKay, F. S. (1925) Mottled enamel: a fundamental problem in dentistry. *Dent. Cosmos,* **67**, 847–860

McKay, F. S. (1928) The relation of mottled teeth to caries. *J. Am. Dent. Assoc.,* **15**, 1429–1437

McKay, F. S. (1933) Mottled teeth: the prevention of its further production through a change in the water supply at Oakley, Idaho. *J. Am. Dent. Assoc.,* **20**, 1137–1149

McNeil, D. R. (1957) *The Fight for Fluoridation,* Oxford University Press, New York

Martin, A. E. (1970) In *Fluorides and Human Health. WHO Monogr. Ser.*, no. 59, WHO, Geneva, pp. 316–318

Medical Research Council (1925) The incidence of dental disease in children. *Med. Res. Counc. Spec. Rep. Ser.* (*Lond.*), no. 97

Minutes of Colorado Springs Dental Society (1908) Cited by McNeil, D. R. (1957), p. 5

Moulton, F. R. (1942) *Fluorine and Dental Health*, American Association for the Advancement of Science, Washington, DC

Parliamentary News (1971) Report of question in the House of Commons on 23 April, 1971. *Br. Dent. J.,* **130**, 412

Report of United Kingdom Mission (1953) *The Fluoridation of Domestic Water Supplies in North America*, HMSO, London

Smith, H. V. and Smith, M. C. (1931) Mottled enamel in Arizona and its correlation with the concentration of fluorides in water supplies. *Bull. Ariz. Agric. Exp. Stn*, no. 32

Smith, M. C. (1931) Account of Tucson Dental Association meeting in Arizona. *Daily Star*, 3 May, 1931, cited by McNeil, D. R. (1957), p. 34

Weaver, R. (1944) Fluorosis and dental caries on Tyneside. *Br. Dent. J.*, **76**, 29–40

Weaver, R. (1950) Fluorine and wartime diet. *Br. Dent. J.*, **88,** 231–239

World Health Organisation (1958) Report of Expert Committee on Water Fluoridation. *WHO Tech. Rep. Ser.*, no. 146

World Health Organisation (1969) Fluoridation and dental health. *WHO Chron.*, **23**, 505–512

World Health Organisation (1970) *Fluorides and Human Health. WHO Monogr. Ser.*, no. 59, Geneva, WHO

Bibliography

Dunning, J. M. (1962) *Principles of Dental Public Health*, Harvard University Press, Cambridge, Mass.

McClure, F. J. (Ed.) (1962) *Fluoride Drinking Waters*, US Department of Health Education and Welfare, National Institute of Dental Research, Bethesda, Md.

McClure, F. J. (1970) *Water Fluoridation*, US Department of Health Education and Welfare, National Institute of Dental Research, Bethesda, Md

McNeil, D. R. (1957) *The Fight for Fluoridation*, Oxford University Press, New York

World Health Organisation (1970) *Fluorides and Human Health. WHO Monogr. Ser.*, no. 59, WHO, Geneva

Young, W. O. and Striffler, D. F. (1964) *The Dentist, His Practice and His Community*, Saunders, Philadelphia

Chapter 3

Water fluoridation and child dental health

In the previous chapter, attention was focused on results reported from fluoride and non-fluoride areas. The purpose of this chapter is to consider in greater detail the impact of water fluoridation on the dental needs of children.

The deciduous dentition

The pre-school child

Very few studies have concentrated on the pre-school child. Tank and Storvick (1964), in the USA, examined 132 children aged 1–6 years, born and brought up in Corvallis (1.0 ppm F in drinking water) and 114 children of similar age from Albany (fluoride-free). The examinations were carried out once a year for 5 years, so although a total of 246 children were involved in the study, some were examined more than once. The results showed that, for each age group, caries experience was lower in Corvallis than in Albany; combining all age groups, the mean caries rate was 56% lower in the fluoride area than in the non-fluoride area. There was no difference between the communities in the number of erupted teeth at each year age group (Table 3.1).

Winter *et al.* (1971) reported the caries rate in 602 pre-school children aged 1–4 years in London, England, a low-fluoride area. The only study giving the caries experience of pre-school children from a high-fluoride area in the UK was carried

Table 3.1 Number of erupted teeth and mean dmft in 1–6-year-old children living in Albany (fluoride-free) and Corvallis (1.0 ppm F) (After Tank and Storvick, 1964)

Age at last birthday (yr)	*No. children examined*		*No. erupted deciduous teeth*		*Mean dfmt*	
	Albany	*Corvallis*	*Albany*	*Corvallis*	*Albany*	*Corvallis*
1	36	96	11.2	11.3	0.14	0.08
2	50	73	17.9	18.1	1.26	0.59
3	53	66	20.0	20.0	4.25	1.44
4	53	52	20.0	20.0	5.51	2.31
5	24	28	19.4	19.4	6.00	3.29
6	13	27	16.5	17.6	7.77	3.19
All ages	229	322	17.5	17.7	4.16	1.82

Table 3.2 Caries experience of pre-school children in Hartlepool and London (After Winter *et al.*, 1971; Murray and Atkinson, 1971)

Age (yr)	*Hartlepool (F = 1.5–2.0 ppm)*			*London (F = 0.2 ppm)*		
	No. children	*Mean dmf*	*Per cent caries-free*	*No. children*	*Mean dmf*	*Per cent caries-free*
1	–	–	–	172	0.04	98
2	45	0.2	93	173	0.8	82
3	148	0.6	77	146	1.4	64
4	223	1.0	63	110	3.1	42
5	32	1.3	50	–	–	–

out in Hartlepool (F = 1.5–2.0 ppm) by Atkinson in 1968 (Murray and Atkinson, 1971). Ten nursery schools and play groups in the town were visited to give elementary oral hygiene instruction to mothers and children. As part of this programme, 448 children aged 2–5 years received a dental examination. The results of these two studies are compared in Table 3.2 and show that the benefits of fluoridation are apparent even from the earliest years.

The primary school child

The early fluoridation studies in America concentrated mainly on the permanent dentition. One of the first studies to highlight in detail the effect of water fluoridation on the deciduous dentition was that reported in the UK by Weaver (1944) in North Shields (F = 0.4 ppm) and South Shields (F = 1.4 ppm). The mean dmf was 41% lower in South Shields than North Shields (3.9 dmf teeth as against 6.6 dmf teeth) and this difference seemed to be distributed fairly evenly throughout the various deciduous teeth (Figure 3.1).

This observation was supported by a ‘cradle to the grave’ study carried out in Hartlepool in 1967–70 (Murray, 1969a,b). Three thousand eight hundred and four children aged 3–18 years, being a stratified random sample of all children born and continuously resident in Hartlepool, were examined, including 500 5-year-old children. A sample of 527 5-year-old children from the low-fluoride town of York (F = 0.25 ppm) were also examined during the same period to provide a control. The mean dmf in Hartlepool was 64% lower than in York (1.5 dmf teeth compared with 4.1 dmf teeth). The number of dmf teeth per 100 erupted teeth for each tooth type is given diagrammatically in Figure 3.2. The percentage number of dmf teeth in York was 20.5; in Hartlepool it was 7.45, giving a York:Hartlepool ratio of 2.75:1. This ratio for all teeth is very similar to the ratios for deciduous molars and for maxillary incisors, which contribute approximately 95% of the total dmf value, and show that deciduous molars and deciduous maxillary incisors benefit approximately equally from water fluoridation. Over half the Hartlepool 5-year-old children were caries-free (51.2%) compared with less than a quarter of the York children (22.4%) (Figure 3.3). Twice as many deciduous molars had to be extracted in York (7.8%) compared with Hartlepool (3.7%).

The first city in the UK to fluoridate was Birmingham in 1964. In 1970, 5-year-olds from non-fluoridated Dudley had 5.1 deft compared with 2.5 deft in the 5-year-olds living in fluoridated Birmingham (Beal and James, 1971). In a later

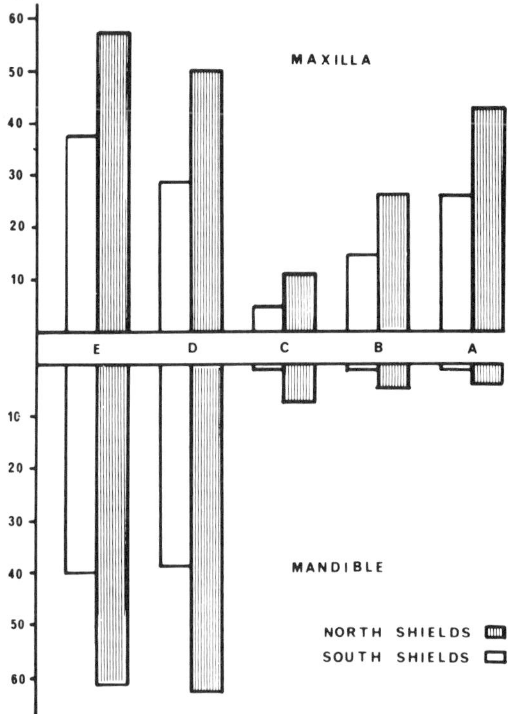

Figure 3.1 Per cent caries experience in each tooth type in 5-year-old children from North and South Shields (From Weaver, 1944)

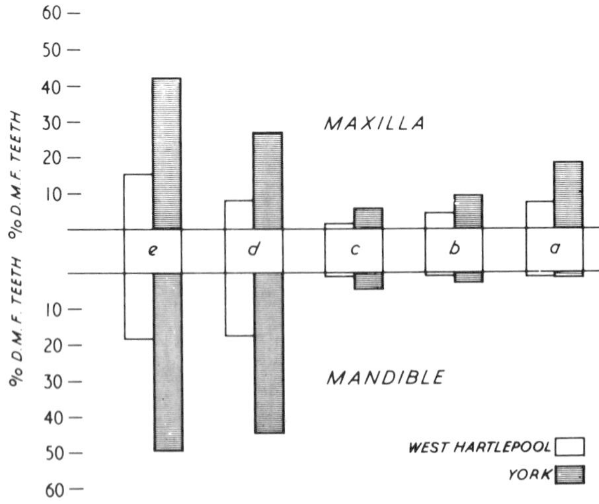

Figure 3.2 Caries experience in each tooth type in 5-year-old children from Hartlepool and York (From Murray, 1969a; reproduced by courtesy of the Editor, *British Dental Journal*)

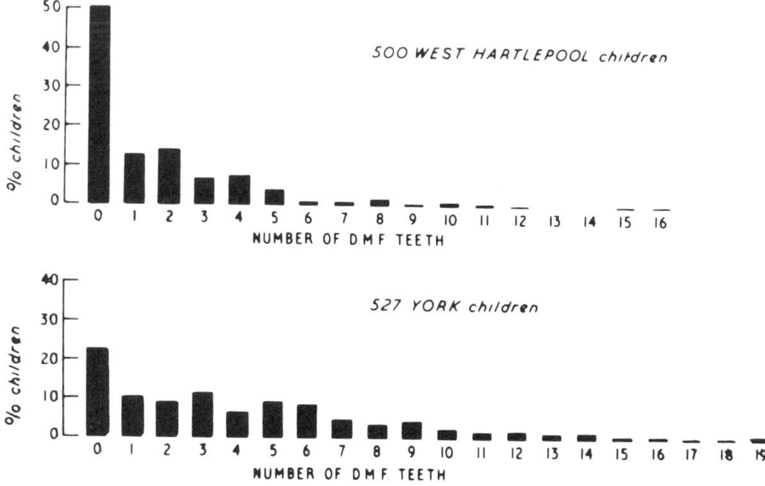

Figure 3.3 Frequency distribution of dmf teeth in 5-year-old children from Hartlepool and York (From Murray, 1969a; reproduced by courtesy of the Editor, *British Dental Journal*)

survey, Whittle and Downer (1979) observed that dmft scores for 4–5-year-old children living in fluoridated Birmingham were 54% less than the dmft scores of 4–5-year-old children living in an area of non-fluoridated Salford, which had been matched with the Birmingham area on socioeconomic factors and dentist:population ratio. Rock, Gordon and Bradnock (1981a) compared the dental health of 6–13-year-old children who had lived continuously in fluoridated Birmingham with children of the same age living in non-fluoridated Wolverhampton. Bitewing radiographs supplemented the clinical examination. The result for deciduous teeth in the 6–9-year-olds showed that the average Wolverhampton child had nearly twice as many decayed teeth, had the same number of filled teeth and had four times as many teeth extracted because of decay, as the average child in Birmingham.

Half of the island of Anglesey was one of the original three test areas for fluoridation in the UK, commencing fluoridation in 1955. However, the non-fluoridated (control) half of Anglesey fluoridated in 1964, so that in a study conducted by Jackson, James and Wolfe (1975) in 1974, the mainland area of Bangor/Caernarvon was used as a control. This study was unique in that children from the fluoridated and non-fluoridated areas were brought to a central site and mixed before examination. The Anglesey 5-year-olds had 2.8 dmft, 38% less than the Bangor/Caernarvon 5-year-olds (4.6 dmft).

Part of west Cumbria fluoridated in October 1969. The caries experience of 5-year-olds living in this area was compared with the caries experience of similarly aged children living in non-fluoridated Cumbria (Jackson, Gravely and Pinkham, 1975). Mean dmft scores for the two areas were 2.4 and 4.4 respectively, a difference in favour of the children living in fluoridated Cumbria of 46%.

Similar results were observed in four districts of Leeds which fluoridated in 1968. A comparison of the caries experience of 5-year-old children living in these districts with the caries experience of similarly aged children in two neighbouring non-fluoridated areas, in 1979, revealed that the children in the former areas had

62% less caries experience than the children in the non-fluoridated areas. Per 1000 children, there were 43 extracted deciduous teeth in the non-fluoridated areas compared with 11 in the fluoridated districts (Jackson, Goward and Morrell, 1980).

The city of Newcastle and areas of Northumberland County fluoridated in June 1969. A total of 771 5-year-olds were included in a study conducted in 1975 where urban fluoridated Newcastle was compared with urban non-fluoridated Ashington, and rural fluoridated Northumberland compared with similar areas of Northumberland which were not fluoridated (Rugg-Gunn *et al.*, 1977). The children in fluoridated Newcastle had 57% less, and children in fluoridated Northumberland 67% less caries experience (deft) compared with their non-fluoridated controls. Twenty-nine per cent of the Newcastle children were caries-free compared with only 11% in Ashington, and 34% of children in fluoridated Northumberland were caries-free compared with only 12% in non-fluoridated Northumberland.

A unique feature of this study is that lifetime experiences of toothache and general anaesthetics for dental extractions were measured. Forty per cent of the Ashington 5-year-olds had suffered from toothache compared with 22% of fluoridated Newcastle children, and 38% of 5-year-olds in non-fluoridated Northumberland had had toothache compared with only 17% in fluoridated Northumberland. General anaesthetic experience was 47% less in Newcastle compared with Ashington and 68% less in fluoridated compared with non-fluoridated Northumberland. The cost of treating the 5-year-olds was £5–6 per child more expensive (1976 NHS scale of fees) in the non-fluoridated areas compared with the fluoridated areas. The reduction in caries was greatest in the approximal surfaces, both in actual surfaces (2.5 per child) and percentage difference (75%) (Figure 3.4). The percentage reduction was lower for fissure sites

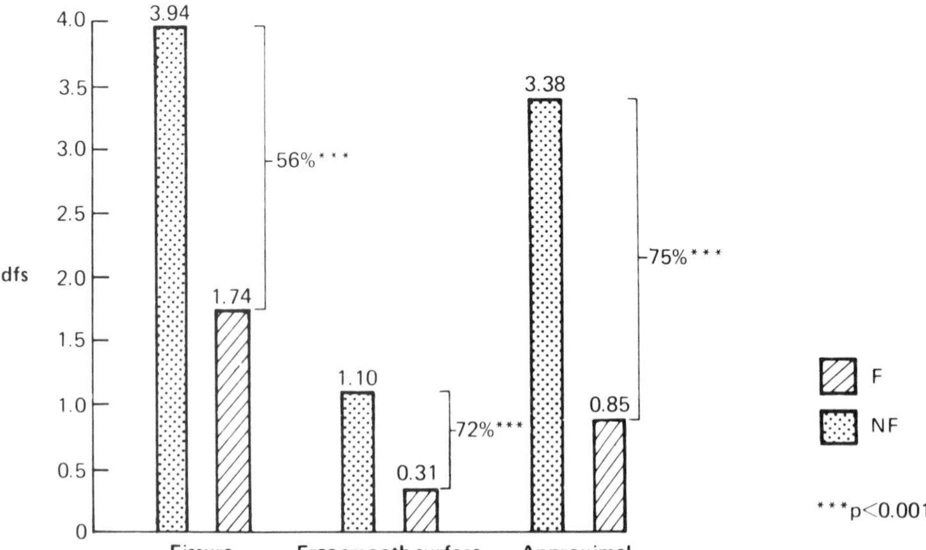

Figure 3.4 Effect of fluoridation on the caries experience (dfs) for each surface type (fissure, approximal and free smooth surface) separately in the deciduous dentition of 5-year-old children in Newcastle and Northumberland (From Rugg-Gunn *et al.*, 1977; reproduced by courtesy of the Editor, *British Dental Journal*)

(56%) compared with free smooth surfaces (72%), but was more important in absolute terms (a difference of 2.2 surfaces compared with 0.8 surfaces per child).

Social class information was available for children in the above study. The differences in caries experience (deft) between children in the fluoridated and non-fluoridated areas were 26% for social classes I and II, 60% for social class III and 71% for social classes IV and V (Table 3.3). Fluoridation appeared to particularly benefit lower social class children and remove intersocial class differences in dental caries experience (Carmichael *et al.*, 1980).

Table 3.3 Caries experience (deft) for 5-year-olds in fluoridated and non-fluoridated Newcastle and Northumberland according to social class (From Carmichael *et al.*, 1980)

Social class	*Area*		*Difference (%)*
	Fluoridated	Non-fluoridated	
I, II	2.5	3.4	0.9 (26)
III	2.4	6.0	3.6 (60)
IV, V	2.0	7.0	5.0 (71)

In addition to the areas artificially fluoridated at 1.0 ppm the North-East of England contains communities receiving natural fluoride levels of 0.2 and 0.5 ppm F. The curve in Figure 3.5 shows the relation between the caries experience of 5-year-old children living in four communities and their water fluoride levels

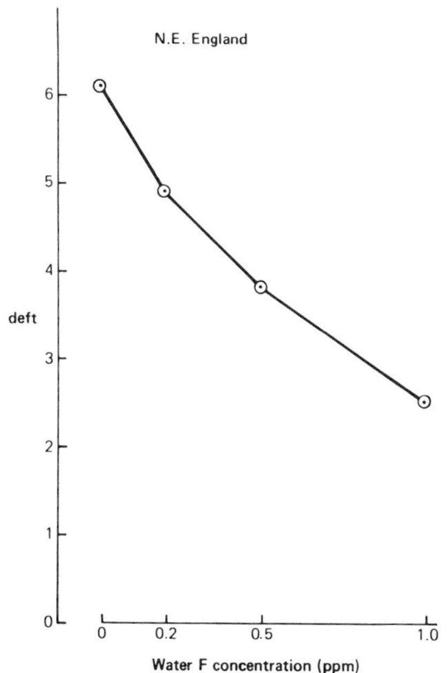

Figure 3.5 Relationship between caries experience (deft) in 1038 5-year-old children living in four areas of North-East England and the fluoride concentration in their drinking water (From Rugg-Gunn *et al.*, 1981; reproduced by courtesy of the Editor, *British Dental Journal*)

(Rugg-Gunn *et al.*, 1981). The slightly curved shape is very similar to those recorded for the permanent dentition by American dental epidemiologists (Figure 3.6).

The effect of water fluoridation in reducing dental caries in the deciduous dentition should not be underestimated. Although in a sense deciduous teeth are 'temporary', approximately 30% of all teeth that decay are deciduous teeth (D. Jackson, 1974, pers. comm.). Thus a reduction in the caries experience of the deciduous dentition is a most important factor when the need for dental treatment in a community is considered. In addition, it has important psychological and social benefits in that far fewer children in a fluoride area are exposed to the unfortunate sequelae of untreated dental caries – pain, sepsis, extraction of teeth – and so are likely to have a more positive attitude to dental treatment in later life.

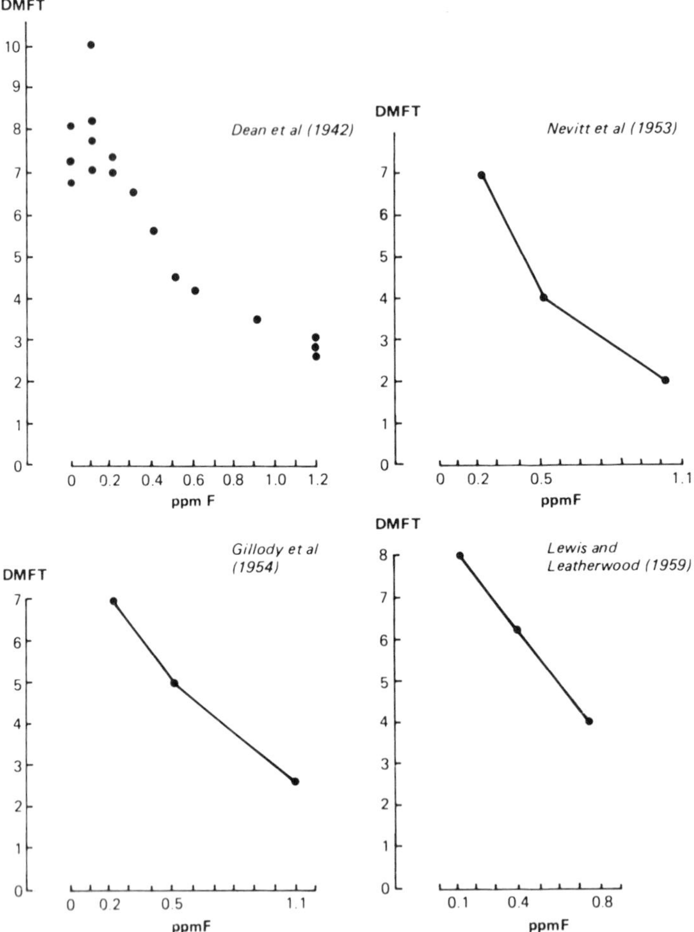

Figure 3.6 Relationship between caries experience (DMFT) and water fluoride concentration (ppm F) in four American studies. (1) Dean *et al.*, 1942; data shown refer to 5963 12–14-year-old children. (2) Nevitt *et al.*, 1953; 318 12-year-old children. (3) Gillody *et al.*, 1954; 311 13-year-old children. (4) Lewis and Leatherwood, 1959; 899 14-year-old children (From Rugg-Gunn *et al.*, 1981; reproduced by courtesy of the Editor, *British Dental Journal*)

The permanent dentition

The early studies by Dean and co-workers in Galesburg and Monmouth and Macomb and Quincy (Dean *et al.*, 1939), in the USA, stressed two important points about the effect of water fluoridation on the pattern of caries attack in the permanent dentition. First, they observed a strikingly low amount of interproximal caries and, secondly, they reported that the mortality rate of first permanent molars was much lower in the fluoride areas (Galesburg 1.8 ppm and Monmouth 1.7 ppm) than in the non-fluoride areas (Macomb and Quincy 0.2 ppm). The data on which these two observations were based are summarized in Tables 3.4 and 3.5. This suggested that, first, fluoride in drinking water had a greater caries-inhibitory effect on approximal or smooth surfaces than on pit and fissure caries and, secondly, that the rate of progression of a carious lesion is much slower in a fluoride area than in a non-fluoride area.

Table 3.4 Approximal surface caries in maxillary incisors of 12–14-year-old children (Galesburg and Monmouth, and Macomb and Quincy, USA) (From Dean *et al.*, 1939)

	*No. children**	*No. approximal surfaces*	*No. carious surfaces*	*Dental caries per 100 surfaces*
Galesburg and Monmouth	342	2718	16	0.59
Macomb and Quincy	354	2814	251	9.00

* The children in this table include only those who have continuously used the municipal water supply throughout life.

Table 3.5 Mortality of first permanent molars in 12–14-year-old children (Galesburg and Monmouth, and Macomb and Quincy, USA) (From Dean *et al.*, 1939)

	No. children	*No. first permanent molars missing or extraction indicated*	*No. missing per 100 children examined*	*Per cent of those examined with one or more missing first permanent molars*
Galesburg and Monmouth	467	56	12.0	8.6
Macomb and Quincy	418	292	70	35.4

Both these observations have been substantiated by subsequent studies. The Tiel–Culemborg water fluoridation experiment was designed specifically to assess the preventive effect of fluoridated drinking water on different tooth surfaces. The study's findings on fluoride's protective effect on all tooth surfaces has been presented previously (page 21) and in Table 2.2.

Backer Dirks (1974) compared the percentage distribution of the various types of carious surfaces in 15-year-old children from Holland and New Zealand (Table 3.6). He concluded that in the fluoridated towns, the relative importance of proximal and gingival lesions is markedly reduced, the pit and fissure lesions constituting more than 65% of all cavities. Thus, not only was a reduction in the total number of cavities achieved, but also there was an important shift towards less complicated restorations. He calculated that if pit and fissure cavities are regarded

Table 3.6 Percentage distribution of the various types of carious surfaces in 15-year-old children consuming drinking water with 0.1 or 1.0 ppm F (Holland and New Zealand) (From Backer Dirks, 1974)

	ppm F	*Pits and fissures*	*Gingival lesions*	*Proximal lesions*	*Total*
Culemborg	0.1	48.1	13.5	38.0	99.6
Tiel	1.0	73.2	4.5	22.3	100
Hastings, 1954	0.1	43.8	8.7	47.5	100
Hastings, 1970	1.0	65.5	2.9	31.6	100

as one treatment unit, gingival cavities as one unit, and the more time-consuming proximal cavities as 1½ units, an assessment of the reduction in treatment time can be made (Table 3.7). These figures show the reduction in treatment time brought about by water fluoridation.

However, because the figures in Table 3.7 have only included time to treat caries, they are likely to be an overestimate of the saving in surgery time. Ast *et al.* (1970) reported that the chair time needed to provide examination, prophylaxis and corrective care was about 1½ times more in non-fluoridated Kingston than in fluoridated Newburgh, USA. Reductions in dental manpower required in

Table 3.7 Units of time necessary for treatment of 15-year-old children consuming water with 0.1 or 1.0 ppm F (Holland and New Zealand) (From Backer Dirks, 1974)

	ppm F		*Difference in treatment time*
	0.1	*1.0*	*(%)*
Hastings, 1954–70	62.7	22.9	63
Culemborg–Tiel	36.7	13.7	63

fluoridated areas have been reported by Denby and Hollis (1966) in New Zealand and by Künzel (1976) in East Germany. Both these areas were fortunate, and perhaps unusual, in having sufficient manpower to meet the dental needs of the children. Denby and Hollis observed that the number of children who were able to be treated by a New Zealand dental nurse was 690 in fluoridated Hastings but only 475 in a non-fluoridated town. Künzel observed that the paedodontist:child ratio increased from 1:1659 in 1959 to 1:3208 in 1971 following the introduction of fluoridation in Karl-Marx-Stadt in 1959. The trend towards a requirement for simpler fillings in fluoridated areas was highlighted by Künzel (1976), who reported that single surface fillings were reduced by 52%, and 2 or more surface fillings by 77% in 6–18-year-olds after 12 years' fluoridation.

Backer Dirks (1974) also summarized data concerning the number of missing first permanent molars in fluoride and non-fluoride areas (Table 3.8) and concluded that in fluoride areas the number of extracted first molars is reduced by at least 75%. He also pointed out that the baseline rate of extractions is very different in the three studies referred to, indicating that apart from dental caries the availability and type of dental treatment must also affect the rate of extractions.

Table 3.8 Number of missing first molars per 100 children consuming drinking water with 0.1 or 1.0 ppm F

	Age	*ppm F*		*Per cent difference*
		0.1	*1.0*	
Kingston–Newburgh	13/14	61	9	85
Evanston, 1946–61	12/14	16	4	75
Culemborg–Tiel	15	44	2	95

Data for 15-year-old children in the Hartlepool–York study also confirmed these observations (Murray, 1969b). The mean DMF was 45% lower in Hartlepool than York (5.0 as against 9.0). The distribution of DMF teeth in the two communities is shown diagrammatically in Figure 3.7. The percentage number of DMF teeth for each tooth type is shown in Figure 3.8. Approximately 95% of first permanent molars in York were carious; the figure for Hartlepool was 65% – a difference of approximately 30%. Twice as many first molars had been extracted in York as in Hartlepool (17.9% as against 8.7%), in spite of the fact that the dentist:population ratio, and hence the availability of dental treatment, was much more favourable in York than it was in Hartlepool.

Maxillary incisors benefited more from exposure to fluoride than first molars and apparently maxillary central incisors were protected to a greater extent than maxillary lateral incisors. This apparent anomaly is because there are far more palatal pit lesions in lateral incisors than central incisors. When only approximal surfaces on these teeth were considered, there were 11 times more approximal lesions in York than in Hartlepool at 15 years of age (Table 3.9).

The greatly reduced occurrence of caries in incisor teeth in fluoridated areas has also been reported in other UK studies. Fifteen-year-old children in fluoridated Anglesey had 82% fewer carious incisor teeth than children in fluoride-low control areas (Jackson, James and Wolfe, 1975). In addition, Whittle and Downer (1979)

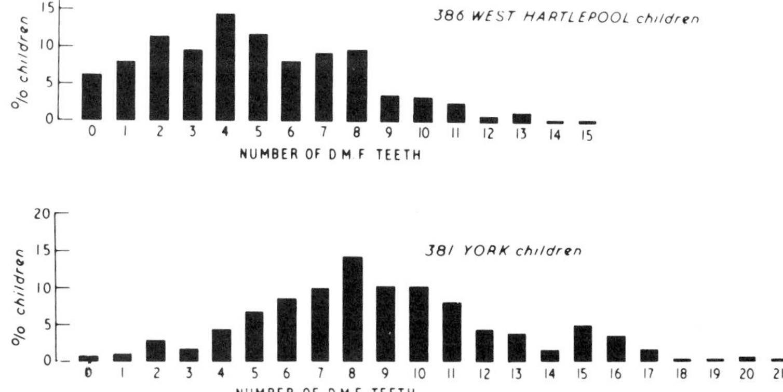

Figure 3.7 Frequency distribution of DMF teeth in 15-year-old children from Hartlepool and York (From Murray, 1969b; reproduced by courtesy of the Editor, *British Dental Journal*)

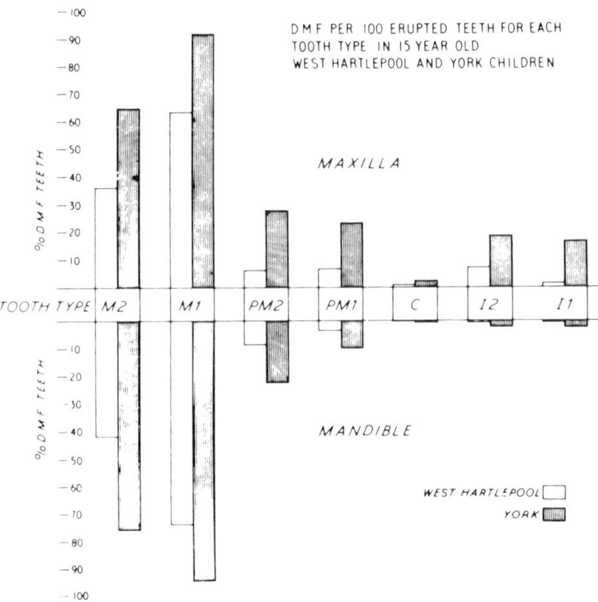

Figure 3.8 Caries experience in each tooth type in 15-year-old children from Hartlepool and York (From Murray, 1969b; reproduced by courtesy of the Editor, *British Dental Journal*)

Table 3.9 Maxillary incisor approximal caries in 15-year-old children in Hartlepool (1.5–2.0 ppm F) and York (0.25 ppm F)

	No. children	*No. DF sites*	*Per cent sites carious*
Hartlepool	386	19	0.6
York	381	200	6.6

reported that the number of carious anterior teeth in 11–12-year-old children living in fluoridated Birmingham was 74% less than in non-fluoridated Salford.

Thus, the effect of living in a fluoridated area is to reduce mean caries experience by 45%, to markedly reduce the need to extract first permanent molars, and to virtually eliminate the need for approximal restorations in maxillary incisors.

Effect of varying concentrations of fluoride on dental caries

Dean's study in 1942 (see Figure 2.2) showed the relationship between caries experience and fluoride content of the water supply to 21 cities in the USA. Dean's original observations have been substantiated by a number of investigations. Møller (1965) showed that data from Denmark and Sweden followed the same trend as that reported from America (Figure 3.9). In addition, studies in the UK, Hungary, Austria and Spain show a decrease in caries experience with increasing fluoride content of the water supply up to about 2 ppm; this information is summarized in Table 3.10 (Naylor and Murray, 1989).

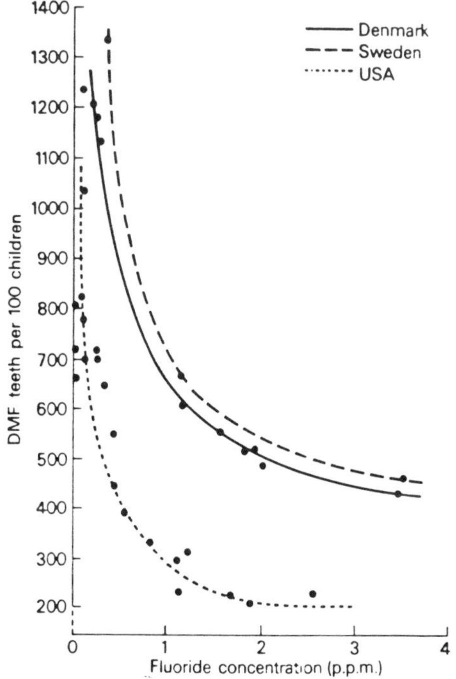

Figure 3.9 Caries experience in 12–13-year-old children from Denmark, Sweden and the USA in relation to concentration of fluoride in water supplies (From Møller, 1965, with permission)

Fluoridation studies in Britain – 1975–90

Studies into the effects of water fluoridation on the prevalence of dental caries in children have been reported at regular intervals throughout the 1980s. It is possible to divide them into four main groups.

1. Reports comparing dmf/DMF rates from fluoride and low-fluoride communities.
2. Effect of fluoridation and the secular trends in caries.
3. The relationship between social class and the effect of water fluoridation.
4. The cessation of fluoridation.

Reports from fluoride and low-fluoride communities

Birmingham was fluoridated in 1964 and Newcastle followed in 1968. Not surprisingly, many of the studies involve one or other of these cities. In 1979, Whittle and Downer carried out a study of infant and secondary school children in two electoral wards, one in Birmingham and one in Salford. Examinations were confined to children in maintained schools who were lifetime residents of each ward and whose parents had consented to their participating. Children were examined under constant conditions in a mobile surgery that visited each school. The results

Table 3.10 Dental caries in 12–14-year-old children in communities with varying concentrations of fluoride in drinking water (From Naylor and Murray, 1989)

Reference	*Country*	*Town*	*F Supply*	*No. children*	*Mean DMF*
Dean (1942)	USA	Michigan City	0.09	236	10.37
		Elkhart	0.11	278	8.23
		Portsmouth	0.13	469	7.72
		Zanesville	0.19	459	7.33
		Middletown	0.2	370	7.03
		Quincy	0.13	330	7.06
		Lima	0.3	454	6.52
		Marion	0.43	263	5.56
		Pueblo	0.6	614	4.12
		Kewanee	0.9	123	3.43
		East Moline	1.2	152	3.03
		Colorado Springs	2.6	404	2.46
		Galesburg	1.9	273	2.36
		Waukegan	0.0	423	8.10
		Oak Park	0.0	329	7.22
		Evanstown	0.0	256	6.73
		Elgin	0.5	403	4.44
		Joliet	1.3	447	3.23
		Aurora	1.2	633	2.81
		Maywood	1.2	171	2.58
		Elmhurst	1.8	170	2.52
Arnold (1948)	USA	Nashville	0.0	662	4.6
		Key West	0.1	95	10.7
		Clarksville	0.2	60	4.6
		Vicksburg	0.2	172	5.87
		Escanaba	0.2	270	8.8
		Hereford	3.1	60	1.47
Galagan (1953)*	USA	Yuma	0.4	29	2.45
		Tempe	0.5	45	2.82
		Tucson	0.7	167	3.48
		Chandler	0.8	42	2.45
		Casa Grande	1.0	22	2.00
		Florence	1.2	34	3.56

Nevitt *et al*. (1953)	USA	Low F	0.08–0.26	311	8.5
		Medium F	0.42–0.68	222	4.8
		High F	0.87–1.32	254	2.1
Lewis and Leatherwood (1959)	USA	Macon	0.11	1182	6.33
		Savanah	0.37	1188	5.22
		Moultrie	0.75	136	3.15
Gillody *et al*. (1954)		Low F	0.1–0.3	114	3.65
		Medium F	0.5	109	2.80
		High F	0.8–1.6	88	1.41
Klein (1948)	USA	Williamstown and Clayton	0.1	81	7.2
		Woodstown, Glassboro and Pitman	1.3–2.2	176	1.9
Forrest (1956)	UK	Saffron Walden and district	0.1	145	6.6
		Stoneleigh and Maldon West	0.1–0.2	114	6.1
		Slough	0.9	119	2.6
		Harwich	2.0	92	1.5
		Burnham-on-Crouch	3.5	62	1.4
		West Mersea	5.8	51	2.8
Adler (1951)	Hungary	Sarretudvari	0.20	166	4.25
		Öcsöd	0.21	222	2.09
		Bekesszentandras	0.21	177	2.43
		Biharnagybajom	0.33	143	3.06
		Kumszentmarton farms	0.72	86	1.29
		Szekszard	0.76	292	0.91
		Kunszentmarton village	0.99	283	1.02
		Komadi	1.09	343	1.31
Binder (1965)	Austria	Low F	0.00	90	4.9
		Umhansen, Silz and Mallnitz	1.0–1.8	82	1.2
Sellman *et al*. (1957)	Sweden	Malmö	0.3–0.5	145	13.3
		Nyvang	1.0		
		Astorp	1.3	149	6.8
		Simrishamm	1.3		
Møller (1965)	Denmark	Vejen	0.05	148	12.5
		Aalestrup	0.2	52	12.2
		St. Heddinge	0.25	43	11.7
		Slagelse	0.34	424	11.2
		Naestved H	1.2	157	6.2
		Praestø	1.6	43	5.5
		Naestved N	1.8	42	5.2
		Naestved G	1.9	150	5.2
		Stroby Egede	2.0	12	4.9
		Tappernøje and Strøby By	3.4	14	4.2

Table 3.10 continued

Reference	*Country*	*Town*	*F Supply*	*No. children*	*Mean DMF*
Vines and Clavero (1968)†	Spain	Aezcoa	0.1	34	6.25
		Valle de Erro	0.1	22	6.02
		Tafalla	0.5	149	5.64
		Pitillas	0.7	21	5.14
		Pamplona	0.7	670	5.03
		Mueillo et Fruito	0.75	37	5.01
		Funes	0.65	66	4.91
		Falces	0.65	93	4.57
		Potasas	0.6	70	4.56
		Tudela	0.6	192	4.49
		Murcia	0.8	462	3.41
		Abanilla	1.5	47	2.35

* These studies were carried out in Arizona, which has a very high mean annual temperature.
† 10–12-year-old children.

Table 3.11 Caries experience in 5- and 12-year-old children from Birmingham and Salford (From Whittle and Downer, 1979)

Age group	*Fluoridated (Birmingham)*	*Low-fluoride (Salford)*	*Per cent difference*
4–5-year-olds			
No. in group	70	76	
Mean dmft	1.64	3.55	54
11–12-year-olds			
No. in group	138	149	
Mean DMFT	2.22	4.00	45

are summarized in Table 3.11. The authors concluded that the relative costs of providing treatment of the caries diagnosed was some 50% lower in the fluoridated area.

Two years later Downer, Blinkhorn and Attwood (1981) measured the effect of fluoridation among Scottish children who were lifetime residents in Stranraer (fluoridated in 1971) and Annan (control). The results (Table 3.12) showed that the cost of dental treatment was nearly 50% lower in Stranraer than Annan.

Table 3.12 Caries experience in 5- and 10-year-old children from Stranraer and Annan (Downer, Blinkhorn and Attwood, 1981)

Age group	*Fluoridated (Stranraer)*	*Control (Annan)*	*Per cent difference*
4–5-year-olds			
No. in group	129	101	
Mean dmft	2.48	4.39	44
9–10-year-olds			
No. in group	147	141	
Mean DMFT	1.66	3.35	56

In the same year, the dental health of Birmingham children was compared with children from Wolverhampton (Rock, Gordon and Bradnock, 1981a). One hundred children were selected at each age from 6 to 13 years inclusive, from Birmingham and Wolverhampton, respectively. A total of 1757 children were examined by two dentists in a mobile caravan that was taken to each school. Bitewing radiographs were taken and used to diagnose approximal caries. The mean DMF values are summarized in Table 3.13.

In a subsequent paper concerned only with caries experience of first molar teeth, Rock, Gordon and Bradnock (1981b) record that DMF rates for all first molars in Birmingham rose from 0.15 at 6 years to 2.34 at age 13. In Wolverhampton, comparable figures were 0.46 and 3.22. By the age of 11 years, 40% of the Birmingham children had all four first molars sound, whereas in Wolverhampton

Table 3.13 Caries experience in Birmingham and Wolverhampton children (From Rock, Gordon and Bradnock, 1981a)

Age	*Mean DMFT*		*Mean DMFS*	
	Birmingham	*Wolverhampton*	*Birmingham*	*Wolverhampton*
6	0.14	0.42	0.18	0.53
7	0.26	0.77	0.29	1.07
8	0.94	1.59	1.19	2.23
9	1.06	2.24	1.61	3.59
10	1.34	3.24	1.74	5.95
11	1.91	3.45	3.14	7.23
12	2.63	5.68	4.46	11.41
13	3.36	5.42	6.06	10.01

only 12% had no first molar caries at this age. Almost four times as many first molars had been extracted in Wolverhampton compared with Birmingham.

Six years later, a study of 14-year-old children from South Birmingham and Bolton (Mitropoulos *et al.*, 1988) reported a DMFT value of 2.26 in the fluoridated area compared with 3.79 in the low-fluoridated area (Table 3.14). In this study it was not possible to ascertain whether the children had resided continuously in the fluoridated area.

Table 3.14 Caries experience in 14-year-old children in Birmingham and Bolton in 1987 (From Mitropoulos *et al.*, 1988)

	Birmingham	*Bolton*
No. in group	234	275
Mean DMFT	2.26	3.79

Although the overall DMFT values are lower than those recorded in Birmingham and Wolverhampton 6 years previously, the percentage difference in favour of Birmingham was 40%.

In 1968 the water supply to four districts of Leeds was fluoridated. In the early part of 1979 a dental examination was made of 5-year-old continuous residents in the fluoridated districts. At the same time a similar study was made of 5-year-old children in two neighbouring low-fluoride districts of Leeds where the water supply contains about 0.1 ppm (Jackson, Goward and Morrell, 1980). The results showed (Table 3.15) a difference of 62% in dmf values in favour of the fluoridated districts.

Table 3.15 Caries experience in 5-year-old Leeds children (From Jackson, Goward and Morrell, 1980)

	Fluoridated area	*Low-fluoride area*
No. in group	470	440
Mean dmf	1.23	3.28

Four times as many deciduous teeth were extracted in the low-fluoride districts compared with the fluoridated communities.

The prevalence of caries in 1003 10-year-old children continuously resident in fluoridated Newcastle and low-fluoride Northumberland was reported by Murray *et al.* (1984). The mean DMFS was 23% lower in Newcastle (2.3) than in Northumberland (3.0), although fluoridation had been sub-optimal between 1977 and 1981 owing to alterations in the water supply system (Figure 3.10).

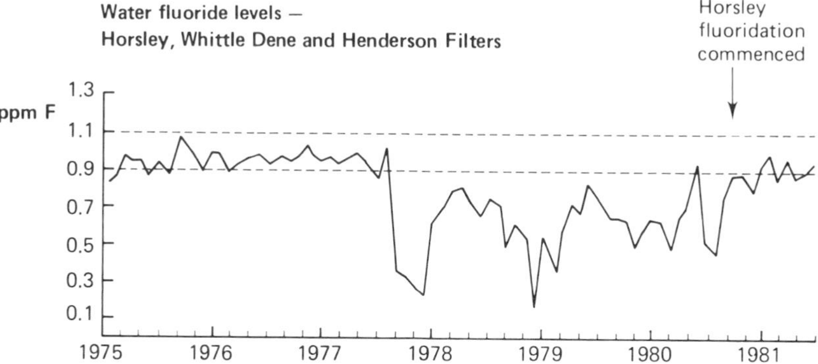

Figure 3.10 Water fluoride levels in Newcastle 1975–81 (From Murray *et al.*, 1984; reproduced with kind permission of the Editor, *British Dental Journal*)

The dental health of 5-year-old Newcastle children was compared with children of similar age from North Manchester by Duxbury *et al.* (1987) (Table 3.16). Caries experience was 60% lower in Newcastle children, and twice as many were caries-free, compared with Manchester children.

A 10% sample of children from both populations was selected by stratified sampling and efforts were made to ensure that the social class make-up of the samples was similar. A total of 18 schools were involved in the study.

Table 3.16 Caries experience in 5-year-old Newcastle and North Manchester children (From Duxbury *et al.*, 1987)

	Newcastle	*North Manchester*
No. in group	219	244
Mean dmf	1.33	3.31

Effect of fluoridation and secular trends in caries

Studies in Anglesey and Newcastle have reported on the effect of fluoridation and secular trends in caries. Anglesey was one of the communities involved in the British fluoridation studies in the 1950s. Part of this island was fluoridated on 17 November 1955. After 11 years of study the whole of the island was fluoridated. Jackson and co-workers reported on epidemiological surveys carried out in 1974 and 1983 (Jackson, James and Wolfe, 1975; Jackson, James and Thomas, 1985). The authors commented that opponents of fluoridation criticized the 1974 study by stating that there was no adequate control community, it was not double blind and the data were analysed in a way that gave opportunities for the results to be altered.

In the 1983 study the investigators went to extraordinary lengths to rebut these criticisms. The sampling was carried out by a Specialist in Community Medicine of Gwynedd Health Authority, letters were sent to parents asking for permission to examine their child or children and information was sought on the child's length of residence, the receipt of fluoride supplements and the availability of water to the household – mains, well or both. Children were brought to a common diagnostic centre and the examiners were kept completely ignorant of the child's residential code.

Two independent referees, Professor B. Hogan, Pro-Vice Chancellor of Leeds at the time, and Dr G. O. Williams, retired Archbishop of Wales, were chosen to look after the coded sheets giving details of each child's residence. The sealed envelope, containing details of the place of residence, was opened in the presence of Mr M. Parkin of the *Guardian* newspaper. The results of the 1983 study (Jackson, James and Thomas, 1985) are summarized in Table 3.17. A comparison of the results from 1974 and 1983 is given in Table 3.18.

Table 3.17 Caries experiences in Anglesey children (From Jackson, James and Thomas, 1985)

Age group	*Mon (fluoridated)*	*Arfon (control)*	*Difference (%)*
5-year-olds			
No. in group	219	128	
Mean dmft	1.58	3.55	55
12-year-olds			
No. in group	115	48	
Mean DMFT	1.84	2.73	42
15-year-olds			
No. in group	121	51	
Mean DMFT	4.73	7.69	38

Table 3.18 Secular change in caries experience of 5- and 15-year-old children from Anglesey (From Jackson, James and Wolfe, 1975; Jackson, James and Thomas, 1985)

Age group		*Mon (fluoridated)*	*Arfon (control)*	*Difference (%)*
5-year-olds				
Mean dmf:	1974	2.83	4.58	
	1983	1.58	3.55	55
Percentage difference		30	22	
15-year-olds				
Mean DMF:	1974	6.37	11.44	
	1983	4.73	7.69	38
Percentage difference		26	33	

Thus there was a fall in caries of between 22% and 23% in both communities between 1974 and 1983, but the lower caries experience in the fluoridated communities was maintained.

Seaman, Thomas and Walker (1989) reported that the mean dmf of 5-year-olds was 0.80 in fluoridated Anglesey compared with 2.26 in non-fluoridated Gwynedd, a difference of 55%. Although the absolute figures from this study, carried out in 1987, are lower than those reported by Jackson and co-workers (Table 13.18) who examined children 4 years earlier, the absolute difference in mean dmft between the fluoride and non-fluoride communities had been maintained (1.46 according to Seaman, Thomas and Walker, 1989; 1.25 according to Jackson, James and Thomas, 1985).

Rugg-Gunn and co-workers have been involved in three surveys of 5-year-old children continuously resident in fluoridated Newcastle and low-fluoride Northumberland (Rugg-Gunn *et al.*, 1977; French *et al.*, 1984; Rugg-Gunn, Carmichael and Ferrell, 1988). The results for the 1987 study are given in Table 3.19. The results of this study were compared with the findings of the 1976 and 1981 surveys (Figure 3.11). Caries experience fell in both areas between 1976 and 1981, but no further decline was observed between 1981 and 1987.

Table 3.19 Caries experiences in 5-year-old Newcastle and Northumberland children in 1987 (From Rugg-Gunn, Carmichael and Ferrell, 1988)

	Newcastle (fluoridated)	*Northumberland (control)*	*Difference (%)*
No. in group	457	370	
Mean dmft	1.8	3.9	54

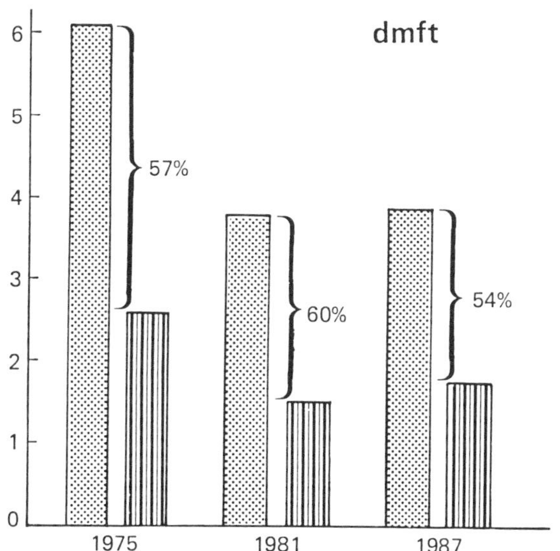

Figure 3.11 Caries experience (mean dmft) of 5-year-old children in the fluoridated (lined columns) and non-fluoridated (stippled columns) areas of N.E. England in 1975, 1981 and 1987 (From Rugg-Gunn, Carmichael and Ferrell, 1988; reproduced with kind permission of the Editor, *British Dental Journal*)

Secular trends of dental caries in the natural fluoride area of Hartlepool can be observed over a 40-year period.

In 1949, Robert Weaver examined 1258 children, aged 5, 12 and 15 years, from West Hartlepool. In 1967, Murray (1969a,b) examined 3804 children aged 3–18 years from West Hartlepool. Twenty years later, Hartlepool children were surveyed again by community dental officers as part of the Northern Region Epidemiological Dental Surveys (Evans and Dowell, 1988, 1990; Dowell and Evans, 1989). The results of these surveys are summarized in Table 3.20.

Table 3.20 Caries experience in Hartlepool children, 1949–90

Age group	*Weaver (1949)*	*Murray (1967)*	*BASCD Surveys (1987–89)*
5-year-olds			
Mean dmf	1.8	1.5	0.8
Percentage caries-free	54	51	67
12-year-olds			
Mean DMF	1.0	2.0	0.7
Percentage caries-free	60	30	59
15-year-olds			
Mean DMF	2.1	4.9	1.7
Percentage caries-free	37	26	39

In spite of the secular change in dental caries that has been referred to so often in the past few years, caries experience in Hartlepool remains one of the lowest recorded of any part of the country.

Relationship between social class and effect of water fluoridation

Another aspect of the 'Newcastle and Northumberland' studies was that they demonstrated the effect of social class on dental caries, at least in the deciduous dentition. In their first paper, Carmichael *et al.* (1980) reported a significant trend towards higher caries experience in lower social classes in the low-fluoride area and a non-significant, less pronounced trend in the other direction in the fluoridated area (Table 3.21). They concluded that fluoridation was having its greatest effect in the lower social class groups and appeared to remove inter-social class differences in dental caries experience.

Table 3.21 Mean dmft values and social class in 5-year-old children from Newcastle and Northumberland (From Carmichael *et al.*, 1980)

Social class	*Newcastle (fluoridated)*	*Northumberland (low-fluoride)*	*Difference (%)*
I, II	2.5	3.4	26
III	2.4	6.0	60
IV, V	2.0	7.0	71

Carmichael and co-workers repeated this type of analysis in 1984 and 1989 (Carmichael *et al.*, 1984; French *et al.*, 1984; Carmichael, Rugg-Gunn and Ferrell, 1989) (Tables 3.22 and 3.23).

Table 3.22 Mean dmf values and social class in 5-year-old children from Newcastle and Northumberland (From Carmichael *et al.*, 1984)

Social class	*Newcastle (fluoridated)*	*Northumberland (low-fluoride)*	*Difference (%)*
I, II	0.98	2.15	54
III	1.54	3.55	57
IV, V	1.54	3.91	61

Table 3.23 Mean dmft values and social class in 5-year-old children from Newcastle and Northumberland (From Carmichael, Rugg-Gunn and Ferrell, 1989)

Social class	*Newcastle (fluoridated)*	*Northumberland (low-fluoride)*	*Difference (%)*
I, II	1.1	2.2	49
III	1.7	3.7	54
IV, V	2.4	5.0	51
Unclassified	2.4	4.5	46

The numbers unclassified were high in the 1989 survey, approximately one-quarter of the sample, and were reported separately, but were more likely to be in the low social class groups or those whose fathers were unemployed. The main findings of the 1984 and 1989 reports were, first, that fluoridation was effective in all social class groupings and, secondly, because caries levels were higher in social classes IV and V, fluoridation brought about greater savings for social classes IV and V children than for social classes I and II children.

Bradnock, Marchment and Anderson (1984) investigated the effects of fluoridation and social background on caries experience of 5-year-old children living in the West Midlands. Their results are summarized in Table 3.24.

The trends demonstrated in this investigation did not correspond with the work carried out in Newcastle/Northumberland, but there were differences in the sampling methods used in the two studies. The sample in the North-East involved 28 schools, which were randomly selected by the Northern Regional Health

Table 3.24 Mean dmft values and socioeconomic grouping (SEG) for 5-year-old children living in the West Midlands (From Bradnock, Marchment and Anderson, 1984)

	No. children	*Fluoride areas*	*No. children*	*Low-fluoride areas*	*Difference (%)*
	174	1.09	179	1.91	43
High SEG	76	0.47	81	0.90	59
Low SEG	98	1.56	98	2.74	43

Authority Statistician's Office. Only children whose parents consented, who had lived since birth in that locality and were Caucasian were included in the study. Parental occupation was obtained from school medical records or parental questionnaires and was coded according to the Registrar General's classification. In the West Midlands, sampling was carried out on a geographical basis by choosing nine schools from electoral wards, stratified as to whether the inhabitants were from predominantly high or low social backgrounds. The children were not necessarily continuously resident in the communities in which they went to school.

Cessation of fluoridation

Mansbridge (1969) reported that after cessation of the fluoridation scheme in Kilmarnock, in 1962 the prevalence of caries had increased, in children aged 3–7 years. By 1968, the proportion of children free from decay approximated to the pre-fluoridation level of 1956 and to that of the control children in Ayr.

Following the Opinion of Lord Jauncey on Fluoridation in Strathclyde in 1983, water fluoridation schemes in Scotland had to be withdrawn.

Stephen, McCall and Tullis (1987) reported the results of clinical and radiographic examinations of 5-year-old children who had been born and raised in the fluoridated town of Wick, compared with similar subjects 5 years after Wick water was defluoridated in 1979 because of a decision taken by Highland Regional Council. The results are summarized in Table 3.25 and show that a substantial rise in dental caries had occurred. The authors concluded that this localized caries increase, which is against all national, local and social class trends, resulted from the 1977 decision to deprive Wick inhabitants of fluoridated water supplies.

Table 3.25 Caries experience in 5-year-old Wick children in 1979 and 1984 (From Stephen, McCall and Tullis, 1987)

	1979	*1984*	*Percentage increase (1979 base)*
No. children	106	126	
Clinical mean dmft	2.63	3.92	49
Clinical and radiographic dmfs	8.42	13.93	67

Attwood and Blinkhorn (1988) reported on the effect of this decision in Stranraer. In 1980, a comparison had been made between the dental health of 10-year-old children in Stranraer, 10 years after the introduction of water fluoridation, and those in Annan, which had a negligible concentration of fluoride in the public water supply. In 1986, the opportunity was taken to examine 10-year-olds again, employing the same diagnostic criteria and one of the examiners involved in the previous study. Only lifetime residents were included in the analysis. The results (Table 3.26) showed that whereas DMFT values had fallen by 16% in Annan, they had risen by 4% in Stranraer after fluoridation had been withdrawn.

The authors concluded that although 10-year-old children in Stranraer may still have some residual benefit from earlier fluoridation, the study suggested that their dental health had started to deteriorate.

Table 3.26 Caries experience in 10-year-old children in Stranraer and Annan, 1980–86 (From Attwood and Blinkhorn, 1988)

Study	*No. children*	*Stranraer (mean DMFT)*	*No. children*	*Annan (mean DMFT)*	*Reduction (%)*
1980	147	1.66	141	3.35	56
1986	127	1.72	105	2.81	39
Percentage difference		+4		−16	

References

Adler, P. (1951) The connections between dental caries experience and water-borne fluorides in a population with low caries incidence. *J. Dent. Res.*, **30**, 368–381

Arnold, F. A. Jr (1948) Fluorine in drinking waters. Its effect on dental caries. *J. Am. Dent. Ass.*, **36**, 28–36

Ast, D. B., Cons, N. C., Pollard, S. T. and Garfinkel, J. (1970) Time and cost factors to provide regular, periodic dental care for children in a fluoridated and non-fluoridated area: final report. *J. Am. Dent. Assoc.*, **80**, 770–776

Attwood, D. and Blinkhorn, A. S. (1988) Trends in dental health of ten-year-old school children in South-West Scotland after cessation of water fluoridation. *Lancet*, 30 July

Backer Dirks, O. (1974) The benefits of water fluoridation. *Caries Res.*, **8**, suppl. 2–15

Beal, J. F. and James, P. M. C. (1971) Dental caries prevalence in 5 year old children following five and a half years of water fluoridation in Birmingham. *Br. Dent. J.*, **130**, 284–288

Bradnock, G., Marchment, M. D. and Anderson, R. J. (1984) Social background, fluoridation and caries experience in a 5-year-old population in the West Midlands. *Br. Dent. J.*, **156**, 127–131

Binder, K. (1965) Karies und fluorreiches Trinkwasser-kritische Betrachtung. *Osterr. Z. Stomat.*, **62**, 14–18

Carmichael, C. L., French, A. D., Rugg-Gunn, A. J. and Furness, J. A. (1984) The relationship between social class and caries experience in five year old children in Newcastle and Northumberland after twelve years' fluoridation. *Comm. Dent. Health*, **1**, 47–54

Carmichael, C. L., Rugg-Gunn, A. J. and Ferrell, R. S. (1989) The relationship between fluoridation, social class and caries experience in 5-year-old children in Newcastle and Northumberland in 1987. *Br. Dent. J.*, **167**, 57–61

Carmichael, C. L., Rugg-Gunn, A. J., French, A. D. and Cranage, J. D. (1980) The effect of fluoridation upon the relationship between caries experience and social class in 5-year-old children in Newcastle and Northumberland. *Br. Dent. J.*, **149**, 163–167

Dean, H. T., Arnold, F. A. and Elvove, E. (1942) Domestic water and dental caries V. Additional studies of the relation of fluoride domestic waters to dental caries experience in 4425 white children aged 12 to 14 years of 13 cities in 4 states. *Public Health Rep.* (*Wash.*), **57**, 1155–1179

Dean, H. T., Jay, P., Arnold, F. A. Jun., McClure, F. J. and Elvove, E. (1939) Domestic water and dental caries, including certain epidemiological aspects of oral *L. acidophilus*. *Public Health Rep.*, **54**, 862–888

Denby, G. C. and Hollis, M. J. (1966) The effect of fluoridation on a dental public health programme. *N.Z. Dent. J.*, **62**, 32–36

DHSS (1969) *The Fluoridation Studies in the United Kingdom and the Results Achieved after Eleven Years, A Report of the Committee on Research into Fluoridation*, Department of Health and Social Security Reports on Public Health and Medical Subjects No. 122, DHSS, London

Dowell, T. B. and Evans, D. J. (1988) The dental caries experience of 14-year-old children in England and Wales. *Commun. Dent. Hlth*, **5**, 395–410

Dowell, T. B. and Evans, D. J. (1989) The caries experience of 5-year-olds in Great Britain. *Commun. Dent. Hlth*, **6**, 271–279

Downer, M. C., Blinkhorn, A. S. and Attwood, D. (1981) Effect of fluoridation on the cost of dental treatment among urban Scottish schoolchildren. *Commun. Dent. Oral Epidemiol.*, **19**, 112–116

Duxbury, J. T., Lennon, A. M., Mitropoulos, C. M. and Worthington, H. V. (1987) Differences in caries levels in 5 year old children in Newcastle and North Manchester in 1985. *Br. Dent. J.*, **162**, 457–458

Evans, D. J. and Dowell, T. B. (1990) The dental caries experience of 12-year-old children in Great Britain. *Commun. Dent. Hlth*, **7**, 307–314

Forrest, J. R. (1956) Caries incidence and enamel defects in areas with different levels of fluoride in the drinking water. *Br. Dent. J.*, **100**, 195–200

French, A. D., Carmichael, C. L., Furness, J. A. and Rugg-Gunn, A. J. (1984) The relationship between social class and dental health in 5 year old children in the North and South of England. *Br. Dent. J.*, **156**, 83–86

French, A. D., Carmichael, C. L., Rugg-Gunn, A. J. and Furness, J. A. (1984) Fluoridation and dental caries experience in 5 year old children in Newcastle and Northumberland in 1981. *Br. Dent. J.*, **156**, 54–57

Galagan, D. J. (1953) Climate and controlled fluoridation. *J. Am. Dent. Ass.*, **47**, 159–170

Gillody, C. J., Heinz, H. W. and Eastman, P. W. (1954) A dental caries and fluoride study of 19 Nebraska cities. *J. Neb. Dent. Assoc.*, **31**, 3–13

Jackson, D., Goward, P. E. and Morrell, G. V. (1980) Fluoridation in Leeds. *Br. Dent. J.*, **149**, 231–234

Jackson, D., Gravely, J. F. and Pinkham, I. O. (1975) Fluoridation in Cumbria. *Br. Dent. J.*, **139**, 319–322

Jackson, D., James, P. M. C. and Thomas, F. D. (1985) Fluoridation in Anglesey 1983: a clinical study of dental caries. *Br. Dent. J.*, **158**, 45–49

Jackson, D., James, P. M. C. and Wolfe, W. B. (1975) Fluoridation in Anglesey. *Br. Dent. J.*, **138**, 165–171

Klein, H. (1948) Dental effects of accidentally fluoridated waters – dental caries experience in deciduous and permanent teeth of school age children. *J. Am. Dent. Ass.*, **36**, 443–453

Künzel, W. (1976) Trinkwasserfluoridierung Karl-Marx-Stadt XIII. *Stomat. DDR*, **26**, 458–465

Lemke, C. W., Doherty, J. M. and Arra, M. C. (1970) Controlled fluoridation: the dental effects of discontinuation in Angigo, Wisconsin. *J. Am. Dent. Assoc.*, **80**, 782–786

Lewis, F. D. and Leatherwood, E. C. (1959) Effect of natural fluorides on caries incidence in three Georgia cites. *Public Health Rep.* (*Wash.*), **74**, 127–131

Mansbridge, J. N. (1969) The Kilmarnock studies. Appendix to: *The Fluoridation Studies in the United Kingdom and Results Achieved After 11 Years*, HMSO, London

Mitropoulos, C. M., Lennon, M. A., Langford, J. W. and Robinson, D. J. (1988) Differences in dental caries experience in 14 year old children in fluoridated South Birmingham and in Bolton in 1987. *Br. Dent. J.*, **164**, 349–350

Møller, I. J. (1965) *Dental fluorose og caries*, Rhodes International Science Publishers, Copenhagen

Murray, J. J. (1969a) Caries experience of five-year-old children from fluoride and non-fluoride communities. *Br. Dent. J.*, **126**, 352–354

Murray, J. J. (1969b) Caries experience of 15-year-old children from fluoride and non-fluoride communities. *Br. Dent. J.*, **127**, 128–131

Murray, J. J. and Atkinson, K. (1971) Caries experience of West Hartlepool children aged 2–18 years. *Dent. Pract. Dent. Rec.*, **21**, 387–388

Murray, J. J., Gordon, P. H., Carmichael, C. L., French, A. D. and Furness, J. A. (1984) Dental caries and enamel opacities in 10 year old children in Newcastle and Northumberland. *Br. Dent. J.*, **156**, 255–258

Naylor, M. N. and Murray, J. J. (1989) *Fluorides and Dental Caries in the Prevention of Dental Disease*, 2nd edn (ed. J. J. Murray), Oxford Medical Publications, Oxford, pp. 141–144

Nevitt, G. A., Diefenbach, V. and Presnell, C. E. (1953) Missouri's fluoride and dental caries study. *J. Mo. State Dent. Assoc.*, **33**, 10–26

Rock, W. P., Gordon, P. H. and Bradnock, G. (1981a) Dental caries experience in Birmingham and Wolverhampton school children following the fluoridation of Birmingham water in 1964. *Br. Dent. J.*, **150**, 61–66

Rock, W. P., Gordon, P. H. and Bradnock, G. (1981b) Caries experience in West Midland school children following fluoridation of Birmingham water in 1964. *Br. Dent. J.*, **150**, 269–273

Rugg-Gunn, A. J., Carmichael, C. L. and Ferrell, R. S. (1988) Effect of fluoridation and secular trend in caries in 5 year old children living in Newcastle and Northumberland. *Br. Dent. J.*, **165**, 359–364

Rugg-Gunn, A. J., Carmichael, C. L., French, A. D. and Furness, J. A. (1977) Fluoridation in Newcastle and Northumberland: a clinical study of 5-year-old children. *Br. Dent. J.*, **142**, 359–402

Rugg-Gunn, A. J., Nicholas, K. E., Potts, A., Cranage, J. D., Carmichael, C. L. and French, A. D. (1981) Caries experience of 5 year old children living in four communities in N.E. England receiving differing water fluoride levels. *Br. Dent. J.*, **150**, 9–12

Seaman, S., Thomas, F. D. and Walker, W. A. (1989) Differences between caries levels in 5-year-old children from fluoridated Anglesey and non-fluoridated mainland Gwynedd in 1987. *Commun. Dent. Hlth,* **6**, 215–221

Sellman, S., Syrrist, A. and Gustafson, G. (1957) Fluorine and dental health in Southern Sweden. *T. Odont. Tskr.*, **65**, 61–93

Stephen, K. W., McCall, D. R. and Tullis, J. I. (1987) Caries prevalence in Northern Scotland before, and 5 years after, water defluoridation. *Br. Dent. J.*, **163,** 324–326

Tank, G. and Storvick, C. A. (1964) Caries experience of children 1–6 years old in two Oregon communities (Corvallis and Albany). 1. Effects of fluoride on caries experience and eruption of teeth. *J. Am. Dent. Assoc.,* **69**, 749–757

Vines, J. J. and Clavero, J. (1968) Investigacion de la relacion entre la incidencia de caries y contenido del ion fluor en las agnas de abastecimiento. *Rev. San. E. Hig. Pub.*, **42**, 401–431

Weaver, R. (1944) Fluorosis and dental caries on Tyneside. *Br. Dent. J.*, **76**, 29–40

Weaver, R. (1950) Original communications on fluorine and wartime diet. *Br. Dent. J.*, **88**, 231–239

Whittle, J. G. and Downer, M. C. (1979) Dental health and treatment needs of Birmingham and Salford schoolchildren. *Br. Dent. J.,* **147**, 67–71

Winter, G. B., Rule, D. C., Mailer, G. P., James, P. M. C. and Gordon, P. H. (1971) The prevalence of dental caries in pre-schoolchildren aged 1–4 years. *Br. Dent. J.,* **130**, 271–277

Chapter 4

Water fluoridation and adult dental health

Although many studies have shown conclusively that water fluoridation is effective in reducing caries in the permanent teeth of children, some doubts have been raised as to whether the observed reductions are due to a delay in the onset of clinical dental caries in the permanent dentition, or whether water fluoridation is having a truly long-term caries-preventive effect. The best way of resolving this problem is to carry out studies on adults continuously resident in fluoride and non-fluoride areas.

Deatherage (1943) made a study of the dental health in 2026 white national service selectees (mainly aged 21–28 years) living in 91 Illinois communities, with public water supplies varying in fluoride content. The communities were graded according to the content of the drinking water as follows:

F = 0.0–0.1 ppm – fluoride-free areas
F = 0.9 ppm – suboptimal fluoride areas
F = 1.0 ppm and over – fluoride areas

The mean DMF of selectees continuously resident in fluoride areas (F = 1.0 ppm) was 6.21 compared with a mean DMF value of 10.79 for selectees who had lived in fluoride-free areas all their lives.

Weaver (1944), in Britain, examined 100 mothers attending Maternity and Child Welfare clinics in North Shields (F = 0.25 ppm) and South Shields (F = 1.2–1.8 ppm). Third molar teeth were not assessed because of their varied eruption pattern. The results are presented in Table 4.1.

Table 4.1 Mean DMF of mothers in North Shields and South Shields (From Weaver, 1944)

North Shields			*South Shields*		
Age (yr)	*No. examined*	*Mean DMF*	*Age* (yr)	*No. examined*	*Mean DMF*
20	1	6	20	4	5
20–24	25	11	20–24	32	7
25–29	33	15	25–29	19	9
30–34	22	17	30–34	20	15
35–39	12	18	35–39	16	17
40+	7	19	40+	9	17

Weaver concluded that the South Shields mothers initially had a delay of caries experience of about 5 years; this delay was not constant and, by 30–34 years, caries experience in South Shields was similar to that in North Shields. The evidence given by Weaver cannot be regarded as conclusive. Apart from the fact that the numbers and selected sample upon which he based his conclusions were too small for adequate analysis, the DMF index cannot be regarded as a true measure of caries experience in adults because of the increasing number of caries-free teeth extracted for periodontal, prosthetic or surgical reasons. The M fraction of the index occupies approximately 85% of the total DMF in Weaver's study: this very high extraction rate would certainly have masked any caries-inhibitory property of fluoride drinking water.

Forrest, Parfitt and Bransby (1951) examined adults from three high-fluoride areas, South Shields (0.82 ppm F), Colchester (1.45 ppm F) and Slough (0.9 ppm F), and three low-fluoride areas, North Shields (0.07 ppm F), Ipswich (0.3 ppm F) and Reading (0.1 ppm F). To obtain groups of like social status, mothers attending antenatal and infant welfare centres were examined. Only those continuously resident in one of the above communities were examined. In all 286 mothers were seen in high-fluoride areas and 296 mothers were seen in low-fluoride areas. An uncorrected DMF index was used: the results are presented in Table 4.2. The authors stated that at each age caries incidence was lower in the high-fluoride areas than in the low-fluoride areas, but that the difference seemed to indicate a delay in onset of dental caries of about 10 years. Even in this study, which was of a highly selected sample, the numbers in the older age groups are too small to allow firm conclusions to be drawn.

Table 4.2 Caries experience of expectant and nursing mothers in low- and high-fluoride communities (From Forrest, Parfitt and Bransby, 1951)

Age (yr)	*No. examined*		*Mean DMF*		*Difference* (%)
	Low F	High F	Low F	High F	
20	22	17	12.5	8.5	33
21–25	92	91	16.2	10.0	38
26–30	107	69	19.3	12.5	35
31–35	40	61	21.5	16.2	25
36–40	30	23	22.8	19.0	16
40+	5	7	26.4	22.0	17

Russell and Elvove (1951), in the USA, also studied the effect of fluoride on dental caries experience in an adult population. Residents in Colorado Springs, Colo. (population 36 789 in 1940) were selected for the investigation, principally because of the long and reliable fluoride history of this town; the water supply contained 2.55 ppm F. Nearby Boulder, Colo. (population 13 000 in 1940) was utilized as a control; in this town there was only a trace of fluoride in the drinking water. Examination lists were based on school census records, birth records, marriage records and city directories. Age limits of 20–44 years were established. When the sample lists were assembled they were found to constitute a random cross-section of all people from the two communities. An attempt was made to examine each listed person; approximately 80% of the actual number of eligible persons agreed to a dental examination. Most of the men were professional or semi-professional workers, business proprietors, skilled craftsmen or students. There were comparatively few unskilled or semi-skilled workers in either group. More than half of the women examined were housewives and the remainder were mostly clerical and sales workers. College graduates constituted a high percentage of each sample – about 40% in Boulder and 20% at Colorado Springs. Both groups had received a high level of dental care and dental hygiene was generally good. For the purpose of this study 'continuous residence' was defined as 'residence unbroken except for periods not exceeding 60 days during the time of development and eruption of the permanent teeth; thereafter more than half the life had to be spent in the respective community'. The results of this study are recorded in Table 4.3. Russell and Elvove concluded that total rates for DMF permanent teeth were about 60% lower in Colorado Springs than in Boulder for each age group. Caries inhibition apparently continued undiminished up to at least 44 years. Boulder residents had lost three to four times as many teeth from dental caries as had those of Colorado Springs.

Table 4.3 Mean number of DMF teeth, together with its standard deviation (SD), in adults from Boulder and Colorado Springs (excluding third molars) (From Russell and Elvove, 1951)

Age (yr)	*Male*	*Female*	*Both*	*Mean DMF*	*±SD*
BOULDER					
20–24	22	29	51	14.0	4.9
25–29	26	15	41	16.5	5.5
30–34	17	12	29	18.3	5.2
35–39	8	14	22	21.8	5.1
40–44	6	6	12	21.7	6.0
20+	79	76	155	17.2	
COLORADO SPRINGS					
20–24	36	36	72	5.4	5.1
25–29	61	40	101	6.5	5.0
30–34	55	27	82	7.1	4.9
35–39	51	24	75	9.2	7.0
40–44	36	19	55	10.3	6.4
20+	239	146	385	7.5	

In a further article concerned with the same study, Russell (1953) assessed the inhibition of approximal caries in adults with lifelong fluoride exposure. He comments that studies of approximal caries in children are complicated by variation in the time risk factor for individual tooth types. This difficulty is minimized when adults are considered, but unfortunately progressive tooth loss in adults prevents the true pattern of surface attack from being determined. Because of this the most desirable age group to study is the oldest in which tooth loss has been minimal. Russell concluded that the optimal age was 35 years and proceeded to group all adults up to this age: there were 68 such persons at Boulder and 183 at Colorado Springs. The mean age of the Boulder group was 29.0 years and of the Colorado group 29.6 years. The mean number of missing teeth was 2.2 and 0.6, respectively; the corresponding mean DMF values were 16.8 and 6.6. In this investigation, approximal tooth areas were used as the unit of estimation. For example, an approximal area was made up of the distal surface of the maxillary first molar and the mesial surface of the maxillary second molars. The results were expressed as a percentage of approximal site areas at risk which were decayed, missing or filled, because of dental caries. In Colorado Springs the prevalence of DMF approximal site areas affected was 61–100% lower than in Boulder.

Englander and Wallace (1962) stated that there was a need to compare the dental caries experience of a large sample of adults who had continuously resided in a city having approximately 1 ppm F in its domestic water with that of a similar sample of adults in a nearby city who had consumed water low in fluoride. The communities they chose for study were Aurora, Illinois (F = 1.2 ppm), and Rockford, Illinois (fluoride-free). The main purpose of the Englander and Wallace study concerned the effect of fluoride on periodontal disease and hence only persons with at least 10 natural teeth present were examined. In each city, local workers telephoned mature residents and asked them to volunteer for examination. Newspapers, television and radio were used to solicit cooperation of all persons who met the residential criteria. A careful review of information received by telephone showed that of all persons over 20 years old contacted, 14% were edentulous in Rockford and less than 2% were edentulous in Aurora. No edentulous persons, or those with fewer than 10 natural teeth, were asked to report for examination. This population was therefore highly selected. A total of 896 continuous residents in Aurora and 935 residents in Rockford were examined. Women constituted 61% of the sample in Aurora and 63% of the sample in Rockford. The number in each age group, and the DMF values, for Aurora and for Rockford, are given in Table 4.4. The authors

Table 4.4 Mean DMF values against age for residents in Aurora (1.2 ppm F) and Rockford (no F) (After Englander and Wallace, 1962)

Age group	*Aurora*		*Rockford*	
	No. in group	*Mean DMF*	*No. in group*	*Mean DMF*
18–19	162	6.05	120	11.27
20–29	188	8.78	223	16.92
30–39	255	11.03	342	17.65
40–49	205	12.41	191	18.00
50–59	86	12.58	59	13.34
All ages	896	10.13	935	16.78

state that dental caries experience was significantly less for Aurora residents than for residents of Rockford. The mean DMF for Aurora was approximately 10 compared with approximately 17 for residents of Rockford. Overall reduction in DMF teeth for Aurorans over residents of Rockford was 40% approximately, in comparison with the reduction of approximately 60% found by Russell. Englander and Wallace suggested that failure to duplicate Russell's reduction was probably due to various factors, such as the elimination of people with fewer than 10 natural teeth, differences in examination techniques, and the inclusion of persons over 45 years of age. In Rockford, the mean DMF value in the 50–59-year age group (13.34) was much lower than that for younger age groups, and this suggests that the persons examined in the oldest age groups belonged to a biased sample. From the figures in the 50–59-year age group the mean DMF values for Aurora (12.58) and Rockford (13.34) are very similar.

Between individuals of similar age, the extent of dental disease varies over a wide range. Because of this, population estimates must be based on large numbers of people. This requirement is easily met in child studies because school children are effectively a captive population. This does not apply to adults, and hence adult studies are far more difficult to carry out. It is almost impossible to obtain a perfect sample of adult residents within any community for the purposes of dental study. Bulman *et al.* (1968) attempted to obtain a random sample of adults in Salisbury and Darlington by taking a sample of adults whose names were selected at random from the electoral registers of the two areas. In the end only 68% of those interviewed in Salisbury and 79% of those interviewed in Darlington were examined. A similar level of cooperation was obtained in the Adult Dental Health Survey of England and Wales (Gray *et al.*, 1970) where 77% of selected samples were examined and interviewed. These studies, however, were not of continuous residents. It would be impossible to ascertain the total pool of continuous residents within a community unless each resident was contacted. Even then, not all the continuous residents would give permission for a dental examination to be carried out. This is a very real problem of dental health studies in fluoride and non-fluoride areas, where it is essential to examine continuous residents.

In 1968–69, 4774 adults from Hartlepool and York were examined to try to measure in greater detail the long-term effect of fluoride in drinking water (Murray, 1971a). The County Borough of Hartlepool, population 100 000, is situated in the south-east corner of County Durham, some 8 miles north of the River Tees. Domestic water is supplied to Hartlepool by the Hartlepool Water Company, founded in 1841; it is a private company and its pipelines are not connected to any of the surrounding local authority water boards. The fluoride concentration in the drinking water is 1.5–2.0 ppm.

The City of York was used as a control town. Domestic water is supplied to the City of York by the York Water Company, which obtains its water from the River Ouse. The fluoride content of the water varies between the limits of 0.15 ppm and 0.28 ppm, depending on whether or not the river is in spate. The mean fluoride concentration is 0.2 ppm. The population of York is 105 000, very similar to that of Hartlepool. The socioeconomic status of active males in the two towns is very similar (1961 Census). Furthermore, caries experience of 5-year-old and 15-year-old York children was found to be very similar to that of the 'national average' for non-fluoride towns in England (Murray, 1968), suggesting that the pattern of caries experience in York was probably very similar to that of other low-fluoride towns. It was for these reasons that York was chosen as a control town.

In order to determine the full effect of fluoride drinking water on the dental structures, it is necessary to examine people who have been born and lived virtually all their lives in a fluoride area. The following definition of 'continuous residence' was adopted: a person who had been born in Hartlepool, had lived all his/her school life in the town (except for holidays) and had been away from the town during his/her life for no more than 6 years. This means that all those people termed 'continuous residents' had been exposed to fluoride drinking water during birth and childhood and had spent nearly all, if not all, of their adult life in the town. The definition was sufficiently flexible to allow people attending colleges, or working in other areas for short periods, or those who had done military service, to be included in the sample.

In order to obtain a sample of Hartlepool adults, large establishments were approached and asked to cooperate in the study. The aims of the project were discussed with the management and representatives of the workers in order to obtain as much cooperation as possible. Once approval had been given, a letter was sent to each person in the factory or establishment explaining the reason for the survey and asking for his/her cooperation. Subsequently arrangements were made for those people who had been born in Hartlepool, and who had agreed to a dental examination, to be seen in the place of work. Thirteen establishments, including all sections of Hartlepool Council, were visited in order to obtain as representative a sample of Hartlepool adults as possible. The number of Hartlepool adults examined in each quinquennial age group is recorded in Table 4.5.

Table 4.5 Number of adults examined in each age group in Hartlepool and York

Age	*Hartlepool*			*York*		
	Male	*Female*	*Total*	*Male*	*Female*	*Total*
15–19	141	450	591	61	102	163
20–24	132	298	430	149	158	307
25–29	107	75	182	199	76	275
30–34	102	77	179	186	56	242
35–39	100	77	177	188	83	271
40–44	86	77	163	225	106	331
45–49	83	80	163	270	123	393
50–54	48	51	99	167	86	253
55–59	55	49	104	185	65	250
60+	34	13	47	132	22	154

Although the sample of people examined cannot be called a true random sample of Hartlepool adults, it included people from all the major places of work in Hartlepool and spanned the whole social scale: directors, professional people, white-collar workers, skilled, semi-skilled and unskilled workers. The percentage of people in each social class in the sample examined is recorded in Table 4.6; 80% of the people examined were in social classes III and IV. It is therefore felt that every effort was made to achieve as representative as possible a sample of Hartlepool adults, concomitant with examining large numbers of people, and bearing in mind the fact that many people, particularly in the older age groups, were excluded from the study because they did not fulfil the criteria for 'continuous residence'.

A similar procedure to that used in Hartlepool was adopted in York to obtain a population sample of a low-fluoride area. Three large establishments agreed to cooperate in this study. The purpose of the survey was explained to representatives of the management and employees in each case. After approval had been given, a letter was sent to each person in the place of work asking for his/her cooperation in the study. Three people who had lived for a time in Hartlepool and one person who was born in Colchester and lived in Mersea (all high-fluoride areas) were excluded from the results.

The number of York adults examined in each quinquennial age group is recorded in Table 4.5 and the number of people in each social group is recorded in Table 4.6. As in Hartlepool, the people examined spanned the whole social scale. The percentage of adults in social classes I, II and III who were examined was slightly higher in York than in Hartlepool and the percentage of adults in social classes IV and V who were examined was slightly lower in York than in Hartlepool. However,

Table 4.6 Social class of adults examined in Hartlepool and York

Class	*Hartlepool*		*York*	
	No.	*Per cent*	*No.*	*Per cent*
I	3	0.1	14	0.5
II	202	9.5	371	14.0
III	899	42.1	1337	50.7
IV	805	37.7	797	30.2
V	226	10.6	120	4.6

in both communities approximately 80% of adults examined were in social classes III and IV, so that overall, the fluoride sample and the non-fluoride sample were fairly well balanced with respect to social class. The mean DMF values for all people examined, including edentulous persons, is shown in Figure 4.1.

Unfortunately, the DMF index is not an accurate measure of caries experience in adults because of the increasing number of caries-free teeth which are extracted (for periodontal and prosthetic reasons) as age advances. In order to try to measure the full caries inhibitory effect of fluoride in the drinking water, it is essential to try to measure more accurately caries experience in an adult population in fluoride and non-fluoride areas. Russell and Elvove (1951) attempted to compensate for the inaccuracy of the DMF index in adults by recording the primary reasons for

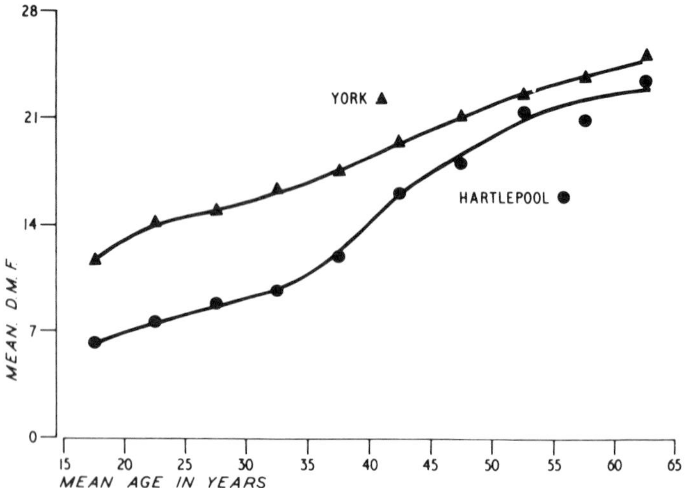

Figure 4.1 Mean DMF values in adults from Hartlepool and York, including edentulous persons (From Murray, 1971a; reproduced by courtesy of the Editor, *British Dental Journal)*

extraction based upon a history of signs and symptoms. Apart from the fact that subjective evidence of this nature is unreliable, a tooth removed for any reason other than caries may have suffered caries attack also. Unless reliable life records are available, an accurate assessment of the cumulative incidence of dental caries over a wide age range would seem to be impossible.

Three different approaches were made in the Hartlepool–York study to try to overcome this problem. First, it can be argued that the greatest error in the DMF index when used in adults is the inclusion of edentulous people in the DMF count, because it is these people who will have had the greatest proportion of caries-free teeth extracted in order to wear full dentures. On the other hand, those people who want to keep their teeth will have had relatively few caries-free teeth extracted and thus a more accurate measure of caries experience would be to calculate the observed DMF (DM_oF) in dentate persons (Figure 4.2). Comparing Figures 4.1 and 4.2, it will be seen that, using the latter index, the difference between the communities is much more clear cut.

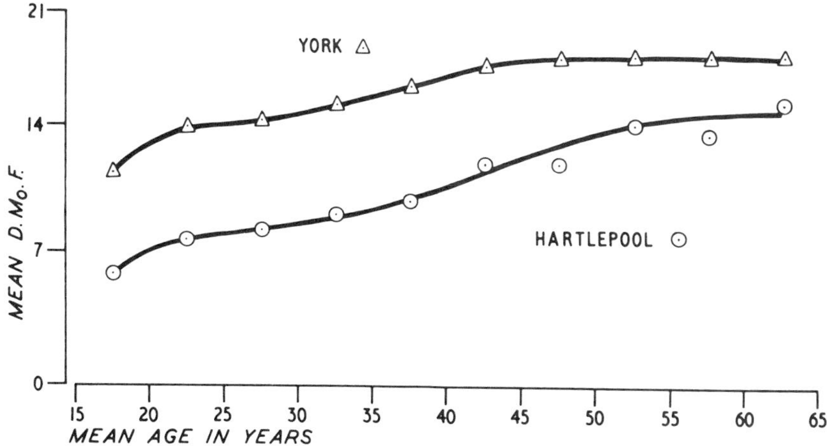

Figure 4.2 Mean DMF values in adults from Hartlepool and York, excluding edentulous persons (From Murray, 1971a; reproduced by courtesy of the Editor, *British Dental Journal*)

A second approach is to use the method put forward by Jackson (1961), who suggested that if, by a sampling survey, the percentage number of extracted teeth which were carious was known for any specific community, it would appear reasonable to apply correction factors to the M fraction of the DMF value at each age group, in order to obtain a more accurate measurement of caries experience in an adult population. This procedure was adopted in order to obtain 'correction factors' for the Hartlepool–York data.

All 7 dental practitioners in Hartlepool and 19 of the dental practitioners in York agreed to cooperate in the study by collecting teeth extracted in their surgeries, over a specified period of time. Ten polythene bottles marked according to the quinquennial age groups used in the study (15–19 years, 20–24 years and so on) were supplied to each practitioner. In Hartlepool only those teeth extracted from people who had been born and lived most of their lives in Hartlepool were collected. This part of the study extended from March 1968 to April 1969 in York and from January 1968 to September 1969 in Hartlepool. The teeth were separated according to age and type and examined for dental caries. A probe was used if caries was not obvious to the naked eye. All filled teeth were presumed to have been carious. In all, 7933 extracted teeth were collected in York and 2958 teeth were collected in Hartlepool. The correction factors for each tooth type and the corrected DMF values (DM_cF) for the total population (including the edentulous) were calculated (Murray, 1971b).

The DM_cF values at any year age group can only be an approximation of true caries experience in the whole population. As a check on the validity of the correction factors, the DM_cF values for the total population were compared with the DM_oF values for the dentate population in each community (Figure 4.3). (The dentate population includes only those people with at least one natural tooth.) The DM_cF values (total population) were effectively identical with the DM_oF values (dentate population) up to the age of 45 years in both communities. Thereafter the

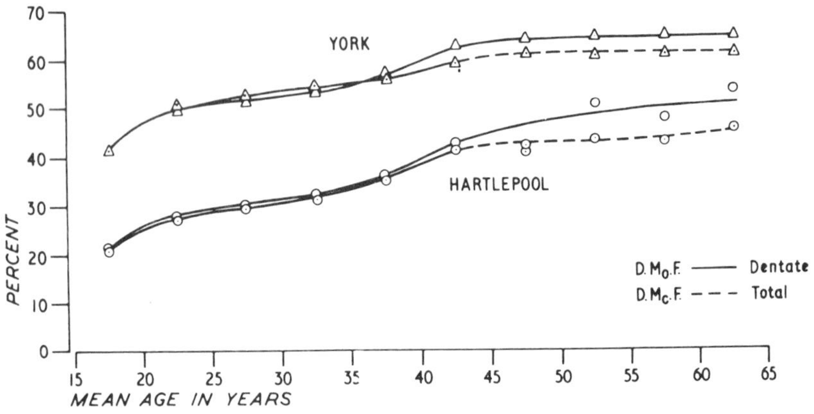

Figure 4.3 Comparison of corrected DMF values (total population) with observed values (From Murray, 1971b; reproduced by courtesy of the Editor, *British Dental Journal*)

DM_oF (dentate) values were slightly higher than the DM_cF (general) values; this is to be expected because even in a dentate population one would imagine that a small proportion of caries-free teeth would have to be extracted for periodontal, prosthetic or surgical reasons. Overall, it is considered that the DM_cF values give a good estimate of caries experience in the population throughout the whole age range in Hartlepool and York. The ceiling DM_cF value in Hartlepool was 45.6% and in York it was 61.0%; this means that the maximum DMF in Hartlepool was 25% lower than it was in York.

Unfortunately, the DMF index gives no indication of the number of surfaces affected by caries. Thus the third approach is to ignore missing teeth altogether and not attempt to apply correction factors or assume that a missing tooth should be counted as 3 or 5 surfaces. Instead the number of decayed or filled surfaces in teeth present in the mouth can be measured and this method gives perhaps the most accurate measure of the extent of caries in adults in different communities. Data using this method have been reported (Jackson, Murray and Fairpo, 1973). Three types of tooth sites were considered: smooth-surface sites (mesial, distal and buccal cervical), occlusal surfaces and pit sites. The increment in caries was virtually nil in persons aged 45 years and above. Thus in this age group permanent differences

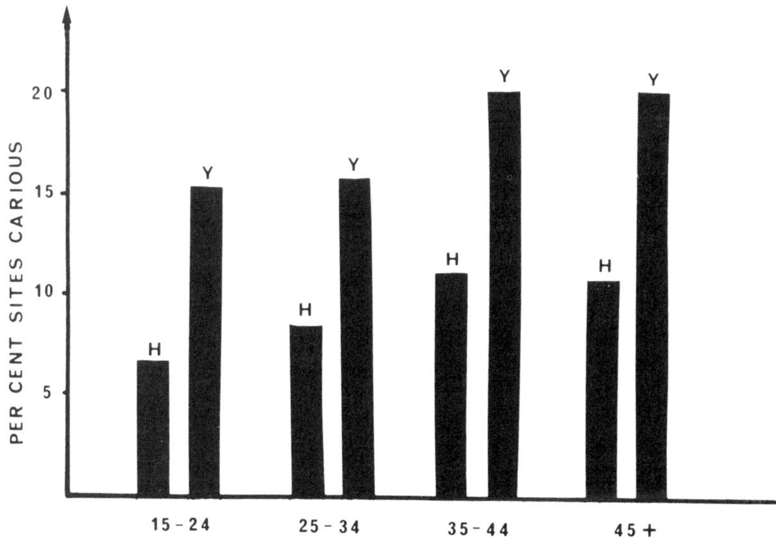

Figure 4.4 Percentage number of decayed/filled sites in teeth present in the mouths of Hartlepool and York adults (From Murray, 1974; reproduced by courtesy of the Editor, *Community Health*)

between Hartlepool and York can be observed. In persons aged 45 years and above, 36 678 specified sites in the York population were examined; of these, 7182 or approximately 20% were carious. In Hartlepool, 17 422 specified sites were examined and of these 1909 or approximately 11% were carious. Thus in dentate persons aged 45 years and above, the number of carious sites was 44% lower in Hartlepool than it was in York. Data for the number of DF sites in standing teeth in 10-year age groups for the two communities are recorded diagrammatically in Figure 4.4. Taking this information as a whole, it can be stated that fluoride in drinking water does not have a merely short-term delaying effect on the appearance of dental caries, but has substantial lifelong caries-preventive effects.

Water fluoridation and the prevalence of root caries

The prevalence of root caries is receiving increased attention as the population ages and yet people retain their teeth longer. A number of studies have been carried out to determine whether fluoride has any effect on root caries in adult populations. Stamm and Banting (1980) reported that 502 adults (average age 40.2 years) examined in naturally fluoridated Stratford (1.5 mg/l) had 0.64 root lesions per person, compared with 1.36 lesions per person in non-fluoridated Woodstock, where the mean age of the 465 adults examined was 42.8 years. The authors concluded that lifetime consumption of fluoridated water is capable of significantly reducing the prevalence of root surface caries.

A similar finding was reported by Burt, Ismail and Eklund (1986), who measured the prevalence of root caries in two New Mexico communities. One community, Deming, has a natural fluoride concentration of 0.7 mg/l in its drinking water, optimum for its climate. The other, Lordsburg, was naturally fluoridated at 3.5 mg/l, five times the optimum. Dental examinations were carried out on 151 adults in Deming (mean age 39.8 years) and 164 in Lordsburg (mean age 43.2 years). Only persons born in the communities were included. The prevalence of root caries was 22.8% in Deming and 7.3% in Lordsburg; mean number of lesions was 0.69 in Deming and 0.08 in Lordsburg. The results by age are summarized in Table 4.7.

Table 4.7 Prevalence of root caries in Lordsburg (optimal fluoride) and Deming (high fluoride) (From Burt, Ismail and Eklund, 1986)

Age group	*Lordsburg (F = 0.7 ppm)*			*Deming (F = 3.5 ppm)*		
	No. in group	*Per cent with root caries*	*Mean no. root lesions*	*No. in group*	*Per cent with root caries*	*Mean no. root lesions*
27–40	81	3.7	0.04	87	11.5	0.15
41–50	37	5.4	0.05	46	34.8	1.35
51–65	46	15.2	0.17	18	55.6	1.61
Total	164	7.3	0.08	151	23.8	0.69

Regression analysis showed that the city of residence was the major predictor of root caries. The authors concluded that, when combined with previous research, their results confirm that root caries experience is directly related to the fluoride concentration in the drinking water.

A recent study (Hunt, Eldredge and Beck, 1989) focused attention on the incidence of new coronal or root caries in adults, based on a longitudinal survey of elderly people living in two rural counties in Iowa, USA. From a random sample of 520 dentate people, 482 adults agreed to participate in the baseline examination and 451 were available for the second examination 18 months later. The results for coronal and root caries incidence (Table 4.8) showed that for coronal caries incidence, there were essentially no differences between residents of non-fluoridated communities and people who had resided in fluoridated communities for 30 years or less (1.93–2.15 surfaces). Beyond 30 years' residence, the increment was approximately one-third less and increasingly less among successively longer term residents (1.67–1.11 surfaces). For root caries incidence, there were minimal differences between residents of non-fluoridated communities and people who had resided in fluoridated communities 40 years or less (1.02–1.24 surfaces). Beyond 40

Table 4.8 Coronal and root caries incidence in 18 months among elderly residents of non-fluoridated (NF) and fluoridated (F) communities, by years of residence (From Hunt, Eldredge and Beck, 1989)

Years of residence	*No. in group*	*Type of community*	*New coronal caries (surfaces)*	*New root caries (surfaces)*
61+	26	F	1.11	0.54
51–60	22	F	1.21	0.55
41–50	29	F	1.52	0.59
31–40	24	F	1.67	1.04
21–30	35	F	2.15	1.02
11–20	75	F	1.93	1.21
5–10	39	F	2.13	1.24
Lifelong	174	NF	1.95	1.11

years' residence, root caries was approximately 50% lower than lifelong residents from the non-fluoridated communities. This difference was statistically significant; the authors concluded that 30 or 40 years' exposure to fluoridated water was beneficial for these elderly adults, even though in many cases the exposure started in adulthood.

References

Bulman, J. S., Slack, G. L., Richards, N. D. and Wilcocks, A. J. (1968) A survey of the dental health and attitudes towards dentistry in two communities. Part 2, Dental data. *Br. Dent. J.*, **124**, 549–554

Burt, B. A., Ismail, A. I. and Eklund, S. A. (1986) Root caries in an optimally fluoridated and a high-fluoride community. *J. Dent. Res.*, **65**(9), 1154–1158

Deatherage, C. F. (1943) Fluoride domestic waters and dental caries experience in 2026 white Illinois selective service men. *J. Dent. Res.*, **22**, 129–137

Englander, H. R. and Wallace, D. A. (1962) Effects of naturally fluoridated water on dental caries in adults. *Public Health Rep.*, **77**, 887–893

Forrest, J. R., Parfitt, G. J. and Bransby, E. R. (1951) The incidence of dental caries among adults and young children in three high and three low fluoride areas in England. *Monthly Bull. Minist. Health*, **10**, 104–111

Gray, P. G., Todd, J. E., Slack, G. L. and Bulman, J. S. (1970) *Adult Dental Health in England and Wales in 1968*. Government Social Survey. Department of Health and Social Security. HMSO, London

Hunt, R. J., Eldredge, J. B. and Beck, J. D. (1989) Effect of residence in a fluoridated community on the incidence of coronal and root caries in an older adult population. *J. Public Hlth Dent.*, **49**(3), 138–141

Jackson, D. (1961) An epidemiological study of dental caries prevalence in adults. *Arch. Oral Biol.*, **6**, 80–93

Jackson, D., Murray, J. J. and Fairpo, C. G. (1973) Lifelong benefits of fluoride in drinking water. *Br. Dent. J.*, **134**, 419–422

Murray, J. J. (1968) *M.Ch.D. thesis*, University of Leeds

Murray, J. J. (1971a) Adult dental health in fluoride and non-fluoride areas. *Br. Dent. J.*, **131**, 391–395

Murray, J. J. (1971b) Adult dental health in fluoride and non-fluoride areas. Part 2. Caries experience in each tooth type. *Br. Dent. J.*, **131**, 437–442

Murray, J. J. (1974) Water fluoridation: a choice for the community. *Community Health*, **6**, 75–83

Russell, A. L. (1953) The inhibition of approximal caries in adults with lifelong fluoride exposure. *J. Dent. Res.*, **32**, 138–143

Russell, A. L. and Elvove, E. (1951) Domestic water and dental caries. VII. A study of the fluoride dental caries relationship in an adult population. *Public Health Rep.*, **66**, 1389–1401

Stamm, J. W. and Banting, D. W. (1980) Comparison of root caries prevalence in adults with life-long residence in fluoridated and non-fluoridated communities. *J. Dent. Res.*, **59** (spec. issue A)

Weaver, R. (1944) Fluorine and dental caries: further investigations on Tyneside and in Sunderland. *Br. Dent. J.*, **77**, 185–193

Chapter 5

Community fluoridation schemes throughout the world

Reductions in dental caries observed in the communities which were the first to fluoridate have been reported and reviewed extensively (Adler, 1970; Backer Dirks, 1974; Murray, 1986). Following the early favourable reports, many other communities decided to fluoridate their public water supplies so that by 1981 approximately 210 million people worldwide were consuming fluoridated water, in addition to the 103 million or so people receiving naturally fluoride-rich water supplies (Murray, 1986).

The Fédération Dentaire Internationale (FDI) has been diligent at collecting information on the status of water fluoridation throughout the world. At the end of 1984, 39 countries had said that they operated artificial fluoridation schemes (Table 5.1). The size of the populations served is often difficult to establish and the figures must be taken as approximate only.

The British Fluoridation Society (1990) has also collected information on the world status of fluoridation and estimated the total population receiving fluoridated water to be 286 million. The numbers in each continent were recorded as: North America 134.5 million, Central America 1.2 million, South America 57.7 million, Africa 0.4 million, Europe 60.3 million, Asia 20.1 million and Oceania 12.2 million.

Dental health has been monitored in many of these countries and the findings of surveys in artificially fluoridated areas will be reviewed, since such information is not readily available because reports are frequently written and published in the language of the country concerned (Table 5.2). This review has been confined to those studies reporting standard caries indices (dmft and DMFT); information on reduction in dental care costs is not so internationally comparable and will be discussed separately in Chapter 19.

The Americas

The world's first artificial fluoridation plant began in Grand Rapids, USA, in 1945. By 1986 over 53% (130 million) of Americans on the piped-water supply received fluoridated water (Brunelle and Carlos, 1990). Four per cent use naturally fluoridated water (Loe, 1986). This percentage of the population served with fluoridated water has increased from 10% in 1980, to 23% in 1960, 39% in 1970 and 51% in 1980 (Bohannan *et al.*, 1985).

The US authorities have been most conscientious at monitoring its effectiveness. The classic Grand Rapids–Muskegon (Arnold *et al.*, 1962), Newburgh–Kingston

Table 5.1 Status of water fluoridation worldwide, showing 39 countries which have artificial fluoridation schemes – the status of natural water fluoridation in these countries is also given (Data by courtesy of the Fédération Dentaire Internationale, London. Status as at 31 December 1984, unless indicated by asterisk)

Country	*Artificial*		*Natural*	
	No. communities	*Pop. served*	*No. communities*	*Pop. served*
*Argentina (1981)	17	349 911†	32	1 100 000†
*Australia	360† (1)	10 065 700 (65%)	66 (2)	128 900
Brazil (1981)	122	7 500 000	?	?
Canada	460	8 383 000	*136 (1981)	174 181
*Chile (1981)	73	4 342 193	2	70 248
*Columbia (1981)	46	8 000 000	0	0
*Cuba (1981)	5	?	?	?
*Czechoslovakia (1981)	70†	3 000 000	10†	15 000†
*Egypt (1981)	1 (2)	?	0	0
Fiji	1	167 000†	0	0
Finland	1	72 000	40†	200 000
*Germany (Dem. Rep.) (1981)	30	1 500 000	?	?
Guatemala	1	1 800 000	?	?
*Guyana (1981)	1 (3)	45 000	8*P	190 000
Hungary	1	2 064 300	15	124 761
*Ireland (1981)	135	1 884 000	1	200 300†
*Israel (1981)	1 (4)	?	3	?
Korea	2	320 000	some	very small
*Libya (1981)	5	400 000	15	1 000 000
Malaysia	107 centres	50–55%	?	?
*Mexico (1977)	4	2 450 000	10 states	5 000 000 (5)
*Netherlands Antilles (P) (1974)	2	200 000	–	–
New Zealand	80	2 000 000†	0	0
*Panama (1974)	8	509 554	0	0
*Papua New Guinea (P) (1975)	1	102 000	1	70 000
*Paraguay (1977)	1	350 000	3	?
*Peru (1981)	3	500 000	6	80 000
Philippines	5	3 000 000†	some	? (6)
*Poland (1977)	20	2 200 000	2	300 000
*Puerto Rico‡ (1974)		1 820 000 (61%)	0	0
*Romania (1977)	1	110 000	?	?
Singapore	1	2 502 000	0	0
*Spain (1981)	1	?	some	?
*Switzerland (1981)	1	200 000	4	20 000
Taiwan	2	600 000†	–	–
*UK	34	5 500 000	9	100 000
USA	8 278 (7)	106 170 149	3 063	9 778 797
*USSR (1977)	85	?	?	15%
*Venezuela (1981)	32	(8)	54	4 562 800 (8)

* No updated information received. The figure in brackets is the year the country updated.
† Estimate only.
‡ Information from other sources.
? Number not known or not given.
P Information provided in March 1975 by the Pan-American Health Organization.

Notes
(1) Towns with over 200 population.
(2) Fluoridation of water supplies is not yet effective due to technical and financial problems. Fluoridation has begun in Alexandria as a pilot study.
(3) Measurements of the fluoride content of a number of public sources have been found to be generally less than 0.5 ppm, but the figures are inconsistent and unreliable.
(4) The major cities will be fluoridated by 1985.
(5) Population with fluorosis: 5 000 000.
(6) Varying degrees of fluorosis have been found in school children in several communities.
(7) Includes school water supply fluoridation.
(8) There are 32 communities with artificially fluoridated water and 54 communities with naturally fluoridated water, serving a total population of 4 562 800.

Table 5.2 Results of surveys into the effectiveness of public water fluoridation schemes throughout the world

Country	*Fluoridated community*	*Reference*	*Year fluoridation began*	*Year of study*	*Age of subjects (yr)*	*Caries index*	*Non-fluoridated community caries experience*	*Caries reduction (%)*	*Type of study*†
USA	Grand Rapids	Arnold *et al*. (1956)	1945	1951	5	deft	5.3	57	CA
	Grand Rapids	Arnold *et al*. (1962)	1945	1960	15	DMFT	12.4	50	CA
	Newburgh	Ast *et al*. (1956)	1945	1955	6–9	DMFT	2.3	58	CA
	Marshall	Taylor and Bertram (1965)	1945	1956	10	DMFT	4.3	67	SC
	Sheboygan	Schreiber (1966)	1946	1950	5	dmft	4.8	45	SC
	Evanston	Blayney and Hill (1967)	1946	1961	14	DMFT	11.7	49	CA
	Lewiston	Young (1958)	1947	1957	10	DMFT	7.0	79	SC
	Oshkosh	Steele (1977)	1948	1975	14	DMFT	9.1	50	SC
	Charlotte	Szwejda (1962)	1949	1961	6	deft	5.3	51	CA
	Charlotte	Szwejda (1962)	1949	1961	11	DMFT	3.3	57	CA
	Antigo	Lemke *et al*. (1970)	1949–1960	1966	5–6	deft	5.3	53	SC
	Newark	Musselman (1957)	1950	1955	6	DMFT	1.1	82	SC
	New Britain	Erlenbach and Tracy (1961)	1950	1961	10	DMFT	3.9	48	SC
	Cleveland, Ohio	Johnsen *et al*. (1986)	1950	1984	3–5	deft	2.8	18	CA
	Milan	Trithart and Denney (1956)	1951	1956	6	deft	6.9	42	CA
	Louisville	Gernert (1958)	1951	1956	6	deft	6.0	46	SC
	Athens	Chrietzberg and Lewis (1958)	1951	1957	6	DMFT	1.2	85	SC
	Iowa	Iowa State DOH (1960)	1951	1958	5	deft	5.1	44	SC
	Tuscaloosa	Klymko (1959)	1951	1959	6	deft	5.6	52	CA
	Tuscaloosa	Klymko (1959)	1951	1959	8	DMFT	2.3	73	CA
	Fort Wayne	Mollenkopf (1963)	1951	1962	10	DMFT	3.7	50	CA
	Columbus	Trubman (1965)	1951	1962	10	DMFT	3.3	47	CA
	Grand Junction	Reger *et al*. (1963)	1951	1962	6	deft	5.3	50	SC
	Grand Junction	Reger *et al*. (1963)	1951	1962	12	DMFT	5.9	68	SC
	Norway	Garcelon (1956)	1952	1955	7	DMFT	2.1	71	SC
	Antioch	Stadt *et al*. (1960)	1952	1957	5	deft	4.1	42	SC
	Orangeburg	Bunch (1959)	1952	1958	6	deft	5.5	47	SC
	Orangeburg	Bunch (1964)	1952	1963	10	DMFT	3.3	41	SC
	Maryland	Russell and White (1961)	1952	1959	5	deft	2.8	65	SC
	Maryland	Russell and White (1961)	1952	1959	7	DMFT	1.1	77	SC
	Baltimore	McCauley *et al*. (1961)	1952	1960	6	DMFT	1.2	68	SC
	Easton	Sogaro (1964)	1952	1962	5	deft	5.0	71	CA
	Easton	Sogaro (1964)	1952	1962	10	DMFT	3.6	53	CA
	Amery	Arra and Lemke (1964)	1952	1962	9	DMFT	3.8	29	CA

Roundup	Anon. (1962)	1952	1962	10	DMFT	4.0	60	CA
Washington, DC	Ostrow (1963)	1952	1962	10	DMFT	2.2	37	SC
Cleveland, Tenn.	Holmes (1963)	1952	1963	6	deft	6.9	57	SC
Cleveland, Tenn.	Holmes (1963)	1952	1963	11	DMFT	7.6	63	SC
Hagerstown	Leonard (1963)	1952	1963	11	DMFT	4.2	62	SC
Rush City	Jordan (1964)	1952	1964	10	DMFT	5.0	50	SC
Providence	Yacovone and Parente (1974)	1952	1972	12	DMFT	7.1	63	SC
Richmond	Crooks and Konikoff (1972)	1952	1972	13	DMFT	7.2	50	SC
Monmouth	Ross *et al*. (1960)	1953	1959	6	DMFT	0.8	50	SC
Milwaukee	Schultz (1969)	1953	1959	5	deft	3.6	35	SC
Milwaukee	Schultz (1969)	1953	1965	10	DMFT	3.6	56	SC
Boseman	Snyder (1964)	1953	1964	10	DMFT	5.0	50	SC
Mystic-Stonington	Erlenbach (1964)	1953	1964	11	DMFT	4.4	35	CA
Corvallis	Tank and Storvick (1964)	1953	*c*.1962	5	deft	6.0	45	CA
Salem	Anon. (1971)	1953	1971	12	DMFT	6.9	67	SC
Philadelphia	Bronstein (1969)	1954	1967	5	deft	3.2	50	SC
Philadelphia	Gordon (1975)	1954	1969–1970	15	DMFT	9.3	52	SC
St Louis	Smith and Paquin (1962)	1955	1961	7	DMFT	0.8	50	SC
Kingsport	Bryan and Smith (1966)	1955	1965	10	DMFT	3.9	62	SC
Albert Lea	Jordan (1970)	1955	1969	6	deft	5.7	42	SC
Albert Lea	Jordan (1970)	1955	1969	12	DMFT	6.2	53	SC
Cleveland	Healy (1963)	1956	1962	5–6	deft	3.4	62	SC
Lebanon	Fishman and Collier (1965)	1956	1964	6	deft	5.4	47	SC
Lebanon	Fishman and Collier (1965)	1956	1964	8	DMFT	2.4	68	SC
Chicago	Weinstein (1972)	1956	1972	14	DMFT	11.6	51	SC
Fayette	Moncrief (1970)	1957	1969	10	DMFT	5.1	63	SC
Mobile	Russell (1965)	1958	1965	6	deft	5.6	32	CA
Mobile	Russell (1965)	1958	1965	7	DMFT	2.0	72	CA
Silver Bay	Jordan *et al*. (1969)	1958	1968	5	deft	4.6	46	SC
Silver Bay	Jordan *et al*. (1969)	1958	1968	10	DMFT	3.6	45	SC
Kalamazoo	Margolis *et al*. (1975)	<1964	1974	4–6	deft	2.4	47	CA
Kalamazoo	Margolis *et al*. (1975)	<1964	1974	7–10	DMFT	1.6	36	CA
Asheville	Dudney *et al*. (1977)	1965	1976	6	dft	3.6	20	SC
Asheville	Dudney *et al*. (1977)	1965	1976	10	DMFT	3.3	59	SC
Winona	Flaven (1977)	1965	1976	5	deft	4.0	74	CA
Winona	Flaven (1977)	1965	1976	10	DMFT	3.4	57	CA
Cudahy	Doherty and Krippene (1972)	1966	1971	5	deft	3.9	56	SC
New Haven	Konick (1979)	1967	1977	10	DMFT	3.5	51	SC
Lincoln*	Knodle (1989)	1970	1984	10	DMFT	5.1	60	SC
Memphis*	Hardison *et al*. (1984)	1970	1982	6	deft	4.3	74	SC
Memphis*	Hardison *et al*. (1984)	1970	1982	10	DMFT	3.0	76	SC

Table 5.2 continued

Country	Fluoridated community	Reference	Year fluoridation began	Year of study	Age of subjects (yr)	Caries index	Non-fluoridated community caries experience	Caries reduction (%)	Type of study
Canada	Brantford	Brown *et al.* (1960)	1945	1959	12–14	DMFT	7.5	57	CA
	Brandon	Connor and Harwood (1963)	1955	1962	6–8	deft	6.5	41	SC
	Brandon	Connor and Harwood (1963)	1955	1962	6–8	DMFT	2.0	74	SC
	Toronto	Lewis (1976)	1963	1975	5	deft	3.9	56	SC
	Toronto	Lewis (1976)	1963	1975	11	DMFT	3.6	35	SC
	Prince George	Hann (1968)	1955	1968	12–14	DMFT	11.2	60	SC
	Edmonton	Payette (1982)	1967	1979	6	dft	4.3	23	CA
	Edmonton	Payette (1982)	1967	1979	11	DMFT	4.4	45	CA
	Windsor	Tessier (1987)	1978	1986	6–7	dmft	5.4	41	CA
Puerto Rico	Puerto Rico	Guzman (1961)	1953	1958	6	DMFT	1.2	66	SC
Cuba	La Salud	Künzel (1982)	1973	1980	7	deft	2.8	68	SC
	La Salud	Künzel (1982)	1973	1980	8–9	DMFT	1.8	72	SC
Brazil	Campinas	Viegas and Viegas (1974)	1962	1972	5	deft	5.5	68	SC
	Campinas	Viegas and Viegas (1974)	1962	1972	10	DMFT	5.1	55	SC
	Barretos	Viegas and Viegas (1985)	1971	1981	10	DMFT	5.1	56	SC
Columbia	San Pedro	Mejia *et al.* (1976)	1965	1972	8	DMFT	3.8	78	CA
	Medellin	Bojanini *et al.* (1981)	1969	1979	10	DMFT	5.4	66	SC
UK	Anglesey	DHSS (1969)	1955	1965	5	deft	4.8	40	CA
	Anglesey	Jackson *et al.* (1975)	1956	1974	15	DMFT	11.4	44	CA
	Watford	DHSS (1969)	1956	1967	5	deft	2.8	43	CA
	Watford	DHSS (1969)	1956	1967	10	DMFT	3.1	35	CA
	Kilmarnock	DHSS (1969)	1956	1961	5	deft	6.9	42	CA
	Balsall Heath	Beal and James (1971)	1964	1970	5	deft	5.2	62	SC
	Northfield	Beal and James (1971)	1964	1970	5	deft	4.9	50	SC
	Birmingham	Whittle and Downer (1979)	1964	1977	5	deft	3.6	54	CA
	Birmingham	Mitropoulos *et al.* (1988)	1964	1987	14	DMFT	3.8	40	CA
	Leeds	Jackson *et al.* (1980)	1968	1979	5	deft	3.3	62	CA
	Scunthorpe	Beal and Clayton (1981)	1968	1975	5	deft	3.5	48	CA
	Cumbria	Jackson *et al.* (1975)	1969	1975	5	deft	4.4	46	CA
	Newcastle upon Tyne	Rugg-Gunn *et al.* (1977)	1969	1975	5	deft	6.1	57	CA
	Newcastle upon Tyne	Murray *et al.* (1984)	1969	1981	10	DMFT	2.0	20	CA
	Northumberland	Rugg-Gunn *et al.* (1977)	1969	1975	5	deft	6.1	67	CA
	Stranraer	Downer *et al.* (1981)	1971	1980	4–5	dmft	4.4	44	CA
	Stranraer	Downer *et al.* (1981)	1971	1980	9–10	DMFT	3.4	50	CA
Ireland	Dublin	O'Hickey (1976)	1964	1969	5	deft	5.8	65	SC

	Limerick	Lemasney *et al.* (1984)	1966	1980	11	DMFT	3.6	42	CA
Netherlands	Tiel	Kwant *et al.* (1973)	1953	1969	15	DMFT	13.9	51	CA
Finland	Kuopio	Nordling and Tulikoura (1970)	1959	1968	7	DMFT	3.1	55	CA
Switzerland	Basel	Gülzow and Maeglin (1979)	1962	1977	15	DMFT	7.2	59	SC
DDR	Karl-Marx-Stadt	Künzel (1968)	1959	1966	5	deft	2.9	76	CA
	Karl-Marx-Stadt	Künzel (1976)	1959	1972	12	DMFT	4.1	66	CA
Czechoslovakia	Tabor	Jirásková *et al.* (1969)	1958	1964	6–7	deft	5.3	36	CA
Poland	Wroclaw	Wigdorowicz-M. *et al.* (1975)	1967	1972	5	deft	5.5	38	SC
	Wroclaw	Wigdorowicz-M. *et al.* (1983)	1967	1980	13	DMFT	5.7	32	SC
Romania	Tirgu-Mures	Csögör *et al.* (1968)	1960	1965	5	deft	3.6	37	CA
	Tirgu-Mures	Csögör *et al.* (1973)	1960	1971	10	DMFT	3.3	52	CA
USSR	Murmansk	Rybakov *et al.* (1978)	1966	1976	10	DMFT	3.0	50	SC
	Monchegorsk	Rybakov *et al.* (1978)	1968	1976	8	DMFT	2.7	54	SC
	Ivan-Frankovsk	Gabovich *et al.* (1972)	1966	1970	8	DMFT	2.2	55	CA
	Leningrad	Strelyukhina *et al.* (1976)	1969	1974	5	deft	4.9	29	CA
	Szczecin	Domzalska *et al.* (1982)	1969	1977	6	dmft	6.7	25	CA
Singapore	Singapore	Wong *et al.* (1970)	1956	1968	7–9	deft	10.7	31	CA
	Singapore	Wong *et al.* (1970)	1956	1968	7–9	DMFT	2.9	31	CA
Malaysia	Kluang	Awang (1973)	1966	1973	7	deft	7.2	37	SC
	Kluang	Awang (1973)	1966	1973	7	DMFT	2.3	75	SC
Hong Kong	Hong Kong*	Evans *et al.* (1987)	1961	1980	6–8	dmft	9.2	57	SC
	Hong Kong*	Evans *et al.* (1987)	1961	1980	9–11	DMFT	4.4	70	SC
Taiwan	Chung-Hsing	Hsieh *et al.* (1979)	1972	1978	5	deft	8.5	26	CA
	Chung-Hsing	Hsieh *et al.* (1986)	1972	1984	12	DMFT	4.3	56	CA
Japan	Yamashina	Minoguchi (1964)	1952	1963	11	DMFT	3.6	33	CA
Australia	Tamworth	Martin and Barnard (1970)	1963	1969	5	deft	5.7	48	SC
	Tamworth	Barnard (1980)	1963	1979	15	DMFT	12.3	78	SC
	Canberra	Carr (1976)	1964	1974	5	deft	5.0	71	SC
	Canberra	Carr (1976)	1964	1974	10	DMFT	4.4	51	SC
	Townville	Videroni *et al.* (1976)	1965	1975	6	deft	5.3	57	CA
	Townville	Videroni *et al.* (1976)	1965	1975	10	DMFT	4.8	54	CA
	Kalgoorlie	Medcalf (1975)	1968	1973	6	deft	6.3	40	SC
	Perth	Medcalf (1978)	1968	1977	6	deft	4.4	48	CA
	Perth	Medcalf (1978)	1968	1977	10	DMFT	3.9	51	CA
	Sydney*	Burton *et al.* (1984)	1968	1982	12	DMFT	8.5	84	SC
New Zealand	Hastings	Ludwig (1965)	1954	1964	5	deft	8.4	52	SC
	Hastings	Ludwig (1971)	1954	1970	15	DMFT	16.8	49	SC
	Lower Hutt	Hollis and Knowsley (1970)	1959	1969	5	deft	8.0	47	SC
	Lower Hutt	Hollis and Knowsley (1970)	1959	1969	10	DMFT	6.2	42	SC

Only surveys reporting deft or DMFT have been included. In studies where results are given for several ages, for deciduous teeth age 5 years was preferred, and age 15 for permanent teeth.
* Control area studies where background caries prevalence is likely to have changed (see page 86).
† CA, 'control area' study; SC, 'self-control' study (see text on p. 86).

(Ast *et al.*, 1956) and Evanston–Oak Park (Blayney and Hill, 1967) studies are well known. Fluoridation has been monitored in well over 100 communities, although some of these reports have only appeared as press articles and many are published in State health department reports and newsletters. It is inevitable, as the effectiveness of fluoridation has been demonstrated repeatedly in the USA and elsewhere, that results of fresh surveys will be published less frequently. In a national survey of US children, a 39% lower caries prevalence was found in 5-year-olds continuously resident in optimally fluoridated communities compared with those living in areas lacking fluoride (Newbrun, 1989).

Canada has a long history of fluoridation, beginning in Brantford in 1945. By 1980, fluoridation was reaching 8.9 million Canadians in 432 communities – 37% of the population or 46% of those on public water systems (Canadian Dental Association, 1981). The results of the Brantford–Sarnia–Stratford study are well known (Brown and Poplove, 1965), but caries experience has also been monitored in Brandon (Connor and Harwood, 1963) and Toronto (Lewis, 1976), fluoridated in 1955 and 1963, respectively. The Toronto survey is one of the best investigations into the effectiveness of water fluoridation as a public health measure and should serve as a guide to other cities which are operating, or planning to introduce, fluoridation schemes.

Approximately 380 million people live in Latin America of whom about 70 million consume fluoridated water (Flanders, 1988). In Central America, most of Puerto Rico is fluoridated and, in 1961, fluoridation reached 93% of the population on piped supply or 63% of the total population (Guzman, 1961). Many countries in Central and South America have water supplies with substantial levels of naturally occurring fluoride (FDI, 1984).

Fluoridation is fairly widespread in South America. The highest proportion occurs in Paraguay (100%) (WHO, 1969), although only one-tenth of the population received a piped supply. On the other hand, about half the people of Chile were on a piped supply and 56% of these received fluoridated water. Fluoridation is also widespread in Panama and Nicaragua. In Brazil, fluoridation began in 1953 in the town of Baixa Guando. In 1967, after 14 years' fluoridation, a caries reduction of 67% was observed. By 1977, some 9.4 million people in 227 Brazilian cities and towns in 18 states received fluoridated water (Goncalves Dinez *et al.*, 1982). There have been only a few reports of the effectiveness of fluoridation in South America.

Europe

In the UK, fluoridation began in 1955 in three trial areas: Watford, Kilmarnock and Anglesey. Apart from these three areas, the dental aspects of fluoridation have been monitored and substantial caries reductions found in Birmingham, Cumbria, Newcastle, Northumberland, Leeds, Scunthorpe and Stranraer.

In Ireland, fluoridation became mandatory in 1960, and by 1987 60% of the population of 3.5 million were receiving fluoridated water (Bell, 1989). Because of widespread fluoridation, the choice of control towns has been difficult, but its effectiveness has been assessed in Cork, Dublin and Limerick. The effect of fluoridation on a country-wide basis has been demonstrated in a national survey of children's dental health (O'Mullane *et al.*, 1988).

In Belgium, the town of Assesse was fluoridated in 1956 with a population of 0.4 million people in 1974, but its effectiveness has not been monitored and no artificial fluoridation existed in 1986 (Vreven, 1987). A pilot fluoridation scheme began in Kassel-Wahlershausen (West Germany) in 1952, but was later discontinued, so that by 1978 there was no fluoridation in that country; detailed data on the effectiveness of fluoridation in Kassel have not been published, although Auermann and Lingelbach (1964) reported a 28% caries reduction. In Norrkoping in Sweden, which was fluoridated only from 1952 to 1962, a 52% reduction in caries in 7-year-old children was observed (Quentin and Lingelbach, 1963).

One of the best studies into the effect of water fluoridation was conducted in Holland, where Tiel fluoridated in 1953. Reports on this well-known study provide detailed information on the effect of fluoridation on different teeth and types of tooth surface (Backer Dirks, Houwink and Kwant, 1961; Kwant *et al.*, 1973). Indeed this study gives almost the only data available on the effect of fluoridation in continuously resident 18-year-olds, showing a 53% reduction, or an absolute difference of 19 cavities per person (Kwant *et al.*, 1974). Fluoridation ceased in Tiel in 1974, at a time when 2.7 million Dutch people (20% of the population) were receiving fluoridated water.

The only Finnish community to fluoridate has been the city of Kuopio, where fluoridation began in 1959, with Jyväskylä as control (Nordling and Tulikoura, 1970). In Switzerland, although the first community to fluoridate was Aigle in 1960, the effects of fluoridation have been studied more thoroughly in Basel (1962) (Gülzow, Kränzlin and Maeglin, 1978; Gülzow and Maeglin, 1979).

In 1972, 10 cities in East Germany (DDR) had fluoridated and by 1981 this had risen to 30, reaching 14% of the population with plans to extend to 35% of the population by 1990 (Künzel, 1983; FDI, 1984). The effectiveness of this measure has been thoroughly studied in Karl-Marx-Stadt by Künzel (1968, 1976): fluoridation began in 1959 with the city of Plauen as control, until 1971 when Plauen itself fluoridated. Examinations were conducted in alternate years on children aged 3–18. Künzel also gives data for each tooth type separately for each age group, confirming that incisor teeth benefit most.

In Hungary, attempts to introduce fluoridation have not been successful: it was started in the town of Szolnok in 1962 but was abandoned one year later. It has been reported that 63% of the population of Bulgaria were drinking fluoridated water in 1974, but no data on its effectiveness could be traced. On the other hand, the effectiveness of water fluoridation in Czechoslovakia, Poland and Romania has been documented. In Czechoslovakia, Tabor has been the main test town, fluoridated in 1958, with Pisek as control. In addition to the 36% caries reduction in Tabor (Jirásková *et al.*, 1969), a small reduction was observed in children in Bialystok after 6 years' fluoridation (Januszko *et al.*, 1977) and a 70% caries reduction in Brunn after 3 years (Auermann and Lingelbach, 1964). In 1972, 36 Czech communities had fluoridated, covering 10% of the population. This had increased to 70 communities in 1984 (FDI, 1984) or 22% of the population (Künzel, 1983).

Progress in fluoridation has been slower in Poland where, by 1974, 3.7% (1.3 million) of the population were receiving fluoridated water. By 1983, the proportion had risen to 8% (Künzel, 1983) involving 20 communities (2.2 million people) (FDI, 1984). The effect has been monitored in the city of Wroclaw which commenced fluoridation in 1967 (Wigdorowicz-Makowerowa *et al.*, 1978, 1983).

The town of Tirgu-Mures in Romania fluoridated its water supplies in 1960, and in 1984 was the only fluoridated community in that country. From 1962 onwards, caries experience has been monitored in 3–14-year-old children (Csögör *et al.*, 1968, 1973), but due to technical difficulties fluoridation has not been continuous and between 1960 and 1971 operated on only 64% of the total possible number of days.

Fluoridation of the public water supplies has advanced rapidly in the USSR since it commenced in Norilsk in 1958 (Aksjuk, 1977). By 1972, 13 million people were receiving fluoridated water in 24 communities, but this had risen to 20 million by 1977, and to 20% of the population in 1983 (Künzel, 1983) in 85 communities (FDI, 1984). Climate differs so markedly in different regions of the USSR that the optimum water fluoride level ranges from 0.6 ppm F in the south to 1.2 ppm F in the north (Murray, 1986). After 7 years of fluoridation, dental caries in Norilsk 7-year-olds had decreased by 43% with an overall reduction in the cost of filling materials in Norilsk by 30%, despite the fact that fluoridation was said to be intermittent (Toth, 1972). Fluoridation began in 1966 in Ivano-Frankovsk, with Dolina as control (Gabovich *et al.*, 1972), and in Leningrad in 1969 with surrounding areas as control (Strelyukhina *et al.*, 1976; Kliachkina *et al.*, 1981). One of the more comprehensive USSR studies has monitored fluoridation in Murmansk, commencing in 1966, and Monchegorsk, commencing in 1968, in the Arctic regions. This has been undertaken by the Central Research Institute of Stomatology (CRIS), Moscow, in collaboration with the World Health Organisation (Rybakov *et al.*, 1978). Suntsov (1985) reported that intermittent and sub-optimal fluoridation in Omsk was having a marked anti-caries effect, but only in the mixed dentition. Sub-optimal levels of fluoride seem to be a feature of artificial fluoridation schemes in the USSR. Abrams (1988) reported that only 3 samples out of 47 taken from fluoridated Moscow and Leningrad collected over a 3-year period had fluoride levels of 0.8 ppm or over and the remaining 44 samples contained 0.3 ppm or less.

Asia

There are few fluoridation schemes operating in Africa or the Middle East. In many of these countries, particularly those associated with the Rift Valley, extensive areas of high naturally occurring fluoride levels exist. In Saudi Arabia, the oil company Aramco has fluoridated the drinking water of its community to 0.7 ppm, the optimum for that climate, and this is said to be very cost-effective (Hammer, 1986). Thirty-eight per cent of the population of Israel receive optimally fluoridated water (Gordon *et al.*, 1990).

By 1975, only one Malaysia state, Johore, had fluoridated its water supplies. Results of dental surveys carried out before and after 7 years of fluoridation in the towns of Johore Bahru and Kluang indicated reductions of 60% and 75%, respectively, in caries experience (Awang, 1973).

In 1954, the Government of Singapore approved adoption of a fluoridation scheme. This commenced in May 1956 and by July 1958 the entire population of 2.5 million people received optimally fluoridated water (at 0.7 ppm) (Teo, 1984). The effect on dental health was reported by Wong, Goh and Oon (1970) and by Lim (1986).

The domestic water supplies in the major metropolitan areas of Hong Kong were fluoridated during 1961 and practically all other urban areas were supplied soon afterwards. The fluoride level was initially set at 0.7–0.9 ppm depending on season, but was increased to 1.0 in 1967 before being reduced to 0.7 ppm in 1978. The history of fluoridation there and changes in caries experience have been reported by Evans, Lo and Lind (1987) and Lo, Evans and Lind (1990).

Fluoridation commenced on an experimental basis in Taiwan in 1972. In the fluoridated village of Chung-Hsing, caries experience in 5-year-olds changed from 6.5 dft in 1971 to 6.3 dft in 1978 after 6 years' fluoridation at 0.6 ppm F. However, caries experience in the control, non-fluoridated village of Tsao-Tun increased from 6.4 dft in 1971 to 8.5 dft in 1978. A similar pattern was observed in the permanent dentition in 1981 and 1984 after 9 and 12 years' fluoridation. In fluoridated Chung-Hsing, the DFMT of 12-year-olds was 1.1 in 1971 and 1.9 in 1984 (a rise of 73%), whereas in non-fluoridated Tsao-Tun, the DMFT was 0.9 in 1971 and 4.3 in 1984 (a rise of 377%). These increases were probably due to a rise in sugar consumption, resulting from increasing economic prosperity (Guo *et al.*, 1984; Hsieh *et al.*, 1986).

There is at present no fluoridation in Japan. The only town to fluoridate, Yamashina, began in 1952 but fluoridation has now ceased. The average caries experience for 11-year-old children was 1.53 DMFT in 1952, but this has increased to 2.39 after 11 years' fluoridation. However, caries experience in the control town of Shugakuin increased even more, from 1.36 to 3.59 DMFT over the same time period, in the same age group. Therefore, if the caries experience in the fluoridated and control town in 1963 are compared, a 33% reduction in caries was observed, although this may be an underestimate as caries experience was higher in Yamashina than in Shugakuin before fluoridation (Minoguchi, 1964; Adler, 1970).

Australasia

Fluoridation has been widely introduced in Australia, so that by 1984, 10.2 million Australians (66% of the population) in some 900 towns and cities were drinking fluoridated water (National Health and Medical Research Council, 1985). One of the first communities to fluoridate was Tamworth, which began in 1963 (Martin and Barnard, 1970; Barnard, 1980), but one of the most thorough investigations into its effectiveness has been conducted in Canberra (Carr, 1976). Areas of Western Australia were fluoridated in 1968 and Medcalf (1971, 1975) reported on its effect upon caries experience in the Kalgoorlie area after 6 years of fluoridation.

Hastings was the first New Zealand community to fluoridate and the reports of its effectiveness are well known (Ludwig, 1965, 1971). The very high caries experience found in New Zealand has meant that, in real terms, a larger number of teeth are prevented from becoming carious in Hastings, for a given percentage reduction, than in other communities. For example, the mean DMFT for 15-year-old children in 1954 was 16.8, which fell to 8.5 by 1970, a percentage reduction of 49% or 8.3 teeth less. The corresponding figures for tooth surfaces were 42.5 DMFS in 1954 and 17.4 in 1970, a 59% reduction or the large difference of 25 tooth surfaces, 15 of which were approximal. Gingival surfaces benefited most (87%), approximal surfaces by 73% and occlusal surfaces least (39%). The effect of 10 years' fluoridation in the city of Lower Hutt has been reported (Hollis and Knowsley, 1970). In 1980, 54% of the total population of New Zealand (or 84% of the population on public water supplies) were receiving fluoridated water (Donaldson, 1980).

Summary

Figure 5.1 has been compiled from the percentage reductions observed in studies of artificial water fluoridation throughout the world, given in Table 5.2. Data for the deciduous and permanent dentitions are presented separately. There were 113 studies in 23 countries: in 66 studies, data were given for deciduous teeth, and in 86 studies, data were given for permanent teeth. Fifty-nine out of the 113 studies took place in the USA. For deciduous teeth, the modal percentage caries reduction was 40–49% (24 out of the 66 studies), and for permanent teeth, the modal percentage caries reduction was 50–59% (33 out of the 86 studies). These results are in line with the oft-quoted statement that 'fluoridation cuts caries by half'.

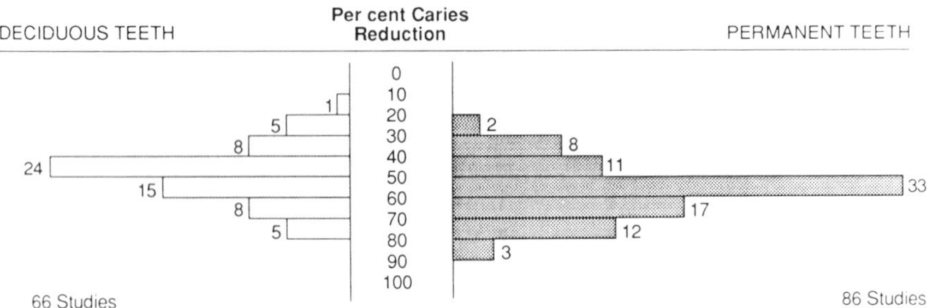

Figure 5.1 Percentage caries reductions observed in 113 studies into the effectiveness of artificial water fluoridation in 23 countries. Sixty-six studies gave results for the deciduous dentition and 86 studies gave results for the permanent dentition

The results given in Figure 5.1 come from different types of study. They were carried out in different countries, by different examiners using different diagnostic criteria on subjects of different ages who were not always continuous residents in the communities investigated. In some areas, caries prevalence was high and in others low. In general, factors such as these do not influence the validity of the results, since they affect the fluoridated and control communities equally. However, one factor which may influence the interpretation of the findings is the choice of control group, which can be either a 'self-control' (SC) or a 'control area' (CA) type. The type of study is listed in the last column of Table 5.2. Where a study presented data from both types of design, preference was given to the CA results. Just over half of the studies were SC studies, where the dental status of the community was measured before introduction of water fluoridation and any change observed subsequently, after water fluoridation, was deemed to be caused by water fluoridation. This retrospective control design is satisfactory so long as no change in the underlying prevalence of the disease has occurred. This assumption is sometimes not justified and, in some studies, fluoridation has been judged against a background rise or fall in caries prevalence. Examples where this is very likely to have occurred are marked with an asterisk in Table 5.2.

A better design is to identify a community similar to the fluoridated (or test) community, so that the test and control communities can be assessed in parallel. It is reasonable to assume that any rise or fall in background caries prevalence will occur in both communities equally and thus not influence assessment of the effectiveness of fluoridation. Sometimes it is not possible to identify a suitable CA

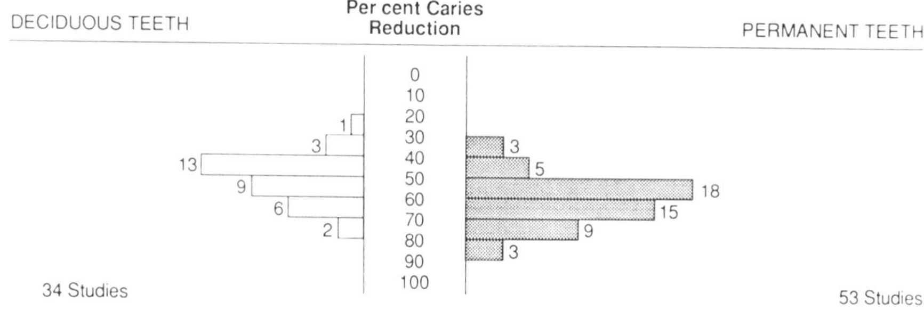

Figure 5.2 Percentage caries reductions observed in studies of the effectiveness of artificial fluoridation. These studies were all self-control (or retrospective control) studies

(because of widespread fluoridation, for example) and reliance has to be placed on a retrospective control data.

Because of the possible influence of choice of control in fluoridation studies, Figures 5.2 and 5.3 were compiled: Figure 5.2 for SC studies only, and Figure 5.3 for CA studies only. There is a slight shift towards higher percentage caries reductions being recorded in SC studies (Figure 5.2), especially for permanent teeth. However, the modal percentage caries reductions are the same: 40–49% for deciduous teeth, and 50–59% for permanent teeth. The statement 'fluoridation cuts caries by half' is still justified.

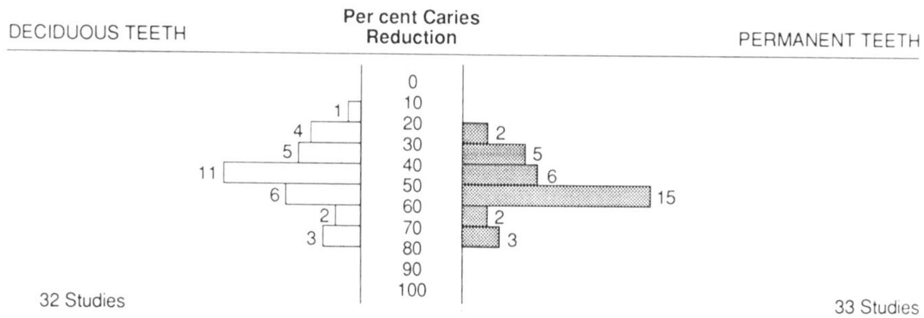

Figure 5.3 Percentage caries reductions observed in studies of the effectiveness of artificial fluoridation. These studies were all control area (or parallel control) studies

The extent of fluoridation varies widely throughout the world, but it is steadily increasing (Murray, 1986). In the USA, New Zealand, Australia, Canada, Ireland, Hong Kong and Singapore most of the population receive fluoridated water, and the results have been well documented. Fluoridation is said to be extensive in Latin America, but there are few data on these schemes. Fluoridation has been expanding fast in eastern Europe and the results are clearly recorded in East Germany (DDR). It would seem that the optimum fluoride level is not always maintained in the extensive schemes in the USSR. In west Europe, fluoridation is limited. While Ireland has extensive fluoridation, only 10% of the UK population receive fluoridated water, and Basel is the only fluoridated city in Switzerland. Increasing caries prevalence is being reported from southern Europe and the Middle East and it could be that fluoridation may be introduced into these regions.

References

Abrams, R. A. (1988) Community water fluoridation in Leningrad and Moscow. *Community Dent. Oral Epidemiol.*, **16**, 129–130

Adler, P. (1970) Fluorides and dental health. In *Fluorides and Human Health*, WHO Monogr. Ser. No. 59, WHO, Geneva, chap. 9

Aksjuk, A. F. (1977) Hygienic aspects of the fluoridation of the drinking water in various climatic-geographic areas of the USSR. *Z. Gesamte. Hyg.*, **23**, 85–87

Anon. (1962) Dental decay reduced by 60 per cent in round-up fluoridation program. *Treasure State Health (Montana)*, **12**, 1

Anon. (1971) Salem dental survey 1971. *J. Oreg. Dent. Assoc.*, **18**, 16–17

Arnold, F. A., Dean, H. T., Jay, P. and Knutson, J. W. (1956) Effect of fluoridated public water supplies on dental caries prevalence. *Public Health Rep.*, **71**, 652–658

Arnold, F. A., Likins, R. C., Russell, A. L. and Scott, D. B. (1962) Fifteenth year of Grand Rapids fluoridation study. *J. Am. Dent. Assoc.*, **65**, 780–785

Arra, M. C. and Lemke, C. (1964) Effects of adjusted fluoridated water on dental caries in school children of Amery, Wis. *J. Am. Dent. Assoc.*, **69**, 460–464

Ast, D. B., Smith, D. J., Wachs, B. and Cantwell, K. T. (1956) Newburgh–Kingston caries-fluorine study XIV. Combined clinical and roentgenographic dental findings after ten years of fluoride experience. *J. Am. Dent. Assoc.*, **52**, 314–325

Auermann, E. and Lingelbach, H. (1964) Status and prospects of fluoridation in Europe. *J. Am. Public Health*, **54**, 1545–1550

Awang, A. R. (1973) *Report of the Results of Seven Years of Fluoridation at Kluang, Johore.* Annual Conference of Directors of Medical and Health Services, Malaysia, Kuala Lumpur, Ministry of Health

Backer Dirks, O. (1974) The benefits of water fluoridation. *Caries Res.*, **8** (suppl.), 2–15

Backer Dirks, O., Houwink, B. and Kwant, G. W. (1961) The results of 6½ years of artificial fluoridation of drinking water in the Netherlands. *Arch. Oral Biol.*, **5**, 284–300

Backer Dirks, O., Künzel, W. and Carlos, J. P. (1978) Caries-preventive water fluoridation. *Caries Res.*, **12** (suppl. 1), 7–14

Barnard, P. D. (1980) Fluoridation in Tamworth after 15 years. *Dent. Outlook*, **6**, 46–47

Beal, J. F. and Clayton, M. (1981) Fluoridation, a clinical survey in Corby and Scunthorpe. *Publ. Health, Lond.*, **95**, 152–160

Beal, J. F. and James, P. M. C. (1971) Dental caries prevalence in 5-year-old children following five and a half years of water fluoridation in Birmingham. *Br. Dent. J.*, **130**, 284–288

Bell, C. J. (1989) Fluoridation of water supplies in Ireland, 1978–1987. *J. Irish Dent. Assoc.*, **35**, 119–121

Blayney, J. R. and Hill, I. N. (1967) Fluorine and dental health. *J. Am. Dent. Assoc.*, **74**, 233–302

Bohannan, H. M., Graves, R. C., Disney, J. A., Stamm, J. W., Abernathy, J. B. and Bader, J. D. (1985) Effect of secular decline in caries on the evaluation of preventive dentistry demonstrations. *J. Publ. Health Dent.*, **45**, 83–89

Bojanini, J. N., Arango, G. C. and Pineda, A. R. (1981) Diez anos de fluoruracion de aguas en Medellin. *Rev. Fed. Odont. Columb.*, **29**, 52–61

British Fluoridation Society (1990) *World Status of Fluoridation*, Briefing Paper, BFS, London

Bronstein, E. (1969) A survey of caries-experience among the pre-school children of Philadelphia. *J. Public Health Dent.*, **29**, 24–26

Brown, H. K., McLaren, H. R. and Poplove, M. (1960) The Brantford–Sarnia–Stratford fluoridation caries study – 1959 report. *J. Can. Dent. Assoc.*, **26**, 131–142

Brown, H. K. and Poplove, M. (1965) The Brantford–Sarnia–Stratford fluoridation caries study. Final survey 1963. *J. Can. Dent. Assoc.*, **31**, 505–511

Brunelle, J. A. and Carlos, J. P. (1990) Recent trends in dental caries in US children and the effect of water fluoridation. *J. Dent. Res.*, **69** (spec. iss.), 723–727

Bryan, E. T. and Smith, C. E. (1966) The results of ten years of continuous fluoridation in Kingsport, Tennessee. *J. Tenn. State Dent. Assoc.*, **46**, 30–34

Bunch, G. A. (1959) Post-fluoridation dental survey. *S. Carolina Dent. J.*, **17**, 3–17

Bunch, G. A. (1964) Results of ten year post-fluoridation survey. *S. Carolina Dent. J.*, **22**, 7–11

Burton, V. J., Rob, M. I., Craig, G. G. and Lawson, J. S. (1984) Changes in the caries experience of 12-year-old Sydney schoolchildren between 1963 and 1982. *Med. J. Austral.*, **140**, 405–407

Canadian Dental Association (1981) Water fluoridation in Canada, a status report 1980. *Canad. Dent. Assoc. J.*, **47**, suppl.

Carr, L. M. (1976) Fluoridation in Canberra. Part III. Dental caries after ten years. *Aust. Dent. J.*, **21**, 440–444

Chrietzberg, J. E. and Lewis, F. D. (1958) An evaluation of caries prevalence after five years of fluoridation. *J. Am. Dent. Assoc.*, **56**, 192–193

Collins, C. K. and O'Mullane, D. M. (1970) Dental caries experience in Cork city schoolchildren aged 4–11 years after 4½ years of fluoridation. *J. Irish Dent. Assoc.*, **16**, 130–134

Connor, R. A. and Harwood, W. R. (1963) Dental effects of water fluoridation in Brandon, Manitoba: second report. *J. Can. Dent. Assoc.*, **29**, 716–722

Crooks, E. L. W. and Konikoff, A. B. (1972) A twenty-year study of the effectiveness of fluoride in the Richmond water supply. *Virginia Dent. J.*, **49**, 24–26

Csögör, L., Guzner, N. and Cristoloveanu, R. (1968) Prophylaxis of dental decay in the town of Tirgu Mures by fluoridation of the drinking water. *Stomatol.* (*Buch.*), **15**, 33–38

Csögör, L., Guzner, N., Cristoloveanu, R. and Shapira, M. (1973) Prophylaxie de la carie dentaire par fluorisation de l'eau potable dans la ville de Tirgu-Mures. *rev. Port. Estomatol. Cir. Maxilofac.*, **14**, 89–98

Department of Health and Social Security (1969) *The Fluoridation Studies in the United Kingdom and the Results Achieved After Eleven Years*, Report No. 122, London, HMSO

Doherty, J. M. and Krippene, B. (1972) Fluoridation in Cudahy – five-year evaluation. *J. Wis. State Dent. Soc.*, Aug., 247–249

Domzalska, E., Opuchlik, E., Janczuk, Z., Lisiecka, K. and Opalko, K. (1982) The state of teeth of children aged 6 years in the city of Szczecin in 1977. *Czas. Stomatol.*, **35**, 421–425

Donaldson, E. W. (1980) New Zealand – fluoridation. *Br. Dent. J.*, **148**, 80

Downer, M. C., Blinkhorn, A. S. and Attwood, D. (1981) Effect of fluoridation on the cost of dental treatment among urban Scottish schoolchildren. *Community Dent. Oral Epidemiol.*, **9**, 112–116

Dudney, G. G., Rozier, R. G., Less, M. F. and Hughes, J. T. (1977) Ten years of fluoridation in Asheville, North Carolina. *N. Carolina Dent. J.*, **60**, 11–16

Erlenbach, F. M. (1964) Mystic-Stonington dental survey. *Conn. Health Bull.*, **78**, 231–234

Erlenbach, F. M. and Tracy, E. T. (1961) Tenth year of New Britain, Connecticut, fluoride study. *Conn. Health Bull.*, **75**, 371–382

Evans, R. W., Lo, E. C. M. and Lind, O. P. (1987) Changes in dental health in Hong Kong after 25 years of water fluoridation. *Community Dent. Health*, **4**, 383–394

Fédération Dentaire Internationale (1984) *World Fluoridation Status: As at 31 December 1984*. FDI, London

Fishman, S. R. and Collier, D. R. (1965) Eight years fluoridation – Lebanon, Tenn. *J. Tenn. State Dent. Assoc.*, **45**, 48–57

Flanders, R. A. (1988) School dental health in Honduras. *J. Publ. Health Dent.*, **48**, 168–171

Flaven, B. M. (1977) *Benefits of Eleven Years of Fluoridated Water – the Winona Report*, Minneapolis, Minnesota Department of Health, Feb. 1977

Gabovich, R. D., Dmitrochenko, A. S. and Stepanenko, G. A. (1972) The effect of fluoridation of water in Ivano-Frankovsk on dental caries in the population. *Stomatol.* (*Mosk.*), **51**, 14–17

Garcelon, A. H. (1956) Fluoridation of water supply; the Norway, Maine study. *New Engl. J. Med.*, **254**, 1072–1077

Gernert, E. B. (1958) Five year report on fluoridation in Louisville, Kentucky. *J. Kentucky Dent. Assoc.*, July, 29–32

Goncalves Dinez, R., Vicente de Araujo, H. and José de Albuquerque, A. (1982) Development of a simplified water fluoridation technique for small communities. *Bull. Pan. Am. Health Organ.*, **16**, 224–232

Gordon, J. J. (1975) *Fluoridation in Philadelphia*, Report to Mr. J. Small, USPHS, Bethesda, Feb.

Gordon, M., Sarnat, H., Sgan-Cohen, H. D. and Mann, J. (1990) Trend of caries prevalence in children and young adults in Israel. *Community Dent. Oral Epidemiol.*, **18**, 108

Gülzow, H.-J., Kränzlin, H. and Maeglin, B. (1978) Ist der Kariesrückgang nach Trinkwasser fluoridierung in Basel auf eine Verzögerung in Zahndurchbruch zurückzuführen? *Schweiz. Monatsschr. Zahnheilkd.*, **88**, 1192–1200

Gülzow, H.-J. and Maeglin, B. (1979) Karioesstatistische Ergebnisse nach 15 jähriger Trinkwasser-fluoridierung. *Dtsch. Zahnärzl. Z.*, **34,** 118–123

Guo, M.-K., Hsiah, C.-C., Hong, Y.-C. and Chen, R.-S. (1984) Effect of water fluoridation on prevalence of dental caries in Chung-Hsing New Village. *J. Formosan Med. Assoc.*, **83**, 1035–1043

Guzman, R. M. (1961) Status of fluoridation in Puerto Rico. *J. Am. Waterwks Assoc.*, **53**, 141–145

Hammer, M. (1986) Fluoridation of Saudi Arabia's water. *Middle East Health*, **10**, 46D–47D

Hann, H. J. (1968) *The Dental Benefits of Water Fluoridation; 1968 Prince George Report*. Prince George, British Columbia, Prince George and District Dental Society and the Northern Interior Health Unit, Oct.

Hardison, J. R., Wicker, J. U. and van Cleave, M. L. (1984) The results of twelve years of continuous fluoridation in Memphis TN. *J. Tenn. Dent. Assoc.*, **64,** 31–35

Healy, T. F. (1963) *Study of the Effects of Fluoride on Teeth of Children in Cleveland Public Schools*, Cleveland Public Schools, Cleveland, Ohio

Hollis, M. J. and Knowsley, P. C. (1970) Ten years of fluoridation in Lower Hutt. *N.Z. Dent. J.*, **66**, 235–238

Holmes, C. B. (1963) Eleven year fluoridation evaluation on dental health status and practice. *J. Tenn. State Dent. Assoc.*, **43**, 223–233

Hsieh, C.-C., Guo, M.-K. and Hong, Y.-C. (1979) Effect of water fluoridation on prevalence of dental caries in Chung-Hsing New Village after six years. *J. Formosan Med. Assoc.*, **78**, 168–176

Hsieh, C.-C., Guo, M.-K., Hong, Y.-C. and Chen, R.-S. (1986) An evaluation of caries prevalence in Chung-Hsing New Village after 12 years of water fluoridation. *J. Formosan Med. Assoc.*, **85**, 822–831

Iowa State Department of Health (1960) *Controlled Fluoridation in Public Water Supplies*. Iowa New Series No. 1822 (Jan. 15) and No. 1850 (Nov. 5). State University of Iowa

Jackson, D., Goward, P. E. and Morrell, G. V. (1980) Fluoridation in Leeds; a clinical survey of 5-year-old children. *Br. Dent. J.*, **149**, 231–234

Jackson, D., Gravely, J. F. and Pinkham, I. O. (1975) Fluoridation in Cumbria; a clinical study. *Br. Dent. J.*, **139**, 319–322

Jackson, D., James, P. M. C. and Wolfe, W. B. (1975) Fluoridation in Anglesey; a clinical study. *Br. Dent. J.*, **138**, 165–171

Januszko, T., Komenda, W., Dobrowolski, J., Smorczewska, B., Szymaniak, E., Zalewska, E. and Kisiel, A. (1977) Evaluation of effectiveness of drinking water fluoridation for prevention of dental caries in children of elementary schools in the city of Bialystok. *Czas. Stomat.*, **30**, 555–560

Jirásková, M. *et al.* (1969) Water fluoridation in Czechoslovakia. *V. Csek. Stomatol.*, **69**, 129–138

Johnsen, D. C., Bhat, M., Kim, M. T., Hagman, F. T., Allee, L. M., Creedon, R. L. and Easley, M. W. (1986) Caries levels and patterns in head start children in fluoridated and non-fluoridated urban and non-urban sites in Ohio, USA. *Community Dent. Oral Epidemiol.*, **14,** 206–210

Jordan, W. A. (1964) The Rush City report – ten years of fluoridated water. *Minn. Dept Health Rep.*, **832**, July

Jordan, W. A. (1970) Fluoridated water benefits continue; Albert Lea's 1969 dental survey. *North-West Dent.*, **49**, 77–80

Jordan, W. A., Pugnier, V. A. and McKee, D. P. (1969) Silver Bay reports, following ten years of fluoridated water. *North-West Dent.*, **48**, 7–10

Kliachkina, L. M., Vinogradova, I. E. and Beliaevskaia, L. A. (1981) Effects of water fluoridation on the prevalence and incidence of caries of the permanent teeth of Leningrad school children. *Stomatologiia* (*Mosk.*), **60**, 52–53

Klymko, M. B. (1959) The effect of artificial water fluoridation on the teeth of Tuscaloosa school children. *J. Ala. Dent. Assoc.*, **43**, 5–9

Knodle, J. M. (1989) Controlled fluoridation benefits after 14 years of implementation. *Clin. Prev. Dent.*, **11**, 21–26

Konick, L. (1979) Dental health survey of New Haven schoolchildren after ten years of fluoridation. *Conn. Health Bull.*, **93**, 32–40

Künzel, W. (1968) Results and prospects of water fluoridation in the German Democratic Republic. *Caries Res.*, **2**, 172–179

Künzel, W. (1976) *Trinkwasserfluoridierung als Kollektive Kariesvorbeugende Massnahme*, 2nd edn, VEB Verlag Volk und Gesundheit, Berlin

Künzel, W. (1982) Reduction in caries after 7 years of water fluoridation under climatic conditions in Cuba. *Caries Res.*, **16**, 272–276

Künzel, W. (1983) Approach to the prevention of oral diseases in the socialist countries of Europe. In *Prevention of Oral Diseases*, Report of a WHO Workshop, held in Erfurt, December, Medical Academy Erfurt, Erfurt, East Germany

Künzel, W. and Patron, F. S. (1983) Zur kariesprotektiven Effectivät fluoridangereicherten Trinkwasser unter den klimatischen Bedingungen Kubas. *Zahn. Mund. Kieferheilkd.*, **71**, 341–348

Kwant, G. W., Groenveld, A., Pot, T. J. and Purdell Lewis, D. (1974) Fluoride-toeveeging aan het drinkwater v; Een vergelijking van de gebitsgezondheid van 17- en 18-jarigen in Culemborg en Tiel. *Ned. Tijdschr. v. Tandheelkd.*, **81**, 251–261

Kwant, G. W., Houwink, B., Backer Dirks, O., Groeneveld, A. and Pot, T. J. (1973) Artificial fluoridation of drinking water in the Netherlands; results of the Tiel–Culemborg experiment after 16½ years. *Neth. Dent. J.*, **80**, suppl. 9, 6–27

Lemasney, J., O'Mullane, D. and Coleman, M. (1984) Effect of fluoridation on dental health in 5- and 11-year-old Irish schoolchildren. *Community Dent. Oral Epidemiol.*, **12,** 218–222

Lemke, C. W., Doherty, J. M. and Arra, M. C. (1970) Controlled fluoridation; the dental effects of discontinuation in Antigo, Wisconsin. *J. Am. Dent. Assoc.*, **80**, 782–786

Leonard, R. C. (1963) Fluoridation in Maryland. *Md. State Dept. Health Month. Bull.*, **35**(5), 1–4

Lewis, D. W. (1976) *An Evaluation of the Dental Effects of Water Fluoridation, City of Toronto 1963–1975*, City Hall, Department of Public Health, Toronto

Lim, L. A. (1986) Dental caries status of children and youth in Singapore. *Ann. Acad. Med. Singapore,* **15**, 275–279

Lo, E. C. M., Evans, R. W. and Lind, O. P. (1990) Dental caries status and treatment needs of the permanent dentition of 6–12 year olds in Hong Kong. *Community Dent. Oral Epidemiol.*, **18**, 9–11

Loe, H. (1986) The fluoridation status of US public water supplies. *Public Health Rep.*, **101**, 157–162

Ludwig, T. G. (1965) The Hastings fluoridation project V – dental effects between 1954 and 1964. *N.Z. Dent. J.*, **61**, 175–179

Ludwig, T. G. (1971) The Hastings fluoridation project VI – dental effects between 1954 and 1970. *N.Z. Dent. J.*, **67**, 155–160

McCauley, H. G., Frazier, T. M. and Rivas, L. P. (1961) Dental caries in Baltimore schoolchildren after seven years of fluoridation of the public water supply. Baltimore Bureau of Statistics. *Q. Statist. Rep.*, **13**, 14–21

Margolis, F. J., Reames, H. R., Freshman, E., McCauley, J. C. and McLaffrey, H. (1975) Fluoride – ten-year prospective study of deciduous and permanent dentition. *Am. J. Dis. Child.*, **129**, 794–800

Martin, N. D. and Barnard, P. D. (1970) Tamworth dental survey results 1963, 1969. *Dental Outlook,* **23**, 6–7

Medcalf, G. W. (1971) First permanent molars of six-year-old children after two and a half years of fluoridation in Western Australia. *Aust. Dent. J.*, **16,** 252–254

Medcalf, G. W. (1975) Six years of fluoridation on the goldfields of Western Austrlia. *Aust. Dent. J.*, **20**, 170–173

Medcalf, G. W. (1978) Ten years of fluoridation in Perth, Western Australia. *Aust. Dent. J.*, **23**, 474–476

Mejia, D. R., Espinal, F., Velez, H. and Aguirre, S. M. (1976) Use of fluoridated salt in four Columbian communities VIII. *Bol. Sanit. Panam.*, **80**, 205–219

Ministry of Health, Scottish Office, Ministry of Housing and Local Government (1962) *The Conduct of the Fluoridation Studies in the United Kingdom and the Results Achieved After Five Years.* Report No. 105. HMSO, London

Minoguchi, G. (1964) Eleventh year of fluoridation study at Yamashina in Kyoto and some problem about the fluoridation of waterworks in Japan. *Bull. Stomatol. Kyoto Univ.*, **4**, 45–124

Mitropoulos, C. M., Lennon, M. A., Langford, J. W. and Robinson, D. J. (1988) Differences in dental caries experience in 14-year-old children in fluoridated South Birmingham and in Bolton in 1987. *Br. Dent. J.*, **164**, 349–350

Mollenkopf, J. (1963) Benefits of fluoridation apparent in Fort Wayne. *Ind. St. Board Health Month. Bull.*, Feb., 6–8

Moncrief, E. W. (1970) Results of eleven years of fluoridation in Fayette, Alabama. *J. Ala. Dent. Assoc.*, **54**, 18–25

Murray, J. J. (1986) Appropriate use of fluorides for human health. In *Community Water Fluoridation*, World Health Organisation, Geneva, pp. 38–73

Murray, J. J., Gordon, P. H., Carmichael, C. L., French, A. D. and Furness, J. A. (1984) Dental caries and enamel opacities in 10 year-old children in Newcastle and Northumberland. *Br. Dent. J.*, **156**, 225–258

Musselman, P. (1957) Report on dental findings in Newark, Delaware children after five years of fluoridation. *J. Am. Dent. Assoc.*, **54**, 783–785

National Health and Medical Research Council (1985) Report of working party on fluorides in the control of dental caries. *Austral. Dent. J.*, **30**, 433–442

Newbrun, E. (1989) Effectiveness of water fluoridation. *J. Publ. Health Dent.*, **49**, 279–289

Nordling, H. and Tulikoura, I. (1970) Results of the fluoridation of drinking water in Kuopio. *Suom. Hammaslääk.*, **17**, 517–524

O'Hickey, S. (1976) Water fluoridation and dental caries in Ireland: background, introduction and development. *J. Irish Dent. Assoc.*, **22**, 61–66

O'Hickey, S. and Pigott, B. (1983) Dental caries experience of Dublin schoolchildren after 10½ years of fluoridation. *J. Irish Dent. Assoc.*, **29**, 5–8

O'Mullane, D. M., Clarkson, J., Holland, T., O'Hickey, S. and Whelton, H. (1988) Effectiveness of water fluoridation in the prevention of dental caries in Irish children. *Community Dent. Health*, **5**, 331–344

Ostrow, A. H. (1963) *Ten Year Fluoridation Report*. Report of the Washington Dept. Public Health, Bureau of Dental Health, 18 March

Payette, M. (1982) Effets de la fluoruration des eaux potables sur la prévalence de la carie dentaire et sur le coût des traitements de la carie résiduelle chez les écolier de 6 à 17 ans de Montréal et d'Edmonton en 1979. *J. Dent. Que.*, **19**, 15–23

Quentin, K.-E. and Lingelbach, H. (1963) Trinkwasserfluoridierung in Europa. In *Advances in Fluorine Research and Dental Caries Prevention* (eds J. L. Hardwick, J. P. Dustin and H. R. Held), Oxford, Pergamon, pp. 23–32

Reger, R. H., Dunn, M. M. and Downs, R. A. (1963) *The effects of 10 years of fluoridation on the teeth of school-age continuous residents of Grand Junction 1951–1962*. Colorado Department of Health, Denver, Colo., Appendix, pp. 4–11

Ross, M. R., Hecht, S. J. and Gleeson, J. C. (1960) Results of five years of fluoridation in 21 Monmouth County municipalities. *J. New J. State Dent. Soc.*, **31**, 14–16

Rugg-Gunn, A. J., Carmichael, C. L., French, A. D. and Furness, J. A. (1977) Fluoridation in Newcastle and Northumberland; a clinical study of 5-year-old children. *Br. Dent. J.*, **142**, 395–402

Russell, A. L. and White, C. L. (1961) Dental caries in Maryland and children after seven years of fluoridation. *Public Health Rep.*, **76**, 1087–1093

Russell, D. L. (1965) Dental caries rate of Mobile County school children; comparison of children in areas supplied by fluoridated and non-fluoridated communal water supplies. *Ala. J. Med. Sci.*, **2**, 381–388

Rybakov, A. I., Pakhomov, G. N., Kuklin, G. S. and Alimsky, A. V. (1978) A decade of experience in drinking water fluoridation and dynamics of caries among schoolchildren in the European part of the USSR beyond the Arctic Circle. Personal communication, World Health Organisation

Schreiber, M. F. (1966) Sheboygan led fluoridation 'war' on tooth decay. Wis. State Board of Health, *Fluoridation News*, **3**(2), 1

Schultz, W. E. (1969) Results of the city of Milwaukee dental surveys 1950, 1959, 1965. *J. Wis. St. Dent. Soc.*, **45**, 195–198

Smith, J. E. and Paquin, O. (1962) The effect of five and one-half years of water fluoridation on the continuous resident child population of St. Louis, Missouri. *J. Missouri Dent. Assoc.*, **42**(7), 10–16

Snyder, J. R. (1964) Benefits of fluoridation in Boseman. Montana State Board of Health, *Treasure State Health*, **13**(11), 4

Sogaro, L. H. (1964) Phillipsburg, N. J.–Easton, Pa. fluoridation study. *J. Am. Dent. Assoc.*, **69**, 295–299

Stadt, Z. M., Blum, H. L., Barney, E. E. and Fletcher, E. (1960) Contra Costa County fluoridation reports. *J. Cal. State Dent. Assoc.* and *Nevada State Dent. Assoc.*, Apr., 109–113

Steele, A. (1977) Oshkosh School dental survey indicates decay decline. Wis. Dept. of Health and Social Services, *Fluoridation News,* **13**(1), 3

Strelyukhina, T. F., Belova, T. A., Belyaevskaya, L. A. and Gromova, E. M. (1976) Influence of water fluoridation on dental caries experience among schoolchildren in Leningrad. *Stomatol. (Mosk.)*, **8**, 66–69

Suntsov, V. G. (1985) Results of the local and general fluorine prophylaxis of caries in the children of Omsk Province. *Stomatologiia (Mosk.)*, **64**, 11–12

Szwejda, L. (1962) Eleven years of fluoridation in Charlotte, N. Carolina. *Dent. Soc. J.,* **45**, 107–113

Tank, G. and Storvick, C. A. (1964) Caries experience of children one to six years old in two Oregon communities. *J. Am. Dent. Assoc.,* **69**, 750–757

Taylor, E. and Bertram, F. P. (1965) Marshall Study credit is due; discussion of the tabular data from the ten-year Marshall, Texas dental fluoridation study. *Texas Dent. J.,* Feb., 30–31

Teo, C. S. (1984) Fluoridation of public water supplies in Singapore. *Ann. Acad. Med. Singapore,* **13**, 247–251

Tessier, C. (1987) Effets de la fluoruration de l'eau à Windsor Qué depuis 7 ans sur les enfants de 6 à 7 ans. *J. Dent. Que.,* **24**, 17–23

Toth, K. (1972) The methods and results of caries prevention with fluorides in Hungary and in Eastern European countries. *Rev. Belge Med. Dent.,* **27,** 521–527

Trithart, A. H. and Denney, R. P. (1956) Study of caries experience rates of 6-yr-old children of Milan, Tenn. after 5 yrs of fluoridation. *J. Tenn. State Dent. Assoc.,* **36**, 156–159

Trubman, A. (1965) Dental caries in Mississippi children; comparison of a fluoride with non-fluoride towns. *J. Miss. Dent. Assoc.,* **21**, 19–23

Videroni, W., Sternberg, G. S. and Davies, G. N. (1976) Effect on caries experience of lifetime residents after 10 years of fluoridation in Townsville, Australia. *Community Dent. Oral Epidemiol.,* **4**, 248–253

Viegas, Y. and Viegas, A. R. (1974) Data analysis of the prevalence of dental caries in Campinas city (S. Paulo, Brazil) after ten years of water fluoridation. *Rev. Saude Publica,* **8**, 399–409

Viegas, Y. and Viegas, A. R. (1985) Data analysis on the prevalence of dental caries in Barretas city (S. Paulo, Brazil) after ten years of water fluoridation. *Rev. Saude Publ. S. Paulo,* **19**, 287–299

Vreven, J. (1987) Dental caries in Belgium, preventive and legal aspects. In *Strategy for Dental Caries Prevention in European Countries According to their Laws and Regulations* (eds R. M. Frank and S. O'Hickey), IRL Press, Oxford, pp. 119–125

Weinstein, H. N. (1972) Effectiveness of fluoridation. *Chicago Board of Health Newsletter,* **12**, 1–2

Whittle, J. G. and Downer, M. C. (1979) Dental health and treatment needs of Birmingham and Salford schoolchildren. *Br. Dent. J.,* **147**, 67–71

Wigdorowicz-Makowerowa, N., Dadun-Sek, A. and Plonka, B. (1978) Comparison of effectiveness of water fluoridation during 5 and 8 years in Wroclaw. *Czas. Stomatol.,* **31**, 817–823

Wigdorowicz-Makowerowa, N., Plonka, B. and Dadun-Sek, A. (1975) Evaluation of water fluoridation effectiveness in children in Wroclaw during 5 years. *Czas. Stomatol.,* **28**, 253–259

Wigdorowicz-Makowerowa, N., Plonka, B. and Dadun-Sek, A. (1983) Effect of water fluoridation during 13 years in Wroclaw on the condition of permanent teeth in schoolchildren. *Czas. Stomatol.,* **36**, 243–249

Wong, M. Q., Goh, S. W. and Oon, C. H. (1970) A ten-year study of fluoridation of water in Singapore. *Dent. J. Malaysia Singapore,* **10**, 20–40

World Health Organisation (1969) *Status of Water Fluoridation in the Americas.* Document No. HP/DH/2. Dental Health Section, Department of Health Services and the Department of Engineering and Environmental Sciences, Pan American Health Organisation, Regional Office of WHO

Yacovone, J. A. and Parente, A. M. (1974) Twenty years of community water fluoridation: the prevalence of dental caries among Providence, R. I. schoolchildren. *R. I. Dent. J.,* June, 3–18

Young, W. O. (1958) Fluorides and dental caries in Idaho V; ten years of fluoridation in Lewiston. *Idaho State Dent Assoc. Newsletter*, Feb.

Chapter 6

Removal of excess fluoride from water supplies

Knowledge that excessive levels of fluoride in drinking water are related to the occurrence of dental fluorosis preceded the unravelling of the fluoride and caries relationship (Chapter 2). Figures 2.1 and 2.2 (pages 15 and 17) clearly show that dental caries decreases but dental fluorosis increases as the concentration of fluoride in drinking water increases. High levels of dental fluorosis are disfiguring and constitute a public health problem, such that drinking water standards in some countries include upper limits for fluoride concentration. The US Public Health Service (1962) Drinking Water Standards list 'optimum fluoride concentrations' and 'upper control limits', which depend on the annual mean maximum daily temperature. At that time, the US Public Health Service estimated that about 4.2 million people lived in 1142 communities served by public water supplies that exceeded the upper control limit for fluoride content. In 712 of these communities, with a combined population of 1.8 million, fluoride levels were at least twice the optimum, which constituted grounds for rejection of the water supply (US Public Health Service, 1962).

Many States in India have ground waters between 1 and 5 mg F/l, and in some areas fluoride concentrations exceed 21 mg F/l. The Ministry of Health, Government of India, have prescribed 1.0 mg/l and 2.0 mg/l as the permissive and excessive limits, respectively, for fluoride in drinking water, while the Indian Standard Specification for Drinking Water gives the desirable limit as 0.6–1.2 mg/l (Indian Standards Institute, 1983; Nanoti and Nawlakhe, 1988). Although not all India's drinking water supplies have been analysed, it was estimated in 1980 that 2240 villages or communities with a population of nearly 2 million appeared to be exposed to high fluoride levels that may require defluoridation.

In many regions of north, west and east and southern Africa drinking water contains high levels of fluoride (Jeboda, 1986). Fluorosis is particularly severe in areas affected by the Rift Valley. Manji (1983) reported that the prevalence of fluorosis was 44% in permanent teeth and 19% in deciduous teeth in a nation-wide survey in Kenya. Fluoride levels over 10 ppm in drinking water are common, with 40 ppm F being recorded in Naivasha (Manji, 1983) and as high as 145 ppm F in Crater (Walvekar and Qureshi, 1982). The situation is similar in Tanzania, with the prevalence of fluorosis reaching 83–95% in the Arusha-Moshi area. Springs, rivers, boreholes and lakes all contain high concentrations of fluoride, the highest being the Maji ya Chai river with 45 ppm F (Mosha, 1984). With low caries levels existing over much of Africa, defluoridation of drinking water is a higher public health priority than fluoridation (Walvekar and Qureshi, 1982; Manji, 1983). However, it is not clear to what extent dental fluorosis is seen as a problem by the communities and how this is weighed against the risk of dental caries with associated pain, infection and loss of teeth.

Methods available for defluoridation of drinking water

The most obvious way of reducing exposure to water-borne fluorides is to change the water supply to one containing an acceptable level of fluoride. Most other methods involve chemical or physicochemical removal of fluoride. These have been reviewed by Møller (1988) and with specific relevance to India by Tewari and Goyal (1986). Examples where these have been tried will be given in the next section.

Activated carbon
This is produced from heated and ground wood, paddy husks, coconut fibre and other carboniferous waste. It is most effective when pH is low, but this is disadvantageous as the pH of the water then has to be raised to make it acceptable for consumption.

Bone
Dried and crushed natural bone and bone char (dried and crushed bone heated to 600°C for 20 min) are efficient removers of fluoride. The latter is preferred since bacterial contamination is reduced and taste is improved compared with natural bone. Bone char can be regenerated with caustic soda. It should be noted that the use of bone is unacceptable to some religious groups.

A 3:1 mixture of bone char and charcoal has been used in Thailand (Phantumvanit, Songpaisan and Møller, 1988) and may be especially useful for household units.

Hydroxyapatite
The affinity of fluoride for hydroxyapatite is an important reason for fluoride's anti-caries effect, and is used as a method for defluoridation. Powdered hydroxyapatite is effective alone or in combination with tri-calcium phosphate.

Lime and aluminium
Lime and aluminium sulphate both have a high affinity for fluoride and can be used for removal of excess fluoride from water, either alone or in combination. On their own, both lime and aluminium have disadvantages. First, control of pH and alkalinity is crucial when lime is used, and the method is only reasonable when removal of both hardness and fluoride is required. Secondly, dosage with aluminium has to be carefully controlled so as to avoid excessive levels of residual aluminium. The combined use of lime and aluminium is the central feature of the Nalgonda technique which was developed at the Indian National Environmental Engineering Research Institute (NEERI) at Nagpur in 1974 (Bulusu, 1988). It was developed for medium size communities but is adaptable down to village level.

Magnesium oxide has also been used as an alternative to calcium oxide, and aluminium chloride is sometimes used together with aluminium sulphate.

Opinya, Pameijer and Grön (1987) investigated the possibilities of using magnesium oxide or bone meal to defluoridate Kenyan drinking water. As far as is known, these studies have not progressed further than the laboratory stage. Both magnesium oxide and bone meal are readily available and inexpensive in Kenya, where water fluoride levels can exceed 9 ppm. Both removed fluoride, but reaction time was faster with the bone meal than with magnesium oxide, and the taste of the water treated with bone meal was also better.

Ion-exchange resins

These are commercially produced resins and, as such, are expensive and uneconomical in most circumstances. The taste of the treated water is sometimes poor. A number of these resins have been proposed (Tewari and Goyal, 1986; Møller, 1988).

Examples of those investigated are: polystyrene resins, strongly basic quarternary ammonium type resins, sulphonated sawdust impregnated with aluminium, defluoron-1 and defluoron-2.

Activated alumina (mainly aluminium oxide) has been investigated in the USA (Horowitz, Maier and Thompson, 1964) and India (Bulusu and Nawlakhe, 1988).

Other methods such as reverse osmosis and electrolysis, although effective, are too expensive to consider further.

Practical experience in defluoridation

Change in water supply

The classical public health experiment of laying a new water pipeline from Carpenter Springs to the village of Oakley, Idaho, USA, in 1925, was described in Chapter 2. Eight years later, McKay (1933) reported a dramatic reduction in the prevalance of brown-stained permanent teeth. Five years later, Dean, McKay and Elvove (1938) reported a reduction in mottled enamel in children 10 years after the water supply of the town of Bauxite, Arkansas, was changed and 1 year later similar results in South Dakota were reported (Dean, Elvove and Poston, 1939).

However, it is not always feasible or practical for a community to replace or dilute its existing water supply. Partial replacement, of a kind, was described by Gerrie and Kehr (1957) where dental fluorosis was prevented by children using low-fluoride bottled water.

Britton, South Dakota, USA

This community of 1430 persons received water containing, on average, 6.7 ppm F. On 20 November 1948 a defluoridation plant became operational using synthetic hydroxyapatite. However, it was only partially effective, reducing the water fluoride level to 3.6 ppm instead of the target level of 1.5 ppm and, because of this and because of an excessive loss of material, the plant was closed after 4 years' use. Bone char replaced the hydroxyapatite and defluoridation recommenced in January 1953, reducing the fluoride level to 2.5 ppm between January 1953 and September 1954, and from September 1954 to 1.6 ppm F. Initially, the cost of the plant was borne by the US Public Health Service, but this was transferred to Britton in 1965.

The dental health of children in Britton was recorded in 1948, 1960 and 1965 (Horowitz, Maier and Law, 1967). In 1948, 100% of children had fluorosis, but this fell to 29% in 1965. Children aged 6–10 years in 1965, almost all of whom had consumed water containing 1.6 ppm exclusively, had a fluorosis index of 0.7, about 72% lower than the score of 2.4 recorded for this age group in 1948.

Bartlett, Texas, USA

Bartlett is a small community with a population of less than 2000 in 1952 when it was decided to defluoridate the public water supply which had one of the highest fluoride levels (8.0 ppm) in the USA. The defluoridation plant was installed by the US Public Health Service and used activated alumina, in an insoluble granular form. The water percolated through the gravity-type contact tank at a maximum rate of 400 US gal/min (1 US gal = 3.78 litres). It was designed to reduce the fluoride level from 8.0 to 1.0 ppm. The alumina was periodically reactivated. The plant cost US$ 15 000 in 1951 and the cost of chemicals was 5.0 cents per 1000 US gal. The plant functioned well: during the first 11 years (1952–63) more than 6500 water samples were obtained from the distribution system indicating an average fluoride level of 1.1 ppm (Horowitz, Maier and Thompson, 1964; Horowitz and Heifetz, 1972).

Dental examinations of children were undertaken in 1952, 1954, 1963 (after 11 years) and 1969 (after 17 years). The prevalence of fluorosis in Bartlett children fell from 96% in 1954 to 18% in 1969. Over the same period, the fluorosis index fell from 2.5 to 0.4 (Horowitz and Heifetz, 1972).

India

India has extensive areas of endemic fluorosis, and there is a need for comprehensive mapping of fluoride levels in drinking water and a programme of defluoridation (Tewari and Goyal, 1986). Much development work has been undertaken by NEERI at Nagpur. Systems which looked promising were investigated in pilot studies. A pilot plant using the ion exchange resins carbion and defluoron-1 (in proportion 8:1) commenced at Gangapur (Rajasthan). Aluminium solution was used as a regenerant, but the system was unsuccessful as most of the defluoron-1 was washed out.

To overcome these problems, defluoron-2 was developed in 1968. It is a sulphonated coal using aluminium solution as regenerant. The life of the medium was found to be 2–4 years. Two plants, each of 20 000 Imp. gal capacity per regeneration (1 Imp. gal = 4.55 litres), have been installed. No details of effectiveness or cost have been obtained, although Tewari and Goyal (1986) reported that defluoron-2 was successful in removing fluorides, but regeneration and maintenance of the plant required skilled operation which was not readily available. In response to this drawback, NEERI developed the Nalgonda technique.

The Nalgonda technique involved adding, in sequence, an alkali (usually lime) and aluminium sulphate and/or aluminium chloride. The choice and dosage of chemicals depends upon the properties of the source water. Descriptions of plant design, tables of dosage schedules and likely costs have been given by Bulusu (1988). A typical plant might serve a population of 5000. One important consideration is the uncertain number of hours of power supply, and the plant was designed to operate on 4 h supply per day. The process is inherently chemical-intensive, although improvements have been made in this respect. The cost of water defluoridated using the Nalgonda technique is about 1.5–3 times the cost of the untreated water, although it is likely to be much cheaper than transporting water over long distances (Bulusu, 1988).

A defluoridation plant using the Nalgonda technique was commissioned in the town of Kadiri in Andhra Pradesh in 1980 to treat water containing 4.1–4.8 mg F/l.

It had a capacity of 2270 m^3/day and served the population of 34 000. Initially, the plant was operated by a research and development team of NEERI, but was given over to the Kadiri Municipality after its performance was judged satisfactory. During the first few years the plant became a model of water treatment technology for defluoridation. The inclusive cost of treating the water was calculated at 1 rupee/m^3. Subsequently, visitors reported that the operation and maintenance of the plant had declined, and this was confirmed by NEERI during two visits in 1984–86. These difficulties highlight the problem of maintenance and staffing – aspects discussed more fully by Nanoti and Nawlakhe (1988).

Conclusions

Fluorosis is endemic in some areas of the world and constitutes a public health problem. Many methods capable of reducing the fluoride content of drinking water to a level optimum for health (about 1 ppm, depending on climate) have been identified. Some of them have been tried, but only in the USA and India. The effectiveness of defluoridation at substantially reducing dental fluorosis has only been reported in the USA. Problems of cost and availability of equipment and materials, and the lack in some areas of trained personnel for plant maintenance, have seemingly prevented more widespread introduction of water defluoridation. Much has been achieved in reducing caries prevalence and severity in many countries by appropriate use of fluorides; now attention also needs to be given to reducing excessive fluoride levels to those optimum for dental and general health.

References

Bulusu, K. R. (1988) Defluoridation for small communities by the Nalgonda technique. In *New Frontiers in Fluoride Studies for Health* (eds A. J. Rugg-Gunn and M. Rahmatulla), COSTED, Singapore, pp. 175–187

Bulusu, K. R. and Nawlakhe, W. G. (1988) Defluoridation of water by activated alumina. In *New Frontiers in Fluoride Studies for Health* (eds A. J. Rugg-Gunn and M. Rahmatulla), COSTED, Singapore, pp. 188–210

Dean, H. T., Elvove, E. and Poston, R. F. (1939) Mottled enamel in South Dakota. *Public Health Rep.*, **54**, 212–228

Dean, H. T., McKay, F. S. and Elvove, E. (1938) A report of a mottled enamel survey of Bauxite (Ark.) ten years after a change in the common water supply. *Public Health Rep.*, **53**, 1736–1748

Gerrie, N. F. and Kehr, F. (1957) Experience in preventing dental fluorosis by using low-fluoride bottled water. *Public Health Rep.*, **72**, 183–188

Horowitz, H. S. and Heifetz, S. B. (1972) The effect of partial defluoridation of a water supply on dental fluorosis; final results in Bartlett, Texas, after 17 years. *Am. J. Public Health*, **62**, 767–769

Horowitz, H. S., Maier, F. J. and Law, F. E. (1967) Partial defluoridation of a water supply and dental fluorosis; results after 11 years. *Public Health Rep.*, **82**, 965–972

Horowitz, H. S., Maier, F. J. and Thompson, M. B. (1964) The effect of partial defluoridation of a water supply on dental fluorosis; results after 11 years. *Am. J. Public Health*, **54**, 1895–1904

Indian Standards Institute (1983) *Indian Standard Specification for Drinking Water* UDC 663.6, IS: 10500-1983. ISI, New Dehli

Jeboda, S. O. (1986) Prospects for fluoridation in Africa. *Odontostomatol. Trop.*, **9**, 147–152

McKay, F. S. (1933) Mottled enamel; the prevention of its further production through a change of water supply at Oakley, Idaho. *J. Am. Dent. Assoc.*, **20**, 1137–1149

Manji, F. (1983) Fluoride supplements in Kenya, a viewpoint. *Odontostomatol. Trop.*, **6**, 157–160

Møller, I. J. (1988) Defluoridation of drinking waters. In *Dental Fluorosis* (eds O. Fejerskov, F. Manji and V. Baelum), Munksgaard, Copenhagen, pp. 90–98

Moshi, H. J. (1984) Endemic dental fluorosis and the possibilities of defluoridation and fluoridation of water supplies in Tanzania. *Odontostomatol. Trop.*, **7**, 89–96

Nanoti, M. V. and Nawlakhe, W. G. (1988) Operational experiences of defluoridation of water with special reference to the defluoridation plant at Kadiri. In *New Frontiers in Fluoride Studies for Health* (eds A. J. Rugg-Gunn and M. Rahmatulla), COSTED, Singapore, pp. 218–228

Opinya, G. N., Pameijer, C. H. and Grön, P. (1987) Simple defluoridation procedures for Kenyan borehole water. *Community Dent. Oral Epidemiol.*, **15**, 60–62

Phantumvanit, P., Songpaisan, Y. and Møller, I. J. (1988) The ICOH-defluoridator; an appropriate technology defluoridation device for individual households. *World Health Forum*, **8**, 85–90

Tewari, A. and Goyal, A. (1986) Fluoride; defluoridation; needs, methods and cost analysis. *J. Indian Dent. Assoc.*, **58**, 487–492

US Public Health Service (1962) *Public Health Service Drinking Water Standards*, P.H.S. Publication No. 956, US Government Printing Office, Washington, p. 8

Walvekar, S. V. and Qureshi, B. A. (1982) Endemic fluorosis and partial defluoridation of water supplies; a public health concern in Kenya. *Community Dent. Oral Epidemiol.*, **10**, 156–160

Chapter 7

Addition of fluoride to school water supplies, salt, milk and fruit juice

Although the importance of fluoride in the prevention of dental caries in the first-half of this century principally concerned fluoride in public water supplies, other vehicles for fluoride have been recommended for almost as long a time. Tablets containing calcium fluoride were recommended for 'the strengthening of teeth' in the last century, as was bone meal, which makes one suspect that, in those early days, calcium was considered to be of at least equal importance to fluoride.

Initially it was thought that, to be effective, the fluoride had to be ingested, absorbed into the body and laid down in the forming tooth enamel. This undoubtedly occurs and has come to be known as the 'systemic' or 'pre-eruptive' method of fluoride administration. Since enamel formation is completed (except for third molars) by about the age of 12 years, fluoride administration was thought to be only effective up to this age.

However, epidemiological studies in the USA in the 1930s and 40s proved otherwise. Analysis of data collected for children entering areas with optimum levels of fluoride, at various ages, indicated that erupted teeth benefited substantially from exposure to fluoride. At the same time, American research workers showed that the amount of fluoride in tooth enamel could be increased by applying fluoride topically to tooth surfaces. This was the birth of the 'topical' mode of action or 'topical' method of applying fluoride.

It should be appreciated that the 'systemic effect' and 'pre-eruptive effect' are not exactly the same. The meaning of pre-eruptive effect is fairly self-evident – the benefit accruing from the ingestion of an adequate level of fluoride while a tooth is forming and before its eruption into the mouth. On the other hand, a systemic effect is that accruing from ingestion and absorption of fluoride, and this can occur post-eruptively via saliva and crevicular fluid. Although most of the systemic effect of fluoride will occur before tooth eruption, the possible post-eruptive systemic effect via these oral fluids should not be ignored.

In Chapters 3–5 the effectiveness of fluoridation of public water supplies was considered. In this chapter, three alternatives will be discussed: fluoridation of school water supplies, and the addition of fluoride to salt and to milk and fruit juice. The effectiveness of fluoride tablets will be discussed in Chapter 8. The addition of fluoride to flour and sugar have been proposed and the possible benefits of adding fluoride to sugar have been discussed by Luoma (1985). Mundorff *et al.* (1988) showed that fluoride added to sugar reduced the cariogenicity of dietary sugars in rats significantly. Apart from this, there is little information on the use of flour or sugar as vehicles for fluoride, and they will not be considered further.

School water fluoridation

Two advantages of water fluoridation are that, first, no effort is required by the recipients and, secondly, that the cost per person is low. However, the cost per person increases as the size of the population served by each fluoridation plant decreases. It was of interest, therefore, to see whether fluoridation of a school's water supply was effective and economical. Unlike other school-based preventive programmes (e.g. fluoride tablets and mouthrinses), no action is required by the children.

The decision to commence trials of school water fluoridation was encouraged by three pieces of information. First, Ast *et al.* (1956), Hill, Blayney and Wolf (1957) and Arnold (1956) observed during the US public water fluoridation studies that children who received fluoridated water for the first time at the age of 6 years benefited substantially. Secondly, children who lived in homes which received water with negligible fluoride levels but attended a school with a water supply containing 3.5 ppm F (naturally occurring) received considerable benefit from this elevated fluoride level at school (Barron and Lewis, 1968). Thirdly, children who first attended school in Bauxite, USA, with 13.7 ppm F in the drinking water, at the age of 6 years, did not develop fluorosis (Kempf and McKay, 1930).

As yet, school water fluoridation has been tested only in the USA, where 40 million people live in areas without community water supplies and many rural schools are supplied by their own well.

By 1983, 500 schools (in 13 States) with a combined enrolment of 213 000 children, operated school water fluoridation schemes (Heifetz, Horowitz and Brunelle, 1983). Seventy-five per cent of these school water fluoridation projects were in the States of North Carolina, Kentucky and Indiana (Ripa, 1985). In the State of Indiana, 91 schools operated such schemes and only 26 schools, which could potentially be fluoridated, had still to do so (Mallat, Beiswanger and Smith, 1987). The cost per child per year, including equipment and labour, has been estimated at $1.50 (Newbrun, 1978).

The first investigation began in 1954 in the Virgin Islands with fluoridation of the water supply at 2 schools at a level of 2.3 ppm F. Because one of the schools was altered and enlarged during the study, and operation of the machinery was intermittent and eventually broke down, the study cannot be considered satisfactory. In 1962, 7–13-year-old children in the school receiving the more consistent supply of fluoridated water (for 8 years) were examined, together with children of similar age in other schools in the same district. The children attending the fluoridated school had about 22% less DMFT than the control children, at least indicating that school water fluoridation might be beneficial (Horowitz, Law and Pritzker, 1965).

Since then three major studies, each planned to last 12 years, have been undertaken in mainland USA. The first two, in Pike County, Kentucky, and Elk Lake, Pennsylvania, began in 1958, while the third in Seagrove, North Carolina, began in 1968. In Elk Lake, the final examinations (after 12 years) took place in 1970, but this was not possible in Pike County where the organization at the two test schools changed and further dental examinations were not conducted after the 8-year follow-up examination in 1966.

In the Pike County schools, water was fluoridated at 3.0 ppm (or 3.3 times the optimum level for public water supplies in the same area), while in the Elk Lake schools the water fluoride level was 5 ppm (or 4.5 times the optimum public water supply level). These levels were chosen because children consume part of their daily water intake at school and only attend school for a maximum of about 200 days per year. In addition, children do not enter school before 6 years, an age when incisor teeth can be considered to be no longer at risk of developing mottled enamel. Since no objectionable mottling was observed in any teeth in the children attending the Pike County and Elk Lake schools, a higher fluoride level (6.3 ppm or 7 times the optimal community water fluoride level) was tested in the third American study in Seagrove. In all three of these studies, children in the test schools were examined before fluoridation of the school's water supply began, and the results of these baseline examinations then served as control data for comparison with the results of the surveys after 4, 8 and 12 years' school fluoridation.

Interim results after 8 years of school fluoridation in Pike County and Elk Lake (Horowitz *et al.*, 1968) showed that children who had continually attended schools in the two study areas had very similar reductions in DMFT of about 33% and 35%, respectively, compared with similarly aged children who attended these schools before fluoridation began.

Results after 12 years of school fluoridation in Elk Lake (5.0 ppm F) and Seagrove (6.3 ppm F) are given in Table 7.1. Substantial savings in absolute terms (5.2 and 5.9 DMFS) and in percentage terms (39.5% and 47.6%) were observed. Benefits were apparent for all ages, but were most marked for children aged 12–17 years (Horowitz, Heifetz and Law, 1972; Heifetz, Horowitz and Brunelle, 1983). Not all teeth benefited equally (Table 7.2). Approximal (mesial and distal) surfaces benefited most both in absolute and percentage terms, and greater preventive effects were observed in late-erupting teeth (canines, premolars and second molars) than in early-erupting teeth (incisors and first molars). This may be because the late-erupting teeth received both a pre- and post-eruptive exposure to fluoride, whereas the early-erupting teeth received only post-eruptive exposure, although difference in length of time exposed to the cariogenic challenge in the mouth may be an additional explanation (Horowitz, 1973). No fluorosis was observed during the dental examinations at any of the schools (Heifetz, Horowitz and Brunelle, 1983).

It should be appreciated that the design of these studies was retrospective, or a self-control design. As discussed in Chapter 5, these designs are susceptible to

Table 7.1 Mean DMF surfaces for children aged 6–17 years, at baseline and after 12 years of school water fluoridation in Elk Lake, Pa (5.0 ppm F) and Seagrove, NC (6.3 ppm F) (From Heifetz *et al.*, 1983)

Study area	*Mean* DMFS*	*Mean* DMFS*	*Difference in mean DMFS*	*Difference from baseline (%)*
Elk Lake	1958 13.12 (*n* = 1030)	1970 7.94 (*n* = 1149)	5.18	39.5
Seagrove	1968 12.39 (*n* = 766)	1980 6.49 (*n* = 758)	5.90	47.6

* Adjusted to combined baseline age distribution at both schools.

changes in the background level of caries in the community. The trials in Pike County and Elk Lake, which ran from 1958 to 1970, were unlikely to be affected by any change in background caries level, but the trial in Seagrove began in 1968 and ended in 1980. During this time, caries prevalence in US children declined – this will have resulted in a slight exaggeration of the observed effects in Seagrove. As Heifetz, Horowitz and Brunelle (1983) pointed out, these differences in background trends in caries in US children preclude making firm conclusions of the superiority of school fluoridation at seven times the optimum compared with 3.3 times or 4.5 times the optimum. Any advantages of the highest level (seven times) would seem to be small, and most school and health authorities have opted to use a fluoride level of 4.5 times the optimum for that area (Mallat, Beiswanger and Smith, 1987).

In summary, fluoridation of school water supplies is technically feasible, results in a substantial reduction in caries experience in school children and the cost of this public health measure is low. The slightly bigger benefit achieved with 6.3 ppm F is not sufficiently greater than that observed with 5 ppm F to warrant the higher fluoride level, and Heifetz, Horowitz and Driscoll (1978) therefore recommend school fluoridation at the lower level of 5 ppm F, or 4.5 times the optimum level of fluoridation of community water supplies in that locality.

Table 7.2 Mean DMF surfaces for school children in Elk Lake, Pa (5.0 ppm F since 1958) and Seagrove, NC (6.3 ppm F since 1968), for different surface types and for early- and late-erupting teeth (From Horowitz *et al.*, 1972, and Heifetz *et al.*, 1983)

	All surfaces	*Occlusal*	*Approximal*	*Buccolingual*
ELK LAKE SCHOOL				
All teeth				
1958	13.5	5.8	4.8	2.9
1970	8.1	3.8	2.2	2.1
% reduction from 1958	40	34	53	29
Early erupting teeth				
1958	9.0	3.2	3.5	2.4
1970	6.2	2.6	1.8	1.8
% reduction from 1958	31	17	47	26
Late erupting teeth				
1958	4.5	2.6	1.3	0.5
1970	1.9	1.2	0.4	0.3
% reduction from 1958	57	54	69	44
SEAGROVE SCHOOL				
All teeth				
1968	11.9	4.2	3.9	3.8
1980	6.3	3.2	1.1	2.0
% reduction from 1968	48	24	73	48
Early erupting teeth				
1968	9.0	2.7	3.2	3.1
1980	4.9	2.2	1.0	1.7
% reduction from 1968	46	19	70	45
Late erupting teeth				
1968	2.9	1.5	0.8	0.7
1980	1.4	1.0	0.1	0.3
% reduction since 1968	51	31	82	60

Fluoridated salt

As a dietary vehicle for ensuring adequate ingestion of fluoride, domestic salt comes second to drinking water; salt's enrichment with iodide already provides an effective means of preventing goitre. Indeed it was a medical practitioner concerned with the prevention of goitre in Switzerland who, over 40 years ago, pioneered the addition of fluoride to salt as a caries-preventive measure (Wespi, 1948, 1950). Fluoridated salt has been on sale in Switzerland since 1955, and by 1967 three-quarters of domestic salt sold in Switzerland was fluoridated at 90 mg F/kg salt (or 90 ppm F). However, it was soon accepted that the original estimates of salt intake, upon which calculations of fluoride concentrations in salt were based, were too high and the ingestion of fluoride too low.

Since 1983 the amount of fluoride added to salt has been 250 mg F/kg salt (250 ppm F). This is available in 23 Swiss cantons with 5.5 million inhabitants and is used voluntarily by 70% of the population (Marthaler, 1983). In contrast to the situation in Switzerland, Toth (1976, 1980) suggested, on the basis of studies of urinary fluoride concentration, that the level of fluoride added in Hungary should be raised from 250 to 350 mg F/kg.

Despite the widespread use of fluoridated salt in Switzerland, its effectiveness is not easily measured since, in many Swiss communities, other preventive programmes (fluoride tablets or fluoride brushing) have been operating in many schools for over 20 years. Salt fluoridation was introduced into the Canton of Vaud (population 500 000) in 1969–70 and since 1970 the level of fluoride addition to salt used in the home and in bakeries has been 250 mg F/kg (250 ppm F) in the form of KF. Distribution of fluoride tablets was compulsory in schools in Vaud since 1953, but this ceased in 1970. In one area of Vaud the annual brushing exercises with fluoride gel (1.2% F), begun in 1965, continued after 1970 for children up to the age of 10 years. The control areas were Romont and Châtel-St-Denis in the Canton of Fribourg, and St. Aubin in the Canton of Neuchâtel. Some of the households in these control communities had been using salt fluoridated to 90 ppm F before 1970 and continued to do so after 1982. In two of the control communities, fluoride tablets were distributed at school, while in one community children brushed annually with fluoride gel (1.2% F) during the study period 1970–82. At this time, 60–80% of toothpastes sold in Switzerland contained fluoride.

Interim results were published by Marthaler *et al.* (1977, 1978), from which they concluded that the caries-preventive effectiveness of fluoridated salt in Vaud was greater than the 25% or so reduction observed following the addition of 90 mg F/kg in other Swiss cantons (Marthaler and Schenardi, 1962). The results after 12 years are given in detail by de Crousaz *et al.* (1985). Dental examinations of 100–200 children in four age groups – 8, 10, 12 and 14 years – were conducted on an examiner-blind basis in 1970, 1974, 1978 and 1982, although the numbers of children aged 14 years in the control area were too small to analyse. Results for DMF sites are given in Table 7.3. The authors concluded that: (a) there was a decline in caries experience in children in the control communities; (b) a similar decline occurred in 12- and 14-year-old children living in the test communities – this was not the case for 8- and 10-year-olds where a low caries prevalence already existed in 1970, probably due to earlier use of fluoride tablets; (c) caries experience was consistently lower in children who consumed salt fluoridated to 250 mg F/kg compared with children in the control communities. Caries experience of children in Vaud in 1982 was similar to those recorded for children in Basle who had

Table 7.3 Mean number of DMF sites per child living in the Canton of Vaud, Switzerland, which had received salt fluoridated to 250 ppm F since 1970, compared with children in a control area (From de Crousaz *et al.*, 1985)

Age (yr)	*Control*					*Test*				
	1970	*1974*	*1978*	*1982*	*% redn*	*1970*	*1974*	*1978*	*1982*	*% redn*
8	3.7	2.5	3.3	1.9	49	2.2	1.9	1.6	1.8	17
10	7.4	6.0	4.4	4.4	40	5.4	3.7	3.6	4.3	19
12	15.4	11.2	8.5	8.2	47	10.4	7.3	6.6	5.0	52
14	–	–	–	–	–	16.2	12.6	10.5	8.2	49

consumed water fluoridated at 1.0 ppm F, and similar to children in Zürich Canton who had benefited from a school-based dental programme which had been operating for the past 16 years (Figure 7.1). The authors concluded that this study provides further evidence of a substantial cariostatic effect of fluoride when added to salt.

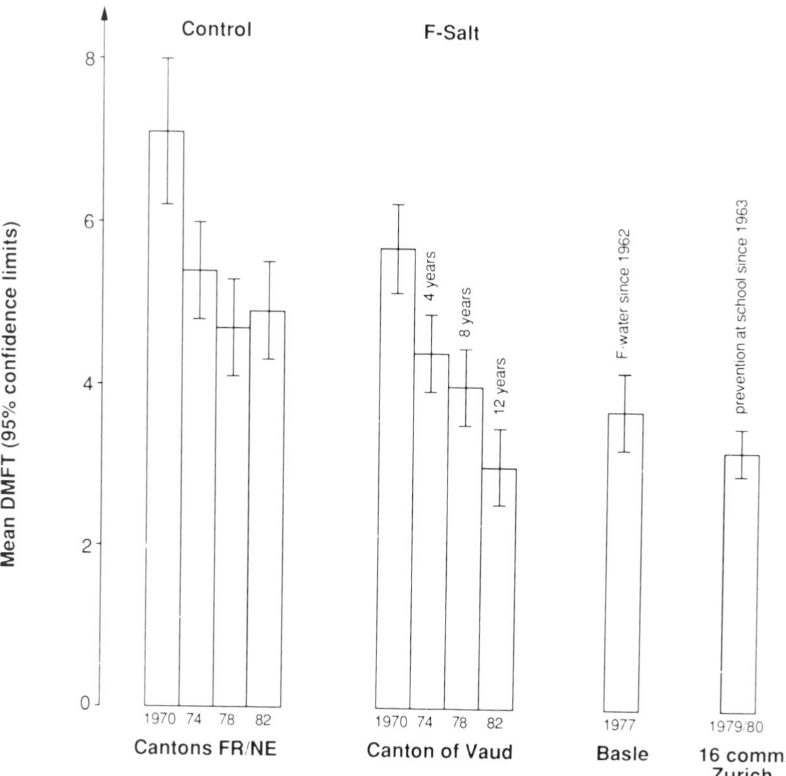

Figure 7.1 Mean DMFT for 12-year-old Swiss children in the control Cantons of Fribourg and Neuchâtel; receiving salt fluoridated to 250 mg F/kg in Vaud; in fluoridated Basle; and in 16 communities in Zürich Canton (After de Crousaz *et al.*, 1985; reproduced with kind permission of the Editor, *Helvetica Odontologica Acta*)

The effect on the dental health of children after 9 years of salt fluoridation at 250 ppm F in the Canton of Glarus was reported by Steiner *et al.* (1986). Caries experience fell in Glarus more rapidly than in other areas, pointing to a cariostatic effect of fluoridated salt.

Toth (1976) reported the effectiveness of 250 mg F/kg salt fluoridation in Hungary after 8 years' use. The results (Table 7.4) indicated a reduction of 39% in deft in 6-year-old children in the test community, while caries experience increased by 7% in the control community children over the same period. Although there was an imbalance in caries experience between the two communities at the start of the experiment in 1966, this alone could not explain the differences observed in 1974.

Table 7.4 Caries experience (deft) for 6-year-old children living in test and control communities in Hungary after 8 years' salt fluoridation (at 250 mg F/kg) (From Toth, 1976)

	Experimental	*Control*
1966	6.8	8.6
1974	4.1	9.2
Difference	−2.7 (−39.5%)	+0.6 (+7.1%)

After 10 years' exposure to salt fluoridation, Toth (1979) observed that 5- to 6-year-olds in the same test community had 2.8 deft, compared with 6.0 deft in the control community, and 1.4 deft in children of the same age living in an area with fluoridated water. These 10-year results indicated that a substantial caries reduction occurred after the introduction of salt fluoridation, but this was less than occurred with water fluoridation.

In 1977, the fluoride level in the test salt was raised to 350 mg F/kg. According to Marthaler (1983), Toth observed caries reductions in 1982 of 53–68% after use of salt with this raised level of fluoride.

In 1964, a study was initiated in four Colombian communities (Mejia *et al.*, 1976). In the village of Montebello, sodium fluoride was added to domestic salt (at 200 mg F/kg), while in Armenia calcium fluoride was added to domestic salt (at 200 mg F/kg), in San Pedro drinking water was fluoridated (at 1 ppm F) and Don Matias remained as the control community. At the end of the project, after 8 years, reductions in caries prevalence and experience in 8-year-old children were large in the three communities receiving fluoride in salt or water, although a small reduction was also observed in the control town (Table 7.5). When all children aged 6–14 years were included in the data analyses, the reduction in DMFT

Table 7.5 Caries experience (DMFT) for 8-year-old children living in three test communities and one control community in Colombia, South America, after 8 years (From Mejia *et al.*, 1976)

	NaF salt	*CaF_2 salt*	*Water F*	*Control*
1964	3.7	3.8	3.8	4.3
1972	1.4	1.1	0.8	3.8
Difference	2.3 (61%)	2.7 (72%)	3.0 (78%)	0.5 (13%)

between 1964 and 1972 was 50% in Montebello (NaF in salt), 48% in Armenia (CaF_2 in salt), 60% in San Pedro (water F) and 5% in the control town Don Matias. Analysis of urine samples throughout the year revealed that fluoride excretion was similar in the two fluoridated salt communities, but excretion levels in the salt communities were 20% lower than those recorded in the fluoridated water town.

Encouraging results were also reported after the addition of NaF to domestic salt in a closed children's institution in Pamplona, Spain (Vines, 1971). Because of the high estimated salt intake, particularly in their special salt bread, the fluoride level was only 112 mg F/kg salt but, after 4 years, reductions in caries experience were observed in all ages in the range 8–13 years.

Subsequently, it was found that mixing was improved by using KF instead of NaF, and wet spraying of KF onto dry salt was the method of choice for big plants. Dry mixing is suitable for small plants (Marthaler, 1983). Potassium fluoride appears to be suitable for addition to salts obtained from many different countries (Marthaler and Sener-Zanola, 1985). In the Columbian study, CaF_2 (which is soluble at 8 ppm F) was as effective in caries prevention as NaF, which is a thousand times more soluble. However, if less than 4–6 ppm F is available in ionic form (as occurs with bread made with 250 ppm F salt), the indispensable topical effect is very much reduced.

The average ingestion of salt amounts to 7–10 g/day per person in several developed countries: about 3–5 g comes from domestic salt, 2–3 g is naturally present in foods and 2–3 g is added during manufacture.

In summary, the caries-preventive effectiveness of fluoridated salt is substantial, approaching that of fluoridated water. This view is based on a comparatively small number of studies (compared with the data on water fluoridation) which have lasted for a maximum of 12 years. Since April 1983, the fluoride content of salt in Switzerland has been 250 ppm F. Urinary fluoride concentration studies have indicated that this concentration may be slightly less than optimal in children but sufficient in adults (Marthaler, 1983). Salt appears to be a safe vehicle for fluoride administration (Mühlemann, 1967; Ruzicka, Mrklas and Rokytova, 1976; Marthaler, 1983). The merits of salt fluoridation as a community preventive measure will be discussed further in Chapter 19.

Fluoridated milk and fruit juices

Both bovine and human milk contain low levels of fluoride – about 0.03 ppm F (Ericsson and Ribelius, 1971). Because milk is recommended as a good food for infants and children, it was considered, over 30 years ago, to be a suitable vehicle for supplementing children's fluoride intake in areas with fluoride-deficient water supplies. Ericsson (1958) showed that fluoride was absorbed in the gut just as readily from milk as from water, refuting the suggestion that the high calcium content of milk would render the fluoride unavailable. More recently, Villa *et al.* (1989) have shown that fluoride absorption from MFP in milk is as high as that from NaF in water. However, the binding of added fluoride to calcium or protein might reduce the topical fluoride effect in the mouth compared with fluoride in water (Duff, 1981).

The results of five clinical trials of fluoridated milk and one trial of fluoridated fruit juice have been published. The study of Rusoff *et al.* (1962) involved 171 children aged 6–9 years from two schools in Louisiana, USA. Children from one school received a half-pint of homogenized milk daily, fortified with 2.2 mg NaF (yielding 1 mg F). The fluoride was added in the form of 0.5 ml NaF solution to each half-pint before sealing. During the summer vacation, parents of children in the study group were given bottles of aqueous sodium fluoride solution so that 8 drops could be added to their 8 oz (225 ml) glass of milk per day. Children in the control group received homogenized milk without fluoride. This pilot study lasted 3½ years, when 65 children aged 9–12 years remained in the fluoride group and 64 children of similar age in the control group. Unfortunately the two groups were not well balanced with respect to first-molar caries experience at the beginning of the experiment. The DMFT in second molars and first and second premolars, after 3½ years' consumption of fluoridated milk, was 0.34 in the fluoride group and 1.70 in the control group. A difference was still apparent 18 months after cessation of the experiment. However, because of the considerable divergence in caries attack on first molars between groups before the study and the small size of the groups, the lower caries rate in the experimental children must be viewed with caution. The data indicated that some of the effect was likely to be topical.

Ziegler (1962) reported his attempts to introduce fluoridated milk in Winterthur, Switzerland. At first, a sealed plastic bottle of 0.22% sodium fluoride solution was made available to the public in pharmacies against a prescription. Each parent then added 1 ml of this fluoride solution to 1 litre of milk to produce 1 ppm F fluoridated milk. Thus the amount of fluoride ingested depended on the amount of milk consumed – a half-litre of milk contained 0.5 mg F. In 1955, school milk was fluoridated at the central dairy in Winterthur; initially 0.2 mg F was placed in 200 ml milk, but this was increased to 0.5 mg in 1961. A little later, the size of milk bottles was increased to 250 ml, which contained 0.625 mg F. The results of clinical surveys indicated that dental caries was lower in children who had consumed the fluoridated milk for 6 years, compared with control children (Wirz and Ziegler, 1964, quoted in WHO, 1970).

Stephen *et al.* (1981, 1984) reported the results of a 5-year study of the effect on young Glaswegian children of consuming fluoridated milk at school. Children entered the study in 1976 at age 4.5–5.5 years, and drank 200 ml of milk containing 1.5 mg F (7 ppm F) each school day (about 200 days per year). The control group drank milk without added fluoride. After 5 years, the 50 children in the test group had developed a mean of 3.8 DMFS compared with 6.6 DMFS in the 56 children in the control group – a difference of 43%. When data analysis was restricted to permanent teeth which erupted during the study, the mean DMFS scores were 3.3 for the test group and 6.3 for the control group – a difference of 48%. The milk was sucked through straws at least 15 min before the mid-morning break.

A 5-year trial was also conducted in Hungary (Banoczy *et al.*, 1983, 1985) between 1979 and 1983. Children aged 3–9 in the children's city of Fót, north of Budapest, participated, and drank 200 ml of milk or cocoa-milk daily for about 300 days per year. Children aged 3–5 years received 0.4 mg F/day and children 6–9 years 0.75 mg F/day. Children living in another closed community formed a control group. They were similar to the children in the test group, with one exception – while the test group children used a fluoride toothpaste consistently, the control children used either a fluoride or non-fluoride toothpaste. Caries experience was reduced in the test group compared with the control group, both in the deciduous and permanent dentitions, but the beneficial effect was especially marked in first permanent molars in the youngest age group (85% less caries), which received the fluoridated milk from 3 years of age.

The results of a study in Louisiana were more variable (Legett *et al.*, 1987). Fluoridated chocolate-flavoured milk was given to young school children for 2 or 3 years. A statistically significant difference was observed in the group who consumed the fluoridated milk for 2 years but not in the group who participated for 3 years compared with the control groups. One explanation for this difference may be the breakdown of the equipment for 9 months in the middle of the trial. The composition of the control group was not clear from the report of this trial.

Fluoridated milk was given for 3 years to children aged 4–7 years attending schools in Bethlehem, Israel. Each school day, children in the test group received 100 ml of reconstituted powdered cow's milk supplemented with 1 mg F as NaF. Consumption took place at 10 a.m. in school at least 15 min before ingestion of other food or drink. The control group received no beverage in school. The caries experience of children at the beginning and end of the study were not given, preventing an assessment of the initial balance of the groups, but substantial differences in the 3-year caries increments for both the deciduous and permanent teeth were recorded. The 3-year caries increments for the test group were: 1.3 deft and 0.2 DMFT, compared with 3.5 deft and 0.55 DMFT for the control group children.

In warm climates, fluoridated fruit juices may be a practical alternative to fluoridated milk. Gedalia *et al.* (1981) have reported a 28% reduction in DMFS increment in 6–9-year-old Israeli children who consumed 1 mg F in 100 ml of pure orange juice (≡10 ppm F) each school day for 3 years. The 111 test-group children developed 2.5 DMFS over 3 years compared with 3.5 DMFS in the 111 control children who had no beverage. However, interpretation of the results was complicated by the observation that a third group of similarly aged children, who consumed 100 ml of orange juice with no added fluoride, developed 2.9 DMFS over the 3-year period. It would appear, therefore, that the fluoride *per se* might have been responsible for only part of the difference between the fluoride drink group and the no-drink group.

Since absorption of fluoride from water and milk would appear to be about equal, it is likely that their systemic caries-preventive effect would be similar. Fluoridated milk has been shown to have a topical caries-preventive effect in rats (Poulsen, Larsen and Larson, 1976) and possibly in humans (Rusoff *et al.*, 1962), although Rugg-Gunn *et al.* (1976) did not find an increase in plaque fluoride after children had consumed milk containing 5 ppm F, and Gedalia *et al.* (1981) and Zahlaka *et al.* (1987) reported no increase in enamel fluoride in children who consumed 100 ml of 10 ppm F for 3 years in fruit juice or milk, respectively. Kempler *et al.* (1977) have reported that, in hamsters, acidulated fluoride beverages have a greater caries-preventive effect than a neutral fluoride beverage. Although this suggests that low pH fruit drinks may be a better vehicle for fluoride than milk (at a neutral pH), these findings await confirmation from comparative human clinical trials, since acidulated fluoride mouthrinses have not been shown to be superior to neutral fluoride mouthrinses in preventing caries in human subjects (see Chapter 10). On the other hand, Zahlaka *et al.* (1987) believe that, from the results of different trials in Israel, milk is a more effective vehicle for fluoride than fruit juice.

In summary, all the reported trials have shown substantial caries-preventive effects, especially when milk consumption began before the eruption of permanent teeth. Clinical data are still limited, however. Milk fluoridation requires considerable logistic effort and, as yet, it has not been introduced on a community basis.

References

Arnold, F. A. (1956) Effect of fluoridated water supplies on dental caries prevalence, tenth year of Grand Rapids – Muskegon study. *Publ. Health Rep.*, **71**, 652–658

Ast, D. B., Kantwell, K. T., Wachs, B. and Smith, D. J. (1956) Newburgh-Kingston caries fluorine study, XIV. Combined clinical and roentgenographic dental findings after ten years of fluoride experience. *J. Am. Dent. Assoc.*, **52**, 514–525

Banoczy, J., Zimmermann, P., Hadas, E., Pinter, A. and Bruszt, V. (1985) Effect of fluoridated milk on caries; five year results. *J.R. Soc. Health,* **105,** 99–103

Banoczy, J., Zimmermann, P., Pinter, A., Hadas, E. and Bruszt, V. (1983) Effect of fluoridated milk on caries; three year results. *Community Dent. Oral Epidemiol.*, **11**, 81–85

Barron, E. G. and Lewis, J. F. (1968) Effect of a school's naturally fluoridated water on the prevalence of carious lesions. *J. Publ. Health Dent.*, **28,** 167–172

de Crousaz, P., Marthaler, T. M., Weisner, V., Bandi, A., Steiner, M., Roberts, A. and Meyer, R. (1985) Caries prevalence in children after 12 years of salt fluoridation in a Canton of Switzerland. *Schweiz. Mschr. Zahnmed.*, **95**, 805–815

Duff, E. J. (1981) Total and ionic fluoride in milk. *Caries Res.*, **15**, 406–408

Ericsson, Y. (1958) The state of fluorine in milk. *Acta Odont. Scand.*, **16**, 51–77

Ericsson, Y. and Ribelius, U. (1971) Wide variations of fluoride supply to infants and their effect. *Caries Res.*, **5**, 78–88

Gedalia, I., Galon, H., Rennert, A., Biderco, I. and Mohr, I. (1981) Effect of fluoridated citrus beverage on dental caries and on fluoride concentration in the surface enamel of children's teeth. *Caries Res.*, **15**, 103–108

Heifetz, S. B., Horowitz, H. S. and Brunelle, J. A. (1983) Effect of school water fluoridation on dental caries; results in Seagrove NC after 12 years. *J. Am. Dent. Assoc.*, **106,** 334–337

Heifetz, S. B., Horowitz, H. S. and Driscoll, W. S. (1978) Effect of school water fluoridation on dental caries: results in Seagrove, NC, after eight years. *J. Am. Dent. Assoc.*, **97**, 193–196

Hill, N., Blayney, J. R. and Wolf, W. (1957) The Evanston dental caries study XV. The caries experience rates of two groups of Evanston children after exposure to fluoridated water. *J. Dent. Res.*, **36**, 208–219

Horowitz, H. S. (1973) School fluoridation for the prevention of dental caries. *Int. Dent. J.*, **23**, 346–353

Horowitz, H. S. and Heifetz, S. B. (1979) Methods for assessing the cost-effectiveness of caries preventive agents and procedures. *Int. Dent. J.*, **29,** 106–117

Horowitz, H. S., Heifetz, S. B. and Law, F. E. (1972) Effect of school water fluoridation on dental caries; final results in Elk Lake, Pa after 12 years. *J. Am. Dent. Assoc.*, **84**, 832–838

Horowitz, H. S., Law, F. E. and Pritzker, T. (1965) Effect of school water fluoridation on dental caries, St. Thomas, V.I. *Publ. Hlth Rep.*, **80**, 382–388

Horowitz, H. S. *et al.* (1968) School fluoridation studies in Elk Lake, Pennsylvania, and Pike County, Kentucky – results after eight years. *Am. J. Public Health,* **50**, 2240–2250

Kempf, G. A. and McKay, F. S. (1930) Mottled enamel in a segregated population. *Publ. Health Rep.*, **45**, 2923–2940

Kempler, D., Anaise, J., Westreich, V. and Gedalia, I. (1977) Caries rate in hamsters given non-acidulated and acidulated tea. *J. Dent. Res.*, **56**, 89

Legett, B. J., Garbee, W. H., Gardiner, J. F. and Lancaster, D. M. (1987) The effect of fluoridated chocolate-flavoured milk on caries incidence in elementary schoolchildren; two and three year studies. *J. Dent. Child.*, **54**, 18–21

Luoma, H. (1985) Fluoride in sugar. *Int. Dent. J.*, **35**, 43–49

Mallat, M. E., Beiswanger, B. B. and Smith, C. E. (1987) Twelve years of Indiana school fluoridation. *J. Indiana Dent. Assoc.*, **66**, 13–15

Marthaler, T. (1983) Practical aspects of salt fluoridation. *Schweiz. Mschr. Zahnmed.*, **93**, 1197–1214

Marthaler, T. M., de Crousaz, Ph., Meyer, R., Regolati, B. and Robert, A. (1977) Fréquence globale de la carie dentaire dans le canton de Vaud, après passage de la fluoruration par comprimés à la fluoruration du sel alimentaire. *Schweiz. Monatsschr. Zahnheilkd.*, **87**, 147–158

Marthaler, T. M., Mejia, R., Toth, K. and Vines, J. J. (1978) Caries-preventive salt fluoridation. *Caries Res.*, **12**, suppl. 1, 15–21

Marthaler, T. M. and Schenardi, C. (1962) Inhibition of caries in children after 5½ years use of fluoridated table salt. *Helv. Odont. Acta,* **6**, 1–6

Marthaler, T. M. and Sener-Zanola, B. (1985) Availability of fluoride added to various brans of alimentary salt used in southern and central America. *Schweiz. Mschr. Zahnmed.*, **95**, 1195–1200

Mejia, D. R., Espinal, F., Velez, H. and Aguirre, S. M. (1976) Use of fluoridated salt in four Colombian communities VIII. Results achieved from 1964 to 1972. *Bol. Sanit. Panam.*, **80**, 205–219

Mühlemann, H. R. (1967) Fluoridated domestic salt; a discussion of dosage. *Int. Dent. J.*, **17**, 10–17

Mundorff, S. A., Glowinsky, D., Griffith, C. J., Stein, J. H. and Gwinner, L. M. (1988) Effect of fluoridated sucrose in rat caries. *Caries Res.*, **22**, 232–236

Newbrun, E. (1978) Cost-effectiveness and practicality features in the systemic use of fluorides. In *Proceedings of a Workshop on the Relative Efficiency of Methods of Caries Prevention in Dental Public Health* (ed. B. A. Burt), University of Michigan Press, Ann Arbor, pp. 27–48

Poulsen, S., Larsen, M. J. and Larson, R. H. (1976) Effect of fluoridated milk and water on enamel fluoride content and dental caries in the rat. *Caries Res.*, **10**, 227–233

Ripa, L. W. (1985) Community- and school-based caries preventive programmes; participation of New York State children. *N.Y. State Dent. J.*, **51**, 408–418

Rugg-Gunn, A. J., Edgar, W. M., Jenkins, G. N. and Cockburn, M. A. (1976) Plaque F and plaque acid production in children drinking milk fluoridated to 1 and 5 ppm F. *J. Dent. Res.*, **55**, D143 (abstr.)

Rusoff, L. L., Konikoff, B. S., Frye, J. B., Johnston, J. E. and Frye, W. W. (1962) Fluoride addition to milk and its effect on dental caries in school children. *Am. J. Clin. Nutr.*, **11**, 94–107

Ruzicka, J. A., Mrklas, L. and Rokytova, K. (1976) The influence of salt intake on the incorporation of fluoride into mouse bone. *Caries Res.*, **10**, 386–389

Steiner, M., Marthaler, T. M., Weisner, V. and Menghini, G. (1986) Kariesbefall bei Schulkindern des Kanton Glarus, 9 Jahre nach Einführung des höher fluoridierten Kochsalzes (250 mg F/kg). *Schweiz. Mschr. Zahnmed.*, **96**, 688–699

Stephen, K. W., Boyle, I. T., Campbell, D., McNee, S. and Boyle, P. (1984) Five year double-blind fluoridated milk study in Scotland. *Community Dent. Oral Epidemiol.*, **12**, 223–229

Stephen, K. W., Boyle, I. T., Campbell, D., McNee, S., Fyffe, J. A., Jenkins, A. S. and Boyle, P. (1981) A 4-year double blind fluoridated school milk study in a vitamin-D deficient area. *Br. Dent. J.*, **151**, 287–292

Toth, K. (1976) A study of 8 years domestic salt fluoridation for prevention of caries. *Community Dent. Oral Epidemiol.*, **4**, 106–110

Toth, K. (1978) Some economic aspects of domestic salt fluoridation. *Caries Res.*, **12**, 110 (abstr.)

Toth, K. (1979) 10 years of domestic salt fluoridation in Hungary. *Caries Res.*, **13**, 101 (abstr.)

Toth, K. (1980) Factors influencing the urinary fluoride level in subjects drinking low fluoride water. *Caries Res.*, **14**, 168 (abstr.)

Villa, A., Guerrero, S., Cisternas, P. and Monckeberg, F. (1989) Fluoride bio-availability from disodium monofluorophosphate fluoridated milk in children and rats. *Caries Res.*, **23**, 179–183

Vines, J. J. (1971) Fluorprofilaxis de la caries dental a traves de la sal fluorurada. *Revta Clin. Esp.*, **120**, 319–334

Wespi, H. J. (1948) Gedanke zur Frage der optimalen Ernährung in der Schwangerschaft. Salz and Brot als Träger zusätzlicher Nahrungsstoffe. *Schweiz. Med. Wochenschr.*, **78**, 153–155

Wespi, H. J. (1950) Fluoriertes Kochsalz zur Cariesprophylaxe. *Schweiz. Med. Wochenschr.*, **80**, 561–564

World Health Organisation (1970) *Fluorides and Human Health.* WHO Monogr. Ser. No. 59, WHO, Geneva

Zahlaka, M., Mitri, O., Munder, H., Mann, J., Kaldavi, A., Galon, H. and Gedalia, I. (1987) The effect of fluoridated milk on caries in Arab children; results after 3 years. *Clin. Prev. Dent.*, **9**, 23–25

Ziegler, E. (1962) Milk fluoridation. *Bull. Schweiz. Akad. Med. Wiss.*, 18

Chapter 8

Fluoride tablets and drops

Effectiveness in caries prevention

During the 1950s, the value of water fluoridation as a way of preventing caries became clear. It was recognized, however, that water fluoridation was not always possible and that a sensible alternative might be to give children an equivalent amount of fluoride as a tablet. One of the first demonstrations of the value of fluoride tablets for caries prevention was given by Arnold, McClure and White (1960). The number of years the children in this study ingested the tablets varied, but the mode was 7 years. The authors concluded that 'The results correspond with what has been observed in the use of drinking waters containing 1 ppm F'. Children over the age of 3 years received 1 mg F/day and this dose has formed the basis for further studies, and for individual and community prevention, for 30 years.

About 57 reports on the effectiveness of fluoride tablets or drops have appeared in the literature, although some of these are difficult to interpret because of the small size of the test group, the short experimental period or inadequate reporting. The remaining investigations fall into two groups: first, those where the fluoride supplements were given daily at home and were started before school age, and secondly, those where tablets have been distributed in school, on school days only, usually without additional supplementations during holidays or before school age. The effectiveness of the use of fluoride tablets at home is very much harder to investigate because it is difficult to choose a comparable control group and there is frequently a marked fall-off in cooperation; these difficulties do not usually arise in school-based trials. An excellent review of the effectiveness of fluoride tablets was given by Driscoll (1974), and Tables 8.1 and 8.2 are based on his report, but with additional recent data.

Deciduous teeth

Summaries of 21 trials into the effect of fluoride tablets on the deciduous dentition are given in Table 8.1. Thirteen were conducted in Europe, 5 in the USA and 3 in Australia. Sodium fluoride was used in all but one study (although the compound was not stated in one further study), sometimes in combination with vitamins.

The initial age of the subjects and the length of time the tablets were taken varied considerably, making it difficult to draw conclusions on effectiveness accurately. Nevertheless it would appear that a caries-preventive effect was observed consistently (about 50–80% reduction) in studies where the initial age was 2 years or younger. In the three studies in which no effect was found, the children were initially aged 3 years or older. In a more thorough analysis of effectiveness in relation to the age at which ingestion of tablets began, Granath *et al.* (1978) suggested that while buccolingual surfaces may benefit if the commencement age is over 2 years, the effect on approximal surfaces is very much less if the commencement age is 2 years or over. This suggests that the topical effect is greater on the more exposed buccolingual surfaces than on the less accessible approximal surfaces (see also Chapter 12).

The study of Hennon, Stookey and Beiswanger (1977) is the only clinical trial of fluoride tablets conducted in an area with an almost optimal water fluoride level (0.6–0.8 ppm F), although the observations of Glenn (1979) and Glenn, Glenn and Duncan (1982) were on children living in a fluoridated community. A substantial preventive effect was observed by Hennon and co-workers in the children taking fluoride tablets, in addition to the benefit that could be expected to be derived from living in an area with a moderate water fluoride level. In their study, one group of children received 0.5 mg F from birth throughout the 5-year trial period, while another group received 0.5 mg F up to 3 years of age and 1 mg for the remaining 2 years. The effect was slightly greater (47% reduction compared with 37%) in the latter group.

The practice of giving to young children, living in areas with optimal levels of fluoride in the water, additional fluoride dietary supplements has been criticized on the grounds that it substantially increases the risk of dental fluorosis (Schrotenboer, 1981; Stookey, 1981).

Permanent teeth

Summaries of the 34 investigations into the effectiveness of fluoride tablets in preventing caries in the permanent dentition are given in Table 8.2; again, most of the studies are European. The initial age of the subjects and the duration of fluoride tablet intake varied widely. In only four of the studies (Hamberg, 1971; Schützmannsky, 1971; Aasenden and Peebles, 1974; Margolis *et al.*, 1975) were fluoride tablets taken from birth for at least 7 years. Reductions ranged from 39% in Schützmannsky's trial to 80% in the trial of Aasenden and Peebles. In the trial of Margolis and co-workers the children who started taking fluoride tablets at birth showed a 58% reduction in DFT compared with only a 14% reduction in the group of children who started at the age of 4 years, suggesting the importance of ingestion in the first few years of life, before the permanent teeth erupted.

In the five studies conducted in school (initial age 6–7 years) and lasting at least 5 years, the following reductions in caries have been reported: 27% (Schützmannsky, 1965), 20–24% (Berner *et al.*, 1967), 36–47% (Marthaler, 1969), 28–29% (Driscoll *et al.*, 1978) and 61% (Allmark *et al.*, 1982).

Three of the 34 studies were conducted in the UK – all were school-based programmes and all reported substantial caries reductions. Stephen and Campbell (1978) reported an 81% reduction in DMFS in a trial in Glasgow lasting 3 years, while Allmark *et al.* (1982) reported a reduction in DMFS of 61% after 6 years use in Portsmouth, and O'Rourke, Attrill and Holloway (1988) reported a 48% reduction in DMFT in Manchester children after 3 years.

Prenatal

Six trials have investigated the effectiveness of the ingestion of prenatal fluoride tablets, although results of only four of these are given in Tables 8.1 and 8.2,

Table 8.1 Caries-preventive effects of fluoride tablets/drops on deciduous teeth (Based on Driscoll, 1974, and Binder *et al.*, 1978)

Study	*F compound*	*Daily dosage* (mg F)	*Initial age of subjects* (yr)	*No. subjects in F group*	*Duration of F intake* (yr)	*Caries reduction (%)*		*Statistical significance*
						deft	*defs*	
Arnold *et al.* (1960)	NaF	0.5–1	Birth–6	121	1–12	'Comparable to water F'		NR
Pollak (1960)[5]	NaF + V	1	3	100	2	80		NR
	NaF + V	1	4	111	2	20		NR
Ziemnowicz-Glowaka (1960)[5]	NaF	0.8	3	139	2		26	S
Lutomska and Kominska (1962)[5]	NaF	0.6	3–4	154	2	'No significant effect'		NR
Kamocka *et al.* (1964)[5]	NaF	0.75[1]	3	64	3	0		NS
	NaF	0.75[1]	4	79	3	0		NS
Leonhardt (1965)[5]	NaF + V	1+	3	Not known	2	38		NR
	NaF + V	1+	4	Not known	2	30		NR
Hennon *et al.* (1966, 1967, 1970)	NaF + V	0.5–1	Birth–5½	85	3		63	S
	NaF + V	0.5–1	Birth–5½	54	4		68	S
	NaF + V	0.5–1	Birth–5½	60	5		66	S
Margolis *et al.* (1975)	NaF + V	0.5–1	Birth	149	4–6	76		S
	NaF + V	0.5–1	4	77	0–2	29		NS
Hoskova (1968)	NaF	0.25–1	Prenatal	78	4	93		S
	NaF	0.25–1	Birth–1	151	4	54		S
Kailis *et al.* (1968)	NaF	?	Prenatal	50	4–6	82		S
	NaF	?	Birth	92	4–6	56		S
Stolte (1968)[5]	?	1	3	130	3	11		NR

Prichard (1969)	NaF	?	Prenatal	176	6–8	70		S
	NaF	?	Birth	282	6–8	40		S
Hamberg (1971)	NaF + V (drops)	0.5	Birth	342	3	57		NR
	NaF + V (drops)	0.5	Birth	342	6	49		NR
Kraemer (1971)[5]	CaF_2	1	4	170	2	22		NR
	CaF_2	1	5	82	2	18		NR
Schützmannsky (1971)	NaF	1	Prenatal	100	<1	13		S
	NaF	0.25–1	Prenatal	100	9	30		S
	NaF	0.25–1	Birth	100	9	14		S
Aasenden and Peebles (1974)	NaF + V[2]	0.5–1	Birth	87	8–11		78	S
Fanning *et al.* (1975)	NaF	?	<1	581	5	33		NR
Andersson and Grahnen (1976)	NaF	0.25–0.5	1	127	5[3]	31		S
Hennon *et al.* (1977)[4]	NaF + V	0.5–1	<1	44	5		47	S
	NaF + V	0.5	<1	47	5		37	S
Granath *et al.* (1978)	NaF	0.25–0.5	<2	48	2–4		46 BL 51 AP	NS S
	NaF	0.25–0.5	2–3	123	1–2		33 BL −1 AP	NS NS
O'Rourke *et al.* (1988)	NaF	1[1]	5	263	3	18		NS

V, Vitamins; S, Statistically significant; NS, Statistically non-significant; NR, No statistical test reported; BL, Buccolingual; AP, Approximal surfaces.

1 Tablets given only on school days.
2 A NaF + V combination was given up to 3 years of age. Beyond this age, some children received NaF + V, while others received only NaF.
3 Aged 8–10 at examination.
4 In F area (0.6–0.8 ppm F).
5 Quoted by Driscoll (1974).

Table 8.2 Caries-preventive effects of fluoride tablets on permanent teeth (Based on Driscoll, 1974, and Binder *et al.*, 1978)

Study	*F compound*	*Daily dosage* (mg F)	*Initial age of subjects* (yr)	*No. subjects in F group*	*Duration of F intake* (yr)	*Caries reduction (%)*		*Statistical significance*
						DMFT	*DMFS*	
Stones *et al.* (1949)	NaF	1.5	6–14	125	2	0		NS
Bibby *et al.* (1955)	NaF	1	5–14	133	1	Nil		NR
	NaF	1	5–14	119	1	Tentative finding: 'possible'		NR
Niedenthal (1957)[4]	NaF	1[1]	6–7	251	3	22		NR
Wrzodek (1959)[4]	NaF	1[1]	6–9	8 381	3	21		NR
	NaF	1[1]	6–9	13 585	4	22		NR
Arnold *et al.* (1960)	NaF	0.5–1	Birth–6	121	1–15	'Comparable to water F'		NR
Krusic (1960)[4]	CaF_2	Not known	8–15	480	1–3	70		NR
Pollak (1960)[4]	NaF + V	1	6–7	300	2	38		NR
Ziemnowicz-Glowaka (1960)[4]	NaF	0.8[1]	3–6	704	2		33	S
	NaF	0.8[1]	5–6	204	3		28	S
Jez (1962)[4]	CaF_2	Not known	7–11	7 200	2½	0		NR
Krychalska-Karwan and Laskowa (1963)[4]	NaF	Not known	Grammar school	134	4		5	NR
Minoguchi *et al.* (1963)	NaF + V	0.25	Birth–6	75	6	36		NR
Grissom *et al.* (1964)	NaF	1[1]	6–11	178	2		34	S
Kamocka *et al.* (1964)[4]	NaF	0.75[1]	3	64	3	17		NS
	NaF	0.75[1]	4	79	3	60		S
Leonhardt (1964)	NaF	1	6	398	4	32		NR
	NaF	1	7	429	3	25		NR
Hippchen (1965)[4]	Not known	1	6	500	3	32		NR
Schützmannsky (1965)	NaF	0.75[1]	6	580	4		25	NR
	NaF	0.75[1]	6	197	6		27	NR

Berner *et al.* (1967)	NaF	0.5–1[1]	5–7	105	3		84 (except 1st molar)	NR
							33 (1st molar)	NR
	NaF	1[1]	7–9	158	4	16		NR
	NaF	1[1]	7–9	160	6	20		NR
	NaF	1[1]	7–9	109	7	24		NR
De Paola and Lax (1968)	APF	1[1]	6–8	130	2		23	S
Girardi-Vogt (1968)[4]	NaF	1	6	Not known	3	31		NR
Stolte (1968)[4]	Not known	1	3	150	3	69		NR
Marthaler (1969)	NaF	0.5–1[1]	7	450	1–8	36	47	S
Hamberg (1971)	NaF + V	0.5	Birth	342	7	70		NR
Schützmannsky (1971)	NaF	1	Prenatal	100	<1	6		NS
	NaF	0.25–1	Prenatal	100	9	43		S
	NaF	0.25–1	Birth	100	9	39		S
Aasenden *et al.* (1972)	APF	1[1]	8–11	109	3		30	S
	NaF	1[1]	8–11	114	3		27	S
Plasschaert and Konig (1974)	NaF	1	7	208	2		38	S
Aasenden and Peebles (1974)	NaF + V[2]	0.5–1	Birth	100	8–11		80	S
Binder (1974)	NaF	0.25–1	Birth–14	3 084	8–14	43		S
Margolis *et al.* (1975)	NaF + V	0.5–1	Birth	56	7–10	58		S
	NaF + V	0.5–1	4	31	3–6	14		NS
Andersson and Grahnén (1976)	NaF	0.25–0.5	1	127	5[3]		40	S
Stephen and Campbell (1978)	NaF	1[1]	5½	54	3		81	S
Driscoll *et al.* (1978)	APF	1[1]	6–7	150	6		28	S
	APF	2[1]	6–7	135	6		29	S
Allmark *et al.* (1982)	NaF	1[1]	6	124	6	59	61	S
O'Rourke *et al.* (1988)	NaF	1[1]	5	263	3	48		S

V, Vitamins; S, Statistically significant; NS, Statistically non-significant; NR, No statistical test reported.

[1] Tablets given only on school days.
[2] A NaF + V combination was given up to 3 years of age. Beyond this age, some children received NaF + V, while others received only NaF.
[3] Aged 8–12 at examination.
[4] Quoted by Driscoll (1974).

because in the remaining two (Feltman and Kosel, 1961; Glenn, 1979; Glenn, Glenn and Duncan, 1982) insufficient data were reported. In all these trials (Tables 8.1 and 8.2) the percentage caries reduction was greater in the children whose mothers received fluoride tablets in pregnancy. But in spite of the apparent greater benefit of prenatal fluoride, Hoskova (1968) concluded that fluoride administration should begin as soon after birth as possible, attributing the greater benefit to better home conditions in the prenatal group. Feltman and Kosel (1961) compared the caries experience of 672 children who had received (a) only prenatal supplements (162 children), (b) prenatal and postnatal supplements (228 children) and (c) only postnatal tablets from varying ages (282 children). Prenatal fluoride appeared to confer benefit additional to that derived from postnatal fluoride exposure. The trial of Schützmannsky (1971) was better reported and also had three groups: a prenatal fluoride-only group, a prenatal and postnatal group (for 9 years) and a postnatal-only group (also for 9 years). The reductions for deciduous teeth were 13%, 30% and 14% respectively (Table 8.1) and 6%, 43% and 39% respectively, for permanent teeth (Table 8.2), suggesting that a small benefit may be derived from prenatal fluoride ingestion, particularly in the deciduous dentition.

Dr Frances Glenn has written extensively on the benefits of prenatal fluoride supplementation (e.g. Glenn, 1981; Glenn, Glenn and Duncan, 1982; LeGeros *et al.*, 1985; Glenn and Glenn, 1987). Glenn (1979) reported caries prevalence in children attending a private practice who had received prenatal fluoride supplements in addition to receiving an optimum water fluoride level. Nineteen of the 24 children aged 5–17 years who received prenatal supplements were caries-free.

Further data were presented at a symposium 'Perspectives on the Use of Pre-natal Fluorides' (Glenn, 1981) and again 1 year later (Glenn, Glenn and Duncan, 1982). The caries status of 492 children were reported: 97% of the 117 children who received prenatal fluoride were caries-free, whereas only 15% of the 375 children who did not receive prenatal fluoride were caries-free. Reasons put forward by Glenn for the very much better dental health of children who received prenatal fluoride included higher levels of fluoride in exfoliated primary teeth (enamel and dentine) (Glenn, Glenn and Duncan, 1984a) and improved occlusal surface morphology (Glenn, Glenn and Duncan, 1984b). The recommended dose, according to Glenn and Glenn (1987), for mothers is between 1 and 4 mg F/day, e.g. 2 mg F (4.4 mg NaF) per day, and this should be started by the twelfth week of pregnancy.

The clinical data upon which Frances Glenn based her recommendations have been criticized (Driscoll, 1981; Schrotenboer, 1981; Stookey, 1981; Stamm, 1981). These authors concluded that there was a lack of adequate data upon which to recommend the prenatal use of fluoride dietary supplements, but they agreed that properly controlled clinical studies should be undertaken. At present most countries permit, but do not encourage, prenatal fluoride supplementation. A government sponsored trial of prenatal fluoride supplementation is currently in progress in the USA.

Fluoride–vitamin combination

Vitamin and fluoride supplementation has been combined in some preparations sold in the USA. This is convenient when both vitamins and fluoride are required. Glenn (1979) suggested that some preparations contain 250 mg of calcium and that there was a danger that this might inactivate the fluoride. However, examination of the results of trials listed in Tables 8.1 and 8.2 seem to show that the effectiveness of fluoride drops/tablets is neither enhanced nor reduced by their combination with vitamins and minerals: Stookey (1981) came to the same conclusion. They are not at present marketed in the UK.

Type of fluoride compound

The results of the three trials testing CaF_2 compounds are very variable (0–70% reduction); all were short-term trials. The impressive result of Krusic (1960) is surprising, since the insolubility of CaF_2 would obviate the likelihood of a topical effect compared with NaF, and a systemic effect would be very unlikely to occur in this short trial in 8–15-year-old children.

From the three trials in which APF compounds were used, the effectiveness would appear to be no greater than that observed in the larger number of NaF trials. APF tablets are considerably more expensive than NaF tablets (Driscoll *et al.*, 1978), and the greater salivary flow caused by the low pH of the APF tablets is likely to reduce the concentration of fluoride around the teeth and hasten its clearance from the mouth. It would appear that to ensure high and long-lasting salivary F levels, tablets should contain NaF rather than APF, disintegrate slowly in the mouth without being sucked, and possess as little flavour as possible, so long as the tablets are acceptable to children (McCall, Stephen and McNee, 1981).

Although it is desirable that fluoride tablets dissolve slowly so that teeth are bathed in high levels of fluoride for a long time, it is important to appreciate that saliva does not flow extensively around the mouth. Weatherell *et al.* (1984) and Primosch, Weatherell and Strong (1986) have shown clearly that fluoride released from a tablet tends to remain highly concentrated at the site of tablet dissolution. There was very little mixing between the sides of the mouth or between vestibules of upper and lower arches. It would seem important, therefore, that the position of tablets in the mouth is changed regularly (Dawes and Weatherell, 1990).

Dosage and effectiveness

Hennon, Stookey and Beiswanger (1977) have conducted the only study in which the effect of varying the daily dosage level has been investigated in deciduous teeth. One group of children received 0.5 mg F from soon after birth onwards, while a second group received 0.5 mg F up to 3 years of age and 1 mg F after the age of 3 years. The effect was slightly greater in the latter group (47% reduction compared with 37% reduction) after 5 years, but the difference between these two test groups was not statistically significant and not observed consistently at all ages. The authors attribute this lack of difference partly to the fact that the subjects lived in an area with moderate (0.6–0.8 ppm F) water fluoride levels.

Driscoll *et al.* (1974, 1977, 1978) conducted a carefully controlled trial in which subjects, initially aged 6½ years, were randomly divided into 2 test groups and 1 control group. One test group chewed and swallowed 1 tablet (containing 1 mg F as APF), while the second group chewed and swallowed 2 such tablets, taking the first in morning school and the second in afternoon school. After 6 years there was no difference in the preventive effect between the groups of children taking 1 or 2 tablets (28% and 29% reduction, respectively). The caries-preventive effect did not diminish, in either of the test groups, 1½ years after the tablet programme ended

(Driscoll, Heifetz and Brunelle, 1979). Benefits still persisted 4 years after the tablet programme ended, but to a lesser degree (Driscoll *et al.*, 1981).

Effectiveness of fluoride tablets compared with other methods

Poulsen, Gradegaard and Mortensen (1981) compared the effectiveness of the daily use of a 1 mg F tablet and the fortnightly rinsing with 0.2% NaF in a school-based programme in Denmark. The results (Table 8.3) indicated that caries increments were lower in the rinsing group than in the tablet group. This difference was seen in both age groups and was statistically significant in teeth erupted at baseline, but not in teeth erupting during the study. Holm *et al.* (1975) found no statistically significant difference in 2-year caries increments between a group of children who received fluoride tablets (0.42 mg F/day) and a group who rinsed fortnightly with 0.2% NaF, although there was a statistically non-significant trend towards lower caries increment in the rinsing group.

Table 8.3 Comparison of the effectiveness of daily use of 1 mg F tablets in school and fortnightly rinsing with 0.2% NaF in school. Three-year mean DMFS data are given for children initially aged 7 years and for children initially aged 11 years (From Poulsen, Gradegaard and Mortensen, 1981)

Age at baseline (yr)	*Group*	*N*	*Teeth erupted at baseline* Mean (s.d.) DMFS	*Teeth erupting during the study* Mean (s.d.) DMFS
7	Tablets	124	1.65 (2.10)	0.30 (0.86)
	Rinses	125	1.09 (1.73)	0.22 (0.58)
11	Tablets	129	1.65 (2.52)	1.48 (1.68)
	Rinses	121	1.55 (2.79)	1.17 (1.58)

Rather contrary results were reported by Heifetz *et al.* (1987). Two-year interim results from this American trial on children initially aged 5–6 years indicated that 331 children who received a 1 mg F tablet each school day developed an average of 2.06 dmfs, which was less than the average of 2.50 dmfs recorded for the 345 children who rinsed weekly in school with 0.2% NaF. The difference was not statistically significant.

Summary of effectiveness of fluoride tablets and drops

From the results of published trials (Tables 8.1 and 8.2) it would seem that there is no doubt that the use of fluoride tablets or drops is effective in preventing dental caries in both the deciduous and permanent dentitions. The effectiveness would seem to be greater the earlier the child begins to take the fluoride supplement – from 40% to 80% reduction being expected in both deciduous and permanent dentitions if supplementation is commenced before 2 years of age. For school-based schemes the effectiveness would appear to be slightly lower and more variable (30–80% reduction) but still substantial. NaF would appear to be the compound of choice. There have been only two trials investigating whether the size of the daily dose influences effectiveness. There was a hint of a positive dose-response relationship in pre-school children but not in school children.

Results of the home-based trials have to be interpreted with caution, for the attitude to dental health of the mothers who gave their children supplements from birth is likely to be more favourable than mothers who began supplementation later or who formed the control group. Previous reviewers of the effectiveness of fluoride tablets have commented upon this problem of interpretation of results (Driscoll, 1981), and the following three studies are relevant.

At the simplest level, Andersson and Grahnén (1976) observed that the percentage caries reduction recorded after use of fluoride tablets was not affected by differences in social class between the test and control group. In a more thorough study, Granath *et al.* (1978) found that two factors – diet and oral hygiene – were important in interpreting such clinical trials. They found that 4-year-old children who had taken fluoride tablets for at least 2 years had 69% less approximal caries and 57% less buccal and lingual caries than children who had not taken tablets. However, when the variables of diet and oral hygiene were kept constant in the analyses, these caries reductions were reduced to 51% and 46%, respectively. In the third study, Tijmistra, Brinkman-Engels and Groeneveld (1978) found that the difference in caries experience of 15-year-old children who had or had not taken fluoride tablets fell from 15% to 3% when the data were standardized on diet, oral hygiene and father's occupation.

It has to be admitted that daily administration of tablets at home from birth (or prenatally) requires a very high level of parental motivation, and campaigns to get parents to give their children fluoride supplements have not been successful in many countries. These practical aspects of encouraging the use of fluoride dietary supplements will be discussed further in Chapter 19.

Discussion of the dosage of fluoride tablets and drops

At least 18 different dosage regimens for fluoride tablets and drops have been published. These range from the high dosage level recommended before 1976 in Australia of 0.5 mg F daily from birth to 12 months and 1.0 mg F from 1 year onwards (McEniery and Davies, 1979), to the low dosage level in Denmark since 1978 of 0.25 mg F from 6 to 24 months and 0.5 mg F from 2 years onwards (Thylstrup *et al.*, 1979). The recommended dosage regimen in Sweden is similar to the Danish schedule, except that the change from 0.25 to 0.5 mg F/day occurs at the age of 18 months (Widenheim, 1985). In the UK, the dosage regimen used to be 0.5 mg F from birth to 2 years and 1 mg F from 2 years onwards (Silverstone, 1973; Murray, 1976), but in recent years there has been a trend to reduce the dosage of daily fluoride supplements in many countries.

In the UK, the current recommended dosage is 0.25 mg F from 6 months to 2 years, 0.5 mg F from 2 to 4 years and 1.0 mg F over 4 years. The schedule given in Table 8.4 is the same as that proposed by Dowell and Joyston-Bechal (1981), except that the commencement of fluoride supplementation is now delayed until 6 months of age. The schedule given in the British National Formulary (1990) does not give an upper age limit for fluoride supplementation and there is really no reason to stop or avoid supplementation in adulthood. Most regimens give sliding scales of dosages depending upon water fluoride levels (British Association for the Study of Community Dentistry, 1988; Health Education Authority, 1989; British National Formulary, 1990). Since there is considerable disagreement between countries on the recommended dosage levels, it is pertinent to discuss the reasons for changes in dosage schedules.

Table 8.4 Fluoride supplements – age-related dosages (mg F/day) (From British Association for the Study of Community Dentistry, 1988)

Age	*Concentration of fluoride in drinking water (ppm F)*		
	<0.3	*0.3–0.7*	*>0.7*
6 mo to 2 yr	0.25	0	0
2–4 yr	0.50	0.25	0
4–16 yr	1.00	0.50	0

The objective of any systemic fluoride administration is to obtain the maximum caries-preventive effect with a low risk of unacceptable enamel mottling. As far as water fluoridation is concerned this is achieved, in temperate climates, where drinking water contains 1 ppm F. In the past, fluoride tablet dosages have been calculated in an attempt to duplicate the fluoride intake which occurs in people receiving optimally fluoridated drinking water.

In this respect, it is necessary to make two comments. Arnold, McClure and White (1960) estimated that the fluoride intake from public water supplies containing 1 ppm F was about 1 mg F/day in children over the age of 3 years and between 0.4 and 0.6 mg F/day in children less than 3 years. It is important to realize, however, that these were estimates (of older children drinking a litre of water per day) based on calculations published by McClure (1943), who in turn used figures of Adolph (1933), and were not based on epidemiological data. A review of the literature, covering the past 40 years, of water consumption by children, revealed that children drink considerably less (about 60–70% less) water from public supplies than previously assumed (Rugg-Gunn *et al.*, 1987). Thus, the earlier estimates that children over 3 years ingest 1 mg F/day from water were almost certainly too high.

The second point is that fluoride from tablets is ingested and absorbed at one time of day and this is physiologically different from ingestion of fluoride from water where absorption is spread throughout the day. Animal experiments have shown that fluoride given once a day is more likely to cause fluorosis than the same amount of fluoride given intermittently throughout the day (Angmar-Mänsson, Ericsson and Ekberg, 1976) but it is unclear whether this applies to man (see Chapter 16). Because of these points, the balance between dosage of fluoride tablets and the occurrence of dental fluorosis needs to be continually reassessed and considered separately from water-borne fluorides. Further aspects of fluorosis will be discussed in Chapter 13.

Some authorities, because they consider that an increase in fluoride tablet dosage is likely to lead to greater caries prevention, recommend higher dosages for special groups (such as the medically or mentally handicapped). Some flexibility, therefore, in the dosage of fluoride tablets prescribed should be accepted.

References

Aasenden, R. and Peebles, T. C. (1974) Effects of fluoride supplementation from birth on human deciduous and permanent teeth. *Arch. Oral Biol.*, **19**, 321–326

Aasenden, R. and Peebles, T. C. (1978) Effects of fluoride supplementation from birth on dental caries and fluorosis in teen-aged children. *Arch. Oral Biol.*, **23**, 111–115

Aasenden, R., De Paola, P. F. and Brudevold, F. (1972) Effects of daily rinsing and ingestion of fluoride solutions upon dental caries and enamel fluoride. *Arch. Oral Biol.*, **17**, 1705–1714

Adolph, E. F. (1933) The metabolism and distribution of water in body and tissues. *Physiol. Rev.*, **13**, 336–371

Allmark, C., Green, H. P., Linney, A. D., Wills, D. J. and Picton, D. C. A. (1982) A community study of fluoride tablets for school children in Portsmouth. *Br. Dent. J.*, **153**, 426–430

Andersson, R. and Grahnén, H. (1976) Fluoride tablets in pre-school age – effect on primary and permanent teeth. *Swed. Dent. J.*, **69**, 137–143

Angmar-Mänsson, B., Ericsson, Y. and Ekberg, O. (1976) Plasma fluoride and enamel fluorosis. *Calcif. Tissue Res.*, **22**, 77–84

Angmar-Mansson, B. and Whitford, G. M. (1982) Plasma fluoride levels and enamel fluorosis in the rat. *Caries Res.*, **16**, 334–339

Arnold, F. A., McClure, F. J. and White, C. L. (1960) Sodium fluoride tablets for children. *Dent. Prog.*, **1**, 8–12

Berner, L., Fernex, E. and Held, A. J. (1967) Study on the anticarious effect of sodium fluoride tablets (Zymafluor). Results recorded in the course of 13 years of observation. *Schweiz. Monatsschr. Zahnheilkd.*, **77**, 528–539

Bibby, G. G., Wilkins, E. and Witol, E. (1955) A preliminary study of the effects of fluoride lozenges and pills on dental caries. *O. Surg. O. Med. O. Pathol.*, **8**, 213–216

Binder, K. (1974) In *Cost and Benefit of Fluoride in the Prevention of Dental Caries* (ed. G. N. Davis), WHO Offset Publication No. 9, WHO, Geneva, p. 64, Table 23

Binder, K., Driscoll, W. S. and Schützmannsky, G. (1978) Caries-preventive fluoride tablet programs. *Caries Res.*, **12**, suppl. 1, 22–30

British Association for the Study of Community Dentistry (1988) The home use of fluorides for pre-school children. A policy statement. BASCD, Cardiff

British National Formulary (1990) *British National Formulary No. 19: 1990–92*, Section 9.5, British Medical Association, London

Dawes, C. and Weatherell, J. A. (1990) Kinetics of fluoride in the oral fluids. *J. Dent. Res.*, **69** (spec. iss.), 638–644

De Paola, P. F. and Lax, M. (1968) The caries-inhibiting effect of acidulated phosphate-fluoride chewable tablets: a two-year double-blind study. *J. Am. Dent. Assoc.*, **76**, 554–557

Dowell, T. B. and Joyston-Bechal, S. (1981) Fluoride supplements – age related dosages. *Br. Dent. J.*, **150**, 273–275

Driscoll, W. S. (1974) The use of fluoride tablets for the prevention of dental caries. In *International Workshop on Fluorides and Dental Caries Prevention* (eds D. J. Forrester and E. M. Schulz), University of Maryland, Baltimore, pp. 25–111

Driscoll, W. S. (1981) A review of clinical research on the use of prenatal fluoride administration for prevention of dental caries. *J. Dent. Child.*, **48**, 109–117

Driscoll, W. S., Heifetz, S. B. and Brunelle, J. A. (1979) Treatment and post-treatment effects of chewable fluoride tablets on dental caries: findings after 7½ years. *J. Am. Dent. Assoc.*, **99**, 817–821

Driscoll, W. S., Heifetz, S. B. and Brunelle, J. A. (1981) Caries-preventive effects of fluoride tablets in schoolchildren four years after discontinuation of treatments. *J. Am. Dent. Assoc.*, **103**, 878–881

Driscoll, W. S., Heifetz, S. B. and Korts, D. C. (1974) Effects of acidulated phosphate-fluoride chewable tablets on dental caries in school children: results after 30 months. *J. Am. Dent. Assoc.*, **89**, 115–120

Driscoll, W. S., Heifetz, S. B. and Korts, D. C. (1978) Effect of chewable fluoride tablets on dental caries in schoolchildren: results after six years of use. *J. Am. Dent. Assoc.*, **97**, 820–824

Driscoll, W. S., Heifetz, S. B., Korts, D. C., Meyers, R. J. and Horowitz, H. S. (1977) Effect of acidulated phosphate-fluoride chewable tablets in schoolchildren: results after 55 months. *J. Am. Dent. Assoc.*, **94**, 537–543

Driscoll, W. S. and Horowitz, H. S. (1978) A discussion of optimal dosage for dietary fluoride supplementation. *J. Am. Dent. Assoc.*, **96**, 1050–1053

Fanning, E. A., Cellier, K. M. and Leadbeater, M. M. (1975) South Australian kindergarten children: fluoride tablet supplements and dental caries. *Aust. Dent. J.*, **20**, 7–9

Feltman, R. and Kosel, G. (1961) Prenatal and postnatal ingestion of fluorides – fourteen years of investigation – final report. *J. Dent. Med.*, **16**, 190–198

Girardi-Vogt, J. (1968) Results of fluoridation in Darmstadt. *Dissertation*, Johan Wolfgang Goethe University, Frankfurt, Germany, p. 127

Glenn, F. B. (1979) Immunity conveyed by sodium-fluoride supplement during pregnancy: part II. *J. Dent. Child.*, **46**, 17–24

Glenn, F. B. (1981) The rationale for the administration of a NaF tablet supplement during pregnancy and postnatally in a private practice setting. *J. Dent. Child.*, **48**, 118–122

Glenn, F. B. and Glenn, W. D. (1987) Optimum dosage for prenatal fluoride supplementation (PNF): part IX. *J. Dent. Child.*, **54**, 445–450

Glenn, F. B., Glenn, W. D. and Duncan, R. C. (1982) Fluoride tablet supplementation during pregnancy for caries immunity: a study of the offspring produced. *Am. J. Obstet. Gynecol.*, **143**, 560–564

Glenn, F. B., Glenn, W. D. and Duncan, R. C. (1984a) Prenatal fluoride tablet supplementation and the fluoride content of teeth: part VII. *J. Dent. Child.*, **51**, 344–351

Glenn, F. B., Glenn, W. D. and Duncan, R. C. (1984b) Prenatal fluoride tablet supplementation and improved molar occlusal morphology: part V. *J. Dent. Child.*, **51**, 19–23

Granath, L.-E., Rootzen, H., Liljegren, E., Holst, K. and Kohler, L. (1978) Variation in caries prevalence related to combinations of dietary and oral hygiene habits and chewing fluoride tablets in 4-year-old children. *Caries Res.*, **12**, 83–92

Grissom, D. K., Dudenbostel, R. E., Cassel, W. J. and Murray, R. T. (1964) A comparative study of systemic sodium fluoride and topical stannous fluoride applications in preventive dentistry. *J. Dent. Child.*, **31**, 314–322

Hamberg, L. (1971) Controlled trial of fluoride in vitamin drops for prevention of caries in children. *Lancet*, **1**, 441–442

Health Education Authority (1989) *The Scientific Basis of Dental Health Education. A Policy Document*, 3rd edn, HEA, London

Heifetz, S. B., Horowitz, H. S., Meyers, R. J. and Li, S.-H. (1987) Evaluation of the comparative effectiveness of fluoride mouthrinsing, fluoride tablets, and both procedures in combination: interim findings after two years. *Pediatric. Dent.*, **9**, 121–125

Hennon, D. K., Stookey, G. K. and Beiswanger, B. B. (1977) Fluoride–vitamin supplements: effects on dental caries and fluorosis when used in areas with suboptimum fluoride in the water supply. *J. Am. Dent. Assoc.*, **95**, 965–971

Hennon, D. K., Stookey, G. K. and Muhler, J. C. (1966) The clinical anti-cariogenic effectiveness of supplementary fluoride-vitamin preparations. Results at the end of three years. *J. Dent. Child.*, **33**, 3–12

Hennon, D. K., Stookey, G. K. and Muhler, J. C. (1967) The clinical anti-cariogenic effectiveness of supplementary fluoride-vitamin preparations. Results at the end of four years. *J. Dent. Child.*, **34**, 439–443

Hennon, D. K., Stookey, G. K. and Muhler, J. C. (1970) The clinical anti-cariogenic effectiveness of supplementary fluoride-vitamin preparations. Results at the end of five and a half years. *J. Pharmacol. Ther. Dent.*, **1**, 1–6

Hippchen, P. (1965) Caries prevention with fluorides in Düsseldorf children. *Zahnaerztl. Mitt.*, **55**, 897–898

Holm, G. B., Holst, J., Koch, G. and Widenheim, J. (1975) Fluoridsugtablett, nytt hjalpmedel: kariesprofylaktiken. *Tandlakartidningen*, **64**, 354–461

Hoskova, M. (1968) Fluoride tablets in the prevention of tooth decay. *Cesk. Pediatr.*, **23**, 438–441

Jez, M. (1962) Izledki mnozicne fluorizacije zobovja solske mladine. *Zobozdrav. Vest.*, **17**, 113–118

Kailis, D. G., Taylor, S. R., Davis, G. B., Bartlett, L. G., Fitzgerald, D. J., Grose, I. J. and Newton, P. D. (1968) Fluoride and caries: observations on the effects of prenatal and postnatal fluoride on some Perth pre-school children. *Med. J. Aust.*, **11**, 1037–1040

Kamocka, D., Sebastyanska, Z. and Spychalska, M. (1964) The effect of administration of 'Fluodar' tablets on the appearance of caries in children of pre-school age in Szczecin. *Czas. Stomatol.*, **17**, 299–303

Kraemer, O. (1971) Results of two years of dental caries prophylaxis by oral administration of fluoride in Bonn kindergartens. *Dissertation*, Rheinische Friedrich Wilhelm University, Bonn, West Germany

Krusic, V. (1960) Our tests in fluoridation with the calcium fluoride 'Fluokalcia' (CaF_2). *Zobozdrav. Vest.*, **15**, 27–31

Krychalska-Karwan, Z. and Laskowa, L. (1963) Use of fluoride tablets in Polish children. *Czas. Stomatol.*, **16**, 201–205

LeGeros, R. Z., Glenn, F. B., Lee, D. D. and Glenn, W. D. (1985) Some physicochemical properties of deciduous enamel of children with and without pre-natal fluoride supplementation (PNF). *J. Dent. Res.*, **64**, 465–469

Leonhardt, H. (1964) Results of fluorine tablet applications in Salzburg school children. In *Advances in Fluorine Research and Dental Caries Prevention*, Vol. 2 (eds J. L. Hardwick, J. P. Dustin and H. R. Held), Pergamon, Oxford, pp. 49–56

Leonhardt, H. (1965) Mulgatum and Mulgatum-Fluoratum in preschool children. *Therapie der Gegenwart,* **104**, 118–133

Lutomska, K. and Kominska, D. (1962) Effect of fluoride tablets. *Czas. Stomatol.*, **15**, 493–501

McCall, D., Stephen, K. W. and McNee, S. G. (1981) Fluoride tablets and salivary fluoride levels. *Caries Res.*, **15**, 98–102

McClure, F. J. (1943) Ingestion of fluoride and dental caries. *Am. J. Dis. Child.*, **66**, 362–369

McEniery, M. and Davies, G. N. (1979) Brisbane dental survey 1977: a comparative study of caries experience of children in Brisbane, Australia over a 20 year period. *Community Dent. Oral Epidemiol.*, **7**, 42–50

Margolis, F. J., Reames, H. R., Freshman, E., Macauley, J. C. and Mehaffey, H. (1975) Fluoride – ten year prospective study of deciduous and permanent dentition. *Am. J. Dis. Child.*, **129**, 794–800

Marthaler, T. M. (1969) Caries-inhibiting effect of fluoride tablets. *Helv. Odontol. Acta,* **13**, 1–13

Minoguchi, G., Ono, T. and Tamai, S. (1963) Prophylactic application of fluoride for dental caries in Japan. *Int. Dent. J.*, **13**, 510–515

Murray, J. J. (1976) *Fluorides in Caries Prevention*, 1st edn, Wright, Bristol

Niedenthal, A. (1957) Caries prophylaxis with sodium fluoride tablets in Offenbach school children. *Zahnaerzto. Mitt.*, **45**, 576–587

O'Rourke, C., Attrill, M. and Holloway, P. J. (1988) Cost appraisal of a fluoride tablet programme to Manchester primary school-children. *Community Dent. Oral Epidemiol.*, **16,** 341–344

Plasschaert, A. J. M. and Konig, K. G. (1974) The effect of information and motivation towards dental health and of fluoride tablets on caries in school children: 1. Increment over the initial 2-year experimental period. *Int. Dent. J.*, **24**, 50–65

Pollak, H. (1960) Caries prophylaxis with Mulgatum F. Result of an investigation over a period of two years in Nordheim-Westphalia. *Dtsch. Zahnaerzteble.*, **14**, 363–365

Poulsen, S., Gradegaard, E. and Mortensen, B. (1981) Cariostatic effect of daily use of a fluoride-containing lozenge compared to fortnightly rinses with 0.2% sodium fluoride. *Caries Res.*, **15**, 236–242

Prichard, J. L. (1969) The prenatal and postnatal effects of fluoride supplements on West Australian school children, aged 6, 7 and 8, Perth, 1967. *Aust. Dent. J.*, **14,** 335–338

Primosch, R. E., Weatherell, J. A. and Strong, M. (1986) Distribution and retention of salivary fluoride from a sodium fluoride tablet following various intra-oral dissolution methods. *J. Dent. Res.*, **65**, 1001–1005

Rugg-Gunn, A. J., Hackett, A. F., Appleton, D. R., Eastoe, J. E., Dowthwaite, L. and Wright, W. G. (1987) The water intake of 405 Northumbrian adolescents aged 12–14 years. *Br. Dent. J.*, **162**, 335–340

Schrotenboer, G. (1981) Perspectives on the use of prenatal fluorides: a reactor's comments. *J. Dent. Child.*, **48**, 123–125

Schützmannsky, G. (1965) Further results of our tablet fluoridation in Halle. *Dtsch. Stomatol.*, **15**, 107–114

Schützmannsky, G. (1971) Fluorine tablet application in pregnant females. *Dtsch. Stomatol.*, **21**, 122–129

Silverstone, L. M. (1973) Preventive dentistry: systemic fluoride part 2. *Dental Update,* **1**, 101–105

Stamm, J. W. (1981) Perspectives on the use of prenatal fluorides: a reactor's comments. *J. Dent. Child.*, **48**, 128–133

Stephen, K. W. and Campbell, D. (1978) Caries reduction and cost benefit after 3 years of sucking fluoride tablets daily at school. *Br. Dent. J.*, **144**, 202–206

Stolte, G. (1968) Results of three years of caries prophylaxis by oral fluoride application in Solingen kindergartens. *Zahnaerztl. Mitt.*, **58**, 380–382

Stones, H. H., Lawton, F. E., Bransby, E. R. and Hartley, H. O. (1949) The effect of topical applications of potassium fluoride and of the ingestion of tablets containing sodium fluoride on the incidence of dental caries. *Br. Dent. J.*, **86**, 264–271

Stookey, G. K. (1981) Perspectives on the use of prenatal fluorides: a reactor's comments. *J. Dent. Child.*, **48**, 126–127

Thylstrup, A., Fejerskov, O., Brunn, C. and Kann, J. (1979) Enamel changes and dental caries in 7-year-old children given fluoride tablets from shortly after birth. *Caries Res.*, **13**, 265–276

Tijmistra, T., Brinkman-Engels, M. and Groeneveld, A. (1978) Effect of socioeconomic factors on the observed caries reduction after fluoride tablet and fluoride toothpaste consumption. *Community Dent. Oral Epidemiol.*, **6**, 227–230

Weatherell, J. A., Robinson, C., Ralph, J. P. and Best, J. S. (1984) Migration of fluoride in the mouth. *Caries Res.*, **18**, 348–353

Widenheim, J. (1985) On fluoride tablets: a retrospective study of intake pattern and the pre-eruptive effect on occurrence of caries, restorations and fluorosis in teeth. *Thesis*, University of Lund, Malmo

Wrzodek, G. (1959) Does the prevention of caries by means of fluorine tablets promise success? *Zahnaerztl. Mitt.*, **47**, 1–5

Ziemnowicz-Glowaka, W. (1960) Prevention of caries by means of 'Fluodar' tablets. *Czas. Stomatol.*, **13**, 719–728

Chapter 9

Fluoride toothpastes and dental caries

Investigations into the effectiveness of adding fluoride to toothpaste have been carried out since 1945, and cover a wide range of active ingredients in various chemical combinations. There have probably been more reports in the literature on the caries-inhibitory property of fluoride in toothpaste than on any other aspect of topical fluoride therapy. Fluoride compounds which have been tested for caries-inhibitory properties when incorporated into a toothpaste include: sodium fluoride, acidulated phosphate fluoride, stannous fluoride, sodium monofluorophosphate and amine fluoride.

In the UK, a dramatic change in the use of a fluoride toothpaste took place in the 1970s, largely as a result of decisions made by manufacturers to improve their product. Before 1970 less than 10% of branded toothpastes contained fluoride; now over 96% of all toothpaste sold contains fluoride (Figure 9.1). In 1975, the British Dental Association endorsed a number of fluoride toothpastes which, on the basis of clinical trials, had been shown to be effective in reducing dental decay.

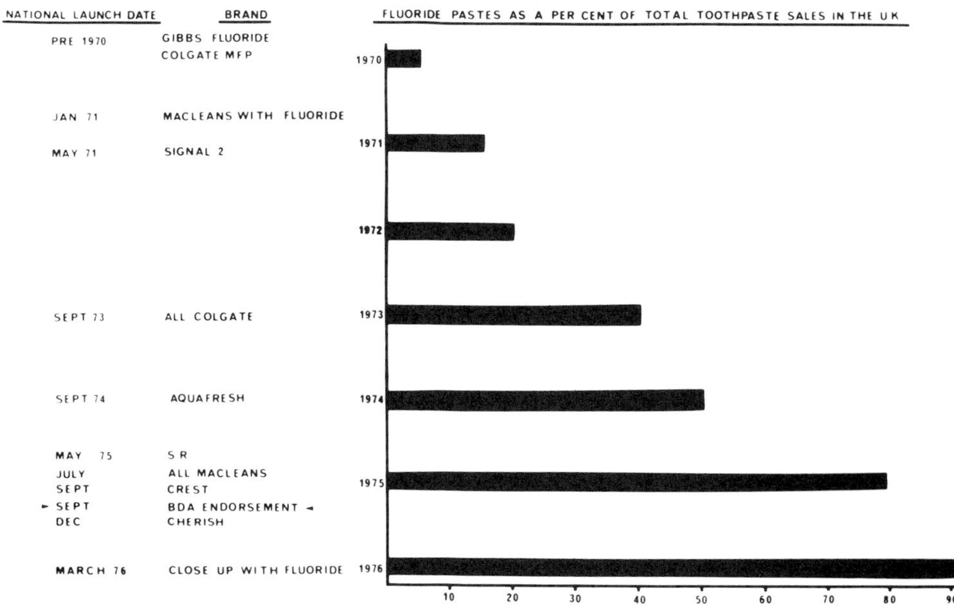

Figure 9.1 Sales of fluoride toothpaste in the UK, 1970–76

Table 9.1 Clinical trials of sodium fluoride dentifrices

Investigators	*% NaF + abrasive*		*Unsupervised (U) or supervised (S) use*	*Duration of trial*	*No. carious surfaces saved per year*	*Reduction in carious surface increment (%)*	*Level of statistical significance*
Bibby (1945)	0.1	$CaCO_3$	S	2 yr	–	–	–
	0.1	$CaCO_3$	U	2 yr	–	–	–
Winkler *et al*. (1953)	0.15	$CaCO_3$	S	18 mo	–	–	–
Muhler *et al*. (1955b)	0.22	Heat-treated Ca orthophosphate	U	1 yr	–	–	–
Kyes *et al*. (1961)	0.2	IMP + 5% anhydrous DCP	U	1 yr	–	–	–
Torell and Ericsson (1965)	0.24	$NaHCO_3$	U	2 yr	1–2	–	0.01
Brudevold and Chilton (1966)	0.22	IMP	U	2 yr	–	–	0.01
	0.22	Sec. Ca phosphate					
Peterson and Williamson (1968)	0.22	IMP	U	2 yr	0.6	14	0.05
Koch (1967a)	0.22	Acrylic	S	3 yr	3.2	40–48	0.001
Koch (1967b)	0.22	Acrylic	U	2 yr	2.1	38	0.01
Weisenstein and Zacherl (1972)	0.22	CaPP	U	21 mo	0.7	25	0.05
Zacherl (1972a)	0.22	CaPP	U	20 mo	1.1	28	0.05
Reed (1973)	0.055	CaPP	U	2 yr	0.15	7.5	
	0.11	CaPP	U	2 yr	0.2	8.5	
	0.22	CaPP	U	2 yr	0.4	20.0	0.05
Forsman (1974)	0.05	SiO_2	U	2 yr	0.2*	10–17*	NS
					0.8†	5–48†	NS

Stookey and Beiswanger (1975)	0.22	CaPP	U	27 mo	0.8	25	0.05
Gerdin (1972b)	0.22 (NaF)	Acrylic	S	2 yr			'Test significantly better than control'
	0.24 (KF)	Acrylic	S				
Reed and King (1975)	0.22	CaPP	U	2 yr	0.65	30	0.05
Edlund and Koch (1977)	0.22	SiO_2	S	3 yr	0.8	23‡	0.05
Ennever *et al*. (1980)	0.22	CaPP	U	28 mo	0.60	37	0.05
	0.22	CaPP (pH10)			0.53	34	0.05
Zacherl (1981)	0.24	SiO_2	U	3 yr	0.82	41	0.05
					(0.35§)	23§	
Beiswanger and Gish (1981)	0.24	SiO_2	U	3 yr	(0.22†)	15§	0.05
Koch *et al*. (1982)	0.1	?	U	3 yr			Positive control
	0.025	?	U	3 yr			Positive control
Lu *et al*. (1987)	0.24	SiO_2	U	3 yr			Positive control
	0.56	SiO_2	U	3 yr		11.8	0.05
Blinkhorn and Kay (1988)	0.32	SiO_2	U	3 yr		No difference between NaF, MFP, and mixed system	
Beiswanger *et al*. (1989)	0.24	SiO_2	U	3 yr	0.2	12‡	0.04

IMP, Insoluble metaphosphate; DCP, Dicalcium phosphate.

* Clinical examination.
† Radiographic examination.
‡ Versus MFP positive control. Placebo not included.
§ Against SnF_2 positive control.

Pastes receiving this 'seal of approval' were Colgate, Crest, Macleans and Signal 2. However, following attempts to involve the British Dental Association (BDA) in competing claims within the dentrifice industry, the BDA has now withdrawn its endorsement, on the grounds that its objective of bringing the advantages of fluoride toothpaste to the notice of the public has been largely achieved (*BDA News*, 1981).

Toothpastes containing sodium fluoride (Table 9.1)

Sodium fluoride was the first fluoride compound to be incorporated in a conventional toothpaste as the active agent. A 2-year study investigating the unsupervised use of such a paste was published by Bibby in 1945. The active ingredient was 0.1% sodium fluoride, but the nature of the abrasive system was not published. It seems reasonable to assume it was of a type used in conventional toothpastes commercially available at that time, probably calcium carbonate. Bibby found no significant reduction in caries increment for the test group using the sodium fluoride paste, in comparison to the use of a placebo paste by a control group. The significance of the study is doubtful in view of the small numbers in the groups, and the wide age range of the study participants. Winkler, Backer Dirks and Van Amerogen (1953), in spite of changing the test formulation, found no significant benefit for supervised use of a 0.15% sodium fluoride paste for 18 months.

Investigations testing the unsupervised use of a paste containing 0.2% sodium fluoride were published introducing alternative abrasive systems. Muhler *et al.* (1955b) investigated a combination of 0.2% sodium fluoride and heat-treated calcium orthophosphate, finding a reduction in caries increment of only 0.3 of a surface for the test group over the 12-month study period. The reduction was neither clinically nor statistically significant.

Kyes, Overton and McKean (1961), using a combination of 0.2% sodium fluoride and 2% sodium N-lauroyl sarcosinate, explored the possibility of using an insoluble sodium metaphosphate abrasive system, but found no significant clinical benefit. Brudevold and Chilton (1966) investigated relative caries-preventive effects for several toothpaste formulas covering a range of active ingredients, including 0.22% sodium fluoride–dicalcium phosphate formula. Two years of unsupervised use gave no statistically significant caries reduction in the test group compared to a control group using a placebo. Thus the early studies tended to suggest that sodium fluoride did not have a caries-preventive effect when incorporated in a toothpaste.

However, in 1961 Ericsson investigated the compatibility of fluoride compounds with conventional constituents of toothpaste and reported that the abrasive systems of calcium carbonate and phosphate inactivate the sodium fluoride by formation of calcium fluoride. He recommended sodium bicarbonate as a compatible abrasive system for sodium fluoride. Subsequently a clinical investigation by Torell and Ericsson (1965) tested the unsupervised use of 0.2% sodium fluoride–sodium bicarbonate formulation and found a cumulative caries reduction of one surface per child for 2 years for the study group.

The clinical value of the abrasive property of a toothpaste is a controversial question. In 1967, Koch published results of a study testing a toothpaste formulation containing 0.22% sodium fluoride, but without a conventional inorganic abrasive. He substituted acrylic particles which are low in abrasivity but allow a maximum of free ionized fluoride, his assumption being that in relation to oral cleanliness, the thoroughness with which one brushes is more relevant than the physical composition of the abrasive. The paste was tested for 3 years of once-a-day brushing at school under supervision. Study participants and their immediate families were supplied with non-fluoridated paste to use at home, to eliminate the possible use of commercial fluoride pastes during the study period. The comparability of the groups initially was good, and the number of reversals of diagnoses recorded was small, and comparable for test and control groups. The cumulative reduction in new carious surfaces for the test groups represented a saving of 7 surfaces per child for the younger group and a saving of 10 surfaces for the older age group. The observed caries reductions in the test groups, as compared to the control groups, were highly significant ($P < 0.001$). The inhibitory effect was sustained over the study period, and increased in magnitude with successive years, until, in the third year, the reduction in new carious surfaces for the test groups was of the order of 50–58% ($P < 0.001$). There was no statistical significance in the difference in caries increments observed between the sexes. The largest relative reduction was noted for the buccal surfaces.

When this trial ended in 1966, a follow-up was organized for 57 children in the younger age study group, to attempt to evaluate the long-term prophylactic effect of 3 years' daily supervised tooth-brushing with a fluoride paste. For the 2-year period immeidately after the study had finished there was a 13% reduction in caries increment for the group who had used the fluoride paste, relative to the control group (Koch, 1970). The reduction in 2 years of 1–2 surfaces per child for the test group was not statistically significant and indicated little long-term practical protection attributable to 3 years' use of a sodium fluoride paste, once regular use of the paste had ceased. This is one of the very few studies reported in the literature which attempts to evaluate whether there is any long-term benefit achieved with use of a fluoride paste. The results of this study suggest that any caries-inhibitory effect of fluoride toothpastes is reliant on regular and sustained applications.

Two trials (Beiswanger and Gish, 1981; Zacherl, 1981) have reported that a 0.243% sodium fluoride–silica abrasive toothpaste (yielding 1000 ppm F) was superior to a 0.4% stannous fluoride–calcium pyrophosphate toothpaste, also yielding 1000 ppm F and marketed as Crest. It has been suggested that the new formulation maintains a higher fluoride ion concentration and allows a greater uptake of fluoride into the outer layers of enamel (Cilley and Haberman, 1981; Mobley and Tepe, 1981). Developments between 1980 and 1990 are considered on pages 144–153.

Toothpastes containing acidulated phosphate fluoride (Table 9.2)

In search of a more potent fluoride agent for caries prevention, it was postulated that the effectiveness of a topical agent was directly related to its ability to deposit fluoride as fluorapatite in enamel. Brudevold *et al.* (1963), while investigating topical applications of fluoride in solution, showed large amounts of fluoride were deposited from high concentrations at a low pH. Unfortunately calcium fluoride was formed in addition to fluorapatite, and was not retained in the enamel as it was soluble in saliva at neutral pH, and washed away within a few hours (Brudevold *et al.*, 1967).

Grøn and Brudevold (1967) postulated a hypothesis that failure to achieve significant results with original neutral sodium fluoride formulations was related

Table 9.2 Clinical trials of acidulated phosphate fluoride dentifrices

Investigators	*Active ingredient (% conc.)*	*Abrasive system*	*pH*	*Duration* (yr)	*Age* (yr)	*Use*	*Statistically significant reductions in carious surfaces*		
							saved	*% redn*	*P*
Brudevold and Chilton (1966)	0.22% NaF +	IMP	4.8–5.3	2	11–17	U	1–2	*	0.01
Peterson and Williamson (1968)	1.5% soluble	IMP	4.8–5.3	2	9–15	U	1	*	*
Slack *et al.* (1971)	orthophosphate	IMP	*	3	11–12	U	–	–	–
Zacherl (1972b)	0.22% NaF	Calc. pyro.	5.5	1⅔	7–14	U	–	–	–

U, Unsupervised use. * Information not given in paper.

not only to the chemical nature of the abrasive but also to the pH values of the formulations. Reports of successful trials of topical acidulated phosphate fluoride solutions encouraged attempts to incorporate this active ingredient into a toothpaste. Brudevold and Chilton (1966) and Peterson and Williamson (1968) published investigations of 2 years' unsupervised use of a formula containing 0.22% sodium fluoride acidulated with 1.5% soluble orthophosphate. The abrasive system used was insoluble sodium metaphosphate which Ericsson (1961) had found did not reduce the amount of available fluoride in sodium fluoride solutions. In both trials the control group did not use a true placebo but a commercially available fluoride-free dentifrice. Caries-reduction effects observed in the test groups were of a similar order (a saving of 1–2 surfaces for each child for the 2-year period). The reduction effects observed in the test group were statistically significant ($P < 0.01$).

Slack, Bulman and Osborn (1971) conducted a 3-year trial of normal home use of the same paste in 11–12-year-olds. Again, a commercially available fluoride-free toothpaste was used for a control paste, while a second control group carried on with normal toothbrushing habits and pastes. No significant difference was found in caries increment for groups using the acidulated phosphate fluoride formulation compared with those for the two control groups over the 3-year period. From the results of these trials, it was not possible to establish whether insoluble metaphosphate was indeed a more suitable abrasive system in combination with fluoride, as the study lacked a true control paste.

A combination of 0.22% acidulated phosphate fluoride and calcium pyrophosphate was investigated by Zacherl (1972b). After unsupervised home use of the test paste for 20 months there was no significant reduction in caries increment observed in the test group compared to similar use of a placebo dentifrice by the control group. The use of a potentially incompatible abrasive system (established by *in vitro* experiments by Ericsson (1961)) and the wide range in age of the study participants could have served to reduce the significance of Zacherl's results. The majority of study participants were known to have regularly used naturally fluoridated well water (F level of 0.8–1.5 ppm), which could have reduced the magnitude of the observed differences between test and control groups.

The clinical value of using acidulated sodium fluoride as an active agent in fluoride toothpastes has not been conclusively established in these published studies. The only investigation using a calcium pyrophosphate abrasive system did not establish any efficacy of this combination. While inadequacy of study design could have clouded the results, the abrasive system may well have been responsible for reduced activity of the paste. In the trials using an insoluble sodium metaphosphate abrasive system, the paste used by the control group was a commercially available fluoride-free paste. The reductions observed in caries increments for test groups could have been attributable to the fluoride ion activity *per se*, but whether the effect of the paste was enhanced by acidulation remains unestablished from these clinical trials. The magnitude of the clinical reductions observed using the same test formula were of a similar order, that is 1–2 surfaces per child for 2 years. A further point for consideration is the possible effect of regular and sustained use of commercially available fluoride toothpastes by participants before the start of any particular trial. While it is known that 33% of the participants in the Brudevold–Chilton study were previous users of fluoride toothpastes, similar information is not available for the Peterson and Williamson study. Slack, Bulman and Osborn (1971) reported that 10% of the participants had previously used a fluoride paste, but felt that this would have no significant reflection on the results. As very few studies have investigated the duration and magnitude of benefit from routine use of a fluoride paste, the magnitude of this effect on the observed results is not known.

Toothpastes containing stannous fluoride (Table 9.3)

Following the initial negative results achieved in clinical trials testing the efficacy of sodium fluoride as an active toothpaste ingredient, attention was turned to other soluble fluorides for possible caries-inhibitory action. Muhler and his associates at Indiana University, USA, having used stannous fluoride as a topical agent, decided to incorporate this compound into a toothpaste, which was manufactured and marketed under licence with the name of Crest in the USA in 1955.

In formulating a stannous fluoride toothpaste compounded in a watery base, attention had to be paid to the known chemical reactivity and instability of stannous fluoride; in solution, tin and fluoride ions are lost by hydrolysis and oxidation (Hefferen, Zimmerman and Koehler, 1966). If the pH is raised, stannous hydroxide is precipitated and a strong stannous fluoride complex is formed (Torell, Hals and Morch, 1958). The conventional abrasive systems of dentrifices at the time were based on calcium salts. However, the chemical affinity of calcium ions for ionic fluoride in solution results in the formation of relatively insoluble calcium fluoride, although the formation of tin fluoride complexes may minimize this change (Torell, Hals and Morch, 1958). Different formulations were tried out by Muhler and his co-workers; the final formulation produced contained 0.4% stannous fluoride and 1% stannous pyrophosphate, in combination with a calcium pyrophosphate abrasive system, formed by treating calcium orthophosphate.

The initial trials began in 1955 and tested a stannous fluoride toothpaste, without the stannous pyrophosphate. The control toothpaste used was of the same composition, but without the active ingredient, and of a pH close to neutrality. Three trials by Muhler and his associates studied the effectiveness of normal home use of this formulation, two of the trials studying children aged 5–15 years for 1 year (Muhler *et al.*, 1955a,b) and a third involving young adults aged 17–36 years (Muhler and Radike, 1957) for 2 years. Reductions in the increment of caries observed in the groups using the test dentifrice for 1 year (compared with the control group) were of the order of 1–1.5 surfaces per child for the study period. The first trial published gave no indication of measures taken to ensure examiner reliability at the examinations and this is reflected in the number of reversals of diagnoses published. For the final examination, the number of reversals for the test group was two and a half times the number recorded for the control group, and these reversals were included in the results. In the second trial there was a loss of two-thirds of the subjects from the groups during the study period, and although there was comparability between the groups at baseline with respect to initial caries experience, there was a lack of this balance at times of re-examination.

The succeeding trials tested a modified formula, containing 1% stannous pyrophosphate, and corresponded to the marketed formula of Crest. Stannous pyrophosphate was added in an attempt to maintain the level of the stannous ion, the hypothesis being that the anti-caries action of fluoride would be augmented by relatively insoluble precipitates formed in enamel by the cation. Subsequent *in vitro* tests have failed to validate this (Brudevold *et al.*, 1967). The evidence now is that there is no cation effect and fluoride is the effective component.

The new formulation was first investigated by Jordan and Peterson (1959). Supervised brushing once a day with the test dentrifice for 2 years, as well as normal home use of the same, resulted in a reduction in caries increment of one surface in 2 years. Another group of the same age (8–11 years) showed no significant reduction in caries increment for normal home use of the test paste. When brushing was supervised three times a day for 10 months, a caries reduction of one surface per child was observed for the study period. The numbers in the groups were small, and trying to relate the results of this special study with the measure of supervision used to potential reduction benefits in a general population would be unrealistic. Muhler (1960), in a 2-year trial of normal home use of the test dentifrice, observed a reduction benefit of 1.5 surfaces in children aged 6–18 years. The initial effect was maintained with time, the test group showing a relatively stable increment of new DMF surfaces, which was lower than that for the control. The only report of a study of 3 years' duration (Muhler, 1962a) observed a reduction of 2 surfaces per child for 3 years of home use of the stannous fluoride dentifrice.

The original stannous fluoride–calcium pyrophosphate Crest formulation has been tested and marketed in many countries, including the USA, Great Britain, Canada and Australia. A summary of over 40 clinical trials is given in Table 9.3, and all have recorded a reduction in caries increment of 1–49%.

In 1964, the Crest formulation was recognized as a therapeutic toothpaste by the Council of Dental Therapeutics of the American Dental Association and was accorded Grade A status. A number of reports referred to the increased staining observed in test groups brushing with a stannous fluoride dentifrice, compared with controls.

Although the stannous fluoride formulation, marketed as Crest, has been subjected to clinical trials for 25 years, it has now been replaced by a sodium fluoride–silica formulation, marketed as Crest Plus.

Toothpastes containing sodium monofluorophosphate (Table 9.4)

Animal experiments (Zipkin and McClure, 1951) and clinical investigations of topically applied solutions containing sodium monofluorophosphate (Hawes, Sonnes and Brudevold, 1954; Goaz, McElwaine and Biswell, 1966) established a caries-inhibitory effect attributable to this agent. *In vitro* investigations by Ericsson (1963), Grøn, Brudevold and Aasenden (1971) and Ingram (1972) have all estimated the uptake of fluoride by intact enamel surfaces to be less from a monofluorophosphate solution than from one of sodium fluoride. At present there are two schools of thought explaining the caries-inhibitory mechanism of the monofluorophosphate ion. One explanation is that it is essentially a fluoride effect (Ericsson, 1963; Grøn, Brudevold and Aasenden, 1971), but the mechanism of fluoride ion release is disputed between these investigators. Ericsson postulates that the monofluorophosphate is deposited in the crystallite lattice and, in subsequent intracrystallite transposition of the deposited monofluorophosphate and apatite hydroxyl groups, fluoride is released and replaces the hydroxyl group in the lattice to form fluorapatite. Grøn and co-workers feel the fluoride ion is released at the solution–crystal interface and is deposited in fluorapatite in the enamel by exchange with the hydroxyl groups in the crystal lattice. Both investigators found that the fluoride ion was also released to the oral environment

Table 9.3 Clinical trials of stannous fluoride dentifrices

Investigators	*% SnF_2 + abrasive*		*Unsupervised (U) or supervised (S) use*	*Duration of trial*	*No. carious surfaces saved per year*	*Reduction in carious surface increment (%)*	*Level of statistical significance*
Muhler *et al*. (1955a)	0.4	CaPP	U	1 yr	1.48	49	0.0001
Muhler *et al*. (1955b)	0.4	CaPP	U	1 yr	0.87	36	0.013
Muhler and Radike (1957) (Adults)	0.4	CaPP	U	2 yr	0.84	34	0.005
Jordan and Peterson (1959)	0.4	CaPP	U	2 yr	0.28	13	NS
			S	2 yr	0.46	21	0.01
Muhler (1961)	0.4	CaPP	U	3 yr	0.6	63*	0.0001
Kyes *et al*. (1961) (Adults)	0.4	CaPP	U	2 yr	0.18	8	NS
Bixler and Muhler (1962)	0.4	CaPP	U	8 mo	1.8	45	0.006
Muhler (1962a)	0.4	CaPP	U	3 yr	0.41	22	0.0062
Muhler (1960)	0.4	CaPP	S	2 yr	1.2	46	–
Finn and Jamison (1963)	0.4	CaPP	S	2 yr	No true placebo	No true placebo	–
Slack and Martin (1964)	0.4	IMP	U	Planned 3–4 yr		Trial not completed	–
Gish and Muhler (1965)	0.4	CaPP	U	1 yr	1.67–3.46	71‡	0.00001
Torell and Ericsson (1965)	0.4	CaPP	U	2 yr	1.16	22	0.01
Bixler and Muhler (1966)	0.4	CaPP	U	3 yr	0.58	37†	0.00001
					0.97	58‡	0.00001
Brudevold and Chilton (1966)	0.4	IMP	U	2 yr	1.08	25	0.05
	0.4	CaPP		2 yr	0.2	4	NS
Halikis (1966)	0.4	IMP	U	15 mo	1.04	27	0.07
Horowitz *et al*. (1966)	0.4	CaPP	U	3 yr	0.33	17	0.01
	0.4	CaPP	S	3 yr	0.42	21	0.01
Thomas and Jamison (1966)	0.4	CaPP	S	2 yr	N/A	36	0.05
	0.4	IMP				37	

Jackson and Sutcliffe (1967)	0.4	CaPP	U	3 yr	0.32	12	NS
James and Anderson (1967)	0.4	CaPP	U	3 yr	1.22	29	
Muhler *et al.* (1967) (Adults)	0.4	CaPP	U	30 mo	1.0	64‡	0.001
Naylor and Emslie (1967)	0.4	IMP	U	3 yr	0.49	14.5	0.001
Slack *et al.* (1967a)	0.4	CaPP	U	3 yr	0.2	7	NS
Slack *et al.* (1967b)	0.4	IMP, SiO_2	U	3 yr	0.0 Clinical	0	NS
					0.3 Radiological	28	0.01
Fanning *et al.* (1968)	0.4	IMP	U	2 yr	1.28	21	0.001
Frankl and Alman (1968)	0.4	CaPP	U	3 yr	–	No true placebo	NS
Mergele (1968a)	0.4	IMP	S	2 yr	0.3	10	0.05
Mergele (1968b)	0.4	CaPP	U	3 yr	0.25	13	NS
(Water F 1.0 ppm)							
Scola and Ostrom (1968)	0.4	CaPP	U	2 yr	1.13	42†	0.001
(Adults)					1.35	48‡	0.001
Muhler (1970)	0.4	CaPP	U	1 yr	1.18	29	0.05
Zacherl and McPhail (1970)	0.4	CaPP	U	30 mo	1.0–0.76	40–44	0.05
Gish and Muhler (1971)	0.4	CaPP	U	5 yr	0.38	29	0.00078
(F water area)							
Slack *et al.* (1971)	0.4	CaPP	U	3 yr	0.76	18	0.01
	0.4	IMP	U	3 yr	1.0	24	0.01
Zacherl (1972a)	0.4	CaPP	U	20 mo	1.1	28	0.05
Zacherl (1972b)	0.4	CaPP	U	2 yr	0.94	22	0.00037
Zacherl (1973)	0.4	CaPP	U	2 yr	0.75	30	0.05
Beiswanger *et al.* (1978)	0.4	CaPP	U	2 yr	No placebo	No placebo*	0.05
Fogels *et al.* (1979)	0.4	SiO_2	U	3 yr	0.41	15	0.01
	0.4	CaPP	U	3 yr	0.40	15	0.01
Ringelberg *et al.* (1979)	0.4	CaPP	U	30 mo	0.44	18	NS
Lu *et al.* (1980) (Adults)	0.4	CaPP	U	1 yr (continuing)	0.23	33	0.05
Zacherl (1981)	0.4	CaPP	U	3 yr	0.44	23	0.05

* Combined with topical F.
† Combined with prophylactic F.
‡ Combined with prophylactic + topical F.

Table 9.4 Clinical trials of sodium monofluorophosphate dentifrices

Investigators	*% MFP + abrasive*		*Unsupervised (U) or supervised (S) use*	*Duration of trial*	*No. carious surfaces saved per year*	*Reduction in carious surface increment (%)*	*Level of statistical significance*
Finn and Jamison (1963)	0.76	IMP	S	2 yr	0.6	26	0.001
Goaz *et al*. (1963)	6.0	Solution	S	14 mo	0.7	39	0.002
Torell and Ericsson (1965)	0.76	$CaCO_3$	S	2 yr	0.7	25	0.001
Naylor and Emslie (1967)	0.76	DCP + $CaCO_3$	U	3 yr	0.6	18	0.001
Frankl and Alman (1968)	0.76	IMP	U	3 yr	0.6	8	0.05
Fanning *et al*. (1968)	0.70	IMP	U	2 yr	1.2	20	0.001
Mergele (1968a) (Houston)	0.76	IMP	U	3 yr	0.3	17	0.05
Mergele (1968b) (Austin)	0.76	IMP	S	22 mo	0.6	20	0.001
Møller *et al*. (1968)	0.76	IMP + DCP	U	30 mo	1.0	19	0.001
Kinkel and Stolte (1968)	0.76	IMP + silica	U	2 yr	–	33	–
Thomas and Jamison (1970)	0.76	IMP	S	2 yr	0.7	34	0.05
Zacherl (1972a)	0.76	Ca pyrophosphate	U	20 mo	0.9	23	0.05
Kinkel and Raich (1972)			–	2 yr	0.7	30.53	0.001
Hargreaves and Chester (1973)	2.0	Al_2O_3	U	3 yr	1.1	23	0.01
Lind *et al*. (1974)	2.0	Al_2O_3	U	3 yr	0.9	38	0.001
Andlaw and Tucker (1975)	0.76	Al_2O_3	U	3 yr	0.6	19	0.001
Downer *et al*. (1976)	0.76	IMP + APF topical applications	S	3 yr	0.8	31	0.001
Peterson *et al*. (1975)	0.76	$CaCO_3$	S	31 mo	0.2	23	0.05
Mainwaring and Naylor (1978)	0.76	IMP	U	3 yr	0.6	17	0.01
Shiere (1976)	0.76	$CaCO_3$	S	2 yr	0.7	23	0.05

Edlund and Koch (1977)	0.76	$CaPO_4 + CaCO_3$	S	3 yr	No placebo group; NaF: SiO_2-containing dentifrice significantly better		
James *et al*. (1977)	2.0	Al_2O_3	U	3 yr	1.2	30	0.01
Howat *et al*. (1978)	0.76	Silica gel	S	3 yr	0.7	26	0.05
Glass and Shiere (1978)	0.76	$CaCO_3$	U	3 yr	0.7	28	0.01
Naylor and Glass (1979)	0.76 + 0.13% CaGP	$CaCO_3$	U	3 yr	0.9	25	0.01
Hodge *et al*. (1980)	0.76 + 0.1% NaF	Al_2O_3	S	3 yr	0.6	22	0.05
Hodge *et al*. (1980)	0.76 + 0.1% NaF		S	3 yr	0.65	24	0.01
Murray and Shaw (1980)	0.76	Al_2O_3 (Low abrasivity)	U	3 yr	0.6	34	0.001
Murray and Shaw (1980)	0.76	Al_2O_3 (Normal abrasivity)	U	3 yr	0.5	27	0.001
Andlaw *et al*. (1983)	0.8	Al_2O_3 (Low abrasivity)	U	3 yr			Positive control
	0.8	Al_2O_3 (Normal abrasivity)	U	3 yr			Positive control
Mitropoulos *et al*. (1984)	0.76	SiO_2	(S)	32 mo	0.3		0.01
	0.19	SiO_2	(S)				(Positive control)
Stephen *et al*. (1988)	0.76	Al_2O_3	U	3 yr			Positive control
	1.2	Al_2O_3	U	3 yr	0.2		0.05
	2.0	Al_2O_3	U	3 yr	0.4		0.001
Conti *et al*. (1987)	0.76	SiO_2	S	3 yr			Positive control
	1.14	SiO_2	S	3 yr	0.17		0.001
Fogels *et al*. (1988)	0.76	SiO_2	S	3 yr			Positive control
	1.14	SiO_2	S	3 yr	0.1	14	0.05

in significant amounts from monofluorophosphate by hydrolysis due to enzymatic action in plaque and saliva. On the other hand, Ingram (1972) has suggested that the anti-cariogenic activity of this compound is a specific monofluorophosphate effect, the MFP ion being incorporated and remaining intact in the crystal lattice by exchange with the phosphate group in the enamel, and as such, the mechanism was less pH dependent than the fluoride reaction with enamel.

In vitro investigations by Ericsson (1961) found no reduction in free fluoride ion activity when sodium monofluorophosphate was combined with abrasives of chalk and insoluble metaphosphate (IMP) which had previously been reported to be a mechanically suitable abrasive for a dentifrice system (Van Huysen and Boyd, 1952). The loss of available fluoride from combinations with silica powder and pumice was very small. However, the loss with calcium pyrophosphate was considerable. Ericsson advised the use of sodium lauroyl sulphate as a compatible detergent for sodium monofluorophosphate, and a binder of carboxymethyl cellulose. In these investigations Ericsson found no marked increase in fluoride uptake by intact enamel with reduction in pH, thus making it easier to formulate an actual paste in relation to the slightly alkaline and highly buffered properties of saliva.

Over 20 trials of toothpastes containing sodium monofluorophosphate (usually in a concentration of 0.8%, yielding 1000 ppm F) have been reported and are summarized in Table 9.4. A variety of abrasives have been used; for example, chalk and 2% aerosil (Torell and Ericsson, 1965), insoluble metaphosphate (Finn and Jamison, 1963; Frankl and Alman, 1968), insoluble metaphosphate with anhydrous dicalcium phosphate and 1% hydrated alumina (Møller, Holst and Sørensen, 1968), dicalcium phosphate dihydrate and chalk (Naylor and Emslie, 1967) and alumina (Hargreaves and Chester, 1973).

Hargreaves and Chester (1973) undertook clinical trials in which they investigated the effect of increasing the concentration of the sodium monofluorophosphate to 2%, the highest fluoride concentration in a toothpaste to date, the assumption being that if the mechanism of effect was that stated by Ingram (1972), by increasing the concentration of monofluorophosphate and using a phosphate-free abrasive system, this would enhance exchange of the monofluorophosphate ions in solution with phosphate in the crystal structure, and help to minimize the inhibitory effect produced by the natural level of phosphate ions present in saliva. The trial investigated 3 years' home use of the paste in three groups of children, aged 5, 8 and 11 years. Home visitors were used to visit each home every 5 weeks to motivate children and families, and maintain interest in the trial. The reductions in caries increments for the test groups relative to the control groups using a placebo paste varied from 1 to 3 surfaces per child over the 3-year period. The observed caries-inhibitory effect did not differ markedly from that observed in studies testing toothpastes containing lower concentrations of monofluorophosphate. The greatest reduction effect was noted on smooth surfaces but worthwhile reductions were recorded in a number of locations where one would expect pit and fissure caries, for example buccal surfaces of the first permanent molars. Similar findings were reported by James *et al.* (1977).

Hargreaves, Chester and Wagg (1974) re-examined 221 children 1 year after the termination of their study. It was reported that a statistically significant difference in DMF increment between active and placebo groups still remained. This suggests that 'carry-over protection', for those children who used the sodium monofluorophosphate toothpaste, continued for at least 1 year after withdrawal of the paste.

Lind *et al.* (1974) carried out a trial in an optimum fluoride area, using a toothpaste of identical formula to that tested by Hargreaves and Chester (1973). After 3 years 1167 children (83% of the original sample) remained in the study. The children were aged 7–12 years initially. The total DMFS increment (clinical and bitewing radiograph scores combined) for the 3-year period was 1.7 surfaces lower in the group receiving the fluoride toothpaste than in the group using the placebo paste (3.71 surfaces as against 5.43 surfaces), a reduction of 32%.

The effectiveness of the fluoride toothpastes in the study by Lind *et al.* (1974) in natural fluoride areas appears to be very similar to that found by Hargreaves and Chester (1973) and James *et al.* (1977) using similar toothpastes in low-fluoride areas.

The effect of the varying abrasiveness of toothpaste containing 0.76 MFP has been reported (Murray and Shaw, 1980). Three toothpastes were used in the trial; one MFP toothpaste with low abrasivity (relative dentine abrasivity (RDA) 60), and MFP dentifrice of normal abrasivity (RDA 110) as positive control, and a placebo non-fluoride low-abrasivity toothpaste (RDA 60).

The children who used the test dentifrices containing 0.8% monofluorophosphate had a lower mean caries incidence than those using the placebo paste without any fluoride additive. The lowest mean caries incidence over the 3-year period was in children who were allocated the low-abrasive fluoride paste. Caries increments for all DMF indices for boys and girls seen by both examiners were consistently lower in this group when compared with the other two groups, but statistical analysis indicated that the difference in caries-inhibitory properties between the fluoride paste with reduced abrasivity and that with conventional abrasivity was not significant. When both groups using the monofluorophosphate pastes were compared with children using the placebo dentifrice, the differences in caries increments were statistically significant.

The reports of two studies state that children using a monofluorophosphate dentifrice exhibited significantly less staining than those using a stannous fluoride paste (Naylor and Emslie, 1967; Fanning, Gotjamanos and Vowles, 1968). This lack of staining associated with use of a monofluorophosphate paste may confer some advantage in acceptability over one containing stannous fluoride. In 1969, a monofluorophosphate dentifrice was recognized by the Council on Dental Therapeutics of the American Dental Association as an accepted dental remedy and was given Grade A status.

A number of agents have been added to MFP toothpastes in an attempt to increase their caries inhibitory effect. Naylor and Glass (1979) detected a consistent, though statistically non-significant trend towards lower caries increment in the group using a toothpaste containing both sodium monofluorophosphate and calcium glycerophosphate. A dentifrice containing both sodium monofluorophosphate and sodium fluoride (1450 ppm F) has been tested (Hodge *et al.*, 1980) and marketed as newly formulated Colgate Dental Cream. It was concluded that the addition of 0.1% sodium fluoride appeared to enhance the effectiveness of a dentifrice containing 0.76% sodium monofluorophosphate. This effect was apparent if the abrasive system was either alumina or dicalcium phosphate. However, in this trial the differences between the positive control (0.76 NaMFP, original Colgate) and the negative (non-fluoride) control were smaller than expected – 13.8% in the DMFT index ($P < 0.05$) and 6.6% (non-significant) in the DFS index. Developments between 1980 and 1990 are considered on pages 144–153.

Toothpastes containing amine fluoride (Table 9.5)

The protection afforded enamel from acid decalcification by aliphatic monoamines in *in vitro* experiments (Irwin, Leaver and Walsh, 1957) led König and Mühlemann (1961) to test the hypothesis that the detergent action of these organic compounds could be combined with the action of fluoride to give an increased measure of protection to hard tooth structures. *In vitro* studies with amine fluorides showed some amine fluoride compounds to be superior to inorganic fluorides in reducing enamel solubility (Mühlemann, Schmid and König, 1957). It was reported by Mühlemann (1967) that amine fluorides were superior to inorganic fluorides in the measure of their caries prevention due to a number of factors. Amine fluorides exhibited a pronounced affinity for enamel, enhancing fluoride uptake by the enamel when used at low concentrations (as in toothpaste). They exhibited a direct anti-enzymatic effect on microbial activity in the plaque by means of the organic moiety of the amine fluoride (Hermann and Mühlemann, 1958; Capozzi *et al.*, 1967). *In vitro* tests established the stability of a formulation with insoluble metaphosphate abrasive (König and Mühlemann, 1961).

Marthaler (1965) published the results of a 3-year double-blind clinical trial with children aged 6–14 years; the mean age of the younger group studied was 7 years and that of the older group was 11–12 years. Tooth-brushing was unsupervised and no organized effort was made to improve the standard of oral cleanliness of the children participating in the trial. The supplies of toothpaste were not delivered to the participants but were available from the local dental clinics, relying on the cooperation of the children to ask for further supplies. The rest of the family were not automatically supplied with the dentifrice being used by the participant. Initially there were three amine fluoride formulations being tested with differing abrasive systems:

Compound amine fluoride dentifrices	*Abrasive system*
A. 297 + 242 (0.125%F)	IMP
B. 297 + 242 (0.125%F)	$BaSO_4$
Single amine fluoride dentifrice	
C. 297 (0.125%F)	$BaSO_4$
Control dentifrices	
D. –	IMP
E. –	$BaSO_4$

After 18 months, because of their low abrasiveness, pastes B and E containing a barium sulphate abrasive system were replaced by pastes A and D. The amine fluoride pastes were compared for clinical efficacy with a control paste containing a conventional detergent, 1% sodium lauroyl sulphate. In the first 3 months of the trial, test pastes were packed in metal tubes in which they were found to lose approximately 20% of their caries-inhibitory potential due to chemical reactivity between the active ingredients in the paste and the tube. Subsequently they were packed in polythene tubes with no evidence of diminishing cariostatic activity, even after 14 months' storage (König and Mühlemann, 1961).

The supply of paste to the participants was subject to interruption after 18 months of the study. This lapse was due to a number of factors. The result of the first 6-month examination had shown no benefit with use of the test pastes. Many children thought the trial had ended after this interval and did not continue to

Table 9.5 Clinical trials of amine fluoride dentifrices

Investigators	*% Fluoride + abrasive*		*Unsupervised (U) or supervised (S) use*	*Duration of trial*	*No. carious surfaces saved per year*	*Reduction in carious surface increment (%)*	*Level of statistical significance*
Marthaler (1965)	297 + 242	IMP	U	3 yr	(*a*)* 3–4	30	0.001
					(*b*)* 4	24	0.05
	297	$BaSO_4$	U	3 yr	–	–	–
Marthaler (1968)	297 + 242	IMP	U	7 yr	5–6	26	0.001
	297	$BaSO_4$	U	7 yr	–	–	–
Patz and Naujoks (1970)	297 + 242 (Elmex)	Not known	U	3 yr	0.25	7	–
Franke *et al.* (1977)	Not known (Elmex)	Not known	U	7 yr	Not known	41†	–
Ringelberg *et al.* (1979)	(1250 ppm F^-)		U	30 mo	0.2	18	NS

* (*a*), *b*) Different age groups.
† Note that this is a combined effect of supervised brushing with fluoride-containing fluid plus unsupervised brushing with toothpaste.

obtain supplies of paste from the clinics. Owing to diminished cooperation, investigators had ceased supply of the pastes to some of the clinics. At 27 months, when results of the 18-month examination showed promising results, the study revived and supplies of paste were received at regular intervals. The mean number of months calculated for the period when the supply of paste had lapsed was 5–7. For some children this period was as long as 12 months.

The statistical planning and design of this study varied from the conventional protocol as suggested by Backer Dirks *et al.* (1967).

Comparisons with the control group were made only for the test groups using the formulations A and B. After 3 years, reductions in the younger age group for children using the test formulation were of the order of 3–4 surfaces per child compared to the control groups ($P < 0.001$). Radiographic evidence showed a reduction of 1 surface per child for the test groups. A higher relative reduction was observed for dentinal lesions, indicating an inhibitory effect on caries progression. Detailed analyses of individual surface reductions showed that almost half the percentage reduction in caries increment between test and control group was clinically diagnosed on the approximal surfaces of anterior teeth. The reduction was of the order of 58% or 1–2 surfaces per child for 3 years. A similar finding was made by Jackson and Sutcliffe (1967) who found a reduction of attack on approximal surfaces of incisor teeth to be of the order of 50% with use of a stannous fluoride–calcium pyrophosphate toothpaste. In the older age group, a total reduction of 4 surfaces per child in the test group was observed for the trial period, while radiographic examination showed a reduction of 1–2 surfaces per child. The strongest reduction effect in the 11–12-year-olds was noted on the buccolingual surface of teeth. There was no caries-inhibitory effect detectable for the occlusal surfaces.

Marthaler (1968) published the results after 7 years for children aged 6–8 years when the study began. The numbers in the group were small. A significant reduction in caries increment for the 7 years was found to be of the order of 5–6 surfaces per child for the test group relative to the control. Radiographic examination revealed a difference in caries increments of the order of 2 surfaces. Approximately 40% of the total increment reduction attributable to the fluoride paste occurred on the approximal surfaces of the buccal segments. The relative reduction effect was greater for dentinal lesions on analysis of radiographic results, indicating a greater inhibitory effect on the progression of early carious lesions to more advanced ones. Interval analysis showed the caries-inhibitory effect of the amine fluoride pastes to be sustained, and even increase, with longer use.

Further studies (Table 9.5) have now been reported. An amine fluoride dentifrice named Elmex is now marketed in a number of European countries, but is not at present on sale in the UK.

Developments in fluoride toothpaste formulation, 1980–90

Fluoride dentifrices play an important part in the 'personal care products' division of a number of multinational companies. It is an intensely competitive market and subject to continuous developments. In the 1980s, research has been concerned with: (a) changing the F concentration; (b) combining more than one fluoride agent; (c) comparing different F formulations; (d) adding other 'active agents'; (e) the effect of F toothpaste on root caries.

Fluoride concentration in toothpaste

The vast majority of fluoride dentifrice trials have involved pastes yielding approximately 1000 ppm (either as 0.76% sodium monofluorophosphate, 0.24% sodium fluoride or 0.4% stannous fluoride (see Tables 9.1, 9.3 and 9.4). A directive from the European Commission suggested an upper limit of 1500 ppm F for toothpastes sold 'over the counter' without prescription (*Directives An Conseil*, Vol. 78–768, 1977), although higher levels of fluoride in a dentifrice were formally recognized by the EEC in 1982 (Council Directive, 1982).

Koch *et al.* (1982) carried out a 3-year clinical trial in 12–13-year-old children to compare the caries prophylactic effect of two dentrifices containing 1000 ppm F and one containing 250 ppm F. The dentifrices were an MFP-based paste yielding 1000 ppm F (Colgate) and two sodium fluoride pastes yielding either 1000 or 250 ppm F. The results (Table 9.6) showed no statistical difference between the three pastes and the authors concluded that regular use of a low-fluoride paste was as effective in controlling caries as a 1000 ppm F paste.

Table 9.6 Three-year mean DFS increments, clinical and radiographic data combined (From Koch *et al.*, 1982)

	Parts per million fluoride		
	250 (NaF)	*1000 (NaF)*	*1000 (MFP)*
No. children	96	96	96
Mean DFS	7.5	7.2	6.7

Mitropoulos *et al.* (1984) compared the relative efficacy of a dentifrice containing 250 ppm F from sodium monofluorophosphate with a similar active control dentifrice containing 1000 ppm F in 725 15–16-year-old subjects over a 32-month period. Their results (Table 9.7) suggest that a dentifrice containing 250 ppm F, from sodium monofluorophosphate, would be significantly less effective in reducing dental caries than a dentifrice containing 1000 ppm F, and that it would be unreasonable to sacrifice efficacy by reducing the fluoride concentration available in the dentifrice.

Table 9.7 Mean DFS increment, clinical and radiographic data combined (From Mitropoulos *et al.*, 1984)

	MFP level as ppm F	
	250	*1000*
No. children	365	360
Mean DFS	4.29	3.61

A number of investigations have been carried out on toothpastes containing higher levels of fluoride.

Stephen *et al.* (1988) carried out a 3-year clinical trial on 3000 12-year-old children in Scotland involving sodium monofluorophosphate yielding 1000, 1500 and 2500 ppm F. The mean 3-year DMFS increments are recorded in Table 9.8 and show a trend to lower caries increment with increasing fluoride content of the toothpaste. The authors concluded that, in the range of the 1000–2500 ppm F, every additional 500 ppm over and above 1000 ppm F would provide a cumulative 6% reduction in caries increment.

Table 9.8 Three-year mean DMFS increments for fluoride groups, clinical and radiographic data combined (From Stephen *et al.*, 1988)

	MFP level as ppm F		
	1000	*1500*	*2500*
No. in group	921	930	466
Mean DMFS	6.80	6.33	5.71

A similar trend was obtained by Conti *et al.* (1988), who evaluated the effectiveness of two MFP dentifrices yielding 1000 and 1500 ppm F in 2415 children aged 8–11 years who completed a 3-year daily supervised brushing programme (Table 9.9).

Table 9.9 Three-year mean DMFS increments, clinical and radiographic data combined (From Conti *et al.*, 1988)

	MFP level as ppm F	
	1000	*1500*
No. in group	1228	1187
Mean DMFS	2.39	1.87

A third study (Fogels *et al.*, 1988) tested two MFP pastes delivering 1000 or 1500 ppm F in children aged 6–11 years. The results (Table 9.10) amounted to a benefit of 0.3 DMFS, over a 3-year period, for the higher fluoride dentifrice.

Table 9.10 Three-year mean DMFS increments, clinical and radiographic data combined (From Fogels *et al.*, 1988)

	MFP level as ppm F	
	1000	*1500*
No. children	950	963
Mean DMFS	2.36	2.02

The longest study so far reported was by Triol *et al.* (1987), who determined the effect of three MFP dentifrices yielding 1000 ppm, 1450 ppm and 2000 ppm F used by children initially aged 9.9 years, over a 4-year period. The results (Table 9.11) showed that the 1450 and 2000 ppm F pastes were significantly superior to the positive control paste.

Table 9.11 Four-year mean DMFS increment (From Triol *et al.*, 1987)

	MFP level as ppm F		
	1000	*1450*	*2000*
No. children	448	470	452
Mean DMFS	3.21	2.95	2.79

The youngest age group involved in a toothpaste trial was studied by Winter, Holt and Williams (1989). Their unique study involved children aged 2 years. A total of 2177 pre-school children were allocated to one of two groups, who used either a conventional MFP paste yielding 1055 ppm F or a low-fluoride paste (0.209 MFP plus 0.060 NaF yielding 550 ppm F). The children were examined 3 years later (Table 9.12) and the authors concluded that the low-fluoride test toothpaste possessed similar anti-caries activity to the control paste and could therefore be recommended for use by young children.

Table 9.12 Mean dmfs (caries-experienced) clinical and radiographic data combined (From Winter *et al.*, 1989)

	Parts per million fluoride	
	550	*1055*
No. children	477	428
Mean dmfs	2.52	2.29

Taking all these studies together, one conclusion can be drawn. In all the studies, the group using the paste with the higher fluoride content showed the lowest caries increment. In Table 9.13, the percentage differences between each of the groups referred to in the above studies are summarized.

Table 9.13 DMF increments and percentage differences reported in caries increments – studies involving mainly sodium monofluorophosphate dentifrices of different concentrations

Study	*Parts per million fluoride (approx.)*				
	250	*500*	*1000*	*1500*	*2000*
Koch *et al.* (1982)	7.5*	– [13.4] →	6.7		
Mitropoulos *et al.* (1984)	4.29	– [18.8] →	3.61		
Winter *et al.* (1989)		2.52† – [10.0] →	2.29		
Triol *et al.* (1987)			3.21 – [8.8] →	2.95	
				2.95 – [5.7] →	2.79
Stephen *et al.* (1988)			6.80 – [7.4] →	6.33	
				6.33 – [10.9] →	5.71
Conti *et al.* (1988)			2.39 – [27.8] →	1.87	
Fogels *et al.* (1988)			2.36 – [16.8] →	2.02	

* NaF dentifrice.
† 0.209 MFP + 0.060 NaF.
[ ] Percentage reduction.

Combining more than one fluoride agent

One of the first studies to use a mixed fluoride system was reported by Hodge *et al.* (1980). Two dentifrices, each containing 0.76% MFP and 0.1% NaF, one having an alumina and the other a dicalcium phosphate abrasive system, were compared with a positive control containing 0.76% MFP in an alumina abrasive system and a non-fluoride negative control with an alumina abrasive system. In all, 799 children aged 14–15 years completed the 3-year clinical trial. The results (Table 9.14) showed that the mixed fluoride systems showed significant reductions in mean caries increments over the positive control. It is not clear from this study whether the improvement was due to the mixture of fluoride agents, or merely to the extra fluoride available from the two test pastes.

Table 9.14 Three-year DFS increment, clinical and radiographic data combined (From Hodge *et al.*, 1980)

	Parts per million fluoride			
	0	*1000*	*1500*	*1500*
No. children	202	194	203	200
Mean DFS	7.83	7.31	5.94	6.08

A second study, by Mainwaring and Naylor (1983), tested a dentifrice containing 0.76% MFP (1000 ppm F) against one in which half the MFP was replaced by sodium fluoride. A non-fluoride, calcium carbonate base dentifrice without other additives acted as a placebo, and a fourth group used 0.76% MFP with 0.13% calcium glycerophosphate. The results (Table 9.15) after 4 years showed that children using the mixed fluoride system had a lower caries increment than those using the MFP paste, although the differences were only statistically significant for smooth surfaces. The lowest caries increment was found in the group brushing with MFP plus calcium glycerophosphate. In contrast to the two previous studies, Juliano *et al.* (1985) concluded there was no difference in efficacy between a NaMFP paste yielding 1000 ppm F or mixed MFP/NaP paste of the same F content.

Table 9.15 Four-year mean DFS increments, clinical and radiographic data combined (From Mainwaring and Naylor, 1983)

	Parts per million fluoride			
	0	*1000 (MFP)*	*1000 (MFP + NaF)*	*1000 (MFP + CaGP)*
No. children	224	230	228	241
Mean DFS	11.00	9.30	8.46	8.17

Further, the report by Ripa *et al.* (1987) concluded that using a mixed fluoride dentifrice (NaF/MFP) at a standard 1000 ppm F concentration or at a 2.5 times standard did not provide superior caries inhibition compared to a conventional MFP paste containing 1000 ppm F (Table 9.16). Although the mixed NaF/MFP pastes showed the lowest caries increments, the reduction of approximately 5%

Table 9.16 Two-year mean DMFS increment, clinical examination only (From Ripa *et al.*, 1987)

	Parts per million fluoride		
	1000 (MFP)	*1000 (MFP + NaF)*	*2500 (MFP + NaF)*
No. children	912	902	955
Mean DMFS	2.54	2.41	2.46

over the positive control was not significant. The authors pointed out that of the households interviewed, 52% admitted that they were using commercial dentifrices for at least part of the time and so it was possible that any small differences in caries protection from the experimental pastes could have been diluted by the subject's use of other brands.

A summary of the four trials in this section is given in Table 9.17.

Comparison of different formulations

The previous section dealt with mixed fluoride systems. A number of research reports have been concerned with a direct comparison between sodium fluoride and sodium monofluorophosphate. Some care must be taken when comparing the various studies in this section. In some cases, experimental formulations have been tested which do not have direct relevance to products eventually launched commercially. A number of different abrasives have been used in formulating a dentifrice and it is essential that constituents do not react with the fluoride compound and reduce its abrasivity. Edlund and Koch (1977) were among the first workers to compare a conventional 1000 ppm MFP dentrifrice (Colgate) with an experimental NaF paste. The results (Table 9.18) for children initially aged 9–11 years, who completed a 3-year supervised brushing programme, indicated that the group brushing with the sodium fluoride paste had the lower caries increment.

Lu *et al.* (1987) compared the anti-caries effects of three fluoride-containing dentifrices – 1100 ppm F as NaF, 2800 ppm F as MFP, 2800 ppm F as NaF – in a 3-year trial and involving initially 4500 school children aged 7–15 years. The results (Table 9.19) showed no significant differences between the 2800 ppm MFP group and the positive control (the 1100 ppm NaF dentifrice) at any point during the 3 years of the study.

The 2800 ppm NaF dentifrice showed significant reductions against the other two pastes after the third year of the study. The estimates of the percentage reductions for this 2800 MFP paste versus the 2800 NaF paste over the 1100 NaF positive control were 4% and 15% respectively. The authors concluded that their clinical findings were supported by laboratory data and emphasized by Stookey (1985), who related the advantage of NaF to its higher uptake by incipient lesions than that of MFP.

In contrast, Blinkhorn and Kay (1988) found no significant differences at the end of a 3-year study into three pastes all yielding 1450 ppm F. The positive control contained 0.76% MFP and 0.10% NaF; the other two pastes contained either 0.32% NaF or 1.1% MFP (Table 9.20).

Table 9.17 Clinical trials of mixed fluoride dentifrices

Investigators	*Fluoride*	*Abrasive*	*Unsupervised (U) or supervised (S) use*	*Duration of trial*	*No. carious surfaces saved per year*	*Reduction in carious surface increment (%)*	*Level of statistical significance*
Hodge *et al*. (1980)	0.76% MFP + 0.1% NaF	Al_2O_3	S	3 yr	0.6	22	0.01
	0.76% MFP + 0.1% NaF	DCP	S	3 yr	0.6	24	0.01
Mainwaring and Naylor (1983)	0.39% MFP + 0.12% NaF	DCP	U	4 yr	0.6	15	0.02
Juliano *et al*. (1985)	0.38% MFP + 0.11% NaF	DCP	S	31 mo	Positive control		
Ripa *et al*. (1987)	0.38% MFP + 0.11% NaF	SiO_2	U	2 yr	Positive control	–	NS against positive control
	0.95% MFP + 0.28% NaF	SiO_2	U	2 yr	Positive control	–	NS against positive control

Table 9.18 Three-year mean DFS increments, clinical and radiographic data combined (From Edlund and Koch, 1977)

	ppm F	
	1000 (MFP)	*1000 (NaF)*
No. children	179	184
Mean DFS	3.2	2.7

Table 9.19 Three-year mean DMFS increments, clinical and radiographic data combined (From Lu *et al.*, 1987)

	ppm F		
	1100 (NaF)	*2800 (NaF)*	*2800 (MFP)*
No. children	703	679	673
Mean DMFS	4.40	3.85	4.37

Table 9.20 Three-year mean DMFS increments, clinical examination only (From Blinkhorn and Kay, 1988)

	ppm F		
	1450 (NaF)	*1450 (MFP)*	*1450 (NaF + MFP)*
No. children	754	736	744
Mean DFS	4.72	4.76	4.52

Koch *et al.* (1988) carried out a study in 1035 11–12-year-old Icelandic children, involving five pastes. Three contained sodium fluoride yielding 1000 ppm F, the fourth contained 250 ppm F from sodium fluoride, and the positive control was an MFP paste yielding 1000 ppm F. The detailed results are not available, but the Abstract recorded that the paste containing 250 ppm was significantly less effective than the other pastes investigated. A test paste with sodium fluoride with a diphosphonic acid derivative (anti-tartar agent) showed the lowest caries increment, but there was no difference in effect between the 1000 ppm MFP paste and the 1000 ppm F NaF paste without diphosphonates.

The last paper to be reviewed in this section is by Beiswanger *et al.* (1989), who carried out a direct comparison of two pastes yielding 1100 ppm F with identical silica abrasive colour match and flavouring, one containing sodium fluoride (Crest) and the other 0.76% sodium monofluorophosphate (Table 9.21). The authors concluded that their study demonstrated that sodium fluoride had greater cariostatic activity than sodium monofluorophosphate. In addition, they reported

Table 9.21 Three-year mean DMF increments, clinical and radiographic data combined, 11–16-year-old children only (From Beiswanger *et al.*, 1989)

	ppm F	
	1100 (NaF)	*1100 (MFP)*
No. children	257	262
Mean dmfs	3.95	4.58

that the scientific literature contains no reports of clinical trials in which the use of MFP dentifrices resulted in significantly greater cariostatic activity. Furthermore, nine out of the 10 trials in which these two fluoride agents were compared found a numerical advantage in favour of sodium fluoride.

Adding other 'active agents'

This section is concerned with the possible effect of other additives on the cariostatic action of fluoride in dentifrices. Andlaw *et al.* (1983) confirmed that a fluoride paste (0.8% MFP) was more effective in reducing caries than a non-fluoride paste containing 3% sodium trimetaphosphate.

The study by Mainwaring and Naylor (1983) has been referred to in a previous section. One of its conclusions was that including 0.13% calcium glycerophosphate to a sodium MFP paste was associated with additional statistically significant reductions in caries increments.

In the early 1980s, Procter and Gamble directed attention to the possible effect of sodium pyrophosphate as an anti-calculus agent. Lu *et al.* (1985) tested a 0.243% NaF paste with soluble pyrophosphate in Taiwanese children aged 8–15 years against a non-fluoride paste with no anti-calculus agent. After 1 year they reported (Table 9.22) that the experimental paste was effective against caries.

Although a number of studies have been reported on the effect of soluble pyrophosphates on dental calculus (Zacherl, Pfeiffer and Swancar, 1985; Mallatt *et al.*, 1985; Lu *et al.*, 1988), no other studies on the effect of adding pyrophosphate to a fluoride paste on caries increments have been reported.

Table 9.22 One-year mean DMFS increments, clinical and radiographic data combined (From Lu *et al.*, 1985)

	ppm F	
	0	*1100 (NaF)*
No. children	573	587
Mean DMFS (examiner 1)	3.78	2.80
No. children	571	585
Mean DMFS (examiner 2)	1.22	0.59

Triol *et al.* (1990) compared the effectiveness, in a 3-year clinical trial, of four dentifrices:

1. 0.76% MFP/silica (Colgate MFP Gel Toothpaste) (positive control).
2. 0.243% NaF/3.3% sol. pyro./1.0% Gantrez/silica (Colgate Tartar Control Toothpaste).
3. 0.243% NaF/2.0% $ZnCl_2$/silica (experimental anti-tartar toothpaste).
4. 0.76% MFP/1.25% zinc oxide/silica (experimental anti-tartar toothpaste).

Final results indicated that there were no significant differences in caries increments among the four groups, suggesting that the experimental pastes were comparable in anti-caries efficacy to the clinically proven positive dentifrice.

The 3-year clinical trial by Stephen *et al.* (1988) confirmed that adding zinc citrate to MFP pastes (as an anti-plaque agent) had no effect on caries increment.

Very recently, Colgate have launched a sodium fluoride paste containing triclosan, a non-ionic antibacterial agent and a co-polymer polyvinylmethyl ether maleic acid (PVM/MA). The addition of the co-polymer has been shown to enhance the retention of triclosan by plaque and saliva. A number of articles on the safety of triclosan and its effect on salivary bacterial counts (DeSalva, Kong and Lin, 1989; Addy, Jenkins and Newcombe, 1989) and plaque formation (Singh *et al.*, 1989) have been reported, but no studies on caries increments have as yet been published.

Effect of fluoride toothpaste on root caries

The vast majority of fluoride dentifrice trials have been carried out on children and adolescents. Little information is available on the effect of fluorides on root surface caries in adults. Jensen and Kohout (1988) carried out a double-blind clinical study of 810 healthy adults aged 54 years and older. Their results (Table 9.23) showed a statistically significant reduction in both coronal and root surface caries in favour of a sodium fluoride dentifrice (1100 ppm) over a placebo paste, after 1 year.

Table 9.23 Root surface caries in adults (From Jensen and Kohout, 1988)

	ppm F	
	0	*1100*
No. adults	406	404
DFS (root surface)	1.24	0.73

Conclusions

The trend in the 1970s, as shown in Figure 9.1 (page 127), was for fluoride pastes (mainly MFP or stannous fluoride) to capture the overwhelming share of the market, in comparison with non-fluoride pastes. This was mainly due to major manufacturers taking a professional decision that the incorporation of fluoride would improve the efficacy of their product, and therefore be of benefit to consumers and be seen to be attractive to them. In the 1980s the trend (Table 9.24)

Table 9.24 Developments in fluoride dentifrices in the 1980s

Year	*Commerical name*	*Fluoride content*		*Other agents*
1980	Colgate	0.76% MFP + 0.1% NaF	≡ 1450 ppm F	
1980	Signal New Formula	1.14% MFP	≡ 1500 ppm F	
1980	Macleans	0.76% MFP	≡ 1000 ppm F	+ 0.13% calcium GP
1981	Crest Plus	0.243% NaF	≡ 1100 ppm F	
1982	Mentadent	0.8% MFP	≡ 1000 ppm F	+ 0.5% zinc citrate trihydrate
1983	Aquafresh 3	0.76% MFP + 0.016% NaF	≡ 1100 ppm F	+ 0.13% calcium GP
1983	Oral B Zendium	0.26% NaF	≡ 1180 ppm F	+ 0.3% glucose oxidase + 1.2% amyloglucosidase
1985	Crest Tartar Control	0.243% NaF	≡ 1100 ppm F	+ soluble pyrophosphate
1986	Colgate Junior	0.76% MFP	≡ 1000 ppm F	
1986	Colgate Tartar Control	0.243% NaF	≡ 1100 ppm F	+ soluble pyrophosphate
1986	Maclean's Milk Teeth Formula	0.40% MFP	≡ 525 ppm F	+ 0.065 calcium GP
1987	Maclean's	0.80% MFP	≡ 1050 ppm F	+ 0.13% calcium GP + 0.215% triclosan
1988	Crest Enamelin Formula	0.32% NaF	≡ 1450 ppm F	
1989	Colgate Gum Protection	0.243% NaF	≡ 1100 ppm F	+ 0.3% triclosan
1989	Crest Gum Health	0.32% NaF	≡ 1450 ppm F	+ 0.3% triclosan + soluble pyrophosphate
1990	Mentadent P	0.8% MFP	≡ 1000 ppm F	+ 0.5% zinc citrate trihydrate + 0.2% triclosan

has been for pastes based on sodium fluoride to capture an increasing share of the market. For one reason or another, major manufacturers such as Beecham's, Colgate and Procter and Gamble have either added sodium fluoride to sodium monofluorophosphate to create a mixed fluoride system in one or more of their products or changed completely to a paste based on sodium fluoride yielding 1100–1450 ppm F.

References

Addy, M., Jenkins, S. and Newcombe, R. (1989) Toothpastes containing 0.3% and 0.5% triclosan. II Effects of single brushings on salivary bacterial counts. *Am. J. Dent.*, **2**, 215–219

Andlaw, R. J., Palmer, J. D., King, J. and Kneebone, S. B. (1983) Caries preventive effects of toothpastes containing monofluorophosphate and trimetaphosphate: a 3-year clinical trial. *Community Dent. Oral Epidemiol.*, **11**, 143–147

Andlaw, R. J. and Tucker, G. J. (1975) A dentrifice containing 0.8 per cent sodium monofluorophosphate in an aluminium oxide trihydrate base. *Br. Dent. J.*, **138**, 426–432

Backer Dirks, O., Baume, L. J., Davies, G. N. and Slack, G. L. (1967) Principal requirements for controlled clinical trials. *Int. Dent. J.*, **17**, 93–103

BDA News (1981) 7 April, p. 2

Beiswanger, B. B., Billings, R. J., Sturzenberger, O. P. and Bollmer, B. W. (1978) The additive anticariogenic effect of an SnF_2–$Ca_2P_2O_7$ dentifrice and APF topical applications. *J. Dent. Child.*, **45**, 137

Beiswanger, B. B. and Gish, C. W. (1981) A three-year study of the effect of a sodium fluoride–silica abrasive dentrifice on dental caries. *Pharmacol. Ther. Dent.*, **6**, 9–16

Beiswanger, B. B., Lehnhoff, R. W., Mallatt, M. E., Mau, M. S. and Stookey, G. K. (1989) Clinical evaluation of the relative cariostatic effect of dentifrices containing sodium fluoride or sodium monofluorophosphate. *J. Dent. Child.*, **56**, 270–276

Bibby, B. G. (1945) Test of the effect of fluoride-containing dentifrices on dental caries. *J. Dent. Res.*, **24**, 297–303

Bixler, D. and Muhler, J. C. (1962) Experimental clinical human caries. *J. Am. Dent. Assoc.*, **65**, 482–488

Bixler, D. and Muhler, J. C. (1966) Effect on dental caries in children in a non-fluoride area of combined use of three agents containing stannous fluoride: a prophylactic paste, a solution and a dentifrice. II. Results at the end of 24 and 36 months. *J. Am. Dent. Assoc.*, **72**, 392–396

Blinkhorn, A. S. and Kay, E. J. (1988) A clinical study in children: comparing the anticaries effect of three fluoride dentifrices. *Clinical Prevent. Dentist.*, **10**(3), 14–16

Brudevold, F. and Chilton, N. W. (1966) Comparative study of a fluoride dentifrice containing soluble phosphate and a calcium-free abrasive. Second year report. *J. Am. Dent. Assoc.*, **72**, 889–894

Brudevold, F., McCann, H. G., Nilsson, R., Richardson, B. and Cocklica, V. (1967) The chemistry of caries inhibition and challenges in topical treatments. *J. Dent. Res.*, **46**, 37–45

Brudevold, F., Savoy, A., Gardiner, D. E., Spinelli, M. and Speirs, R. (1963) A study of acidulated fluoride solutions, I. In vitro effects on enamel. *Arch. Oral Biol.*, **8**, 167–177

Capozzi, L., Brunetti, P., Negri, P. L. and Migliorini, E. (1967) Enzymatic mechanism of action of some fluorine compounds. *Caries Res.*, **1**, 69–77

Cilley, W. A. and Haberman, J. P. (1981) Fluoride in enamel and correlation to caries. *J. Dent. Res.*, IADR Abstr, 1069

Conti, A. J., Lotzkar, S., Daley, R., Cancro, L., Marks, R. G. and McNeal, D. R. (1988) A 3-year clinical trial to compare efficacy of dentifrices containing 1.14% and 0.76% sodium monofluorophosphate. *Community Dent. Oral Epidemiol.*, **16**, 135–138

DeSalva, S. J., Kong, B. M. and Lin, Y. J. (1989) Triclosan: a safety profile. *Am. J. Dent.*, **2**, 185–196

Downer, M. C. (1974) Aspects of the validity of diagnosis in the epidemiology of dental caries. *Ph.D. thesis*, University of Manchester

Downer, M. C., Holloway, P. J. and Davies, T. G. H. (1976) Clinical testing of a topical fluoride caries preventive programme. *Br. Dent. J.*, **141**, 242–247

Edlund, K. and Koch, G. (1977) Effect on caries of daily supervised toothbrushing with sodium monofluorophosphate and sodium fluoride dentifrices after three years. *Scand. J. Dent. Res.*, **85**, 41–45

Ennever, J., Peterson, J. K., Hester, W. R., Segreto, V. A. and Radike, A. W. (1980) Influence of alkaline pH on the effectiveness of sodium fluoride dentifrices. *J. Dent. Res.*, **59**(4), 658–661

Ericsson, Y. (1961) Fluorides in dentifrices. Investigations using radioactive fluorine. *Acta Odontol. Scand.*, **19**, 41–77

Ericsson, Y. (1963) The mechanism of monofluorophosphate action on hydroxyapatite and dental enamel. *Acta Odontol. Scand.*, **21**, 341–358

Fanning, E. A., Gotjamanos, T. and Vowles, N. J. (1968) The use of fluoride dentifrices in the control of dental caries: methodology and results of a clinical trial. *Aust. Dent. J.*, **13**, 201–206

Finn, S. B. and Jamison, H. C. (1963) A comparative clinical study of three dentifrices. *J. Dent. Child.*, **30**, 17–25

Fogels, H. R., Alman, J. E., Meade, J. J. and O'Donnell, J. P. (1979) The relative caries-inhibiting effects of a stannous fluoride dentifrice in a silica gel base. *J. Am. Dent. Assoc.*, **99**, 456–459

Fogels, H. R., Meade, J. J., Griffith, J., Miragliuolo, R. and Cancro, L. P. (1988) A clinical investigation of a high-level fluoride dentifrice. *J. Dent. Child.*, May–June, 210–215

Forsman, B. (1974) Studies on the effect of dentifrices with low fluoride content. *Community Dent. Oral Epidemiol.*, **2**, 166–175

Franke, von W., Künzel, W., Treide, A. and Blüthner, K. (1977) Karieshemmung durch Aminfluorid nach 7 jahren Kollektiv angeleiteter Mundhygiene. *Stomatol. DDR*, **27**, 13–16

Frankl, S. N. and Alman, J. E. (1968) Report of a three-year clinical trial comparing a toothpaste containing sodium monofluorophosphate with two marketed products. *J. Oral Ther. Pharmacol.*, **4**, 443–450

Gerdin, P. O. (1972a) Studies in dentifrices, VIII: clinical testing of an acidulated, non-grinding dentifrice with reduced fluorine content. *Swed. Dent. J.*, **67**, 283–297

Gerdin, P. (1972b) Studies in dentifrices, VI: the inhibiting effect of some grinding and nongrinding fluoride dentifrices on dental caries. *Swed. Dent. J.*, **65**, 521–532

Gish, C. W. and Muhler, J. C. (1965) Combined use of three agents containing stannous fluoride: a prophylactic paste, a solution and a dentifrice. *J. Am. Dent. Assoc.*, **70**, 914–920

Gish, C. W. and Muhler, J. C. (1971) Effectiveness of a stannous fluoride dentifrice on dental caries. *J. Dent. Child.*, **38**, 211–214

Glass, R. L. and Shiere, F. R. (1978) A clinical trial of a calcium carbonate base dentifrice containing 0.76% sodium monofluorophosphate. *Caries Res.*, **12**, 284–289

Goaz, P. W., McElwaine, L. P. and Biswell, H. A. (1966) Anticariogenic effect of a sodium monofluorophosphate solution in children after 21 months of use. *J. Dent. Res.*, **45**, 286–290

Goaz, P. W., McElwaine, L. P., Biswell, H. A. and White, W. E. (1963) Effect of daily applications of sodium monofluorophosphate solution on caries rate in children. *J. Dent. Res.*, **42**, 965–972

Grøn, P. and Brudevold, F. (1967) The effectiveness of sodium fluoride dentifrices. *J. Dent. Child.*, **34**, 122–127

Grøn, P., Brudevold, F. and Aasenden, R. (1971) Monofluorophosphate interaction with hydroxyapatite and intact enamel. *Caries Res.*, **5**, 202–214

Halikis, S. E. (1966) A pilot study on the effectiveness of a stannous fluoride dentifrice on dental caries in children. *Aust. Dent. J.*, Oct., 336–337

Hargreaves, J. A. and Chester, C. G. (1973) Clinical trial among Scottish children of an anticaries dentifrice containing 2 per cent sodium monofluorophosphate. *Community Dent. Oral Epidemiol.*, **1**, 41–46

Hargreaves, J. A., Chester, C. G. and Wagg, B. J. (1974) Assessment of children in active and placebo groups, one year after termination of a clinical trial of a 2% sodium monofluorophosphate dentifrice. European Organization for Caries Research. Preprinted Abstract

Hargreaves, J. A., Chester, C. G. and Wagg, B. J. (1975) An assessment of children in active and placebo groups, one year after termination of a clinical trial of a 2 per cent sodium monofluorophosphate dentifrice. *Caries Res.*, **9**, 291 (abstr.)

Hawes, R. R., Sonnes, S. and Brudevold, F. (1954) Pilot studies of three topical fluoride application procedures. *J. Dent. Res.*, **3**, 661

Hefferen, J. J., Zimmerman, M. and Koehler, H. M. (1966) Reactions of stannous fluoride with some inorganic compounds. *J. Dent. Res.*, **45**, 1395–1402

Hermann, U. and Mühlemann, H. R. (1958) Inhibition of salivary respiration and glucolysis by an organic fluoride. *Helv. Odontol. Acta*, **2**, 28–33

Hodge, H. C., Holloway, P. J., Davies, T. G. H. and Worthington, H. V. (1980) Caries prevention by dentifrices containing a combination of sodium monofluorophosphate and sodium fluoride. *Br. Dent. J.*, **149**, 201–204

Horowitz, H. S., Law, F. E., Thompson, M. B. and Chamberlain, S. R. (1966) Evaluation of a stannous fluoride dentifrice for use in dental public health programs – basic findings. *J. Am. Dent. Assoc.*, **72**, 408–421

Howat, A. P., Holloway, P. J. and Davies, T. G. H. (1978) Caries prevention by daily supervised use of a MFP gel dentifrice. *Br. Dent. J.*, **145**, 233–235

Ingram, G. S. (1972) The reaction of monofluorophosphate with apatite. *Caries Res.*, **6**, 1–15

Irwin, M., Leaver, A. G. and Walsh, J. P. (1957) Further studies on the influence of surface active agents on decalcification of the enamel surface. *J. Dent. Res.*, **36**, 166–172

Jackson, D. and Sutcliffe, P. (1967) Clinical testing of a stannous fluoride–calcium pyrophosphate dentifrice in Yorkshire schoolchildren. *Br. Dent. J.*, **123**, 40–48

James, M. C. and Anderson, R. J. (1967) Clinical testing of a stannous fluoride–calcium pyrophosphate dentifrice in Buckinghamshire schoolchildren. *Br. Dent. J.*, **123**, 33–39

James, P. M. C., Anderson, R. J., Beal, J. F. and Bradnock, G. (1977) A 3-year clinical trial of the effect on dental caries of a dentifrice containing 2 per cent sodium monofluorophosphate. *Community Dent. Oral Epidemiol.*, **5**, 67–72

Jensen, M. E. and Kohout, F. (1988) The effect of a fluoridated dentifrice on root and coronal caries in an older adult population. *J. Am. Dent. Assoc.*, **117**, 829–832

Jordan, W. A. and Peterson, J. K. (1959) Caries inhibiting value of a dentifrice containing stannous fluoride. Final report of a two-year study. *J. Am. Dent. Assoc.*, **58**, 42–44

Juliano, G. F., Yraola, B., Cano-Arevalo, M., Triol, C. W. and Volpe, A. R. (1985) Clinical study comparing the anticaries effect of two fluoride dentifrices. *IADR/AADR*, Abs. 131

Kinkel, H. J. and Raich, R. (1972) Zur Wirking einer Na_2FPO_3 – Zahnpasta auf die Karies bei Kindern. *Schweiz. Monatsschr. Zahnheilkd.*, **82**, 169–175

Kinkel, H. J. and Stolte, G. (1968) Zur Wirkung einer natrium monofluorophosphat – und bromchlorophenhaltigen Zahnpasta im chronischen Tierexperiment und auf die Karies bei Kindern wahrend eines Zwei Jahre langen unüberwachten Gebrauches. *Dtsch. Zahnaerztebl.*, **9**, 455

Koch, G. (1967a) Effect of sodium fluoride in dentifrice and mouthwash on the incidence of dental caries in school children. *Odontol. Revy*, **18**, 48–66

Koch, G. (1967b) Effect of sodium fluoride in dentifrice and mouthwash on the incidence of dental caries in school children. *Odontol. Revy*, **18**, 67–71

Koch, G. (1970) Long-term study of the effect of supervised toothbrushing with a sodium fluoride dentifrice. *Caries Res.*, **4**, 149–157

Koch, G., Karlsson, R., Bergman-Arnadottir, I., Bjarnason, S., Finbogason, S. and Höskuldsson, O. (1988) A three-year comparative double-blind clinical trial on caries-preventing effect of fluoride dentifrices. *Abstracts from 35 ORCA Congress*, No. 110

Koch, G., Petersson, L. G., Kling, E. and Kling, L. (1982) Effect of 250 and 1000 ppm fluoride dentifrice on caries: a three-year clinical study. *Swed. Dent. J.*, **6**, 233–238

König, K. G. and Mühlemann, H. R. (1961) Caries inhibiting effect of amine fluoride containing dentifrice tested in an animal experiment and a clinical study. In *The Present Status of Caries Prevention by Fluorine-containing Dentifrices* (eds H. R. Mühlemann and K. G. König), Huber, Berne, pp. 126–130

Kyes, F., Overton, N. J. and McKean, T. W. (1961) Clinical trials of caries inhibitory dentifrices. *J. Am. Dent. Assoc.*, **63**, 189–193

Lind, O. P., Møller, I. J., von der Fehr, F. R. and Larsen, M. J. (1974) Caries-preventive effect of a dentifrice containing 2 per cent sodium monofluorophosphate in a natural fluoride area in Denmark. *Community Dent. Oral Epidemiol.*, **2**, 104–113

Lu, K. H., Hanna, J. D. and Peterson, J. K. (1980) Effect on dental caries of a stannous fluoride-calcium pyrophsophate dentifrice in an adult population: one-year results. *Pharmacol. Ther. Dent.*, **5**, 11–16

Lu, K. H., Ruhlman, C. D., Chung, K. and Adams, A. (1988) A clinical comparison of anticalculus dentifrices over 4 months of use. *J. Indiana Dent. Assoc.*, **67**, 2

Lu, K. H., Ruhlman, C. D., Chung, K. L., Sturzenberger, O. P. and Lehnhoff, R. W. (1987) A three-year clinical comparison of a sodium monofluorophosphate dentifrice with sodium fluoride dentifrices on dental caries in children. *J. Dent. Child.*, July–Aug., 241–244

Lu, K. H., Yes, D. J. C., Zacherl, W. A., Ruhlman, C. D., Sturzenberger, O. P. and Lehnhoff, R. W. (1985) The effect of a fluoride dentifrice containing an anticalculus agent on dental caries in children. *J. Dent. Ch.*, **52**, 449–451

Mainwaring, P. and Naylor, M. N. (1978) A three-year clinical study to determine the separate and combined caries inhibiting effects of sodium monofluorophosphate toothpaste and an acidulated phosphate fluoride gel. *Caries Res.*, **12**, 202–212

Mainwaring, P. J. and Naylor, M. N. (1983) A four-year clinical study to determine the caries-inhibiting effect of calcium glycerophosphate and sodium fluoride in calcium carbonate base dentifrices containing sodium monofluorophosphate. *Caries Res.*, **17**, 267–276

Mallatt, M. E., Beiswanger, B. B., Stookey, G. K., Swancar, J. R. and Hennon, D. K. (1985) Influence of soluble pyrophosphate on calculus formation in adults. *J. Dent. Res.*, **64**(9), 1159–1162

Marthaler, T. M. (1965) The caries-inhibiting effect of amine fluoride dentifrices in children during three years of unsupervised use. *Br. Dent. J.*, **119**, 153–163

Marthaler, T. M. (1968) Caries inhibition after seven years of an amine fluoride dentifrice. *Br. Dent. J.*, **124**, 510–515

Mergele, M. (1968a) Reports I – a supervised brushing study in state institution schools. *Acad. Med. New J. Bull.*, **14**, 247–250

Mergele, M. (1968b) Report II – an unsupervised brushing study on subjects residing in a community with fluoride in the water. *Acad. Med. New J. Bull.*, **14**, 251–255

Mitropoulos, C. M., Holloway, P. J., Davies, T. G. H. and Worthington, H. V. (1984) Relative efficacy of dentifrices containing 250 or 1000 ppm F in preventing dental caries – report of a 32-month clinical trial. *Community Dental Health*, **1**, 193–200

Mobley, M. J. and Tepe, J. H. (1981) Fluoride uptake from in situ brushing with an SnF_2 and an NaF dentifrice. *J. Dent. Res.*, IADR Abstr., 653

Møller, I. J., Holst, J. J. and Sørensen, E. (1968) Caries reducing effect of a sodium monofluorophosphate dentifrice. *Br. Dent. J.*, **124**, 209–213

Mühlemann, H. R. (1967) Die kariesprophylaktische Wirkung der Aminfluoride – 10 Jahre Erfahrungen. *Die Quintessenz*, 18, Ref. 3192, Issues 5–8

Mühlemann, H. R., Schmid, H. and König, K. G. (1957) Enamel solubility reduction studies with inorganic and organic fluorides. *Helv. Odontol. Acta*, **1**, 23–33

Muhler, J. C. (1960) Combined anticariogenic effect of a single stannous fluoride solution and the unsupervised use of a stannous fluoride-containing dentifrice, II. Results at the end of two years. *J. Dent. Res.*, **39**, 955–958

Muhler, J. C. (1961) A practical method for reducing dental caries in children not receiving the established benefits of communal fluoridation. *J. Dent. Child.*, **28**, 5–12

Muhler, J. C. (1962a) Effect of a stannous fluoride dentifrice on caries reduction in children during a three year study period. *J. Am. Dent. Assoc.*, **64**, 216–224

Muhler, J. C. (1962b) Effect of a stannous fluoride dentifrice on caries reduction in children during a three-year study period. *J. Am. Dent. Assoc.*, **64**, 216–224

Muhler, J. C. (1970) A clinical comparison of fluoride and antienzyme dentifrices. *J. Dent. Child.*, **37**, 501–513

Muhler, J. C. and Radike, A. W. (1957) Effect of a dentifrice containing stannous fluoride on dental caries in adults, II. Results at the end of two years of unsupervised use. *J. Am. Dent. Assoc.*, **55**, 196–198

Muhler, J. C., Radike, A. W., Nebergall, W. H. and Day, H. G. (1955a) Effect of a stannous fluoride-containing dentifrice on caries reduction in children. II. Caries experience after one year. *J. Am. Dent. Assoc.*, **50**, 163–166

Muhler, J. C., Radike, A. W., Nebergall, W. H. and Day, H. G. (1955b) A comparison between the anticariogenic effect of dentifrices containing stannous fluoride and sodium fluoride. *J. Am. Dent. Assoc.*, **51**, 556–559

Muhler, J. C., Spear, L. B., Bixler, D. and Stookey, G. K. (1967) The arrestment of incipient dental caries in adults after the use of three different forms of SnF_2 therapy: results after 30 months. *J. Am. Dent. Assoc.*, **75**, 1402–1406

Murray, J. J. and Shaw, L. (1980) A 3-year clinical trial of the effect of fluoride content and toothpaste abrasivity on the caries inhibitory properties of a dentifrice. *Community Dent. Oral Epidemiol.*, **8**, 46–51

Naylor, M. N. and Emslie, R. D. (1967) Clinical testing of stannous fluoride and sodium monofluorophosphate dentifrices in London schoolchildren. *Br. Dent. J.*, **123**, 17–23

Naylor, M. N. and Glass, R. L. (1979) A 3-year clinical trial of calcium carbonate dentifrice containing calcium glycerophosphate and sodium monofluorophosphate. *Caries Res.*, **13**, 39–46

Patz, von J. and Naujoks, R. (1970) Die kariesprophylaktische Wirkung einer amidfluoridhaligen Zahnpaste bei jugendlichen nach dreijährigen unüberwachten Gebrauch. *Dtsch. Zahnaertzl. Zeitschr.*, **25**, 617–625

Peterson, J. K. (1979) A supervised brushing trial of sodium monofluorophosphate dentrifices in a fluoridated area. *Caries Res.*, **13**, 68–72

Peterson, J. K. and Williamson, L. (1968) Three-year caries inhibition of a sodium fluoride acid orthophosphate dentifrice compared with a stannous fluoride and a non-fluoride dentifrice. International Association for Dental Research. Preprinted Abstract No. 255, p. 101

Peterson, J., Williamson, L. and Casad, R. (1975) Caries inhibition with MFP-calcium carbonate dentifrice in fluoridated area. *J. Dent. Res.*, **54** (special issue), L85, Abstr. L338

Reed, M. W. (1973) Clinical evaluation of three concentrations of sodium fluoride in dentifrices. *J. Am. Dent. Assoc.*, **87**, 1401–1403

Reed, M. W. and King, J. D. (1975) A clinical evaluation of a sodium fluoride dentifrice. *Pharmacol. Ther. Dent.*, **2**, 77–82

Ringelberg, M. L., Webster, D. B., Dixon, D. O. and LeZotte, D. C. (1979) The caries-preventive effect of amine fluorides and inorganic fluorides in a mouth-rinse or dentifrice after 30 months of use. *J. Am. Dent. Assoc.*, **98**, 202–208

Ripa, L. W., Leske, G. S., Sposato, A. and Varma, A. (1987) Clinical comparison of the caries inhibition of two mixed $NaF–Na_2PO_3F$ dentifrices containing 1000 and 2500 ppm F compared to a conventional Na_2PO_3F dentifrice containing 1000 ppm F: results after two years. *Caries Res.*, **21**, 149–157

Scola, F. P. and Ostrom, C. A. (1968) Clinical evaluation of stannous fluoride when used as a constituent of a compatible prophylactic paste, as a topical solution, and in a dentifrice in naval personnel. II. Report of findings after 2 years. *J. Am. Dent. Assoc.*, **77**, 594–597

Shiere, F. R. (1976) *The Massachusetts Study. Report of a clinical trial designed to determine the caries inhibition effect of a dentifrice containing 0.76 per cent sodium monofluorophosphate*, 7/15/76. Beecham Products, New Jersey, USA

Singh, S. M., Rustogi, K. M., Volpe, A. R., Petrone, M., Kirkup, R. and Collins, M. (1989) Effect of a dentifrice containing triclosan and a copolymer on plaque formation: a 6-week clinical study. *Am. J. Dent.*, **2**, 225–230

Slack, G. L., Berman, D. S., Martin, W. J. and Hardie, J. M. (1967a) Clinical testing of a stannous fluoride-calcium pyrophosphate dentifrice in Essex schoolgirls. *Br. Dent. J.*, **123**, 26–33

Slack, G. L., Berman, D. S., Martin, W. J. and Young, J. (1967b) Clinical testing of a stannous fluoride-insoluble metaphosphate dentifrice in Kent schoolgirls. *Br. Dent. J.*, **123**, 9–16

Slack, G. L., Bulman, J. S. and Osborn, J. F. (1971) Clinical testing of fluoride and non-fluoride containing dentifrices in Hounslow school-children. *Br. Dent. J.*, **130**, 154–158

Slack, G. L. and Martin, W. J. (1964) The use of a dentifrice containing stannous fluoride in the control of dental caries. *Br. Dent. J.*, **117**, 275–280

Stephen, K. W., Creanor, S. L., Russell, J. I., Burchell, C. K., Huntingdon, E. and Downie, C. F. A. (1988) A 3-year oral health dose-response study of sodium monofluorophosphate dentifrices with and without zinc citrate: anti-caries results. *Community Dent. Oral Epidemiol.*, **16**, 321–325

Stookey, G. K. (1985) Are all fluoride dentifrices the same? In *Clinical Use of Fluoride* (ed. S. H. Y. Wei), Lea and Febiger, Philadelphia

Stookey, G. K. and Beiswanger, B. B. (1975) Influence of an experimental sodium fluoride dentifrice on dental caries incidence in children. *J. Dent. Res.*, **54**(1), 53–58

Thomas, A. E. and Jamison, H. C. (1966) Effect of stannous fluoride dentifrices on caries in children: two year clinical study of supervised brushing in children's homes. *J. Am. Dent. Assoc.*, **73**, 844–852

Thomas, A. E. and Jamison, H. C. (1970) Effect of a combination of two cariostatic agents in children: a three year clinical study of supervised brushing in children's homes. *J. Am. Dent. Assoc.*, **81**, 118–124

Torell, P. and Ericsson, Y. (1965) Two year clinical tests with different methods of local caries-preventive fluoride application in Swedish schoolchildren. *Acta Odontol. Scand.*, **23**, 287–322

Torell, P., Hals, E. and Morch, T. (1958) Effect of topically applied agents on enamel. *Acta Odontol. Scand.*, **16**, 329–341

Triol, C. W., Graves, R. C., Webster, D. B. and Clarke, B. J. (1987) Anticaries effect of 1450 and 2000 ppm F dentifrices. *J. Dent. Res.*, **66** (Spec. Issue), 216 (Abstr. 879)

Van Huysen, G. and Boyd, T. M. (1952) Cleaning effectiveness of dentifrices. *J. Dent. Res.*, **31**, 575–581

Weisenstein, P. R. and Zacherl, W. A. (1972) A multiple examiner clinical evaluation of a sodium fluoride dentifrice. *J. Am. Dent. Assoc.*, **84**, 621–623

Winkler, K. C., Backer Dirks, O. and Van Amerogen, J. (1953) A reproducible method for caries evaluation. Test is a therapeutic experiment with a fluoridated dentifrice. *Br. Dent. J.*, **95**, 119–124

Winter, G. B., Holt, R. D. and Williams, B. F. (1989) Clinical trial of a low-fluoride toothpaste for young children. *Int. Dent. J.*, **39**, 227–235

Zacherl, W. A. (1972a) Clinical evaluation of neutral sodium fluoride, stannous fluoride, sodium monofluorophosphate and acid fluoride–phosphate dentifrices. *J. Can. Dent. Assoc.*, **38**, 35–38

Zacherl, W. A. (1972b) Clinical evaluation of an aged stannous fluoride–calcium pyrophosphate dentifrice. *J. Can. Dent. Assoc.*, **38**, 155–157

Zacherl, W. A. (1973) A clinical evaluation of a stannous fluoride and a sarcosinate dentifrice. *J. Dent. Child.*, **40**, 451–453

Zacherl, W. A. (1981) A three-year clinical caries evaluation of the effect of a sodium fluoride–silica abrasive dentifrice. *Pharmacol. Ther. Dent.*, **6**, 1–7

Zacherl, W. A. and McPhail, C. W. B. (1970) Final report on the efficacy of a stannous fluoride–calcium pyrophosphate dentifrice. *J. Can. Dent. Assoc.*, **36**, 262–264

Zacherl, W. A., Pfeiffer, H. J. and Swancar, J. R. (1985) The effect of soluble pyrophosphates on dental calculus in adults. *J. Am. Dent. Assoc.*, **110**, 737–738

Zipkin, I. and McClure, F. J. (1951) Complex fluorides: caries reduction and fluoride retention in the bones and teeth of white rats. *Public Health Rep.*, **66**, 1523–1532

Chapter 10

Fluoride mouthrinsing and dental caries

In the early 1940s it was appreciated that tooth enamel could take up fluoride ions from water solutions and that this rendered the enamel more resistant to acid solution. Over the next 50 years this topical method has proved very successful at preventing dental caries, and many permutations and combinations of the concentration of fluoride in the solution, the type of fluoride compound used, and the frequency and mode of application have been studied. Concentrated fluoride solutions have to be applied by trained personnel, usually in a surgery (see Chapter 11), but weak solutions may be applied by the individuals themselves as a dentifrice (Chapter 9) or as a mouthrinse. This chapter will discuss fluoride mouthrinses.

As with most of the early investigations into fluoride and caries, the first trials of fluoride mouthrinses were carried out in the USA. Since then, results of clinical trials in at least 14 different countries have been reported, and the results of the main studies are given in Tables 10.1 and 10.2. These trials have been sufficiently favourable for dental public health officials to adopt fluoride mouthrinshing as the main alternative to water fluoridation in community prevention in many areas of the world, e.g. Sweden, Norway, Denmark, Eire, USA and Cuba. Heifetz (1978) ranked fluoride mouthrinsing as the most cost-effective community procedure out of six alternatives for topical fluoride therapy and most recent articles have been concerned with this aspect (see Chapter 19).

Clinical trials of fluoride mouthrinsing

Tables 10.1 and 10.2 give the results of 32 studies into the effectiveness of fluoride mouthrinsing where the results were expressed as reduction in DMFS increments in permanent teeth. The way in which these trials were organized varied. In the best organized, the children were randomly distributed to control and test groups within each school and class, and the active and control rinses had similar appearance and taste. In some trials, the unit for allocation to groups was the school or class, which allows the possibility of interschool or interclass factors influencing the results. Most studies lasted 2–3 years, and those lasting less than 1 year have been omitted.

In nearly all the trials listed in Tables 10.1 and 10.2, parallel control groups were used. Children were randomly allocated to test or control groups at the start of the trial and caries increments in these groups were measured in parallel over the same time period. In a small number of trials, retrospective control data have been used instead of parallel controls. The disadvantage of the retrospective control design is

Table 10.1 Results of clinical trials of mouthrinsing with fluoride solutions containing sodium fluoride (NaF)

Study	*F concentration* (ppm)	*Rinsing frequency*	*Test group*		*Length of trial* (mo)	*DMFS caries increment*		*Caries reduction* (%)
			Age at baseline	*No. completing trial*		*Control*	*Test*	
Bibby *et al*. (1946)	1000*	3/wk	18–21	31	12	5.6	6.1	9 (increase)
Roberts *et al*. (1948)	45*	2/wk	12	187	12	2.4	3.0	25 (increase)
Torell and Ericsson (1965)	225	1/day	10	160	24	10.0	5.1	49
Torell and Ericsson (1965)	900	1/2 wk S	10	172	24	10.0	7.9	22
Koch (1967)	2225	1/2 wk S	10	85	36	21.1	16.1	23
Koch (1967)	2225	3.7/yr S	7	117	36	6.2	4.6	25
Koch (1967)	225	2.9/yr S	8–10	114	24	4.9	4.8	2
Horowitz *et al*. (1971)	900	1/wk S	6	129	20	1.3	1.1	16
Horowitz *et al*. (1971)	900	1/wk S	11	117	20	2.9	1.7	44
Brandt *et al*. (1972)	900	2/wk S	11–12	94	21	7.0	4.0	43
Moreira and Tumang (1972)	450	3/wk S	7	50	24	7.5	4.0	47
Moreira and Tumang (1972)	450	1/wk S	7	50	24	7.5	5.7	25
Moreira and Tumang (1972)	450	1/2 wk S	7	50	24	7.5	5.8	23
Aasenden *et al*. (1972)	200†	1/day S	8–11	114	36	12.3	9.0	27
Heifetz *et al*. (1973)	3000	1/wk S	10–12	126	24	7.5	4.7	38
Rugg-Gunn *et al*. (1973)	225	1/day S	11–12	222	34	10.2	6.6	36

Gallagher *et al*. (1974)	1800	1/wk S	10–11	306	24	4.4	2.9	34
Maiwald and Padron (1977)	900	1/2 wk S	6	100	88	11.6	5.1	56
De Paola *et al*. (1977)	1000‡	1/day S	10–12	158	24	7.6	4.4	41
Luoma *et al*. (1978)	200§	1/day S	11–15	32	24	6.3	4.2	32
Ripa *et al*. (1978)	900	1/wk S	7–12	750	24	3.2	2.6	20
Ringelberg *et al*. (1979)	250	1/day S	11	179	30	6.3	4.8	23
Triol *et al*. (1980)	112**	1/day S	10–13	509	30	6.3	5.7	9
Triol *et al*. (1980)	225**	1/day S	10–13	532	30	6.3	5.6	11
Triol *et al*. (1980)	450**	1/day S	10–13	545	30	6.3	5.8	8
Heifetz *et al*. (1982)	225	1/day S	10–12	107	34	4.4	2.9	34
Heifetz *et al*. (1982)	900	1/wk S	10–12	102	34	4.4	3.4	24
Driscoll *et al*. (1982)	225	1/day S	12–13	180	30	1.9	1.0	50
Driscoll *et al*. (1982)	900	1/wk S	12–13	158	30	1.9	0.9	55
Poulsen *et al*. (1984)	900	1/2 wk S	7–10	365	36	2.8	2.5	12
Brodeur *et al*. (1988)	900	1/wk S	9–11	271	20	1.0	0.5	47
Brodeur *et al*. (1988)	900	1/wk S	9–11	401	20	2.3	2.1	8
Petchel and Mello (1982)	900	1/wk S	11††	62	40	3.0T	2.3T	23
Leverett *et al*. (1985)	900	1/wk S	11††	c.100	60	5.2	2.0	61
Leske *et al*. (1986)	900	1/wk S	12††	126	84	5.7	1.8	69

S, School only; T, DMFT.

* pH 4.0.
† Rinse swallowed (1 mg F).
‡ pH 4.4.
§ With buffer (pH 5.9).
** After brushing with MFP toothpaste.
†† Retrospective control trial.

Table 10.2 Results of clinical trials of mouthrinsing with fluoride solutions containing acidulated phosphate fluoride (APF), stannous fluoride (SnF_2), ammonium fluoride and amine fluoride (amine F)

Study	*F compound*	*F concentration* (ppm)	*Rinsing frequency*	*Test group*		*Length of trial* (mo)	*DMFS caries increment*		*Caries reduction* (%)
				Age at baseline (yr)	*No. completing trial*		*Control*	*Test*	
Frankl *et al*. (1972)	APF	200*	1/day S	14	246	24	8.7	6.8	22
Aasenden *et al*. (1972)	APF	200*	1/day S	8–11	109	36	12.3	8.7	30
Heifetz *et al*. (1973)	APF	3000	1/wk S	10–12	133	24	7.5	5.5	27
Kani *et al*. (1973)	APF	500	1/day S	10	95	36	7.5	5.9	21
Packer *et al*. (1975)	APF	200	1/day S	8	80	28	2.7	1.9	27
Packer *et al*. (1975)	APF	1000	1/wk S	8	108	28	2.7	1.6	41
Laswell *et al*. (1975)	APF†	200	1/day S	8	106	28	1.6	1.3	23
Laswell *et al*. (1975)	APF†	1000	1/wk S	8	120	28	1.6	0.9	46
Finn *et al*. (1975)	APF	100	2/day	8–13	150	26	6.9	5.6	18
Finn *et al*. (1975)	APF	200	2/day	8–13	142	26	6.9	4.9	29
Ashley *et al*. (1977)	APF	100	1/day S	12	245	24	5.6	4.8	14
Radike *et al*. (1973)	SnF_2†	250	1/day S	8–13	348	20	2.9	1.8	38
McConchie *et al*. (1977)	SnF_2	100	1/day S	10	248	24	5.8	4.6	20
McConchie *et al*. (1977)	SnF_2	200	1/day S	10	248	24	5.8	4.8	17
De Paola *et al*. (1977)	NH_4F	1000‡	1/day S	10–12	159	24	7.6	4.4	42
Ringelberg *et al*. (1979)	Amine F	250§	1/day S	11	162	30	6.3	4.9	22

S, In school only.

* Rinse swallowed (1 mg F).
† In F area.
‡ pH 5.0.
§ pH 4.4.

that any change in caries experience in the population due to other causes (so-called 'secular trends' in caries) interferes with the analyses of the trial. An underlying decrease in caries experience in the population would lead to an overestimate of the effectiveness of the test agent. The trials of Petchel and Mello (1982), Leverett, Sveen and Jensen (1985) and Leske, Ripa and Green (1986) are of retrospective control design (and indicated as such in Table 10.1) and were conducted at a time when caries was declining in US children. These results should be interpreted cautiously, although Leske and co-workers maintain that most of the secular decline occurred before their trial began.

The effectiveness of fluoride mouthrinsing on the primary dentition has not been properly investigated because it is difficult to conduct such studies on pre-school children. Ripa, Leske and Varma (1984) investigated, in a retrospective control study, the effect of mouthrinsing with a 0.2% NaF solution on the primary dentition of children aged 6–8 years in New York State. After 1–3 years of continuous participation, the children showed a 33% decline in dfs compared with baseline findings. Using the same retrospective control design in children of the same age, Petchel and Mello (1982) reported a reduction in deft of 21% at the age of 11 years after rinsing for 3.5 years, and Leverett, Sveen and Jensen (1985) reported a reduction in dfs per hundred surfaces of 28% after 3 years' use.

Efficacy related to type of fluoride compound used

Sodium fluoride has been the most frequently tested fluoride compound (Table 10.1): such solutions would tend to have a neutral pH. Two early studies (Bibby *et al.*, 1946; Roberts, Bibby and Wellock, 1948) suggested that acidified sodium fluoride solutions were ineffective in preventing caries. It was not until Brudevold *et al.* (1963) had shown that acidulated phosphate fluoride (APF) solutions were likely to prevent caries that these solutions, with low pH, were tested as mouthrinses (Table 10.2). Only two trials have provided direct comparisons of NaF and APF mouthrinses (Aasenden, De Paola and Brudevold, 1972; Heifetz, Driscoll and Clayton, 1973). While in the first trial the effectiveness of the NaF and APF rinses was very similar, the trial of Heifetz and co-workers indicated that NaF was slightly more effective but the difference between NaF and APF was not statistically significant. From these studies, and a comparison of Tables 10.1 and 10.2, it can be concluded that APF mouthrinses have not been shown to be superior to those containing NaF.

Stannous fluoride-containing mouthrinses have been tested in two trials, but no direct comparison with other compounds has been made. They do not appear to be superior to NaF-containing rinses. De Paola *et al.* (1977) compared directly a daily rinse containing ammonium fluoride (NH_4F, pH 5.0) with a NaF rinse acidulated to pH 4.4. Caries reductions were high and virtually the same (42% and 41%, respectively). Likewise, caries reductions after using a daily mouthrinse containing amine fluoride appeared to be as effective as a rinse containing NaF at neutral pH – 22% and 23%, respectively (Ringelberg *et al.*, 1979). No reports of rinses containing sodium monofluorophosphate (the most common fluoride compound in toothpaste sold in the UK) appear to have been published.

The possibility of enhancing the effectiveness of NaF mouthrinses by the addition of ions such as Al, Mn, Fe, Mg, Zr and K has been studied by Swedish research workers for over 20 years (Fjaestad-Seger *et al.*, 1961; Nyström *et al.*, 1961; Torell and Siberg, 1962; Gerdin and Torell, 1969; Torell and Gerdin, 1977; Torell, Gromark and Edward, 1983). Although some results suggest effectiveness may be increased by the presence of various combinations of the above ions, their superiority to simple NaF mouthrinses has not been clearly established.

In the most recent trial (Torell, Gromark and Edward, 1983), application with a ferric–aluminium fluoride solution increased the effectiveness of fortnightly rinsing with neutral 0.2% NaF. The trial was conducted in children aged 6–9 years attending the public dental service in Gothenburg, Sweden. Children were randomly assigned to a group which received topical application of neutral 0.2% NaF or to a group which received an application of Fe–Al–F solution. The concentration of fluoride was similar in the two solutions which were applied three times during the first 2 weeks and then every 4 months subsequently. All children continued to receive their fortnightly fluoride rinses in school. The children who received the Fe–Al–F solution developed fewer new carious lesions than the group who received topical NaF. More recently, treating enamel with dicalcium phosphate dihydrate (DCPD) has been studied in the USA, but no data from clinical trials are yet available (Hong, Chow and Brown, 1985).

In summary, alternative compounds to NaF have a less pleasant taste, necessitate careful formulation of flavouring agents, are more expensive and have not been shown to be more effective than neutral NaF solution. Sodium fluoride, therefore, is the compound of choice at present.

Efficacy related to fluoride concentration

The concentration of fluoride in the mouthrinses tested in the trials listed in Tables 10.1 and 10.2 varied between 45 ppm F (Roberts, Bibby and Wellock, 1948) to 3000 ppm F (Heifetz, Driscoll and Creighton, 1973): 3000 ppm F is 0.3% F. Although, in general, the fluoride concentration in mouthrinses tends to vary inversely with rinsing frequency because of the hazard in frequent swallowing of concentrated solutions, five trials have tested different F concentrations but with the same frequency of rinsing. Koch (1967) found, with very infrequent rinsing (3 times per year), a 25% caries reduction with high F concentration (2225 ppm F) and no reduction with low F concentration (225 ppm F) compared with no rinsing. On the other hand, Forsman (1974) found that there was no difference in effectiveness between a 900 ppm F and a 110 ppm F rinse when the rinsing frequency was once a week in school. She suggested that since the efficacy was the same, rinses with lower F concentration might be particularly suitable for pre-school children.

The trial of Finn *et al.* (1975) suggested that doubling the F concentration from 100 to 200 ppm F, in an APF rinse which was used twice a day all year, resulted in greater caries reduction (29% compared with 18%). However, McConchie *et al.* (1977) reported that this direct relationship between concentration and efficacy did not apply to SnF_2 rinses since caries reductions were similar in the two groups rinsing each day in school with either a 100 ppm F or a 200 ppm F rinse.

Triol *et al.* (1980) reported a 30-month clinical trial with four groups: one group of children brushed each school-day, under supervision, with a fluoride dentifrice (0.76% MFP), and the other three groups brushed with the same dentifrice and also rinsed with either 0.025%, 0.05%, or 0.10% NaF solution. All mouthrinses provided an effect additional to that given by the fluoride dentifrice, but there was no difference in effectiveness between the groups using rinses with different concentrations.

Efficacy related to fluoride concentration and frequency of rinsing

In Table 10.3, percentage caries reductions obtained in the trials listed in Tables 10.1 and 10.2 have been categorized according to fluoride concentration and rinsing frequency. The negative results of the pioneering trials of Bibby *et al.* (1946) and Roberts, Bibby and Wellock (1948), and results from the three retrospective control trials of Petchel and Mello (1982), Leverett, Sveen and Jensen (1985) and Leske, Ripa and Green (1986), have been excluded. Although throughout this review, and in Table 10.3 in particular, effectiveness in caries prevention has often been expressed as percentage caries reduction (PCR), this is largely because PCR is a convenient single statistic. For a fuller assessment of the effectiveness of a preventive measure, the absolute values for test and control increments and the difference between them in the number of tooth surfaces prevented should be examined. This is important because factors such as age of subjects, level of caries experience in that community, the proportion of caries occurring in anterior teeth and the diagnostic standards of the examiner can all influence the percentage

Table 10.3 Percentage caries reductions (DMFS) obtained in clinical trials of fluoride mouthrinsing according to fluoride concentration of the rinse (ppm F) and rinsing frequency

Rinsing frequency	*Fluoride concentration* (ppm F)			
	100	*200–250*	*450–1000*	*1800–3000*
Daily, all year	18*	49		
		29*		
Daily, at school	14*	27	21*	
	20†	30*	41*	
	9	22*	42‡	
		36*	8	
		38†	24	
		32	55	
		23		
		27*		
		23*		
		17†		
		22§		
		11		
		34		
		50		
3/wk			47	
2/wk			43	
1/wk			44	27*
			16	38*
			25	34*
			20	
			41*	
			46*	
			47	
			8	
1/2 wks			22	23
			23	
			56	
			12	
3–4/yr		2		25

* APF. † SnF_2. ‡ NH_4F. § Amine F.

reductions obtained. However, despite its limitations, the PCR remains a useful and often quoted statistic for comparing results of clinical trials.

So far as fluoride concentration in the rinse is concerned, the equivocal findings presented in the previous section appear to be supported, to some extent, by the data presented in Table 10.3. The variation in the size of the percentage caries reductions was large and there was only a moderate trend towards increasing effectiveness with increasing fluoride concentration especially within the most popular range, 200–1000 ppm F.

The frequencies of rinsing tested have varied widely – from twice per day (Finn *et al.*, 1975) to 3 times per year (Koch, 1967). Only two trials have tested more than one frequency with other factors (e.g. F concentration) remaining constant. Koch (1967) found that a 2225 ppm F mouthrinse was equally effective if taken once every 2 weeks in school (17 times per year) as when taken 3–4 times per year. On the other hand, Moreira and Tumang (1972) found a 47% caries reduction in children rinsing 3 times per week compared with reductions of 25% and 23% in children rinsing once a week or once every 2 weeks, respectively. With the exception of the very long study of Maiwald and Padron (1977) in Cuba, data presented in Table 10.3 suggest that a rinsing frequency of once a week (or more frequently) would lead to a greater caries-preventive effect than rinsing every 2 weeks (or less frequently).

The results of the three trials in which both F concentration and rinsing frequency have been varied have been contradictory. Torell and Ericsson (1965) found that a 225 ppm F NaF rinse used daily at home resulted in a 49% reduction, over twice the reduction found after rinsing with a stronger solution every 2 weeks in school. However, Packer *et al.* (1975) and Laswell, Packer and Wiggs (1975) found the reverse trend with an APF rinse.

Heifetz, Meyers and Kingman (1982) reported that rinsing weekly with 0.2% NaF was slightly less effective than daily rinsing with 0.05% NaF in a school-based clinical trial, whereas in a similarly designed trial, also in America, Driscoll *et al.* (1982) concluded that there was no difference in effectiveness between rinsing with 0.2% NaF weekly or 0.05% NaF daily in school.

In conclusion, rinsing frequency would appear to be important and the concentration of fluoride slightly less important than frequency. Rinsing once a week or more is likely to be more effective than less frequent rinsing. The cost of a rinsing programme is a major consideration and the cost-effectiveness of daily, weekly and fortnightly rinsing will be considered in Chapter 19.

Duration of rinsing, quantity of rinse and swallowing

In most trials, the duration of rinsing was either 1 or 2 min; sometimes this period was subdivided into two or three rinses of shorter duration. Ten ml was the most commonly used quantity of rinse which was then expectorated into a cup, although in the trials of Aasenden, De Paola and Brudevold (1972) and Frankl, Fleisch and Diodati (1972) 5 ml was dispensed and swallowed after rinsing for 1 min.

Ten ml of a 1000 pm F solution contain 10 mg fluoride; even so, if this quantity was swallowed every day, the fluoride ingested from this source would be less than occurs in some high-fluoride areas, e.g. Bartlett in Texas (see Chapter 16). Mouthrinses are, in the main, for topical fluoride therapy and should not be swallowed. The most susceptible age group is 6 years and under, since the aesthetically important incisor teeth may be at risk of developing fluorosis up to this age. Because of this risk, several workers have investigated the amount of rinse swallowed by children of different ages. Ericsson and Forsman (1969) concluded that below 3 years of age swallowing reflexes were inadequate and rinsing was not recommended. Between ages 4 and 7 years F retention was 22–24% (Table 10.4), although the under 5-year-olds could rinse for only 30 s. Very similar findings were published by Forsman (1974), reinforcing the recommendation of Ericsson and Forsman (1969) that rinsing with a 110 ppm F (0.025% NaF) rinse every week should be completely free from risk in children above 4 years of age.

Table 10.4 Retention of fluoride from NaF mouthrinses by children in two studies

Age (yr)	*No. children*	*Rinsing time* (s)	*F retention* (mg)	*F retention* (%)
		Ericsson and Forsman (1969): 7 ml of 245 ppm F rinse		
4–5	10	30	0.42	24
5–7	20	60	0.35	22
		Forsman (1974): 7 ml of 110 ppm F rinse		
4	5	30	0.17	22
4	5	60	0.23	29
6	10	60	0.16	20

Birkeland (1973) found that 10–11-year-old children retained significantly less fluoride after rinsing with 7 ml than after rinsing with 10 ml, and concluded from these, and F activity studies, that 7 ml was the most suitable quantity. The F retention in his study was 14%, the same figure as that obtained from analysis of 406 returned rinses during a 3-year clinical trial of daily rinsing with 7.5 ml of solution in 12–15-year-old children (Rugg-Gunn, Holloway and Davies, 1973). Hellström (1960) found that 19% of fluoride in 10 ml of rinse was retained in 7–15-year-olds, while Parkins (1972) recorded a 7% retention after adults had rinsed with 5 ml of solution.

A rinsing time of 1–2 min would appear suitable for all ages above 5 years. Five ml may be a sufficient amount of rinse for young children, 7 ml for 10–15-year-olds, while older children and adults may require 10 ml. Rinsing is not suitable for children under 4 years, and caution is needed when recommending rinsing for 4–6-year-old children.

Caries prevention in different teeth and types of tooth surface

It is well established that the percentage reduction in caries following water fluoridation is greater in free smooth surfaces (buccal and lingual) and least in fissure surfaces (see Chapters 2 and 3). This pattern has also been observed in fluoride mouthrinsing trials. The caries increment recorded in the different types of tooth surface in adolescent school children who have rinsed daily in school for 3 years with a 225 ppm F rinse is shown in Figure 10.1. The percentage caries reductions were highest for free smooth surfaces and anterior approximal surfaces (55% and 56%, respectively). However, because the incidence of caries in these surfaces is so much lower, the number prevented from becoming carious is small in

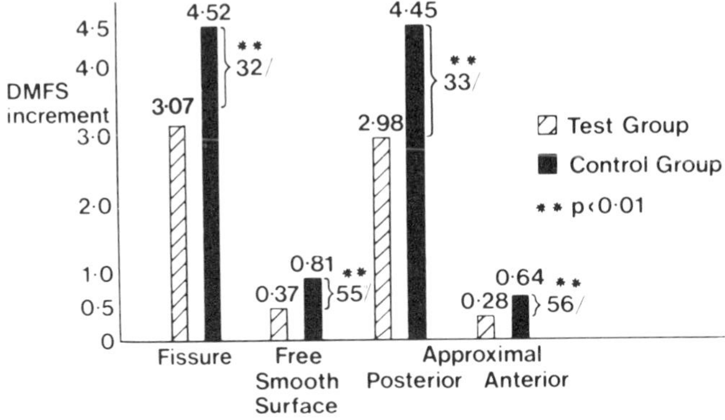

Figure 10.1 Three-year DMFS increments for all children taking part in a clinical trial of daily rinsing with 0.05% NaF, given for each surface type separately (From Rugg-Gunn *et al.*, 1973; reproduced by kind permission of the Editor, *British Dental Journal*)

comparison with fissure or posterior approximal surfaces. The percentage reduction for fissure caries is 32%.

In the same trial, the effect of fluoride mouthrinsing was assessed in the quarter of the children with the highest DMFS scores at baseline. The caries reduction in free smooth and anterior approximal surfaces was very high (72% and 67%), but the reduction on fissure surfaces was low (18%) and non-significant (Figure 10.2). This may be due in part to the high caries prevalence in fissure surfaces, tending towards caries saturation in these surfaces. The majority of caries prevention occurred on posterior approximal surfaces (nearly 1 DMFS per subject per year).

Horowitz, Creighton and McClendon (1971) and Ripa *et al.* (1983) also found substantial caries reductions in all types of tooth surface after weekly rinsing with a

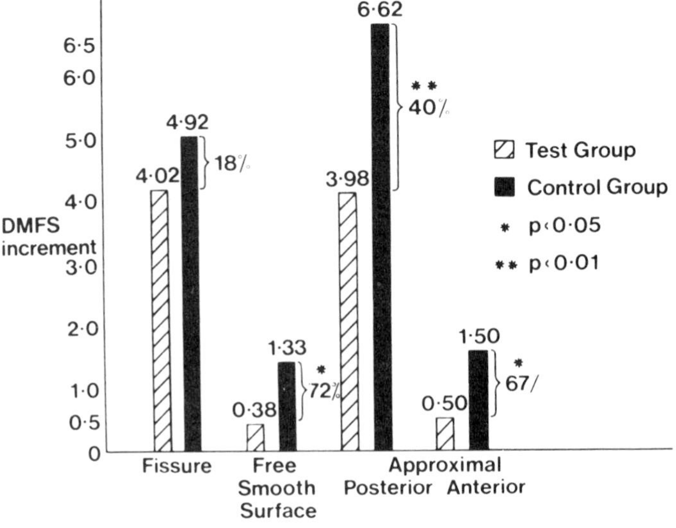

Figure 10.2 Three-year DMFS increments for the quarter of children with the highest initial DMFS at the beginning of a clinical trial of daily rinsing with 0.05% NaF, given for each surface type separately. (From Rugg-Gunn *et al.*, 1973; reproduced by kind permission of the Editor, *British Dental Journal*)

900 ppm F rinse, whereas in children with very high caries increment Koch (1967) observed no reduction in fissure surfaces but substantial reductions in other surfaces. Ashley *et al.* (1977) also found only 5% caries reduction in fissure surfaces compared with 54% reduction in other surfaces.

Ripa *et al.* (1983) reported a 69% reduction for approximal surfaces compared with 56% for occlusal surfaces, but the size of the absolute differences was reversed with 0.8 occlusal surfaces saved, at the age of 13 years, compared with 0.1 approximal surfaces. These findings have implications for public health programmes involving fissure sealing and fluoride mouthrinsing (Ripa, Leske and Sposato, 1985) (see Chapter 19).

Koch (1967) observed that anterior teeth benefit most from fluoride mouthrinsing, but his observation that caries reduction was greater in lower teeth (28%) than in upper teeth (19%), possibly due to pooling of rinse in the floor of the mouth, was not substantiated by Rugg-Gunn, Holloway and Davies (1973), who found equal reductions in both jaws. They were aware of Koch's results and urged the children to rinse thoroughly. The distribution of fluoride in the mouth following rinsing with 1000 ppm F has been studied by Weatherell *et al.* (1986): clearance of fluoride was slowest in the upper vestibular area.

In addition to a 30% reduction in carious cavities, Rugg-Gunn and co-workers also found an 18% reduction in the increment of pre-cavitation carious lesions. Fluoride's action will be discussed further in Chapter 15, but suffice it to say that it is uncertain whether this reduction in pre-cavitation carious lesions resulted from an increased rate of healing of these lesions in the fluoride group or a decreased rate in their formation, or both. Nevertheless, Hirschfield (1978) concluded that regular use of fluoride mouthrinses appeared to be effective at reducing decalcification of teeth undergoing orthodontic treatment. In this respect, SnF_2 mouthrinses were found to be more effective than MFP rinses by Dyer and Shannon (1982) in a limited trial involving 22 patients.

There has been some discussion whether the presence of plaque on the tooth surfaces enhances the caries-preventive action of fluoride (Luoma *et al.*, 1978). It would appear likely that the beneficial effect of plaque as a 'biological fluoride applicator', resulting in higher enamel fluoride levels in plaque-covered areas, is likely to be at least equalled by the detrimental effect of plaque as an essential ingredient in the aetiology of caries and gingivitis. This view is, to some extent, supported by Aasenden, De Paola and Brudevold (1972) who found that although caries increment was correlated with debris score in both control and test groups, the percentage caries reductions following the use of a fluoride mouthrinse were approximately the same in subjects with low, medium or high debris scores. In other words, the presence of plaque appeared neither to enhance nor diminish the effectiveness of fluoride mouthrinses.

Short-term clinical studies have suggested that SnF_2 may have antimicrobial properties (Tinanoff, 1985). In one clinical trial, 22 subjects regarded as potentially caries-active rinsed twice a day with either acidulated NaF (pH 4.0) or SnF_2, both containing 200 ppm F. After 12 months, there was a selective reduction in *S. mutans* counts in the 12 subjects using the SnF_2 but no selective reduction in *S. mutans* was observed in the 10 subjects using the acidulated NaF rinse (Tinanoff *et al.*, 1983).

In another trial, over 300 children aged 12–15 years rinsed daily for 28 months with either 0.05% NaF or 0.1% SnF_2. At the end of the study there was no difference between groups in the level of plaque or gingivitis (Leverett, McHugh and Jensen, 1984).

Possible lack of continuing effect after rinsing ceases

Only Koch (1969), McConchie *et al.* (1977) and Leske, Ripa and Green (1986) have re-examined subjects who took part in fluoride mouthrinse trials a year or two after the trials had ceased. Koch (1967, 1969) observed a 22% reduction in caries (4.4 tooth surfaces) during the 3 years of the trial, but in the next 2 years, during which the children did not rinse, the test group developed slightly more caries than the control group children (Table 10.5). This finding has been frequently quoted as indicating that protection conferred by fluoride mouthrinsing is transitory and lost as soon as the rinsing ceases. However, four factors should be mentioned. First,

Table 10.5 Number of new carious tooth surfaces in 69 test and 71 control group children during a 3-year clinical trial of fortnightly mouthrinsing with a 0.5% NaF (2225 ppm F) solution, and during the subsequent 2 years (From Koch, 1969)

	Test	*Control*	*Difference*	*Difference (%)*
During 3 yrs of trial	15.7	20.0	4.4	22
During 2 subsequent yrs	13.7	13.1		
During all 5 years	29.3	33.1	3.8	11

that the children in Koch's trial were 10 years old at the beginning of the study and premolars, second molars and upper canine teeth are likely to have erupted towards the end of the 3-year rinsing period. Most British trials are timed to begin 2 years later, with children aged 12 years, to coincide with the eruption of these teeth. Secondly, caries increments were very high in this trial (nearly 7 new carious surfaces per year per child): the caries challenge would therefore seem to be overpowering, a view supported by the fact that no protection was conferred on fissure surfaces during the 3-year trial in contrast to the findings from other trials. Thirdly, since the test group children developed less caries than those in the control group during the 3-year trial, they had more sound surfaces at risk of attack during the next 2 years. Fourthly, at the end of the 5-year period, children in the test group still had lower caries experience than those in the control group.

McConchie *et al.* (1977) examined children one year after they had completed a 2-year trial testing daily rinsing with stannous fluoride. The level of caries inhibition (16–22%) observed during the 2 years was maintained at the end of the third year. However, the one-year post-trial period is short for adequate evaluation of the permanency or otherwise of the caries-preventive effect of fluoride mouthrinses.

More recently, Leske, Ripa and Green (1986) have reported on the post-treatment effect related to supervised school-based fluoride rinsing in the USA. Their results showed that for periods up to 2.5 years, the effect of fluoride rinsing was still maintained when rinsing ceased at the age of 13 years. These results differ from those of Koch (1969) and this difference could be due to the widespread use of fluoride toothpastes by children in the later American trial which was sufficient to maintain the caries-preventive effect after rinsing ceased.

Using data from the extensive fluoride rinsing schemes in Norway, Haugejorden, Lervik and Riordan (1985) reported a persistence of benefit from participation in such programmes after 6–7 years' discontinuation (at age 21 years).

Adverse effects from fluoride mouthrinsing

Koch and Lindhe (1967) reported that fortnightly mouthrinsing with a 2225 ppm F solution by children in the test group of a clinical trial (Koch, 1967) resulted in a higher level of gingival inflammation compared with the control children who rinsed with distilled water. However, these comparisons should be interpreted with caution since no baseline gingival data were available.

Subsequently at least six reports have found no increase in gingival inflammation resulting from fluoride mouthrinse therapy, although none of these tested fluoride levels as high as 2225 ppm F. Frandsen *et al.* (1972) and Birkeland, Jorkjend and von der Fehr (1973) found no detrimental effect after children had rinsed weekly with a 900 ppm F solution. Rugg-Gunn, Holloway and Davies (1973) and Ashley *et al.* (1977) also found no difference in gingival inflammation between children taking part in their fluoride mouthrinsing clinical trials. The possibility that amine fluoride rinses might reduce plaque quantity and therefore gingival inflammation has been investigated by Ringelberg and Webster (1977) and Stoller, Cohen and Yankell (1977). In both studies, subjects rinsed with 250 ppm F solutions. While Stoller and co-workers found significantly less inflammation in subjects who rinsed twice a day, no difference was found by Ringelberg and Webster when the subjects rinsed once a day. No case of allergy to fluoride in mouthrinses has been substantiated (Torell and Ericsson, 1974).

It is recognized that stannous fluoride solution may occasionally stain teeth. Radike *et al.* (1973) reported that some yellow stain was observed on the teeth of children with poor oral hygiene and that this was somewhat more noticeable in test group children. McConchie *et al.* (1977) also reported staining of teeth in a very small proportion of children taking part in a trial of daily rinsing with SnF_2 mouthrinses (100 and 200 ppm F), but did not mention whether the children were in either of the two active groups or the placebo group.

Comparison of effectiveness with other methods of fluoride therapy

The classical 2-year study of Torell and Ericsson (1965) in Sweden indicated that fluoride mouthrinsing is likely to be among the most effective methods of topical fluoride therapy (Figure 10.3). Caries reductions were greater in the children who rinsed than in children who received clinical topical application of fluoride or who used a fluoride toothpaste. Ringelberg *et al.* (1979) also found that mouthrinses were more effective than toothpastes.

Two trials have compared the relative effectiveness of fluoride rinsing and fluoride varnishes. Bruun *et al.* (1985) found no difference in caries increment between groups of Danish children who received topical application of fluoride varnish every 6 months, compared with fortnightly rinsing with 0.2% NaF. On the other hand, Seppä and Pöllänen (1987) reported that fluoride varnish application every 6 months was more effective than fortnightly rinsing. Holm *et al.* (1975) found that daily chewing of a fluoride tablet was no more effective than weekly fluoride rinsing. However, the trend which they observed in favour of the rinsing programme was supported by Poulsen, Gadegaard and Mortensen (1981), who found that fortnightly rinsing in school with 0.2% NaF was more effective than daily use of a 0.5 mg F tablet at school.

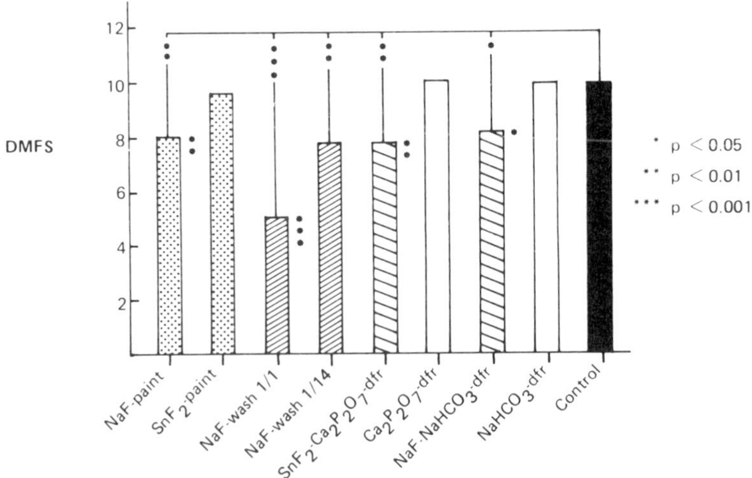

Figure 10.3 Two-year DMFS increments in groups of children in Göteborg, Sweden, who received a variety of fluoride preventive measures both in school and at home. NaF-paint, Topical application of 2% NaF by Knutson's method; SnF_2-paint, Single topical application of 10% SnF_2; NaF-wash 1/1, Daily mouthrinse with 0.05% NaF; NaF-wash 1/14, Fortnightly mouthrinse with 0.2% NaF; SnF_2–$Ca_2P_2O_7$–dfr, Home use of dentifrice containing SnF_2 and calcium pyrophosphate; $Ca_2P_2O_7$–dfr, Control for above SnF_2 dentifrice; NaF–$NaHCO_3$–dfr, Home use of dentifrice containing NaF and sodium bicarbonate; $NaHCO_3$–dfr, Control for above NaF dentifrice; Control, Main control group. (From Torell and Ericsson, 1965; reproduced by kind permission of the Editor, *Acta Odont. Scand.*)

Contrary findings were reported by Heifetz *et al.* (1987), where children aged 6–8 years who had chewed a 1.0 mg F tablet every school-day developed 18% less caries after 2 years than children who rinsed weekly in school with 0.2% NaF. Ollinen (1966) and Rosenkrantz (1967) recorded that rinsing or brushing with the same concentration of fluoride solution performed in school with the same frequency was of equal effectiveness. Ashley *et al.* (1977) observed that the effectiveness of daily supervised brushing with a dentifrice in school or rinsing in school was apparently equal, although Koch (1967) found that supervised daily brushing with fluoride toothpaste in school was twice as effective as fortnightly mouthrinsing in school.

In summary, it would appear that mouthrinsing is at least as effective as alternative methods of topical fluoride therapy. Its effectiveness may be greater than other methods if rinsing is performed frequently (e.g. daily).

Effectiveness of fluoride mouthrinses in combination with other methods of caries prevention

The percentage caries inhibition does not appear to be reduced when mouthrinsing is performed in fluoridated areas (Radike *et al.*, 1973; Laswell, Packer and Wiggs, 1975; Brodeur *et al.*, 1988), although the absolute number of tooth surfaces saved by the rinsing alone is likely to be less. Ashley *et al.* (1977), Ringelberg *et al.* (1979) and Triol *et al.* (1980) observed a small additional effect in children who used both a fluoride dentifrice and a fluoride mouthrinse. Ringelberg and co-workers also found a slight additive effect with a fluoride mouthrinse and twice yearly brushing with an APF prophylactic paste, whereas Heifetz *et al.* (1987) reported that daily use of fluoride tablets and weekly rinsing in school reduced caries by 19% compared with tablets alone and by 33% compared with rinsing alone.

It would appear, therefore, that combinations of types of fluoride therapy increase the preventive effect, but the benefit is less than the sum of effects of the individual methods.

Summary

A wide range of types of fluoride compound, concentration of fluoride and frequency of rinsing has been tested in many areas of the world. From the results it can be concluded that fluoride mouthrinses are among the most effective methods of topical fluoride therapy. As with other topical methods, effectiveness may diminish after rinsing ceases, but this is less likely now that fluoride toothpastes are used widely. Neutral sodium fluoride has been the most commonly tested compound, and because of its effectiveness, ease of formulation, low cost, ease of storage, and lack of taste or possible staining, it is the agent of choice. Effectiveness increases with frequency of rinsing, but substantial reductions are observed with weekly rinses. Fluoride concentrations between 200 and 100 ppm F would seem effective and safe, although rinsing with concentrations around 110 ppm F might be preferable for children under 6 years. Gingival inflammation is unaffected by rinses at concentrations less than 2225 ppm F. Because the organization of mouthrinsing programmes in schools is relatively easy (Little, 1969; Horowitz, 1973; Leske and Ripa, 1977), they have become the method of choice in many community preventive programmes (see Chapter 19). However, in some communities even this level of cooperation may not be forthcoming.

References

Aasenden, R., De Paola, P. F. and Brudevold, F. (1972) Effects of daily rinsing and ingestion of fluoride solutions upon dental caries and enamel fluoride. *Arch. Oral Biol.*, **17**, 1705–1714

Ashley, F. P., Mainwaring, P. J., Emslie, R. D. and Naylor, M. N. (1977) Clinical testing of a mouthrinse and a dentifrice containing fluoride. *Br. Dent. J.*, **143**, 333–338

Bibby, B. G., Zander, H. A., McKelleget, M. and Labunsky, B. (1946) Preliminary reports on the effect on dental caries of the use of sodium fluoride in a prophylactic cleaning mixture and in a mouthwash. *J. Dent. Res.*, **25**, 207–211

Birkeland, J. M. (1973) Intra- and interindividual observations on fluoride ion activity and retained fluoride with sodium fluoride mouthrinses. *Caries Res.*, **7**, 39–55

Birkeland, J. M., Jorkjend, L. and von der Fehr, F. R. (1973) The influence of fluoride mouth rinsing on the incidence of gingivitis in Norwegian children. *Community Dent. Oral Epidemiol.*, **1**, 17–21

Brandt, R. S., Slack, G. L. and Waller, D. F. (1972) The use of sodium fluoride mouthwash in reducing the dental caries increment in eleven year old English school children. *Proc. Br. Paedodont. Soc.*, **2**, 23–25

Brodeur, J.-L., Simard, P. L., Demers, M., Contandriopoulos, A.-P., Tessier, G., Lepage, Y. and Lachapelle, D. (1988) Comparative effects of FMR programs in fluoridated and unfluoridated communities. *J. Can. Dent. Assoc.*, **54**, 761–765

Brudevold, F., Savory, A., Gardner, D. E., Spinnelli, M. and Spiers, R. (1963) A study of acidulated fluoride solutions – 'In vitro' effects on enamel. *Arch. Oral Biol.*, **8**, 167–177

Bruun, C., Bille, J., Hansen, K. T., Kann, J., Qvist, V. and Thylstrup, A. (1985) Three-year caries increments after fluoride rinses or topical applications with a fluoride varnish. *Community Dent. Oral Epidemiol.*, **13**, 299–303

De Paola, P. F., Soparker, P., Foley, S., Bookstein, F. and Bakkhos, Y. (1977) Effect of high concentration ammonium and sodium fluoride rinses on dental caries in schoolchildren. *Community Dent. Oral Epidemiol.*, **5**, 7–14

Driscoll, W. S., Swango, P. A., Horowitz, A. M. and Kingman, A. (1982) Caries-preventive effects of daily and weekly fluoride mouthrinsing in a fluoridated community: final results after 30 months. *J. Am. Dent. Assoc.*, **105**, 1010–1013

Dyer, J. R. and Shannon, I. L. (1982) MFP versus stannous fluoride mouthrinses for prevention of decalcification in orthodontic patients. *J. Dent. Child.*, **49**, 19–21

Ericsson, Y. and Forsman, B. (1969) Fluoride retained from mouthrinses and dentifrices in preschool children. *Caries Res.*, **3**, 290–299

Finn, S. B., Moller, P., Jamison, H., Regattier, L. and Manson-Ling, L. (1975) The clinical cariostatic effectiveness of two concentrations of acidulated phosphate fluoride mouthwash. *J. Am. Dent. Assoc.*, **90**, 398–402

Fjaestad-Seger, M., Norstedt-Larsson, K. and Torell, P. (1961) Försök med enkla metoder för klinisk fluorapplikation. *Sver. Tandläk-Förb. Tidn.*, **53**, 169–180

Forsman, B. (1974) The caries preventing effect of mouthrinsing with 0.025% sodium fluoride solution in Swedish children. *Community Dent. Oral Epidemiol.*, **2**, 58–65

Frandsen, A. M., McClendon, B. J., Chang, J. J. and Creighton, W. E. (1972) The effect of oral rinsing with sodium fluoride on the gingiva of children. *Scand. J. Dent. Res.*, **80**, 445–448

Frankl, S. N., Fleisch, S. and Diodati, R. R. (1972) The topical anticariogenic effect of daily rinsing with an acidulated phosphate fluoride solution. *J. Am. Dent. Assoc.*, **85**, 882–886

Gallagher, S. J., Glassgow, I. and Caldwell, R. (1974) Self-application of fluoride by rinsing. *J. Public Health Dent.*, **34**, 13–21

Gerdin, P.-O. and Torell, P. (1969) Mouthrinses with potassium fluoride solutions containing manganese. *Caries Res.*, **3**, 99–107

Haugejorden, O., Lervik, T. and Riordan, P. J. (1985) Comparison of caries prevalence 7 years after discontinuation of school-based fluoride rinsing or toothbrushing in Norway. *Community Dent. Oral Epidemiol.*, **13**, 2–6

Heifetz, S. B. (1978) Cost-effectiveness of topically applied fluorides. In *The Relative Efficiency of Methods of Caries Prevention in Dental Public Health* (ed. B. A. Burt), University of Michigan, Ann Arbor, pp. 69–104

Heifetz, S. B., Driscoll, W. C. and Creighton, W. E. (1973) The effect on dental caries of weekly rinsing with a neutral sodium fluoride mouthwash. *J. Am. Dent. Assoc.*, **87**, 364–368

Heifetz, S. B., Horowitz, H. S., Meyers, R. J. and Li, S.-H. (1987) Evaluation of the comparative effectiveness of fluoride mouthrinsing, fluoride tablets, and both procedures in combination: interim findings after two years. *Pediatr. Dent.*, **9**, 121–125

Heifetz, S. B., Meyers, R. J. and Kingman, A. (1982) A comparison of the anticaries effectiveness of daily and weekly rinsing with sodium fluoride solutions: final results after three years. *Pediatr. Dent.*, **4**, 300–303

Hellström, I. (1960) Fluorine retention following sodium fluoride mouthwashing. *Acta Odontol. Scand.*, **18**, 263–278

Hirschfield, R. E. (1978) Control of decalcification by the use of fluoride mouthrinses. *J. Dent. Child.*, **45**, 458–460

Holm, G.-B., Holst, K., Koch, G. and Widenheim, J. (1975) Fluoridtuggtablett nytt hjalpmedel i karies-profylaktiken. *Tandläkartidningen*, **67**, 354–361

Hong, Y. C., Chow, L. C. and Brown, W. E. (1985) Enhanced fluoride uptake from mouthrinses. *J. Dent. Res.*, **64**, 82–84

Horowitz, H. S. (1973) The prevention of dental caries by mouthrinsing with solutions of neutral sodium fluoride. *Int. Dent. J.*, **23**, 585–590

Horowitz, H. S., Creighton, W. E. and McClendon, B. J. (1971) The effect on human dental caries of weekly oral rinsing with a sodium fluoride mouthwash. *Arch. Oral Biol.*, **16**, 609–616

Kani, M., Fujioka, M., Nagamine, Y., Fuji, K., Kani, T. and Matsumura, T. (1973) The effect of mouthwash on human dental caries during three years of regular usage with acidulated sodium fluoride solution. *J. Dent. Health* (*Jap*), **23**, 244–250

Koch, G. (1967) Effect of sodium fluoride in dentifrice and mouthwash on incidence of dental caries in schoolchildren. *Odontol. Revy,* **18**, suppl. 2

Koch, G. (1969) Caries increment in schoolchildren during and two years after end of supervised rinsing of the mouth with sodium fluoride solution. *Odontol. Revy,* **20**, 323–330

Koch, G. and Lindhe, J. (1967) The effect of supervised oral hygiene on the gingiva of children. The effect of sodium fluoride. *J. Periodont. Res.,* **2**, 64–69

Laswell, H. R., Packer, M. W. and Wiggs, J. S. (1975) Cariostatic effects of fluoride mouthrinses in a fluoridated community. *J. Tenn. St. Dent. Assoc.,* **55**, 198–200

Leske, G. S. and Ripa, L. W. (1977) Guidelines for establishing a fluoride mouthrinsing caries preventive program for school children. *Public Health Rep.,* **92**, 240–244

Leske, G. S., Ripa, L. W. and Green, E. (1986) Post-treatment benefits in a school-based fluoride mouthrinsing program: final results after 7 years of rinsing by all participants. *Clin. Prev. Dent.,* **8**, 19–23

Leverett, D. H., McHugh, W. D. and Jensen, O. E. (1984) Effect of daily rinsing with stannous fluoride on plaque and gingivitis: final report. *J. Dent. Res.,* **63**, 1083–1086

Leverett, D. H., Sveen, O. B. and Jensen, O. E. (1985) Weekly rinsing with a fluoride mouthrinse in an unfluoridated community: results after seven years. *J. Public Health Dent.,* **45**, 95–100

Little, E. J. (1969) A system of fluoride mouthrinsing in schools. *J. Irish. Dent. Assoc.,* **15**, 103–105

Luoma, H., Murtomaa, H., Nuuja, T., Nyman, A., Nummikoski, P., Ainamo, J. and Luoma, A.-R. (1978) A simultaneous reduction of caries and gingivitis in a group of schoolchildren receiving chlorhexidine-fluoride applications; results after 2 years. *Caries Res.,* **12**, 290–298

McConchie, J. M., Richardson, A. S., Hole, L. W., McCombie, F. and Kolthammer, J. (1977) Caries-preventive effect of two concentrations of stannous fluoride mouthrinse. *Community Dent. Oral Epidemiol.,* **5**, 278–283

Maiwald, H.-J. and Padron, F. S. (1977) The results of collective caries prevention by mouth-rinsing with a 0.2% sodium fluoride solution after 88 months. *Stomatol. DDR,* **27,** 835–840

Moreira, B.-H. W. and Tumang, A. J. (1972) Prevencao da carie dentaria atraces de bochechos com solucoes de fluoreto de sodio a 0.1%. *Rev. Bras. Odontol.,* **29**, 37–42

Nyström, S., Bramstang, S. and Torell, P. (1961) Munsköljning med zirkoniumfluorid- eller jarnfluoridlösingar. *Sven. Tandläk. Tidskr.,* **54**, 217–220

Ollinen, P. (1966) Munsköljning eller borstning med olika fluoridlösingar. *Sver. Tandläk-Förb. Tidn.,* **58**, 913–918

Packer, M. W., Laswell, H. R., Doyle, J., Naff, H. H. and Brown, F. (1975) Cariostatic effects of fluoride mouthrinses in a non-fluoridated community. *J. Tenn. State Dent. Assoc.,* **55**, 22–26

Parkins, F. M. (1972) Retention of fluoride with chewable tablets and a mouthrinse. *J. Dent. Res.,* **51**, 1346–1349

Petchel, K. A. and Mello, A. F. (1982) School-based weekly sodium fluoride rinse program: results after three and one-half years. *Clin. Prev. Dent.,* **4**, 21–23

Poulsen, S., Gadegaard, E. and Mortensen, B. (1981) Cariostatic effect of daily use of fluoride-containing lozenge compared to fortnightly rinses with 0.2% sodium fluoride. *Caries Res.,* **15**, 236–242

Poulsen, S., Kirkegaard, E., Bangsbo, G. and Bro, K. (1984) Caries clinical trial of fluoride rinses in a Danish Public Child Dental Service. *Community Dent. Oral Epidemiol.,* **12**, 283–287

Radike, A. W., Gish, C. W., Peterson, J. K., King, J. D. and Segreto, V. A. (1973) Clinical evaluation of stannous fluoride as an anticaries mouthrinse. *J. Am. Dent. Assoc.,* **86**, 404–408

Ringelberg, M. L., Conti, A. J. and Webster, D. B. (1976) An evaluation of single and combined self-applied fluoride programs in schools. *J. Public Health Dent.,* **36,** 220–236

Ringelberg, M. L. and Webster, D. B. (1977) Effects of an amine fluoride mouthrinse and dentifrice on the gingival health and the extent of plaque of schoolchildren. *J. Periodontol.,* **48**, 350–353

Ringelberg, M. L., Webster, D. B., Dixon, D. O. and LeZotte, D. C. (1979) The caries-preventive effect of amine fluorides and inorganic fluorides in a mouthrinse or dentifrice after 30 months of use. *J. Am. Dent. Assoc.,* **98**, 202–208

Ripa, L. W. and Leske, G. S. (1979) Two years' effect on the primary dentition of mouthrinsing with a 0.2% neutral NaF solution. *Community Dent. Oral Epidemiol.,* **7**, 151–153

Ripa, L. W., Leske, G. S. and Levinson, A. (1978) Supervised weekly rinsing with a 0.2% neutral NaF solution: results from a demonstration program after two school years. *J. Am. Dent. Assoc.*, **97**, 793–798

Ripa, L. W., Leske, G. S. and Sposato, A. (1985) The surface-specific caries pattern of participants in a school-based fluoride mouthrinsing program with implications for the use of sealants. *J. Public Health Dent.*, **45**, 90–94

Ripa, L. W., Leske, G. S., Sposato, A. and Rebich, T. (1983) Supervised weekly rinsing with a 0.2 percent neutral NaF solution: final results of a demonstration program after six school years. *J. Public Health Dent.*, **43**, 53–62

Ripa, L. W., Leske, G. S. and Varma, A. (1984) Effect of mouthrinsing with a 0.2 percent neutral NaF solution on the deciduous dentition of first to third grade school children. *Pediatr. Dent.*, **6**, 93–97

Roberts, J. F., Bibby, B. G. and Wellock, W. D. (1948) The effect of an acidulated fluoride mouthwash on dental caries. *J. Dent. Res.*, **27**, 497–500

Rosenkrantz, F. (1967) Kariesprophylaktischer Vergleich zwischen Mundspülen und Zähneputzen mit Natrium fluoridlösung. *Odontol. Tidskr.*, **75**, 528–534

Rugg-Gunn, A. J., Holloway, P. J. and Davies, T. G. H. (1973) Caries prevention by daily fluoride mouthrinsing. *Br. Dent. J.*, **135**, 353–360

Seppä, L. and Pöllänen, L. (1987) Caries preventive effect of two fluoride varnishes and a fluoride mouthrinse. *Caries Res.*, **21**, 375–379

Stoller, N. H., Cohen, D. W. and Yankell, S. L. (1977) Clinical evaluations of an amine fluoride mouthrinse on gingival inflammation and plaque accumulation. *J. Periodontol.*, **48**, 650–653

Tinanoff, N. (1985) Stannous fluoride in clinical dentistry. In *Clinical Uses of Fluorides* (ed. S. H. Y. Wei), Chap, 3, Lea and Febiger, Philadelphia, pp. 25–34

Tinanoff, N., Klock, B., Camosci, D. A. and Manwell, M. A. (1983) Microbiologic effects of SnF_2 and NaF mouthrinses in subjects with high caries activity: results after one year. *J. Dent. Res.*, **62**, 907–911

Torell, P. and Ericsson, Y. (1965) Two-year clinical tests with different methods of local caries-preventive fluorine application in Swedish school-children. *Acta Odontol. Scand.*, **23**, 287–322

Torell, P. and Ericsson, Y. (1974) The potential benefits derived from fluoride mouth rinses. In *International Workshop on Fluoride and Dental Caries Reductions* (eds D. J. Forester and E. M. Schultz), University of Maryland, Baltimore, Md, pp. 113–166

Torell, P. and Gerdin, P.-O. (1977) Fortnightly fluoride rinsing combined with topical painting of fluoride solutions containing Al-, Fe-, and Mn-ions. *Scand. J. Dent. Res.*, **85**, 38–40

Torell, P., Gromark, P.-O. and Edward, S. (1983) Fortnightly fluoride rinsing combined with topical paintings with a fluoride solution containing Fe- and Al-ions. *Swed. Dent. J.*, **7**, 23–31

Torell, P. and Siberg, A. (1962) Mouthwash with sodium fluoride and potassium fluoride. *Odontol. Revy.*, **13**, 62–71

Triol., C. W., Kranz, S. M., Volpe, A. R., Frankl, S. N., Alman, J. E. and Allard, R. L. (1980) Anticaries effect of a sodium fluoride rinse and an MFP dentifrice in a non-fluoridated water area: a thirty-month study. *J. Clin. Prev. Dent.*, **2**, 13–15

Weatherell, J. A., Strong, M., Robinson, C. and Ralph, J. P. (1986) Fluoride distribution in the mouth after fluoride rinsing. *Caries Res.*, **20**, 111–119

Chapter 11

Topical fluorides and dental caries

Topical fluorides have been used as caries-preventive agents in dental practice for nearly 50 years. During this period, four main types of preparations have been advocated: neutral sodium fluoride solutions, stannous fluoride solutions, acidulated phosphate fluoride agents, and varnishes containing fluoride. Results of clinical trials concerning the effectiveness of the various fluoride agents in reducing the incidence of dental caries will be reviewed and consideration will be given to the benefits of combining different types of topical fluoride treatments and to the effect of topical fluoride therapy for high-risk groups. The effectiveness of incorporating fluoride into prophylactic pastes will be considered. Recently, increasing emphasis has been placed on the fluoride-releasing properties of dental materials and their potential to act as a reservoir of fluoride, providing long-term, slow-release topical treatment. The concluding section will review these developments.

Neutral sodium fluoride solution

In 1940, Volker and colleagues showed that *in vitro* the solubility of enamel could be appreciably reduced by treating it with a fluoride solution. The first clinical study was started by Bibby in 1941 using a 0.1% aqueous NaF solution. After prophylaxis and drying of teeth, applications for 7–8 min were made 3 times a year at 3–4-monthly intervals. One year later the caries increment in the experimental quadrant was 45% lower than that found in the opposing control quadrant (Bibby, 1943).

In 1942, Knutson began a series of clinical trials using a different technique which required four visits within a short period. After prophylaxis and drying, a 2% aqueous NaF solution was applied for 3 min. Knutson concluded that maximum reduction in caries was achieved from four treatments at weekly intervals and suggested that the series of applications should be carried out at the ages of 3, 7, 10 and 13 years to coincide with the eruption of teeth (Knutson, 1948). A 2% aqueous NaF solution has generally been used, although Galagan and Knutson (1948) showed that a 1% NaF solution was equally effective. Many of the subsequent studies have followed Knutson's technique; nearly all reported a reduction in caries varying from 4.9% (Jordan, Snyder and Wilson, 1959) to 58% (Davies, 1950). A few reports (Arnold, Dean and Singleton, 1944; Kutler and Ireland, 1953) produced negative findings, but these studies were carried out on adults.

An important question to ask of the Knutson technique is whether the reduction in caries is only a short-term reduction of a year or so or whether it has a long-term preventive effect. In 1942, Knutson and Armstrong began a study involving children aged 7–15 years. The results after 3 years were published in 1946 and are summarized in Table 11.1. The percentage reduction in DF surfaces between study and control teeth was 33%. However, the procedure of working out the percentage

Table 11.1 Results of a 3-year study of 242 children aged 7–15 years treated with sodium fluoride (From Knutson and Armstrong, 1946)

Quadrant	*No. caries-free teeth (1942)*	*New DF teeth (1945)*	*DF surfaces in new DF teeth*	*DF surfaces in previous DF teeth*	*Total new DF surfaces*	*Difference* in DF surfaces (%)*
Treated	1870	214	287	216	503	32.8
Untreated	1888	338	464	284	748	

* The percentage difference between total new DF surfaces in treated and untreated quadrants has been calculated without reference to the total number of teeth treated.

reduction between study and control quadrants does not take into account the total number of teeth involved. If the number of new carious teeth is given as a percentage of the total number of teeth present in treated and untreated quadrants (Table 11.2), the difference in caries incidence between treated and untreated teeth amounts to 8%.

Table 11.2 Results of a 3-year study of 242 children aged 7–15 years treated with sodium fluoride (From Knutson and Armstrong, 1946)

Quadrant	*Total no. teeth*	*New DF teeth*	*Percentage new DF teeth**
Treated	2086	430	20.6
Untreated	2172	622	28.6

* The new DF teeth are expressed as percentages of the total number of teeth in treated and untreated quadrants.

Sundvall-Hagland *et al.* (1959) studied the effectiveness of Knutson's technique on caries incidence in the deciduous dentition. Their findings after 3 years are given in Table 11.3, from which it will be seen that there was a marked fall-off in inhibition of caries. After 3 years, the reduction in mean DMF surfaces increment between the control and experimental sides was 7.5%. In contrast, Bergman (1953), in a study of 11–12-year-old children, concluded that caries inhibition on the treated side after 3 years was 43%.

Table 11.3 Results of a 3-year study of 102 children aged 2½ years treated with sodium fluoride (From Sundvall-Hagland *et al.*, 1959)

Period (yr)	*No. children*	*Mean DMF surfaces increment on treated side*	*Mean DMF surfaces increment on control side*	*Percentage in DMF surfaces*
1	107	4.6	5.7	19
2	104	7.5	8.7	14
3	102	9.9	10.7	7.5

Stannous fluoride solution

In vitro studies

Buonocore and Bibby (1945) conducted a series of experiments to determine which fluoride salt was the most effective in reducing enamel solubility; they concluded that lead fluoride was appreciably more effective in reducing enamel solubility than was sodium fluoride. However, Muhler and van Huysen (1947) carried out *in vitro* studies of a similar nature using many different reagent solutions and concluded that tin fluoride was the most effective and that lead fluoride and sodium fluoride had about the same absorption qualities for enamel. Much of the work on stannous fluoride has been carried out by Muhler and his colleagues at the University of Indiana, following the finding that stannous fluoride in a concentration of 10 ppm in drinking water given to rats fed on a cariogenic diet was superior to 10 ppm of sodium fluoride in reducing caries (Muhler and Day, 1950). It was also claimed that stannous fluoride was three times more effective than sodium fluoride in preventing dissolution of calcium and phosphorus from enamel by dilute acids (Muhler, Boyd and van Huysen, 1950). Since that time, however, later work using the electron microscope has shown that stannous ions form a coating on the enamel surface (Scott, 1960); this coating has no protective action against the carious process and it has been suggested that stannous ions may actually reduce fluoride uptake (Brudevold *et al.*, 1967).

Clinical studies

The recommended procedure for application of stannous fluoride solution begins with a thorough prophylaxis and drying of the teeth. A freshly prepared 8% solution of stannous fluoride is applied continuously to the teeth with cottonwool so that the teeth are kept moist for 4 min. Gish, Howell and Muhler (1957) studied 554 7-year-olds in Montgomery County, Indiana. After 8 months, children who had received one application of SnF_2 had an average DMF teeth increment of 0.60 compared with an average DMF teeth increment of 0.76 in children who had received four applications of 2% NaF. This gave a 21% difference, although in absolute terms a difference of 0.16 DMF teeth is clinically insignificant. However, Gish and co-workers considered that the results indicated a considerable advantage in using 8% SnF_2, as only one treatment was required and this could be fitted in more conveniently with the patient's recall appointments. Over a 5-year period (1957–62) Muhler, working with Gish and Howell, compared single, annual applications of 8% SnF_2 with a series of four applications of 2% NaF every 3 years. Over the 5-year period the caries increment in the SnF_2 group was approximately 35% less than the increment in the NaF group. No control group was examined, although Gish, Muhler and Howell (1962) suggested that the caries increment in the SnF_2 group was 56% lower than the 'national average' increment for the USA.

Other investigators have found stannous fluoride to be effective, although the percentage reductions reported have generally been less than that obtained by Muhler and his co-workers. On the other hand, some studies in America and Sweden have reported negative results. These studies are tabulated in Table 11.4.

The study by Houwink, Backer Dirks and Kwant (1974) involved 22 pairs of monozygotic twins. The teeth of one child were treated twice yearly with SnF_2 solution (yielding 1% F) over a period of 9 years. When the children were 16 years old, the result was that treated children had 37% fewer lesions than the controls.

Table 11.4 Comparison of the results of stannous fluoride studies

Author	*Study period* (yr)	*Reduction in DMF surfaces* (%)
Compton *et al.* (1959)	1	28
Jordan *et al.* (1959)	2	38
Law *et al.* (1961)	1	24
Mercer and Muhler (1961)	1	51
Burgess *et al.* (1962)	2	29
Harris (1963)	1	23
Torell (1965)	1	None
Wellock *et al.* (1965)	1	None
Horowitz and Lucye (1966)	2	None
Houwink *et al.* (1974)	9	37

Five years after the last application, 18 pairs were examined once more. In 3 pairs the controls had received full dentures. The caries experience of the remaining 15 pairs is summarized in Table 11.5. Although during the period without treatment the study group had a very slightly higher mean annual increment than the control group, the effect of the 9 years' treatment was still apparent 5 years after treatment had stopped. The increment over the 14-year period was still 23.8% lower in the study group than in the control. Thus, there is a divergence of opinion as to the

Table 11.5 DFS increment in 15 pairs of monozygotic children during SnF_2 treatment (1957–66) and during 5 years without treatment (1966–71) (From Houwink, Backer Dirks and Kwant, 1974)

	Period with treatment		*Period without treatment*		*Total DFS 1957–71*	
	Mean DFS	*Mean DFS/yr*	*Mean DFS*	*Mean DFS/yr*	*Total*	*Mean DFS/yr*
Study	14.8	1.6	12.7	2.5	27.5	2.0
Control	24.6	2.7	11.5	2.3	36.1	2.6

effectiveness of stannous fluoride as a caries-preventive agent. A disadvantage of stannous fluoride is that it causes brown pigmentation of teeth, particularly in hypocalcified areas and around margins of restorations. It can also cause gingival irritation. Because stannous fluoride is unstable in aqueous solution it has to be freshly prepared for each treatment.

Acidulated phosphate agents

In vitro studies

As far back as 1947 Bibby reported that as the pH of the solution was lowered fluoride was absorbed into enamel more effectively. Brudevold *et al.* (1963) studied the effect of prolonged exposure of enamel to sodium fluoride in acid sodium phosphate solutions. They concluded that the fluoride concentration in enamel increased with decrease in the pH of the solution. Mellberg (1966) reported that after a 10-min exposure of a cut tooth section to an acid phosphate fluoride solution there was a high fluoride concentration in the inner layers of enamel.

Clinical studies

Acidulated phosphate solutions, containing 1.23% available fluoride in 0.1 M phosphoric acid at pH 2.8, are applied in a similar manner to stannous fluoride solution. The first clinical trial was started in 1961 by Wellock and Brudevold (1963). After 2 years, children in the study group had approximately 66% fewer carious surfaces than children in the control group. Bitewing radiographs were used to aid diagnoses.

Parmeijer, Brudevold and Hunt (1963), in a study of 77 children aged 4–10 years, compared the effectiveness of a solution of neutral sodium fluoride with an acidulated phosphate fluoride (APF) solution used on opposite sides of the mouth. On the right side (APF), 45 new DMF surfaces were recorded, whereas on the left side (NaF), 92 new surfaces were found; it was therefore concluded that APF was 50% more effective than neutral NaF as a caries-preventive agent. Further studies (Wellock, Maitland and Brudevold, 1965; Cartwright, Lindahl and Bawden, 1968) have reported reductions of 44–49% in new DMF teeth in children given annual or bi-annual applications of APF solution compared with control groups receiving treatment with tap water only.

One of the problems of carrying out the topical fluoride applications so far described is that the teeth must be kept moist for 4 min, which means that the solution must be applied with cottonwool to each tooth approximately every 30 s. To overcome this problem, workers experimented with wax or plastic trays in which blotting paper soaked in the solution could be applied to the teeth which would then be continuously surrounded by the fluoride agent. Other workers introduced a gelling agent (usually methyl cellulose or hydroxyethyl cellulose) which removed the need for the blotting-paper inserts. The disadvantage of using trays is that one can never be absolutely sure that all the surfaces of the teeth, particularly the approximal areas, have been completely covered by the fluoride agent. Gentle pressure should be maintained on the tray to force the gel approximally. The gels are thixotropic, that is they convert to a solution and flow more easily under pressure.

Szwejda, Tossy and Below (1967) carried out the first published clinical trial of APF gels on 7-year-old children. They observed no reduction in caries increment after 1 year. In contrast, Bryan and Williams (1968) reported a 45% reduction in DMF teeth after a single application of APF gel in foam rubber trays. The results of these two studies are summarized in Table 11.6. Ingraham and Williams (1970) carried out a 2-year study to compare the effectiveness of APF solutions and gels in reducing caries experience. Their results are shown in Table 11.7. It was concluded that the greatest reduction in caries experience occurred using the APF gels (over 50%); the APF solutions were approximately only half as effective as the gels.

Table 11.6 Results of two 1-year studies of APF gels

Authors	*Age of children* (yr)		*No. children*	*DMF teeth increment*	*Reduction in DMF teeth* (%)
Szwejda *et al.* (1967)	7	Test	182	0.67	
		Control	188	0.65	–
Bryan and Williams (1968)	8–11	Test	121	0.93	
		Control	122	1.69	45.0

Table 11.7 Results of a 2-year study of 238 children aged 6–11 years treated with APF agents (From Ingraham and Williams, 1970)

	Description of group	*No. children*	*Baseline DMF teeth*	*Percentage difference in baseline DMF teeth (from 4A)*	*DMF teeth increment*	*Percentage reduction in DMF teeth*
1.	Prophylaxis only	63	1.49	31	1.76	–
2.	APF solution on cottonwool	57	1.58	39	1.44	18.2
3.	APF solutions in trays with paper inserts	62	1.27	11	1.34	23.9
4A.	APF gel in beeswax trays	28	1.14	–	0.86	51.1
4B.	APF gel in foam rubber trays	28	1.43	25	0.82	53.4
4.	A + B	56	1.29	13	0.84	52.3

However, one of the aspects of this study which makes it rather difficult to interpret is the difference between the groups in baseline DMF teeth values. Although the authors state that there was no statistical difference between the groups at the start of the study, Table 11.7 indicates that there was a 0.44 difference between groups 2 and 4A in the baseline DMF teeth values.

The largest APF study so far carried out is that by Horowitz and Doyle (1971). After 3 years, a total of 681 Hawaiian children aged 10–12 years had taken part continuously in the study. A summary of the results is given in Table 11.8. The

Table 11.8 Results of a 3-year study of 681 children aged 10–12 years treated with APF agents (From Horowitz and Doyle, 1971)

Description of group	*No. in group*	*Baseline DMF teeth*	*DMF teeth increment*	*Percentage reduction in DMF teeth after 3 years*
1. Control: annual prophylaxis only	170	5.15	3.62	–
2. Annual prophylaxis plus APF gel	182	4.96	3.06	15.6
3. Annual prophylaxis plus APF solution	167	5.05	2.68	26.8
4. Bi-annual prophylaxis plus APF solution	162	4.93	2.24	40.3

greatest reduction in caries increment was obtained with the APF solutions rather than the APF gels, in contrast to the findings of Ingraham and Williams (1970). The caries increment in the gel group was 15% lower than that in the control group which was not statistically significant. In absolute terms this meant a difference in DMF teeth increment of 0.6 teeth over a 3-year period, or a caries prevention of 0.2 teeth per person per year. The results for the APF solutions were more favourable; a bi-annual prophylaxis and APF solution application achieved a 40% reduction compared with that in the children in the control group who received an annual prophylaxis only. However, Horowitz (1969), in a discussion of the findings after 2 years, suggested that the extra work involved in carrying out 6-monthly applications may not be justified in terms of the extra caries reduction achieved. He reported that it would be necessary to treat approximately 6 children with the solution twice a year rather than once a year to prevent one more decayed tooth or surface. As each prophylaxis and application took approximately 30 min this means that one dentist or dental hygienist would have to work 3 extra hours a year to prevent one more decayed tooth or surface among 6 children.

The study by Horowitz and Doyle (1971) involved a large number of children from Hawaii, was meticulously reported, and lasted for a longer period of time than any previous topical fluoride study so far published. However, one aspect of the procedure which may have influenced the results was that after the prophylaxis and prior to the fluoride application the teeth were not thoroughly dried with cottonwool or air; instead the gel was applied to the teeth in wax trays after the children had removed as much saliva as they could from their mouths by rapid inspiration of air through clenched teeth. Initially this investigation involved approximately 1100 children aged 10–12 at the start of the study. By the third year the number of children who had been seen at each yearly examination had fallen to 681. Although the fluoride applications ceased at the end of the third year, a further series of examinations was carried out in 397 children 2½–3 years after the last fluoride treatment had been given in order to measure the long-term caries-preventive effect of APF agents. It was concluded that there was only a slight fall-off in caries protection throughout the post-treatment period (Horowitz, Doyle and Kan, 1971). This is the only study so far reported which has attempted to measure the long-term effect of APF agents applied topically either annually or semi-annually.

On the other hand, two studies have reported that application of aqueous NaF, acidulated APF or stannous fluoride produced insignificant reductions in caries increments compared with control groups. Averill, Averill and Ritz (1967), in a 2-year study in Rochester, New York, compared the caries-preventive effect of a 2% aqueous sodium fluoride solution, a 4% stannous fluoride solution and a 2% acidulated phosphate-buffered sodium fluoride solution (pH 4.4) used for topical application in 483 children initially aged 7–11 years old. Each agent was applied twice yearly. Children in the control group received topical applications of distilled water flavoured with wintergreen. The DMFS increment over the 2-year period was 4.4 in the control group, 3.9 in the aqueous NaF group, 4.1 in the SnF_2 group and 4.5 in the APF group.

Similar findings were reported by Cons, Janerich and Senning (1970), who carried out a 3-year study on 1948 7–8-year-old children from Albany, New York. The children were divided into five groups. Children in the control group had distilled water applied for 30 s; those in the stannous fluoride group had 8% SnF_2 applied for 4 min. Two APF agents were used, a solution and a gel; both contained 1.23% NaF at pH 3 in 0.1 M phosphoric acid and were applied for 4 min. All these children first received a prophylaxis with pumice, the teeth were then dried with compressed air and isolated cottonwool holders and salivary ejectors. The agent was applied annually and after treatment the children were asked to avoid eating, drinking or rinsing for 30 min. Children in the fifth group received a prophylaxis and then one series of four applications of 2% aqueous sodium fluoride after the method described by Knutson. At the end of the third year, 1412 children remained in the study. The results (Table 11.9) showed that, for DMF teeth only, the differences between gel and control groups were statistically significant ($P < 0.05$),

Table 11.9 Number of children, mean net increment and difference from control by group for permanent teeth and first molar surfaces, over a 3-year period (From Cons, Janerich and Senning, 1970)

Group	*No.*	*Increment*	*Difference*	*P*
TEETH				
Control	311	1.99	–	–
NaF	270	1.66	0.33	*
SnF_2	273	1.83	0.16	*
APF sol.	280	1.66	0.33	*
APF gel	278	1.50	0.49	<0.05
FIRST PERMANENT MOLAR SURFACES				
Control	311	3.82	–	–
NaF	270	3.41	0.41	*
SnF_2	273	3.52	0.30	*
APF sol.	280	3.88	−0.06	*
APF gel	278	3.14	0.68	*

* $P > 0.05$.

but the magnitude of the difference was less than 0.5 teeth per child, over the 3-year period. None of the treated groups differed significantly from the control when DMFS increments for first permanent molars were compared (Figure 11.1).

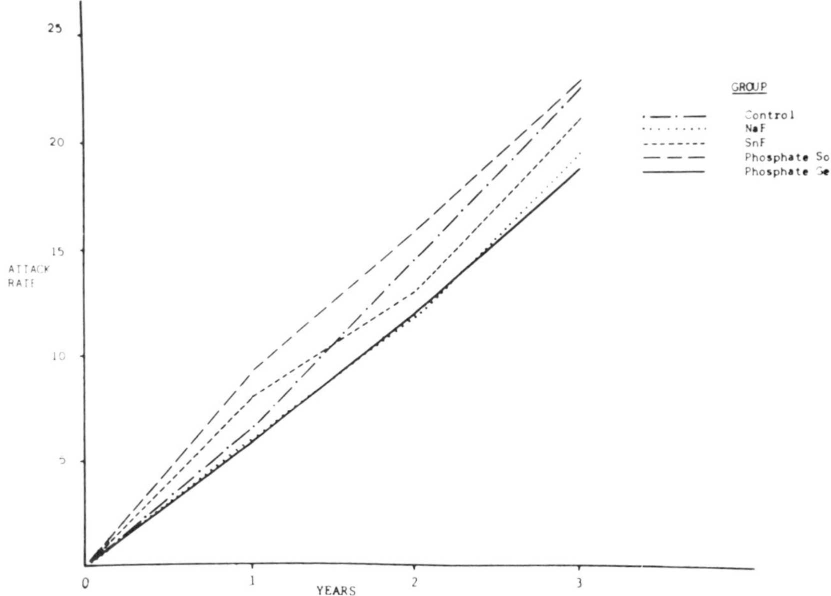

Figure 11.1 Percentage number of first permanent molar surfaces affected by caries over a 3-year period (From Cons *et al.*, 1970) (Copyright by the American Dental Association. Reprinted by permission)

The authors concluded that, considering their own results, together with a large number of other reports on topical fluoride, it was obvious that the mechanism by which topical fluoride retards cavitation is not yet fully understood. They suggested that additional laboratory and clinical research would be necessary to establish the superiority of any given fluoride preparation and the scheduling of topical applications. This conclusion is in accord with that reached by Horowitz and Heifetz (1970), who remarked that the results of the various studies using acidulated phosphate fluoride agents show that it can reduce the incidence of dental caries. However, further long-term studies are needed to determine the exact degree of caries reduction conferred by these agents and the best method and frequency of applying them. APF agents are stable in plastic containers and cause no tooth discoloration or gingival irritation.

Fluoride varnishes

In recent years, varnishes incorporating fluoride have been produced in an attempt to maintain the fluoride ion in intimate contact with the enamel surface for a longer period of time than is achieved by APF agents. Three materials have been used in clinical trials: Duraphat, Elmex Protector and Epoxylite 9070.

Fluoride lacquer, or Duraphat, was first used by Heuser and Schmidt (1968). This fluoride varnish yields 2.26% F^- from a suspension of sodium fluoride in an alcoholic solution of natural varnish substances. The manufacturers claim that it is remarkably water tolerant, so that it covers even moist teeth with a well-adhering film of varnish. Riethe and Weinmann (1970), using 75 Osborne–Mendel rats, reported that both Duraphat and an amine fluoride gel showed similar short-term caries-inhibitory properties in rats. Amine fluoride 297, similar to that used in Reithe and Weinmann's study, had a self-polymerizing polyurethane varnish added to it and was marketed under the name of Elmex Protector. Although amine fluoride has been shown to have caries-inhibitory properties when incorporated in a toothpaste (Marthaler, 1968), no large-scale clinical studies have been carried out to determine whether Elmex Protector has a caries-preventive effect. Rock (1974), in a 2-year study involving 100 children aged 11–13 years, concluded that this material was ineffective as a caries-preventive agent; after 2 years 19.3% of test teeth and 20.5% of control teeth became carious.

Epoxylite 9070 has been described as a long-lasting topical fluoride coating. The type of fluoride used in this preparation is disodium monofluorophosphate, which is incorporated into a soft, flexible, polyurethane-based adhesive coating. Before the Epoxylite 9070 coating is applied, a normal prophylaxis is carried out and then the tooth surfaces should be cleaned with an acid-based cleanser, Epoxylite Cavity Cleanser 9070-C. Although it has been claimed that Epoxylite 9070 has shown a reduction in caries in laboratory rats of up to 60% (Lee, Ocumpaugh and Swartz, 1972), Rock (1972), in a 1-year study of 11–13-year-old children, reported that Epoxylite 9070 produced no significant reduction in the incidence of occlusal caries between test and control group.

Duraphat

Following the early work on Duraphat by Heuser and Schmidt (1968), at least 80 articles on its properties have been published, mainly in the German literature, over the past 20 years.

In addition to the clinical trials of Duraphat as a caries-preventive agent, there have been a series of studies evaluating its effect from a physiological point of view, particularly measuring the fluoride uptake in enamel treated with Duraphat.

A variety of investigations have been concerned with fluoride uptake by enamel following Duraphat application. They can be divided into three groups:

1. *In vitro* studies. Non-carious teeth are extracted and experimental procedures carried out in the laboratory.
2. *In vivo–in vitro* studies. Teeth due to be extracted for orthodontic reasons have had Duraphat applied *in vivo*. After a varying time interval, the teeth are extracted and then F enamel investigations are carried out in the laboratory.
3. *In vivo* studies. Enamel biopsies, usually on the buccal surface of premolar teeth, are taken following Duraphat application.

In vitro studies

The uptake of fluoride by enamel exposed to a fluoride-containing varnish – Duraphat – for 1, 3, 6 and 12 h was studied *in vitro* by Koch and Petersson (1972). The experiment was carried out on 20 non-carious premolars extracted for orthodontic reasons. The enamel was etched with perchloric acid and the fluoride content measured with a specific ion electrode. The highest concentrations of fluoride were found in the outermost layer. In the experimental group, the mean concentration ranged between 2200 ppm F and 3800 ppm F, while the control group showed a value of 1150 ppm F.

The authors reported that the application of sodium fluoride in relatively high concentrations predisposes to the formation of readily soluble calcium fluorides on the surface of the enamel. The calcium fluoride formed has a strong tendency to be eliminated fairly soon – within 24 h – but the residual calcium fluoride may be gradually converted to fluoride apatite, particularly if the enamel is isolated from the oral environment for 16–24 h. Thus, over 18 years ago, one important property of Duraphat was recognized; because of its sticky varnish characteristic it could remain closely adhered to the surface for a long period. This observation was confirmed by Arends, Lodding and Petersson (1980) and Retief *et al.* (1983).

In vitro and *in vivo* studies

The problem of all *in vitro* studies is whether the laboratory studies are clinically relevant. In order to minimize this problem some investigators have applied a topical fluoride agent, allowed a short time period for excess topical material to be brushed away, then had the teeth extracted and subjected to analysis. Most studies of this type (Bang and Kim, 1973; Petersson, 1975, 1976; Grobler *et al.*, 1983; Ogaard *et al.*, 1984) reported an increase in fluoride concentration in enamel, up to a depth of 100 µm, following application of Duraphat.

In vivo studies

The third method of measuring fluoride uptake by enamel is the *in vivo* technique whereby enamel biopsies are taken, usually on the buccal aspect of premolar teeth. One of the first studies of this type involving Duraphat was carried out by Stamm (1974). He pointed out that the interaction between fluoride and human enamel is complex and not fully clarified. Generally, it is thought that one of two reactions takes place so that either fluorapatite or calcium fluoride are formed:

1. $Ca_{10}(PO_4)_6(OH)_2 + 2F\ Ca_{10}(PO_4)_6F_2 + 2OH^-$
2. $Ca_{10}(PO_4)_6(OH)_2 + 2OF\ 10CaF_2 + 6PO_4^3 + 2OH^-$

Most topical fluoride agents have a fluoride ion concentration of between 10 000 and 20 000 ppm which causes the second reaction to predominate forming crystals of calcium fluoride, while the first reaction, although more beneficial to the tooth, proceeds at a far slower rate.

The potential of Duraphat varnish was tested by Stamm (1974) using 35 dental students. Using random numbers, the subject's right or left maxillary arch was selected for treatment with the fluoride varnish; the untreated side acted as a control. The quadrant to be treated received a light prophylaxis with a non-fluoride paste and Duraphat applied. Warm air was blown for a few seconds onto the coated teeth and the patient was instructed not to brush his teeth for the next 12 h. After 5 weeks, the patient was recalled and received a light prophylaxis on both sides of the maxillary arch and an *in vivo* enamel biopsy was carried out. The results of the fluoride measurements showed that subjects differed greatly in their ability to incorporate fluoride into the outer layers of enamel. Overall, there was a mean increase of 591 ppm F on the treated side compared with the control side, 5 weeks after the topical application.

In summary, all studies measuring fluoride in enamel in patients treated with Duraphat have shown increases in fluoride concentration.

Clinical studies

The first human clinical investigations into the effect of Duraphat on caries incidence was published in 1968 by Heuser and Schmidt and this has been followed by many clinical trials over the past 20 years. The majority have been carried out in Germany and the Scandinavian countries; there has been one study from England and one from India, but none from the USA. Schmidt (1981) provided summary tables of Duraphat applications to deciduous and permanent teeth. These are reproduced in modified form (Tables 11.10 and 11.11) and give an overview of the scale of the studies and the range of caries reductions obtained. All the studies are of limited duration, usually 1–2 years.

Table 11.10 Duraphat varnish: summary of clinical studies on deciduous teeth

Reference	*Country*	*No. patients*	*Age* (yr)	*No. applications per year*	*Duration of study*	*Caries reduction* (%)
Hochstein *et al.* (1975)	GDR	94	3–4	1.5	2 yr	34
Murray *et al.* (1977)	England	302	5–6	2	2 yr	7.4
Holm (1979)	Sweden	225	3	2	2 yr	44
Treide *et al.* (1980)	GDR	110	pre-school	4	21 mo	26
Ulvestad (1978)*	Norway	103	7–11	2	2 yr	56*
Grodzka *et al.* (1982)	Poland	322	3	2	2 yr	9
Clark *et al.* (1985)	Canada	703	6–7	3	20 mo	7

* Includes first permanent molars – percentage reduction of approximal surfaces only.

Table 11.11 Duraphat varnish: summary of clinical studies on permanent teeth

Reference	*Country*	*No. patients*	*Age* (yr)	*No. applications per year*	*Duration of study*	*Caries reduction* (%)
Heuser and Schmidt (1968)	FRG	224	13–14	1	15 mo	30
Maiwald and Geiger (1973)	GDR	82	11	1	23 mo	10
		97	11	3	23 mo	46
Hetzer and Irmisch (1973)	GDR	139	9–10	2	3 yr	18–43
Winter (1975)	FRG	165	6	1	2 yr	37
Koch and Petersson (1975)	Sweden	60	15	2	1 yr	75
Murray *et al.* (1977)	England	302	5–6	2	2 yr	37
Leiser and Schmidt (1978)	FRG	366	10–12	2	3 yr	58
Maiwald *et al.* (1978)	Cuba	350	6–12	2	4½ yr	39
Koch and Petersson (1979)	Sweden	200	14	2	2 yr	30*
Seppa *et al.* (1982)	Finland	62	11–13	2	3 yr	30
Holm *et al.* (1984)	Sweden	109	5	2	2 yr	56†
Tewari *et al.* (1984)	India	645	6–12			73

* 30% reduction compared with a positive control group using a 0.2% NaF mouthrinse weekly.
† 65% reduction in fissure caries in first permanent molars.

Heuser and Schmidt (1968) concluded that a 30% reduction occurred in the incidence of caries 15 months after a single application of Duraphat. A contrary result was reported by Maiwald and Geiger (1973) who tested Duraphat in 179 children aged 11 years. A total of 174 children of similar age acted as a control. After 23 months they reported that the varnish had no effect on caries incidence if applied once a year, but a reduction of 45% was obtained when the varnish was used every 4 months. Koch and Petersson (1975) studied the effect of semi-annual applications of Duraphat to the teeth of 60 15-year-old children over a period of 1 year. Sixty-two children of similar age acted as a control group. All these children were exposed to the local dental health programme of mouthrinsing with 0.2% NaF solution every fortnight. Before the varnish was applied, all teeth were cleaned with pumice and rubber cap and the approximal surfaces were also cleaned with dental floss and toothpicks. A clinical and radiographic examination of all children was performed immediately prior to the first application of varnish and repeated 1 year later. In the test group, the mean DMFS score was 31.0 at baseline and this increased to 31.9 at the first-year examination. The baseline score for the control group (27.4) was lower than the test group, but increased to 31.3 by the end of the first year. The mean percentage reduction in caries increment was approximately 75%. The percentage reduction of occlusal surfaces was similar to that recorded on approximal and free smooth surfaces. The authors suggested that the excellent effects on the occlusal surfaces might be the result of the adhesiveness of the varnish and concluded that the short time needed for application, and the low application frequency, make the varnish practical as a preventive measure.

Murray, Winter and Hurst (1977), in a 2-year study, measured the effect of Duraphat applied to the teeth of 446 children initially aged 5 years. The results showed an 8.4% reduction in the deciduous dentition and a 33% reduction in the permanent dentition.

The first 2-year study to be reported from Scandinavia appeared in 1979. Koch, Petersson and Ryden (1979), in Sweden, compared the caries increment in school children exposed to Duraphat every 6 months and in children receiving the conventional weekly fluoride mouthrinsing programme with 0.2% sodium fluoride over a 2-year period. Two hundred 14-year-old children, divided into test and control, participated in the study and were examined clinically and radiographically every year. The caries increment was 30% lower in the Duraphat group compared with the mouthrinsing group (the traditional preventive method being used in Sweden at that time).

Holm (1979) studied the effect of Duraphat applied to 112 3-year-old children every 6 months; 113 children of similar age acted as controls. No placebo treatment was performed in the control group. Annual caries examinations were carried out and bitewing radiographs were taken. The results after 2 years showed an average increment of 2.1 surfaces in the test group and 3.7 in the control group, a difference of 44%.

A further study on the effectiveness of Duraphat when applied to 6–7-year-old children was carried out in Canada (Clark *et al.*, 1985). A total of 703 children were divided into three groups – a Duraphat group, a Fluor Protector group and a control. The study was double blind – neither the examiners nor the participants were aware of group assignment. Clinical procedures were performed by four dental hygienists working specially for the project. Results after 20 months showed that both varnishes had a similar effect compared with the control. Results for deciduous molars showed a 6.9% reduction for Duraphat. These authors also commented: 'The use of fluoride varnishes in Europe is widespread but in North America acceptance has been slow. Based on consideration of effectiveness, safety and practicality one might anticipate increased interest in these agents in North America as the scientific evidence continues to document their effectiveness in caries prevention.'

In summary, the results from 16 clinical studies on children aged 3–15 years suggest that: (a) all studies where Duraphat has been applied more than once a year have shown a caries inhibitory effect; (b) caries reduction achieved has been at least as good as with any other topical fluoride; (c) nearly all the studies have been of limited duration.

Comparison of Duraphat and mouthrinsing

Kirkegaard *et al.* (1986), from Denmark, compared the effect of applying Duraphat every 6 months with a fluoride rinse every second week during the school year, over a 5-year period. Children assigned to have Duraphat applied used a placebo rinse fortnightly; children using a fluoride rinse had a placebo varnish applied every 6 months. For teeth erupted at baseline, after 5 years a 7% difference in favour of the fluoride-rinsing group was found (2.96 DMFS compared with 2.77 DMFS). For teeth erupting during the trial, a 4% difference in favour of the fluoride varnish was found.

A different result was reported by Seppa and Pollanen (1987) from Finland. In their 2-year study, the DMFS increment was markedly lower for the Duraphat group (6.38) compared with the rinsing group (10.37). No placebo was used in this study, so children were randomized by school classes, which resulted in an imbalance between the groups at baseline. The authors pointed out that the caries increments in this study were exceptionally high and therefore the difference between the groups would probably have been smaller in children with lower caries activity. Nevertheless, because the varnish application requires less cooperation, it may be more suitable for caries-risk children.

Combinations of topical fluoride therapy

Combinations of fluoride toothpaste with mouthrinses (Ashley *et al.*, 1977; Triol *et al.*, 1980) and topical gel applications (Lind *et al.*, 1974; Luoma *et al.*, 1978; Mainwaring and Naylor, 1978) have been investigated. The effect on 2-year dental caries increment of a 0.02% APF rinse (100 ppm F^-) (Ashley *et al.*, 1977) and a sodium monofluorophosphate toothpaste (0.76% MFP, yielding 1000 ppm F^-) was assessed, both alone and in combination, in a double-blind controlled clinical trial in a low-fluoride community. Although the greatest reduction in caries (27%, 1.5 DFS/child) occurred in the group receiving both fluoride toothpaste and fluoride rinse, there was no statistical difference among the three experimental groups (fluoride toothpaste alone showed a saving of 1.2 DFS/child and fluoride mouthrinses alone gave a saving of 0.8 DFS/child over the 2-year period).

A 2½-year trial involving the use of an MFP toothpaste in combination with a range of mouthrinses containing 0, 0.025, 0.05 or 0.1% sodium fluoride concluded that there was an additive effect (Triol *et al.*, 1980). The greatest reduction occurred with the most concentrated fluoride rinse, but the difference among the three fluoride mouthrinsing groups was not statistically significant.

Two 3-year studies concluded that the unsupervised use of Na MFP toothpaste was as effective in reducing caries as twice annual, professionally applied, treatments of APF gel. Further, the reductions in caries obtained by the combined use of fluoride toothpaste and gel applications were not significantly greater than the use of fluoride toothpaste or gel applications alone (Lind *et al.*, 1974; Mainwaring and Naylor, 1978). In contrast a 2-year study, involving the use of stannous fluoride alone, annual APF application alone and both treatments in combination (but no placebo group), concluded that there was no difference between the single therapy groups, but that the combined therapy produced significantly less caries and therefore had an additive effect (Luoma *et al.*, 1978). All these studies were carried out in low-fluoride areas.

Horowitz (1980) gave information on studies conducted by the National Institute of Dental Research into combinations of fluoride procedures. One study concerned a combination of APF gel self-application and NaF fluoride rinsing in a fluoride area. The children in the test group applied APF gel (1.23% F) in custom-fitted trays on 5 consecutive days, three times during the first year of the study – a total of 15 gel-tray treatments. In addition, they rinsed for 1 min once a week in school for 3 school years with a 0.2% NaF solution. Children in the control group engaged only in mouthrinsing with a placebo solution (Heifetz *et al.*, 1979). After 30 months, 131 children in the test group had developed 30% fewer DMF surfaces, in teeth present in the mouth at the time of the baseline examination, than 135 children in the control group. It was concluded that although the gel-tray procedure used was expensive and may lack economic practicality, the findings of the study corroborate the effectiveness of self-administered topical fluoride procedures in an optimally fluoridated community.

Horowitz (1980) concluded that 'there is increasing evidence that various combinations of fluoride agents produce additive anticariogenic effects. In order to achieve maximal caries protection, additional studies should be done to determine other effective combinations of fluoride and to verify the effects of those that have already been tested. It is also important to learn the contribution of the various components of the combinations to the total cariogenic effect'. It must be borne in mind that as sales of fluoride toothpastes presently comprise 80% of total toothpaste sales in the USA and over 95% in the UK, all current studies of various fluoride combinations inherently represent evaluations of combined fluoride therapies, assuming that the participants continue to use a dentifrice of their choice.

Topical fluoride therapy for high-risk groups

The need to target professionally applied topical fluoride therapy to patients at increased risk of developing dental caries has been considered by a number of authors (e.g. Shannon, 1982; Katz, 1982). Two groups – the orthodontic patients undergoing fixed appliance treatment, and patients who have received radiotherapy for head and neck malignancy – have been recognized. The need for meticulous oral hygiene and topical fluoride therapy has frequently been stated, but there have been relatively few studies measuring the effectiveness of topical fluoride therapy in such high-risk groups.

Thirty-five cancer patients who had been treated with radiotherapy to the head and neck, supplemented in some cases by chemotherapy, were divided into three groups (Katz, 1982):

Group 1 received topical application of 1% NaF + 1% chlorhexidine, at weekly intervals for 4 weeks. In addition, they were instructed to rinse daily for 1 min with 0.05% NaF–0.2% chlorhexidine mouthrinse.
Group 2 used the same rinse as group 1, but received no topical application.
Group 3 received four topical applications of APF gel and also used a 0.05% NaF mouthrinse daily.

The patients' oral health at the start of radiotherapy was not good – all groups had evidence of untreated caries (Table 11.12).

Table 11.12 Oral health status of patients undergoing radiotherapy (From Katz, 1982)

Group	*No. patients*	*Mean age* (yr)	*Caries status at start of radiotherapy*		*Caries increment after 6–10 months topical therapy*	
			DMFT	*DT*	*DMFT*	*DFS*
1	16	46.8	15.9	5.1	−1.44	−1.81
2	8	52.6	16.0	4.6	0.12	0.12
3	11	53.8	14.4	2.7	1.45	1.91

At the end of the study it was concluded that four applications of a combined sodium fluoride–chlorhexidine solution, plus daily rinses with a combined solution, prevented radiation caries completely and also resulted in the remineralization of incipient existing lesions. Use of the chlorhexidine–fluoride rinses alone also stopped radiation caries but did not permit remineralization to occur. Use of a fluoride gel and daily rinses with a 0.05% sodium fluoride solution was not sufficient to prevent radiation caries.

Wright *et al.* (1985) describe a sequence of dental care for patients who are receiving radiation or chemotherapy at the National Institute of Dental Research clinic. Patients scheduled to receive head and neck radiation therapy are routinely provided with custom vinyl trays to deliver self-applied topical fluoride to the teeth. Daily applications of 1.1% sodium fluoride or 0.4% stannous fluoride to the teeth for 5 min during the 5–6-week radiation treatment period is recommended. The frequency of F-gel application may be reduced to two or three times a week after therapy is completed. Although no data are presented, the authors concluded that a variety of potential oral sequelae associated with cancer therapy can be prevented, reduced in severity or palliatively alleviated when the dental team has an opportunity to participate in the patient's care.

Gorelick, Geiger and Gwinnett (1982) measured the incidence of white spot formation in patients receiving fixed appliance orthodontic treatment and compared them with children who had not received any orthodontic treatment. Twenty-four per cent of children, and 3.6% of teeth, in the control group, had slight white spot formation. In comparison, 50% of children, immediately after debonding, had white spot formation on at least one tooth and 10.8% of teeth had white spots. Maxillary lateral incisors showed the highest incidence of decalcification. None of these children had received topical fluoride therapy. Mizrahi (1982), in a cross-sectional study, also concluded that orthodontic treatment with multi-banded appliances contributed to the development of enamel demineralization. A number of workers then introduced a topical fluoride programme for patients undergoing fixed appliance therapy in order to try to reduce the problem of demineralization.

Geiger *et al.* (1988) examined the effect of a fluoride programme initiated for all their fixed appliance orthodontic patients following their 1982 study. APF gel was applied in the surgery about 3 min after brackets had been bonded and was allowed to remain on the teeth for 3–5 min. The gel was then removed by a spray or rinse of 0.05% NaF solution. The sodium fluoride solution was prescribed as a mouthrinse to be used at night, just before bedtime. There were 101 subjects involved in the study, one-third of whom had one or more teeth with white spot formation. Of the 1567 teeth examined, 117 (7.5%) had some white spots. Lack of compliance in the fluoride programme was associated with an increase in the occurrence of white spot lesions (Table 11.13).

Table 11.13 Number of subjects with white spots after fixed appliance therapy with varying degrees of compliance in a topical fluoride programme (From Geiger *et al.*, 1988)

	Participation in a topical fluoride programme			
	Excellent	*Partial*	*Poor*	*Total*
No. in group	27	21	53	101
No. with white spots	4	9	21	34
Per cent	17	43	40	34

The authors concluded that the single application of topical fluoride immediately after bonding had little or no beneficial effect, but that there was a need for a fluoride rinse to be used continuously during treatment.

The problem of white spot lesions following orthodontic treatment was emphasized by Ogaard (1989). In a study of 19-year-olds, he showed that white spot lesions were significantly higher in the orthodontic group than in the untreated group, and furthermore, these lesions may present an aesthetic problem even more than 5 years after treatment. All orthodontic patients were asked to rinse daily with a 0.05% NaF solution and to use a fluoride toothpaste, but no supervised programmes were carried out.

These studies highlight the fact that white spot lesions associated with fixed appliance therapy may be very resistant to remineralization. If topical fluoride therapy is to be of any value for orthodontic patients, excellent cooperation is required and a systematic fluoride preventive regimen should be followed (Saloum and Sondhi, 1987).

Fluoride prophylactic pastes and dental caries

In vitro investigations have shown that small but significant amounts of enamel (approximately 4 μm) can be removed when a thorough prophylaxis is carried out with commercially available prophylactic pastes containing the usual abrasive systems (pumice, silica dioxide, zirconium silicate, alumina) (Vrbic, Brudevold and McCann, 1967; Vrbic and Brudevold, 1970; Stearns, 1973). This loss of surface enamel is undesirable because the surface enamel contains the highest concentrations of fluoride. Fluoride compounds have been incorporated into prophylactic pastes to try to maintain a high fluoride concentration in the surface enamel and to determine whether, in combination with topical fluoride applications, an additional caries-inhibitory effect can be obtained. The following agents have been incorporated into prophylactic pastes: sodium fluoride, stannous fluoride, acidulated phosphate fluoride, stannous hexafluorozirconate.

Pastes containing sodium fluoride

Investigations of fluoride prophylactic pastes can be traced to 1946. Bibby *et al.* (1946) evaluated a paste containing 1% NaF and pumice in a small group of children and reported a caries increment reduction of 25–43%, depending on the number of treatments given. A second study by the same investigator (Bibby, 1948), with 250 participants in a 1-year study with the above formula, did not confirm the findings.

Pastes containing stannous fluoride

With the development of stannous fluoride as a recognized anti-cariogenic agent, investigations were carried out to determine its effectiveness when incorporated in a prophylactic paste. Initial *in vitro* experiments carried out at Indiana University in the USA reported significant reductions in enamel solubility with application of stannous fluoride–pumice prophylactic pastes (Mericle and Muhler, 1963; Whitehurst, Stookey and Muhler, 1968). The reduction in enamel solubility when a stannous fluoride paste was applied was confirmed by tests investigating an alternative abrasive system of silex–silicone (Segreto, Harris and Hester, 1961; Wolf, 1964). A clinical study to evaluate the effectiveness of this formulation showed that the paste was as effective in preventing dental caries as an 8% topical stannous fluoride solution, but no added benefit resulted from following the prophylaxis by a topical application (Peterson, Jordan and Snyder, 1963). The investigators suggested that the failure to achieve additional benefits by combined use of the agents might be due to the silicone in the paste forming an anti-wetting film on the tooth surface, thus serving as a barrier to the action of the subsequent topical applications.

Another abrasive, lava pumice, was said to be superior as a cleansing agent and more compatible chemically with stannous fluoride than previously tried abrasive systems (Dudding and Muhler, 1962; Mericle and Muhler, 1963). Using an 8.9% stannous fluoride–lava pumice paste, Bixler and Muhler (1966) reported average reductions of 34% of DMF increments at the end of 1 year for children aged 5–18 years receiving two applications of this prophylactic paste at 6-monthly intervals. Another group in the same study, who were treated with a topical application of an 8% stannous fluoride solution as well as the stannous fluoride prophylactic paste, demonstrated an even greater reduction (approximately 45% DMF surfaces) when the results of the two examiners were averaged. Scola and Ostrom (1968) also investigated semi-annual application of the prophylactic paste followed by a topical application of a 10% stannous fluoride solution and routine use of a 0.4% stannous fluoride dentifrice, in US Navy personnel. They reported a significant reduction in caries increment with combined use of applications. However, in the group treated with only stannous fluoride–lava pumice prophylactic paste, a minimal reduction (12% fewer DMF surfaces) was reported which was not statistically significant.

In contrast, Horowitz and Lucye (1966) failed to demonstrate the preventive effect of a stannous fluoride–lava pumice paste or a combination of the paste and topical application of an 8% solution of stannous fluoride in a 2-year study using annual applications for children aged 8–10 years. Independent laboratory investigations by Vrbic, Brudevold and McCann (1967) demonstrated minimal uptake of the fluoride ion by enamel from pastes of stannous fluoride–pumice, due to fluoride complexing. These results were confirmed by Mellberg and Nicholson (1968) in further *in vitro* investigations. These workers also observed a rapid loss of available free fluoride ion with time, and an associated increase in pH to approximate neutrality when using this formulation.

A further abrasive system, zirconium silicate, was shown in clinical and laboratory studies to have superior cleaning properties to pumice and subsequent polishing of the tooth surface treated (Muhler, Dudding and Stookey, 1964; Stookey, Hudson and Muhler, 1966). Its superior reliability as an abrasive system was reported to be related to its action being self-limiting owing to particle size reduction during the period of application. Mellberg and Nicholson (1968) found a smaller loss in available free fluoride and increase in pH when zirconium silicate was used in combination with stannous fluoride, as opposed to lava pumice.

In 1970, Muhler and colleagues published results of an investigation of annual self-application of a 9% stannous fluoride–zirconium silicate prophylactic paste in children aged 6–14 years (Muhler *et al.*, 1970). The paste was applied with a soft toothbrush under supervision of a dentist. Results after 1 year reported a statistically significant reduction in caries increment for the test group of one surface per child despite large losses of subjects, particularly in the test group. Lang *et al.* (1970) reported reductions of 2 surfaces per child in 18 months with 6-monthly self-applications of the same formula for children aged 6–10 years living in an area with an optimum level of fluoride in the water. In contrast, Gunz (1971), using the same technique and formulation of prophylactic paste as Muhler *et al.* (1970), found no difference in caries increment between the test and control groups after one application. The examination was carried out 14 months after the application, but it is unlikely that the slightly greater length of time between application and re-examination explained the negative findings.

Mellberg and Nicholson (1968) considered further the problem of a compatible abrasive system. The results of their *in vitro* study suggested that an abrasive system of insoluble metaphosphate was not associated with any loss of free fluoride ions from the formula, nor any increase in pH values. Vrbic and Brudevold (1970) found this abrasive system removed significantly less enamel when used in a prophylactic paste. However, while it is less deleterious to the tooth surface than all the other abrasives tested, it is inadequate in practice for the removal of all exogenous tooth stains, and would necessitate the use of two pastes – one with a more abrasive quality for heavy stain removal, and an insoluble metaphosphate paste for routine use.

More recently, 3 studies testing the effectiveness of twice-yearly self-application of 9–10% SnF_2 prophylactic paste have been published (Gish *et al.*, 1975; Woodhouse, 1978; Beiswanger *et al.*, 1980). Each study lasted 3 years. While Gish and colleagues reported statistically significant reductions of 25% (1.3 surfaces) for children living in a fluoridated area and 37% (2.0 surfaces) for children living in a low-fluoride area, the reductions in caries increment were lower (16% reduction in DMFS) in the trial of Woodhouse, and no caries reduction was recorded by Beiswanger and co-workers.

In 1969, 250 000 Californian schoolchildren began a school-based preventive programme which involved annual 'brush-ins' with 9% SnF_2 (Zircate) prophylactic paste. The effectiveness of the programme was monitored by Horowitz and Bixler (1976) over a 3-year period. They state that 'the findings of this study are inconclusive and neither fully refute nor support the efficacy of annual self-application of a stannous fluoride–zirconium silicate paste in preventing dental caries.' Zircate (9% SnF_2) paste has now been withdrawn from the market (Beiswanger *et al.*, 1980).

Pastes containing acidulated phosphate fluoride

Following evidence documenting the efficacy of professionally applied acidulated phosphate fluoride in solution and gel forms, Peterson *et al.* (1969) conducted a 2-year study with children aged 11–13 years in a fluoridated and non-fluoridated community to determine the caries-inhibitory effectiveness of freshly prepared acidulated phosphate fluoride–lava pumice prophylactic paste applied annually. The active agent used was potassium fluoride dihydrate giving a concentration of 2.1% fluoride ions. Two examiners independently examined the entire study population: both consistently found only slightly smaller caries increments in the treated groups than in the control groups in both communities. The differences between test and control groups were not statistically significant except those recorded by one examiner in the non-fluoride area only, who found a reduction of one surface per child in 2 years for the test group relative to the control group ($P < 0.05$). The authors suggested this minimal caries inhibition might be attributed to the neutralization of the acid phosphate fluoride reduction in the paste by the pumice abrasive.

In vitro studies by Mellberg and Nicholson (1968), to determine a stable formulation with good cleaning properties and fluoride deposition in enamel, found a formulation of silicone dioxide paste incorporating (in the liquid phase) 1.2% fluoride ion and having a pH of 3.2 to be adequate. An investigation of this paste was reported by de Paola and Mellberg (1973). The paste was applied semi-annually by dental hygienists for children aged 10–13 years for 2 years. The teeth were given a thorough prophylaxis with a placebo paste prior to application of the fluoride paste which was applied and left for 4 min. The active ingredient in the paste was ammonium fluorosilicate giving 1.2% fluoride, and 0.1 M phosphate from monobasic sodium phosphate. At the end of the first year, significant reductions of half a surface of a tooth per child were observed in the test group, while at the end of 2 years a reduction of one surface per child was found. For teeth erupting during the study, a reduction in caries increment in the test group of half a surface per child over the 2-year period was reported.

The results of 1 year's use of the same ammonium silicofluoride (1.2% F) paste (pH 3.0) were reported by Schutz, Forrester and Balis (1974). The subjects of the study were 3–5-year-old children living in fluoridated Baltimore attending a dental clinic for twice-yearly applications of the APF paste. A 9% (0.14 surface) reduction was reported after 1 year.

Pastes containing hexafluorozirconate

Researchers at Indiana University developed a new compound, stannous hexafluorozirconate, which was reported to be effective in reducing the acid solubility of enamel and reducing dental caries. The original data from preliminary *in vitro* and laboratory experiments have not been published. Independent *in vitro* investigations of this compound by Shannon (1969) confirmed that hexafluoro-zirconate did reduce enamel solubility. Results of two preliminary investigations with children who received semi-annual topical applications of stannous hexafluorozirconate showed decided reduction in dental caries (Muhler, Bixler and Stookey, 1968). Concentrations of 16% and 24% stannous hexafluorozirconate in solution with semi-annual applications showed a 16% lower incidence of DMF surfaces for the latter concentration after 12 months. However, the number and magnitude of negative incremental caries scores that appear in the data are disconcerting. Results have not been substantiated by independent investigators.

Horowitz and Heifetz (1970) have reported toxic reactions after use of stannous hexafluorozirconate in a zirconium silicate prophylactic paste. Irritation and subsequent inflammation of the gingiva occurred, and in extreme cases frank necrosis of the soft tissue was produced (Peterson *et al.*, 1967). Muhler, Bixler and Stookey (1968) reported no toxic reactions in study participants with application of the same formula, provided that there was careful preparation of the solution, allowing complete dissolution of the compound to permit part of the tin to be chemically stabilized by forming complexes with zirconium. Muhler maintained that lack of care in preparation of stannous hexafluorozircinate gave a high concentration of tin in the paste, which was responsible for the adverse soft-tissue reactions.

Pilot studies of self-administration of stannous fluoride–zirconium silicate pastes in the USA as a public health measure have reported that 48% of the children who treated themselves with the paste experienced disturbing systematic reactions, such as nausea, vomiting and headaches (Horowitz and Heifetz, 1970).

Controlled professional applications of prophylactic pastes have reported few toxic reactions. As with all topical applications of stannous fluoride, a prophylactic paste containing this compound was found to give transitory blanching and minor irritation of the gingivae in some studies, as well as a degree of staining of the teeth. As one of the major functions of a prophylactic paste is cleansing and stain removal, this latter side-effect detracted from the acceptability of this active ingredient, unless staining effects were modified. The results of the clinical trials with fluoride prophylactic pastes published to date (summarized in Table 11.14) have not established beyond doubt that 6-monthly or yearly prophylaxes with these agents result in caries inhibition.

Incorporation of fluoride into restorative materials

In 1969, Hallsworth and Weatherell examined sections cut from two upper permanent incisors with silicate restorations. They reported that sound enamel directly exposed to the material had a very high fluoride content, whereas that separated from the silicate by even a thin barrier of dentine tended to possess the low concentrations typical of interior enamel (Figure 11.2). They concluded that their findings supported the suggestion that silicate cements have cariostatic properties, probably due to their fluoride content which can be as high as 130 000 ppm.

Table 11.14 Clinical trials of prophylactic pastes containing fluoride

Investigators	*Active ingredient*	*Abrasive system*	*Duration*			*Application*	*Statistically significant reductions*		
			pH	(yr)	*Age*		*Tooth surfaces*	%	*P*
Bibby *et al.* (1946)	1% NaF + H_2O_2	Pumice	4.0	1	(a) 6–15	(a) Semi-annual	*	25	*
					(b) 6–14	(b) 3 times/year	*	42	*
Bibby (1948)	1% NaF + H_2O_2			1	6–15	3 times/year	–	–	–
Gish and Muhler (1965)	8.9% SnF_2	Lava pumice	*	1	6–14	Annual	1–2	39–41	<0.0001
Bixler and Muhler (1966)	8.9% SnF_2		*	3	5–18	Semi-annual	3–4	29–38	0.001
Horowitz and Lucye (1966)	8.9% SnF_2		*	2	8–10	Annual	–	–	–
Peterson *et al.* (1963)	17.5% SnF_2	Silex		2		(a) Semi-annual	*	42	*
						(b) Annual	*	34	*
Scola and Ostrom (1968)	17.5% SnF_2	Lava pumice	*	2	19–20	Semi-annual	–	–	–
Muhler *et al.* (1970)	9% SnF_2	Zirconium silicate	*	1	6–14	Annual	1	64	<0.001
Lang *et al.* (1970)	9% SnF_2			1½	6–10	Semi-annual	2	38–42	
Gunz (1971)	9% SnF_2			1⅙		Annual	–	–	–
Peterson *et al.* (1969)	Potassium fluoride dihydrate (2.1% F) + 4.6% orthophosphoric acid	Lava pumice	*	2	11–13	Annual			
						(a) Fluoride area	(a) –	–	–
						(b) Non-fluoride area	(b) 1	21	0.05
de Paola and Mellberg (1973)	Ammonium fluorosilicate (1.2% F) + 0.1 M phosphate solution	Silica	3.2	2	10–13	Semi-annual	1	21	<0.01

* Data not given.

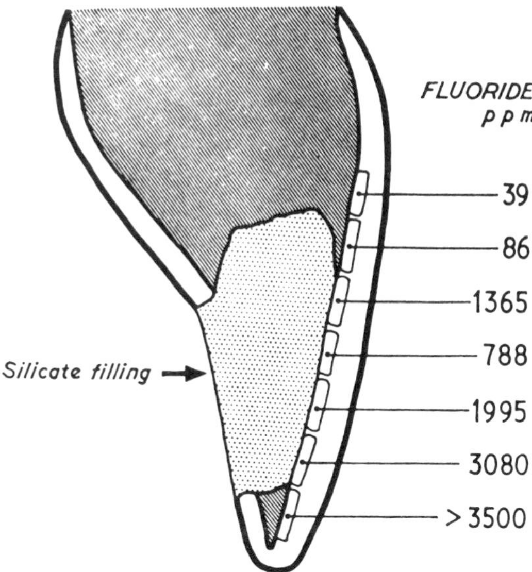

Figure 11.2 Distribution of fluoride in the interior enamel of an upper central permanent incisor from a 17-year-old female. The fluoride concentration of enamel in contact with the silicate restoration was relatively high (From Hallsworth and Weatherell, 1969, by permission)

A comparison of fluoride release from glass ionomer fillings and luting cements, against silicate cement and polycarboxylate cement, was made by Swartz, Phillips and Clark (1984). They found (Figures 11.3 and 11.4) that fluoride released from the glass ionomer cements throughout the 1-year period was similar, both in quantity and pattern, to that released by the silicate cement, whereas the amount of fluoride released by the polycarboxylate cement was negligible after the first few days. They concluded that glass ionomer cements probably possess anti-cariogenic properties similar to those of silicate cement. Broadly similar findings were reported by Meryon and Smith (1984) and Muzynski *et al.* (1988).

Fluoride has also been added to amalgam with the hope of reducing secondary caries around amalgam restorations. Heintze and Mörnstad (1980) suggested that there was less evidence of demineralization around fluoride-containing amalgam restorations, as against cavities restored with conventional or dispersed amalgam. These studies were on extracted teeth, subjected to acidified gelatin gel for 10 weeks. Petersson *et al.* (1985) carried out a 1-year prospective clinical trial of 196 fillings placed in contralateral cavities in primary and permanent teeth. Half the cavities were restored with amalgam containing stannous fluoride yielding 0.5% F and half with a conventional non γ 2 amalgam. The restorations were observed for 4 years, after which no significant differences were found between the two test amalgams. However, the low number of cases of secondary caries occurring during the test period prevented any conclusion about the possible preventive effect of fluoride-supplemented amalgam from being drawn.

More recently, Skartveit *et al.* (1990) reported the results of six primary teeth that had been restored with fluoride-containing materials. These teeth exfoliated naturally and so it was possible to register and compare the amount of fluoride assimilated and retained in the cavity walls. Two of the teeth had been restored

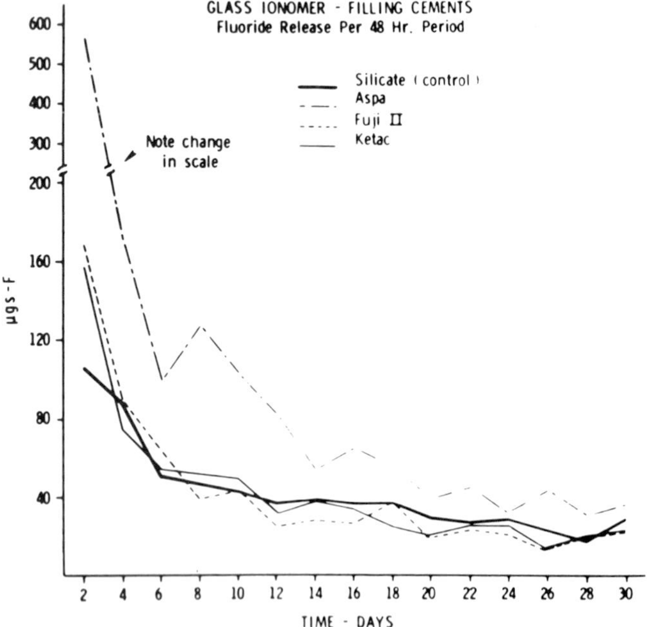

Figure 11.3 Average fluoride release from filling cements during each 48 h over a 30-day period immediately following specimen preparation (From Swartz, Phillips and Clark, 1984, by kind permission of the Editor, *Journal of Dental Research*)

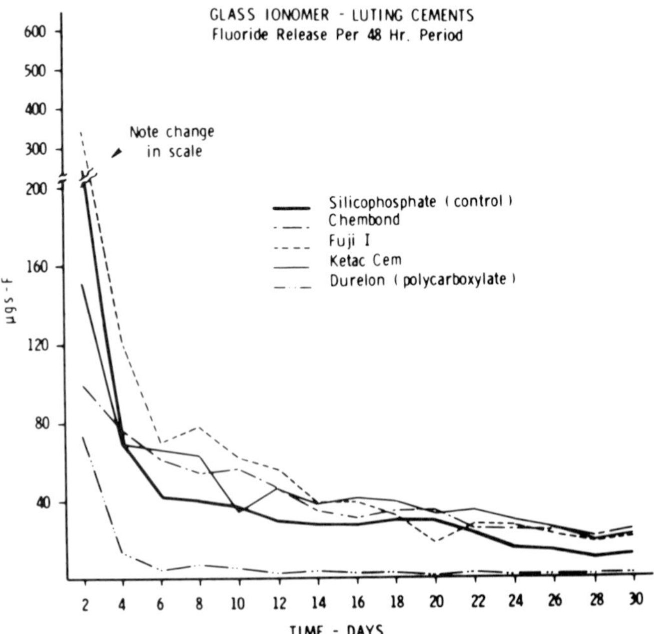

Figure 11.4 Average fluoride release from luting cements during each 48 h over a 30-day period immediately following specimen preparation (From Swartz, Phillips and Clark, 1984, by kind permission of the Editor, *Journal of Dental Research*)

with fluor alloy which contains 1% stannous fluoride; the other four teeth were restored with glass ionomer cement (Fuji III) which contains 11.3% fluoride in the powder. Three primary molars restored with conventional fluoride-free amalgam were collected as a control. In the glass ionomer group, the fluoride concentration ranged from 1.2% to 3.8% in dentine, compared with 0.6–0.9% for the fluoride amalgam group. In the control group none of the specimens showed fluoride concentrations exceeding the detection limit, which was 0.15% by weight.

An authoritative summary of the subject was prepared by Phillips (1988) for the Council on Dental Materials, Instruments and Equipment of the American Dental Association. He pointed out that the mere presence of fluoride in a product will not in itself be effective as there must be a fluoride-release mechanism in the restorative formulation to act in a caries-resistance mode. One of the drawbacks in using *in vitro* data as predictors for an anti-cariogenic effect is that the precise minimal amounts of fluoride uptake or of fluoride leach necessary to achieve caries resistance have not been established. Phillips continued: 'Furthermore, addition of fluoride should not compromise the desirable properties of the material. For example, the fluoride leach could influence essential properties such as strength or solubility of a cement or resin, or the corrosion resistance of an alloy. Ultimately, a meaningful evaluation of the anti-caries capability of fluoride additives invariably awaits the augmentation of *in vivo* documentation.'

References

Arends, J., Lodding, A. and Petersson, L. G. (1980) Fluoride uptake in enamel. *Caries Res.,* **14**, 403–413

Arnold, F. A. Jun., Dean, H. T. and Singleton, D. W. Jun. (1944) Effect on caries incidence of a single topical application of a fluoride solution to the teeth of young adult males of a military population. *J. Dent. Res.,* **23**, 155

Ashley, F. P., Mainwaring, P. J., Emslie, R. D. and Naylor, M. N. (1977) Clinical testing of a mouthrinse and a dentifrice containing fluoride. *Br. Dent. J.,* **143**, 333–338

Averill, H. M., Averill, J. E. and Ritz, A. G. (1967) A two year comparison of three topical fluoride agents. *J. Am. Dent. Assoc.,* **74**, 996–1001

Bang, S. and Kim, Y. J. (1973) Electron microprobe analysis of human tooth enamel coated *in vivo* with fluoride-varnish. *Helv. Odontol. Acta,* **17**, 84–88

Beiswanger, B. B., Mercer, V. H., Billings, R. J. and Stookey, G. K. (1980) A clinical caries evaluation of a stannous fluoride prophylactic paste and solution. *J. Dent. Res.,* **59**, 1386–1391

Bergman, G. (1953) The caries inhibiting action of sodium fluoride. Experimental studies. *Acta Odontol. Scand.,* **11**, suppl. 12

Bibby, B. G. (1943) The effect of sodium fluoride applications on dental caries. *J. Dent. Res.,* **22**, 207

Bibby, B. G. (1947) A consideration of the effectiveness of various fluoride mixtures. *J. Am. Dent. Assoc.,* **34**, 26

Bibby, B. G. (1948) Fluoride mouthwashes, fluoride dentifrices and other uses of fluorides in control of caries. *J. Dent. Res.,* **27**, 367–373

Bibby, B. G., Zander, H., Mckelleget, M. and Labunsky, B. (1946) Preliminary reports on the effects on dental caries of the use of sodium fluoride in a prophylactic cleaning mixture and in a mouthwash. *J. Dent. Res.,* **25**, 207–211

Bixler, D. and Muhler, J. C. (1966) Effect on dental caries in children in a nonfluoride area of combined use of three agents containing stannous fluoride: a prophylactic paste, a solution, and a dentifrice. II. Results after 24 and 36 months. *J. Am. Dent. Assoc.,* **72**, 392–396

Brudevold, F., McCann, H. G., Nilsson, R., Richardson, B. and Coklica, V. (1967) The chemistry of caries inhibition problems and challenges in topical treatments. *J. Dent. Res.,* **46**, 37

Brudevold, F., Savory, A., Gardner, D. E., Spinelli, M. and Speirs, R. (1967) A study of acidulated fluoride solutions I. *In vitro* effects on enamel. *Arch. Oral Biol.,* **8**, 167

Bryan, E. T. and Williams, J. E. (1968) The cariostatic effectiveness of a phosphate-fluoride gel administered annually to schoolchildren. *J. Public Health Dent.*, **28,** 182

Buonocore, M. G. and Bibby, B. G. (1945) Effects of various ions on enamel solubility. *J. Dent. Res.*, **24**, 103

Burgess, R. C., Mondrow, T. G., Nikiforuk, G. and Compton, F. H. (1962) Topical stannous fluoride as a caries preventative for pre-school children. *J. Can. Dent. Assoc.*, **28**, 312

Cartwright, H. V., Lindahl, R. L. and Bawden, J. W. (1968) Clinical findings on the effectiveness of stannous fluoride and acid phosphate fluoride as caries reducing agents in children. *J. Dent. Child.*, **35**, 36

Clark, D. C., Stamm, J. W., Chin Once, T. and Robert, G. (1985) Results of the Sherbrooke-Lac Mégantic fluoride varnish study after 20 months. *Commun. Dent. Oral Epidemiol.*, **13**, 61–64

Compton, F. H., Burgess, R. C., Mondrow, T. G., Grainger, R. M. and Nikiforuk, G. (1959) The Riverdale pre-school dental project. *J. Can. Dent. Assoc.*, **25,** 478

Cons, N. C., Janerich, D. T. and Senning, R. S. (1970) Albany topical fluoride study. *J. Am. Dent. Assoc.*, **80**, 777–781

Davies, G. N. (1950) Dental caries control and the general practitioner. *N.Z. Dent. J.*, **46**, 25

Dudding, N. J. and Muhler, J. C. (1962) Technique of application of stannous fluoride in a compatible prophylactic paste and as a topical agent. *J. Dent. Child.*, **24,** 219–224

Galagan, D. J. and Knutson, H. W. (1948) Effect of topically applied fluoride on dental caries experience, VI. Experiments with sodium fluoride and calcium chloride; widely spaced applications; use of different solution concentrations. *Public Health Rep.*, **63**, 1215

Geiger, A. M., Gorelick, L., Gwinett, A. J. and Griswold, P. G. (1988) The effect of a fluoride program on white spot formation during orthodontic treatment. *Am. J. Orthod.*, **93**(1), 29–37

Gish, C. W., Howell, C. L. and Muhler, J. C. (1957) A new approach to the topical application of fluorides for the reduction of dental caries in children. *J. Dent. Res.*, **36**, 784

Gish, C. W., Mercer, V. H., Stookey, G. K. and Dahl, L. O. (1975) Self-application of fluoride as a community preventive measure: rationale, procedures and 3-year results. *J. Am. Dent. Assoc.*, **90**, 388–397

Gish, C. W. and Muhler, J. C. (1965) Effect on dental caries in children in a natural area of combined use of three agents containing stannous fluoride, a prophylactic paste, a solution and dentifrice. *J. Am. Dent. Assoc.*, **70**, 914–920

Gish, C. W., Muhler, J. C. and Howell, C. L. (1962) A new approach to the topical application of fluorides for the reduction of dental caries in children. Results at the end of five years. *J. Dent. Child.*, **29**, 65

Gorelick, L., Geiger, A. M. and Gwinett, A. J. (1982) Incidence of white spot formation after bonding and banding. *Am. J. Orthod.*, **81**(2), 93–98

Grobler, S. R., Ogaard, B. and Rölla, G. (1983) Fluoride uptake after *in vivo* fluoride varnish application. *Tydskr. Tandheelkd. Ver. S. Afr.*, **38**(2), 55–58

Grodzka, K., Augustyniak, L., Budny, J., Czarnocka, K. *et al.* (1982) Caries increment in primary teeth after application of Duraphat® fluoride varnish. *Commun. Dent. Oral Epidemiol.*, **10**, 55–59

Gunz, G. M. (1971) The effect of self-applied fluoride paste. *J. Public Health Dent.*, **31**, 177–181

Hallsworth, A. S. and Weatherell, J. A. (1969) The microdistribution, uptake and loss of fluoride in human enamel. *Caries Res.*, **3**, 109–118

Harris, R. (1963) Observations on the effect of eight per cent stannous fluoride on dental caries in children. *Aust. Dent. J.*, **8**, 335

Heifetz, S. B., Franchi, G. J., Mosley, G. W. *et al.* (1979) Combined anticariogenic effect of fluoride gel-trays and fluoride mouthrinsing in an optimally fluoridated community. *Clin. Prev. Dent.*, **1**, 21–23, 28

Heintze, U. and Mörnstad, H. (1980) Artificial caries-like lesions around conventional, fluoride-containing and dispersed amalgams. *Caries Res.*, **14,** 414–421

Hetzer, G. and Irmisch, B. (1973) Kariesprotektion durch Fluorlack (Duraphat) – Klinische ergebnisse und erfahrungen. *Dtsch. Stomatol.*, **23**, 917–922

Heuser, H. and Schmidt, H. F. M. (1968) Deep impregnation of dental enamel with a fluorine lacquer for prophylaxis of dental caries. *Stoma,* **21**, 91–100

Hochstein, H. K., Hochstein, U. and Breitung, L. (1975) Erfahrungen mit dem Fluorlack Duraphat. *ZWR,* **1**, 26–28

Holm, A. K. (1979) Effect of a fluoride varnish (Duraphat) in pre-school children. *Commun. Dent. Oral Epidemiol.,* **7**, 241–245

Holm, G. B., Holst, K. and Mejàre, I. (1984) The caries-preventive effect of a fluoride varnish in the fissures of the first permament molar. *Acta Odontol. Scand.,* **42**, 193–197

Horowitz, H. S. (1969) Effect on dental caries of topically applied acidulated phosphate-fluoride: results after two years. *J. Am. Dent. Assoc.,* **78**, 568

Horowitz, H. S. (1980) Established methods of prevention. *Br. Dent. J.,* **149**, 311–318

Horowitz, H. S. and Bixler, D. (1976) The effect of SnF_2-$ZrSiO_4$ prophylactic paste on dental caries: Santa Clara County, Calif. *J. Am. Dent. Assoc.,* **92**, 369–373

Horowitz, H. S. and Doyle, J. (1971) The effect on dental caries of topically applied acidulated phosphate-fluoride: results after 3 years. *J. Am. Dent. Assoc.,* **81**, 166

Horowitz, H. S., Doyle, J. and Kan, M. C. W. (1971) Retained anti-caries protection from topically applied acidulated phosphate fluoride: 30 and 36 month post treatment effects. *IADR Abstr.,* **213**, No. 642

Horowitz, H. S. and Heifetz, S. B. (1970) The current status of topical fluorides in preventive dentistry. *J. Am. Dent. Assoc.,* **81**, 166–177

Horowitz, H. S. and Lucye, H. S. (1966) A clinical study of stannous fluoride in a prophylaxis paste and as a solution. *J. Oral Ther.,* **3**, 17–25

Houwink, B., Backer Dirks, O. and Kwant, G. W. (1974) A nine year study of topical applications with stannous fluoride in identical twins and the caries experience five years after ending the applications. *Caries Res.,* **8**, 27

Ingraham, R. Q. and Williams, J. E. (1970) An evaluation of the utility of application and cariostatic effectiveness of phosphate-fluorides in solution and gel states. *J. Tenn. Dent. Assoc.,* **50**, 5

Jordan, W. A., Snyder, J. R. and Wilson, V. (1959) A study of a single application of eight per cent stannous fluoride. *J. Dent. Child.,* **26**, 355

Jordan, W. A., Wood, O. B., Allison, J. A. and Irwin, V. D. (1946) Effects of various numbers of topical applications of sodium fluoride. *J. Am. Dent. Assoc.,* **33**, 1385

Katz, S. (1982) The use of fluoride and chlorhexidine for the prevention of radiation caries. *J. Am. Dent. Assoc.,* **104**, 164–170

Kirkegaard, E., Petersen, G., Poulsen, S., Holm, S. A. and Heidmann, J. (1986) Caries-preventive effect of Duraphat® varnish applications versus fluoride mouthrinses: 5-year data. *Caries Res.,* **20**, 548–555

Knutson, J. W. (1948) Sodium fluoride solutions: technic for application to the teeth. *J. Am. Dent. Assoc.,* **36**, 37

Knutson, J. W. and Armstrong, W. D. (1946) The effect of topically applied sodium fluoride on dental caries experience. III. Report of findings for the third study year. *Public Health Rep.,* **61**, 1683

Koch, G. and Petersson, L. G. (1972) Fluoride content of enamel surface treated with a varnish containing sodium fluoride. *Odont. Revy,* **23**, 437–446

Koch, G. and Petersson, L. G. (1975) Caries preventive effect of a fluoride-containing varnish (Duraphat) after 1 year's study. *Commun. Dent. Oral Epidemiol.,* **3**, 262–266

Koch, G. and Petersson, L. G. (1979) Effect of fluoride varnish (Duraphat) treatment every six months compared with weekly mouth-rinsing with 0.2 per cent NaF solution on dental caries. *Swed. Dent. J.,* **3**, 39–44

Koch, G., Petersson, L. G. and Ryden, H. (1979) Effect of fluoride varnish (Duraphat®) treatment every six months compared with weekly mouthrinses with 0.2 per cent NaF solution on dental caries. *Swed. Dent. J.,* **3**, 39–44

Kutler, B. and Ireland, R. L. (1953) Effect of sodium fluoride application on the dental caries experience in adults. *J. Dent. Res.,* **32**, 458

Lang, L. A., Thomas, H. G., Taylor, J. A. and Rothar, R. E. (1970) Clinical efficacy of a self-applied stannous fluoride prophylactic paste. *J. Dent. Child.,* **37**, 211–216

Law, F. E., Jeffreys, M. H. and Sheary, H. C. (1961) Topical applications of fluoride solutions in dental caries control. *Public Health Rep.,* **76**, 287

Lee, H., Ocumpaugh, D. E. and Swartz, M. L. (1972) Sealing of developmental pits and fissuress, II. Fluoride release from flexible fissure sealers. *J. Dent. Res.*, **51,** 183

Lieser, O. and Schmidt, H. F. M. (1978) Kariesprophylaktische Wirkung von Fluorlack nach mehrjähringer Anwendung in der Jugendzahnpflege. *Dtsch. Zahnärztl. Zeitschr.*, **33**, 176–178

Lind, O. P., Möller, I. J., Fehr, F. R. von der and Larsen, M. J. (1974) Caries preventive effect of a dentifrice containing 2 per cent sodium monofluorophosphate in a natural fluoride area in Denmark. *Commun. Dent. Oral Epidemiol.*, **2**, 104–113

Luoma, H., Murtomaa, H., Nuuja, T. *et al.* (1978) A simultaneous reduction of caries and gingivitis in a group of schoolchildren receiving chlorhexidine-fluoride applications: results after 2 years. *Caries Res.*, **12**, 290–298

Mainwaring, P. J. and Naylor, M. N. (1978) A three year study to determine the separate and combined caries-inhibiting effects of sodium monofluorophosphate toothpaste and an acidulated phosphate-fluoride gel. *Caries Res.*, **12**, 202–212

Maiwald, J. H. and Geiger, L. (1973) Topical application of a fluoride protective varnish for caries prophylaxis. *Dtsch. Stomatol.*, **23**, 56

Maiwald, H. J., Miyares, S. R. and Banos, F. D. (1978) Result del estudio de aplicación de laca de flúor. *Rev. Cub. Est.*, **15**, 109–114

Marthaler, T. M. (1968) Caries inhibition after seven years of unsupervised use of an amine fluoride dentifrice. *Br. Dent. J.*, **124**, 510

Mellberg, J. R. (1966) Fluoride uptake by intact human tooth enamel from acidulated fluoride phosphate preparations. *J. Dent. Res.*, **45**, 303

Mellberg, J. R. and Nicholson, C. R. (1968) *In vitro* evaluation of an acidulated phosphate fluoride prophylaxis paste. *Arch. Oral Biol.*, **13**, 1223–1234

Mercer, V. H. and Muhler, J. C. (1961) Comparison of a single application of stannous fluoride with a single application of sodium fluoride or two applications of stannous fluoride. *J. Dent. Child.*, **28**, 84

Mericle, M. R. and Muhler, J. C. (1963) Studies concerning the antisolubility effectiveness of different stannous fluoride prophylaxis paste mixtures. *J. Dent. Res.*, **42**, 21–27

Meryon, S. D. and Smith, A. J. (1984) A comparison of fluoride release from three glass ionomer cements and a polycarboxylate cement. *Int. Endodont. J.*, **17**, 16–24

Mizrahi, E. (1982) Enamel demineralization following orthodontic treatment. *Am. J. Orthod.*, **82**(1), 62–67

Muhler, J. C., Bixler, D. and Stookey, G. K. (1968) The clinical effectiveness of stannous hexafluorozirconate as an anticariogenic agent. *J. Am. Dent. Assoc.*, **76,** 558–563

Muhler, J. C., Boyd, T. M. and van Huysen, G. (1950) Effect of fluorides and other compounds on the solubility of enamel, dentine and tri-calcium phosphate. *J. Dent. Res.*, **29,** 182

Muhler, J. C. and Day, H. C. (1950) Effects of SnF_2, NaF on incidence of dental lesions in rats fed caries producing diets. *J. Am. Dent. Assoc.*, **41**, 528

Muhler, J. C., Dudding, N. J. and Stookey, G. K. (1964) The clinical effectiveness of a particular size distribution of zirconium silicate for use as a cleaning and polishing agent for oral hard tissues. *J. Periodontol.*, **35,** 481–485

Muhler, J. C. and van Huysen, G. (1947) Solubility of enamel protected by sodium fluoride and other compounds. *J. Dent. Res.*, **26**, 119

Muhler, J. C., Kelley, G. E., Stookey, G. K., Linds, F. I. and Harris, N. O. (1970) The clinical evaluation of a patient-administered stannous fluoride hexafluorozirconate prophylactic paste on children. I. Results after one year in the Virgin Islands. *J. Am. Dent. Assoc.*, **81**, 142–145

Murray, J. J., Winter, G. B. and Hurst, C. P. (1977) Duraphat fluoride varnish: a 2-year clinical trial in 5-year-old children. *Br. Dent. J.*, **143**, 11–17

Muzynski, B. L., Greener, E., Jameson, L. and Malone, W. F. P. (1988) Fluoride release from glass ionomers used as luting agents. *J. Prosthet. Dentist.*, **60**(1), 41–44

Ogaard, B. (1989) Prevalence of white spot lesions in 19-year-olds: a study on untreated and orthodontically treated persons 5 years after treatment. *Am. J. Orthod.*, **96**(5423), 427

Ogaard, B., Rölla, G. and Helgeland, K. (1984) Fluoride retention in sound and demineralized enamel *in vivo* after treatment with a fluoride varnish (Duraphat). *Scand. J. Dent. Res.*, **92**(3), 190–197

de Paola, P. F. and Mellberg, J. R. (1973) Caries experience and fluoride uptake in children receiving semi-annual prophylaxis with an acidulated prophylaxis fluoride paste. *J. Am. Dent. Assoc.*, **87**, 155–159

Parmeijer, J. H. N., Brudevold, F. and Hunt, E. E. (1963) A study of acidulated fluoride solutions, III. The cariostatic effect of repeated topical sodium fluoride applications with and without phosphate. A pilot study. *Arch. Oral Biol.*, **8**, 183

Peterson, J. K., Horowitz, H. S., Jordan, W. A. and Pugnier, V. (1967) Effectiveness of acidulated phosphate fluoride and stannous zirconium hexafluoride in prophylactic pastes. Abstracted International Association of Dental Research Programs and Abstracts of Papers, No. 277 (March)

Peterson, J. K., Horowitz, H. S., Jordan, W. A. and Pugnier, V. (1969) Effectiveness of an acidulated phosphate fluoride-pumice prophylactic paste: a two year report. *J. Dent. Res.*, **48**, 346–350

Peterson, J. K., Jordan, W. A. and Snyder, J. R. (1963) Effectiveness of stannous fluoride-silex-silicone prophylaxis paste: two year report. *Northwest Dent.*, **42**, 276–278

Petersson, L. G. (1975) On topical application of fluorides and its inhibiting effect on caries. *Odontol. Revy,* **26**, suppl. 34

Petersson, L. G. (1976) Fluorine gradients in outermost surface enamel after various forms of topical application of fluoride *in vivo*. *Odont. Revy,* **27**, 25–50

Petersson, L. G., Rasmusson, C. G., Hagborg, S. and Isacsson, P. (1985) Fluoride supplemented and non γ 2 amalgam. A comparative clinical study into the primary and permanent dentition in children. *Swed. Dent. J.,* **9**, 49–53

Phillips, R. W. (1988) Restorative materials containing fluoride. Report to Council on Dental Materials, Instruments and Equipment. *J. Am. Dent. Assoc.*, **116**, 762–763

Retief, D. H., Bradley, E. L., Holbrook, M. and Switzer, P. (1983) Enamel fluoride uptake, distribution and retention from topical fluoride agents. *Caries Res.*, **17**, 44–51

Riethe, P. and Weinmann, K. (1970) Caries inhibition with fluoride gel and fluoride varnish in rats. *Caries Res.*, **4**, 63

Rock, W. P. (1972) Fissure sealants: results obtained with two different sealants after only one year. *Br. Dent. J.*, **133**, 146

Rock, W. P. (1974) Fissure sealants: further results of clinical trials. *Br. Dent. J.*, **136**, 317

Saloum, F. S. and Sondhi, A. (1987) Preventing enamel decalcification after orthodontic treatment. *J. Am. Dent. Assoc.*, **115**, 257–261

Schmidt, H. F. M. (1981) Fluorid-Applikation zur Kariesprophylaxe und Behandlung überempfindlicher Zahnhälse. *Kariesprophylaxe,* **3**, 117–123

Schutz, H. J., Forrester, D. J. and Balis, S. B. (1974) Evaluation of a fluoride prophylaxis paste in a fluoridated community. *J. Can. Dent. Assoc.*, **40**, 675–683

Scola, F. P. and Ostrom, C. A. (1968) Clinical evaluation of stannous fluoride when used as a constituent of a compatible prophylactic paste, as a topical solution and in a dentifrice in naval personnel, II. Report of findings after two years. *J. Am. Dent. Assoc.*, **77**, 594–597

Scott, D. B. (1960) Electron-microscope evidence of fluoride-enamel reaction. *J. Dent. Res.,* **39**, 1117

Segreto, V. A., Harris, N. O. and Hester, W. R. (1961) A stannous fluoride, silex, silicone dental prophylaxis paste with anticariogenic potentialities. *J. Dent. Res.*, **40**, 90–96

Seppa, L. and Pollanen, L. (1987) Caries preventive effect of two fluoride varnishes and a fluoride mouthrinse. *Caries Res.*, **21**, 375–379

Seppa, L., Tuutti, H. and Luoma, H. (1982) Three year report on caries prevention using fluoride varnish for caries risk children in a community with fluoridated water. *Scand. J. Dent. Res.*, **96**, 89–94

Shannon, I. L. (1969) Stannous hexafluorozirconate and enamel solubility. *J. Dent. Child.*, **36**, 175–180

Shannon, I. L. (1982) Fluoride treatment programs for high-caries-risk patients. *Clin. Prev. Dent.*, **4**(2), 11–20

Skartveit, L., Tveit, A. B., Totdal, B., Ovrebo, R. and Raadal, M. (1990) *In vivo* fluoride uptake in enamel and dentine from fluoride-containing materials. *J. Dentist. Child.*, **58**, 97–100

Stamm, J. W. (1974) Fluoride uptake from topical sodium fluoride varnish measured by an *in vivo* enamel biopsy. *J. Can. Dent. Assoc.*, **40**, 501–505

Stearns, R. I. (1973) Incorporation of fluoride by human enamel, III. *In vivo* effects of non-fluoride and fluoride prophylactic pastes and APF gels. *J. Dent. Res.*, **52**, 30–35

Stookey, G. K., Hudson, J. R. and Muhler, J. C. (1966) Studies concerning the polishing properties of zirconium silicate in enamel. *J. Periodontol.*, **37**, 200–207

Sundvall-Hagland, I., Brudevold, F., Armstrong, W. D., Gardner, D. E. and Smith, F. A. (1959) Comparison of the increment of fluoride in enamel and the reduction in dental caries resulting from topical fluoride applications. *Arch. Oral Biol.*, **1**, 74

Swartz, M. L., Phillips, R. W. and Clark, H. E. (1984) Long-term F release from glass ionomer cement. *J. Dent. Res.*, **63**(2), 158–160

Szwejda, L. F., Tossy, C. V. and Below, D. M. (1967) Fluorides in community programmes: results from a fluoride gel applied topically. *J. Public Health Dent.*, **27**, 192

Tewari, A., Chawla, H. S. and Utreja, A. (1984) Caries preventive effect of three topical fluorides (1½ years clinical trial in Chandigarh schoolchildren of North India). *J. Int. Ass. Dent. Child.*, **15**, 71–81

Torell, P. (1965) Two year clinical tests with different methods of local caries-preventive fluorine application in Swedish schoolchildren. *Acta Odontol. Scand.*, **23**, 287

Treide, A., Hebenstreit, W. and Gunther, A. (1980) Kollective Kariespravention in Vorchulatter unter Verwendung eines Fluoridhaltingenlackes. *Stomat. DDR*, **30**, 734

Triol, C. W., Kranz, S. M., Volpe, A. R., Frankl, S. N., Alman, J. E. and Allard, R. L. (1980) Anticaries effect of a sodium fluoride rinse and an MFP dentifrice in a non-fluoridated area: a thirty-month study. *Clin. Prev. Dent.*, **2**, 13–15

Ulvestad, H. (1978) Applisering av Duraphat fluorlakk. *Norw. Dent. J.*, **88**(5), 207

Volker, J. F., Hodge, H. C., Wilson, H. J. and van Voorkis, S. N. (1940) The absorption of fluorides by enamel, dentine, bone and hydroxyapatite as shown by the use of the radioactive isotope. *J. Biol. Chem.*, **134**, 543–548

Vrbic, V. and Brudevold, F. (1970) Fluoride uptake from treatment with different fluoride prophylaxis pastes and from the use of pastes containing soluble aluminium salt followed by a topical application. *Caries Res.*, **4**, 158–167

Vrbic, V., Brudevold, F. and McCann, H. G. (1967) Acquisition of fluoride by enamel from fluoride pumice pastes. *Helv. Odontol. Acta*, **11**, 21–26

Wellock, W. D. and Brudevold, F. (1963) A study of acidulated fluoride solutions, II. The caries inhibiting effect of single annual applications of an acidic fluoride and phosphate solution. A two year experience. *Arch. Oral Biol.*, **8**, 179

Wellock, W. D., Maitland, A. and Brudevold, F. (1965) Caries increments, tooth discoloration, and state of oral hygiene in children given single annual applications of acid phosphate and stannous fluoride. *Arch. Oral Biol.*, **10**, 453

Whitehurst, V. E., Stookey, G. K. and Muhler, J. C. (1968) Studies concerning the cleaning, polishing and therapeutic properties of commercial prophylactic pastes. *J. Oral Ther.*, **4**, 181–191

Winter, K. (1975) Kariesprophylaxe durch Lokalapplikation von Natriumfluorid-Lack. *Zahnärztl. Mitt.*, **65**, 215–226

Wolf, R. G. (1964) Effect of stannous fluoride prophylaxis paste on enamel solubility. *J. Dent. Res.*, **43**, 168–174

Woodhouse, A. D. (1978) A longitudinal study of the effectiveness of self applied 10% stannous fluoride paste for secondary schoolchildren. *Austral. Dent. J.*, **23**, 422–428

Wright, W. E., Haller, J. M., Harlow, S. A. and Pizzo, P. A. (1985) An oral disease prevention program for patients receiving radiation and chemotherapy. *J. Am. Dent. Assoc.*, **110**, 43–47

Chapter 12

Pre-eruptive effect of fluoride

Historical introduction

Epidemiological studies in the USA during the first half of this century linked the occurrence of dental enamel mottling to the public water supply and, subsequently, to the fluoride content of the drinking water. Enamel mottling only occurred when excessive amounts of fluoride were ingested during the period of enamel formation: for most teeth this was from birth to 12 years. In Chapter 6, on defluoridation of drinking water, it was noted that the occurrence of enamel opacities was prevented if water containing high fluoride levels was not consumed during childhood, i.e. during tooth development. When, a few years later, the link between dental caries experience and the fluoride content of drinking water was recognized, it is perhaps not surprising that an adequate level of fluoride during tooth formation was considered of foremost importance so that the optimum amount of fluoride might be incorporated into the forming tooth and the tooth be better able to resist caries attack. The early results of artificial fluoridation supported this belief, since children born and reared in fluoridated Grand Rapids had much lower caries experience than children living in the control communities, after 6½, 10 and 15 years (see Chapter 2). Indeed, in the early days of fluoridation it was stated: 'It is not essential for fluorides to be continuously present in the diet for more than the first 8 years of life in order that caries be inhibited' (Arnold, 1945); and 'It is not necessary to continue use of fluoridated water after the enamel has been calcified' (McKay, 1952).

Laboratory studies gave support to the idea that increasing the level of fluoride in the forming tooth was a sensible aim. Gron *et al.* (1963) showed that incorporation of fluoride increases the size of apatite crystals as well as assisting in the formation of more perfectly formed crystals. Larger well-formed crystals would have a lower surface:volume ratio than smaller poorly formed crystals and would be likely to dissolve more slowly. Healy and Ludwig (1966) demonstrated that teeth from people in fluoride areas were less soluble than teeth from low-fluoride areas. In addition, epidemiologists commented on the well-rounded cusps and shallow fissures of human teeth from fluoride areas (Ockerse, 1949; Forrest, 1956). These arguments dominated discussions on the action of fluoride in the early days of fluoridation and were used to explain the clinical findings which appeared at that time.

However, as fluoridation studies progressed, and indeed even before they began, a few epidemiologists reported that some inhibition of caries occurred in teeth only exposed to fluoride post-eruptively. Deatherage (1943a,b) noted that the DMFT of males aged 24–26 years who received water containing 1 mg F/litre from age 8 years onward was lower than the DMFT of men who had lived continuously in low-fluoride areas, although higher than for men who had received fluoridated water from birth. Similarly, Weaver (1944) observed that the first permanent molars of children in South Shields, Sunderland and Jarrow in England derived some caries-preventive effect from water containing 1.4 mg F/litre even though these 11–14-year-old children had arrived in the area after these teeth had erupted.

Klein (1945, 1946) observed the development of caries in relocated Japanese children 8–14 years of age, between 1943 and 1945. All the children had previously consumed low-fluoride water, but one group moved to an area with drinking water containing 3 mg F/litre, while another group continued to receive low-fluoride water. Caries development in teeth which were erupted and caries-free in 1943 was 60% less in the former group, suggesting a post-eruptive effect from fluoridated water. Klein also concluded that teeth which had erupted most recently were protected the most.

Klein (1948) went on to examine several groups of 15–19-year-olds in New Jersey (1.3–2.2 mg F/litre) and Hagerstown and Williamstown-Clayton (both low-fluoride areas). Children who had consumed fluoridated water from birth onward showed the greatest reduction in dental caries. Migrant children were classified according to the age at which the consumption of fluoridated water started (0, 5, 10 and 15 years). Caries reduction decreased as the age of commencing consumption of fluoridated water increased. By analysing differences in caries experience for each type of tooth separately, it was clear that both a post-eruptive and a pre-eruptive effect existed.

In another study in America, Russell (1949) recorded caries experience in groups of children who had received fluoridated water for different periods of their lives. He observed both a post-eruptive and a pre-eruptive caries-preventive effect, but he also highlighted the importance of exposure to fluoride just after tooth eruption, and the necessity for the continuing exposure of the erupted tooth to fluoride.

In the UK, the post-eruptive effect of water fluoridation is clearly shown in the study by Hardwick, Teasdale and Bloodworth (1982), which was conducted in two communities in Cheshire, England, between 1975 and 1979. Baseline examinations were undertaken before fluoridation (at 1.0 mg F/litre) began in one of the localities, and then annually for 4 years. Children in the control area (<0.1 mg F/litre) were examined at the same time by one examiner who did not know which of the two localities the children came from. After 4 years, the DMFS increments for all teeth were 6.7 in the fluoride area and 9.2 in the control area (27% less in the fluoride area) (Table 12.1). The percentage difference was greatest (40%) for teeth which erupted after fluoridation began, but a substantial difference (25% or 1.9 DMFS) was observed in teeth already erupted when fluoridation began, indicating a solely post-eruptive or topical effect of water fluoridation.

Thus, it has become clear during the past 40 years that fluoride in drinking water has a post-eruptive as well as a pre-eruptive effect. The mechanisms by which fluoride acts post-eruptively have been studied extensively and are thought to fall into three broad categories: (a) elevated levels of fluoride in plaque fluid and in enamel fluid decrease apatite solubility; (b) fluoride encourages re-mineralization; and (c) fluoride affects plaque organisms so that less acid is produced and the microbial composition is changed (see Chapter 15).

The relative importance of the various pre- and post-eruptive modes of action of fluoride have been debated during recent years. While there is general agreement

Table 12.1 Mean DMFS scores for children aged 12 years at the start of fluoridation (baseline) living in fluoridated and non-fluoridated areas of Cheshire, England. Four-year caries increments given for all teeth, teeth which erupted during the study and teeth which were already erupted at baseline (From Hardwick, Teasdale and Bloodworth, 1982)

	Baseline DMFS	*Four-year DMFS increment*		
		All teeth	*Erupting teeth*	*Erupted teeth*
Fluoride	6.6	6.7	0.85	5.9
Control	7.3	9.2	1.41	7.8
Difference	0.7	2.5 (27%)	0.56 (40%)	1.9 (25%)
Stat. sig.	NS	$P < 0.001$	$P < 0.01$	$P < 0.01$

that the post-eruptive action of fluoride is very important, there is less agreement concerning the pre-eruptive effect. Some dental scientists have suggested that pre-eruptive fluoride administration is ineffective and therefore unnecessary and, indeed, is undesirable. The rest of this chapter will consider this debate.

Before leaving this historical introduction, it is worth discussing the terms 'systemic' and 'topical', which are sometimes used synonymously with 'pre-eruptive' and 'post-eruptive'. Topical action of fluoride occurs by direct contact with the surface of an erupted tooth in the mouth. A systemic effect, however, can occur not only before, but also after eruption. Fluoride is absorbed via the gastrointestinal tract into the body fluid system where it may be incorporated into developing (unerupted) tooth enamel, and also reach the enamel of erupted teeth via saliva and gingival crevicular fluids. Thus, some of the benefit of fluoride from drinking water may be due to a systemic effect via saliva and crevicular fluids. From the epidemiologist's viewpoint it is sensible to use the terms 'pre-eruptive' and 'post-eruptive' when considering caries-preventive effects, rather than 'systemic' and 'topical'.

Post-eruptive effect

There is no doubt of the very great importance of the post-eruptive effect, or local intra-oral effect or topical effect, of fluoride in preventing dental caries. In the previous section, it was noted that during the 1940s and 1950s, epidemiologists began to realize that fluoride in drinking water could give a substantial post-eruptive effect. At that time, research workers were experimenting in applying fluoride solutions topically to teeth, in order to investigate further fluoride's remarkable ability to prevent caries.

Volker *et al.* (1940) demonstrated that enamel solubility could be reduced, *in vitro*, by treating enamel with a fluoride solution and, a few years later, Bibby (1943) reported the first clinical trial of topical fluoride application (see Chapter 11). A very large number of trials have shown that clinical topical applications of fluoride (usually containing about 1% F) reduces caries increments by about 20–40%. If applications are very frequent, the caries-preventive effect is higher: Englander *et al.* (1967) reported an 80% reduction in DMFS increment in 11–14-year-old children who applied 1.1% NaF gel each school-day for 21 months.

Bibby, a New Zealander by birth but who has worked for nearly 60 years in the USA, was not slow to investigate other methods of applying fluoride to erupted teeth. But, while his first trial of clinical topical application of fluoride produced a positive result (a 45% reduction after 1 year), his clinical trials of a sodium fluoride mouthrinse (Bibby *et al.*, 1946) and a sodium fluoride dentifrice (Bibby, 1945) showed no caries-preventing effect.

Despite these early setbacks, fluoride mouthrinsing and fluoride dentifrices have subsequently been shown to be very effective and efficient caries-preventive agents (see Chapters 10 and 9, respectively). Although it is probable that some mouthrinse and dentifrice is swallowed, especially by young children, it must be concluded that the caries-preventive effect of clinical topical application, mouthrinses and dentifrices is topical, on teeth already erupted. The extent to which fluoride ingested from dentifrices by young children and incorporated into their forming teeth (i.e. a pre-eruptive effect) contributes to the overall, substantial, caries-preventive effectiveness of dentifrices has never been quantified. Until epidemiological data become available (and such studies would be very difficult to undertake), it must be assumed that the mode of action of fluoride dentifrices is post-eruptive.

During the 1970s, dental caries prevalence and severity declined in many countries. In Western Europe, North America and Australasia the decline was dramatic and substantial. Two reports (Glass, 1982; Fédération Dentaire Internationale, 1985) agree that the greater use of fluorides was the most likely reason for the decline. While at the beginning of the 1970s very few dentifrices in the UK contained fluoride, by the end of the 1970s nearly all did so (see Chapter 9). In Scandinavia and Switzerland, rinsing or brushing with fluoride solutions in school has been extensive. All these methods give principally a post-eruptive, topical effect and so it must be concluded that the dramatic decline in caries which occurred during the 1970s was very largely due to the post-eruptive exposure to fluoride. This does not infer that pre-eruptive exposure to fluoride did not contribute to the decline – there was some expansion in the use of water fluoridation worldwide and salt fluoridation began in Switzerland – but that its contribution, overall, seems likely to be small in comparison with the post-eruptive effect.

Pre-eruptive effect

At the beginning of this chapter, the general agreement of the very great importance of the post-eruptive effect of fluoride, but disagreement of the pre-eruptive role of fluoride in caries prevention, was noted. Examples of the extreme view that ingestion of fluoride is unnecessary and undesirable can be seen in Fejerskov *et al.* (1988). For example, when discussing salt fluoridation they say that 'the addition of fluoride is based entirely on a mistaken belief that the ingestion is necessary for the prevention of caries. As we have discussed elsewhere, the anti-cariogenic properties of fluoride are principally due to its presence in the mouth when and where decay is taking place, whereas the toxic effects will inevitably be manifest if ingested during the period of the development of the teeth'.

A more balanced view is taken by Ekstrand, Fejerskov and Silverstone (1988) who say in their final chapter:

In reviewing these statements, and combining them with discussions from earlier chapters, certain observations can be made which point to the fact that caries reduction in humans is *not* dependent upon: fluoride being administered via a systemic route; having high levels of fluoride in sound enamel; or having fluoride affect either the bacterial metabolism or bacterial colonization of enamel. The caries reduction, however, is predominantly affected by fluoride being present during active caries development at the plaque–enamel interface where it will directly alter the dynamics of mineral dissolution and reprecipitation. This is not to say that fluoride incorporated into enamel apatite does not reduce its rate of dissolution, but this factor as the only factor responsible for caries reduction can by no means explain the caries reduction data.

Thylstrup (1990) has recently reviewed the evidence that fluoride exerts a negligible pre-eruptive effect. He, first, stressed the importance of combining evidence from epidemiology and laboratory studies. From this he concluded that the most important period for any tooth is between its emergence into the oral environment and its full eruption, and that this is the period during which provision of fluoride is important. The early fluoridation studies and clinical trials of topical fluoride were discussed, in particular regarding the role of fluoride just after tooth eruption. The lack of clear correlation between the concentration of fluoride in enamel and caries experience is taken as further proof that fluoride given pre-eruptively is ineffective. He concluded that 'Both the clinical and laboratory data combine to support the view that the relative importance of pre-eruptive fluoride to human caries progression is of borderline significance compared with the more important post-eruptive effect'.

Thylstrup (1990) and other proponents of the view that pre-eruptive fluoride is unnecessary (Fejerskov *et al.*, 1988) have been hampered by lack of epidemiological data to support their argument. They rely principally on a study by Thylstrup, Bille and Bruun (1982) which presented trends in dental caries in four communities in Denmark between 1973 and 1980. The four communities were: Vordingborg, a stable rural population (20 000) which received water with a natural fluoride content of 1.2 ppm F; Ballerup and Hvidovre, two suburbs of Copenhagen each with expanding populations of 50 000 in 1972; and Skibby, with a small rural and stable population of 5500. Since Child Dental Health Services were introduced in Skibby much later than in the other areas, this small community was omitted from the main comparisons. School-based fluoride rinsing programmes operated in Ballerup and Hvidovre (which received drinking water containing 0.4 ppm F) since 1966 and, in addition, children with high-caries activity received topical application of 2% NaF. Topical fluorides were not given in Vordingborg. Over 80% of dentifrices in Denmark contained fluoride during the study period. The cross-sectional data show (Figure 12.1) that while caries experience fell only slightly in Vordingborg, a marked decline in caries experience was observed in Ballerup and Hvidovre. The results were broadly similar for children aged 7, 13 and 15 years. The authors concluded that the convergence of the DMFS scores was due to topical (post-eruptive) fluoride and that it was reasonable to reconsider water fluoridation in such communities. Beltran and Burt (1988) criticized the Danish study of Thylstrup, Bille and Bruun (1982), pointing out, first, that the comparison between rural Vordingborg and the two suburban communities was hardly valid and, secondly, that the investigation presented no evidence to negate a pre-eruptive effect from drinking water.

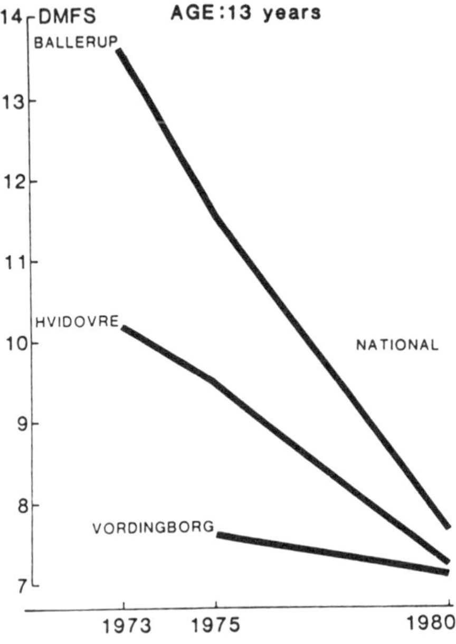

Figure 12.1 Mean DMFS of 13-year-olds living in three communities in Denmark, between 1973 and 1980. Vordingborg received water containing 1.2 ppm F, while children in Ballerup and Hvidovre received school-based topical fluoride therapy (From Thylstrup *et al.*, 1982; reproduced by kind permission of the Editor, *Caries Research*)

One of the most thorough reviews of the epidemiological data concerning the pre-eruptive effect of fluorides has been written by Marthaler (1979). He discussed data from the major long-term studies of water fluoridation in the USA, Canada, New Zealand and The Netherlands. Data in Table 12.2 are taken from his publication, and provide evidence of a pre-eruptive effect from water fluoridation. Permanent teeth usually do not erupt before 6 years of age, so that the difference between the DMFS of 13-year-olds first exposed to fluoridation at the age of 5 years (5.9 DMFT) and the DMFT of 13-year-olds exposed to fluoridation from birth (3.9 DMFT) can be taken as an indication of the benefit of exposure to fluoridation between birth and 5 years of age (a benefit of 2.0 DMFT).

Table 12.2 DMFT of 9- and 13-year-olds in Grand Rapids, USA, who were exposed to fluoridated water for different periods of time (From Marthaler, 1979; compiled from Arnold *et al.*, 1956, 1962)

	Years of exposure to fluoridation prior to examination			
	0	*3*	*8*	*13*
9-year-olds	3.9	3.1	2.0	–
(age at fluoridation)	(9)	(6)	(1)	–
13-year-olds	9.7	8.5	5.9	3.9
(age at fluoridation)	(13)	(10)	(5)	(0)

Marthaler (1979) found a similar benefit of pre-eruptive exposure to fluoridation on analysis of data from Kingston (USA), Oak Park (USA), Sarnia (Canada) and Hastings (New Zealand). Fewer data exist for deciduous teeth but, after examining data from Grand Rapids, Kingston and Albany (USA), he concluded 'that fluoridation should start at birth to provide optimal protection to the deciduous teeth' (Marthaler, 1979).

Marthaler recognized drawbacks with the above types of analysis: data for all types of tooth were combined, and data for the three different types of tooth surface (fissure, approximal and free smooth surface) were combined. Tooth-specific and surface-specific data were reported in the Netherlands fluoridation trial and, from analyses of these data, Marthaler (1979) concluded that all surface-types benefited from pre-eruptive exposure to water fluoridation, but particularly fissure surfaces. Marthaler also concluded that pre-eruptive exposure to fluoride dietary supplements or to school fluoridation led to enhanced effectiveness, although data were limited.

Because of the self-selective nature of many of the clinical studies of fluoride dietary supplements (see Chapter 8), it is more difficult to estimate the effect of pre-eruptive exposure to this fluoride therapy than is the case with water fluoridation (Marthaler, 1979; Thylstrup, 1990). One of the best attempts to do so has been reported by Widenheim (1985) and Widenheim *et al.* (1986). The aim of their investigation was to estimate the pre-eruptive caries-reducing effects of NaF on caries in approximal surfaces of permanent molars and premolars. About 50 12–17-year-old children took part in Lund, Sweden, where the concentration of fluoride in the drinking water is 0.2 mg F/litre. In order to limit the effect of the self-selective nature of the study, information on the following factors was collected for each subject – dietary habits, gingivitis, plaque, salivary *Streptococcus mutans* and salivary lactobacilli levels – and these 'confounding variables' were taken into account in the data analysis. The children, who were all born in 1967 and dentally examined in 1979, 1980, 1981 and 1984, were divided into those who had never taken fluoride tablets and those who had taken them for a minimum of 5 years between 6 months and 6 years of age. Caries experience was lower in those who had taken the fluoride tablets. This amounted to a difference in DFS of 34% in 14-year-olds ($P = 0.01$), but when these data were corrected for confounding factors the difference fell to 24% (about 1 DFS) and was no longer statistically significant. The authors concluded that fluoride (from tablets) does have a pre-eruptive effect which is observable in adolescence. It is possible that some first permanent molars would have received post-eruptive exposure at the age of 6 years. However, the authors reported that excluding the first permanent molars did not alter their results or conclusions.

The most thorough investigation into the relative importance of pre- and post-eruptive exposure to fluoride was undertaken by van Eck (1987). He used the very extensive data collected during the Tiel–Culemborg fluoridation study in The Netherlands (see Chapter 2). The water supply of Tiel was fluoridated continuously from March 1953 to December 1973. Culemborg was the control (low-fluoride) town. Children were examined clinically and radiographically between 1952 (just before fluoridation) and 1986 (13 years after discontinuation of fluoridation). The state of eruption of each tooth was recorded at each examination. Not all children of all ages were examined every year and no examinations took place between 1973 and 1979. These exclusions limit the value of these data to some extent in their ability to differentiate between pre- and post-eruptive effects of fluoride, although

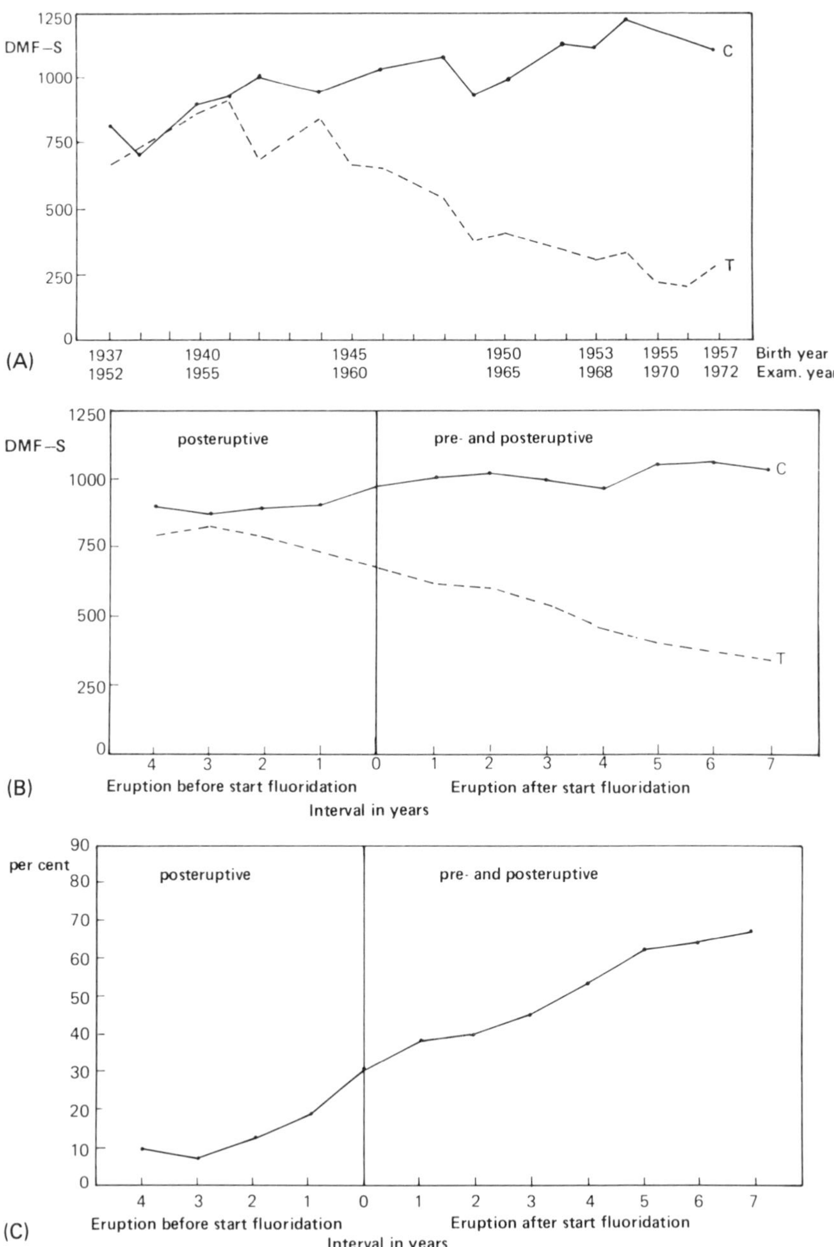

Figure 12.2 DMFS data collected at the beginning of the Tiel (T) and Culemborg (C) fluoridation study which demonstrates the effect of post-eruptive exposure to fluoride, and the effect of exposure to fluoride both pre- and post-eruptively. Data for approximal surfaces of premolars, molars and upper incisors only, in 15-year-olds

(A) Raw data (DMFS per 100 children) obtained at examinations between 1952 and 1972
(B) Data standardized according to time interval between tooth eruption and start of fluoridation in Tiel
(C) Percentage caries reduction in these surfaces in Tiel compared with Culemborg

not for the primary purpose of the study which was to investigate the effectiveness of water fluoridation. Data for Culemborg was collected in parallel, which was important since caries experience rose in Culemborg until 1969 and then declined from 1969 to 1984. Data were, therefore, always expressed as percentage less caries in Tiel compared with Culemborg. The three types of tooth surface (pit and fissure, free smooth surface and approximal) were considered separately.

Figures 12.2 and 12.3 are given to demonstrate the way in which the data were analysed. It is important to realize that at the beginning of fluoridation (1953) data were collected for children of various ages so that it was possible to estimate the effectiveness of fluoride exposure: (a) post-eruptively only, and (b) both pre- and post-eruptively (Figure 12.2). It was not possible to estimate the effect of

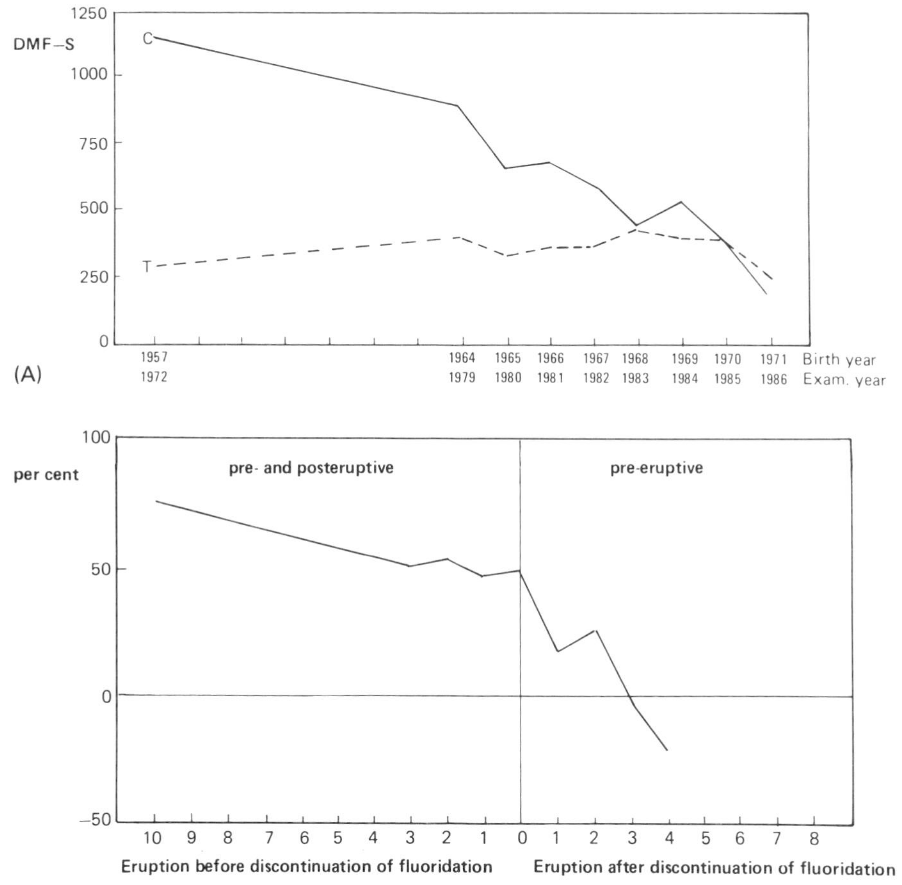

Figure 12.3 DMFS data collected at the end of the Tiel (T) and Culemborg (C) fluoridation study which demonstrates the effect of pre-eruptive exposure to fluoride, and the effect of exposure to fluoride both pre- and post-eruptively. Data for first permanent molars only are given, for 15-year-olds

(A) Raw data (DMFS per 100 children) obtained at examinations between 1972 and 1986
(B) Percentage caries reduction in these surfaces in Tiel compared with Culemborg when data were standardized according to the time interval between tooth eruption and discontinuation of fluoridation in Tiel

pre-eruptive fluoridation only, at the start of fluoridation, except by subtraction of percentage reductions. However, at the termination of fluoridation (1973), it was possible to estimate the effects of (a) pre-eruptive exposure only, and (b) both pre- and post-eruptive exposure (Figure 12.3), but not to directly estimate post-eruptive exposure only.

It can be seen in Figure 12.2C (data obtained at the beginning of fluoridation) that the maximum percentage caries reduction in these surfaces was about 65% (fluoridation began 7 years before tooth eruption), whereas only about 30% reduction was observed in teeth which erupted in the same year as fluoridation began (and the teeth subjected to post-eruptive fluoride only). Percentage caries reduction was only 10% in teeth which had erupted 4 years before fluoridation began (limited post-eruptive exposure).

Figure 12.3B (data obtained at the end of fluoridation) indicate that the maximum percentage caries reduction in these surfaces was about 75% (when fluoridation ceased 10 years after these teeth erupted), whereas only about a 50% reduction was recorded when fluoridation ceased in the same year as these teeth erupted (and therefore subjected to pre-eruptive fluoride only).

Van Eck's conclusions from data analyses *at the beginning of fluoridation* were (van Eck, 1987):

Approximal surfaces

> . . . the use of fluoridated water from birth on causes a mean caries reduction of about 70% at the age of 15 years.
>
> . . . the use of fluoridated water during the post-eruptive period only, causes a reduction which is 45% of the maximal reduction in proximal surfaces at the age of 15 years. This maximal reduction is obtained if consumption extends during the whole pre- and post-eruptive period.

Free smooth surfaces. If, for the first permanent molar,

> . . . the start of consumption of fluoridated water shifts from two years after to two years before eruption, the reduction increases from 36% to 63%.

Pit and fissure surfaces

> . . . the use of fluoridated water has only then a reducing effect on caries in fissures and pits if it is consumed from before the eruption . . . . The maximum effect is only attained if the consumption starts before the calcification period, that is for the first molar from birth. . . . Data for extractions and occlusal fillings, obtained from bitewing radiographs, do not contradict this statement.

His summary of the analyses *at the end of fluoridation* were:

> . . . the use of fluoridated water during the pre-eruptive period still has a reducing effect on caries experience, even if it is not followed by post-eruptive use. However, post-eruptive use increases substantially the effect. The degree of the pre-eruptive effect has an inverted relationship to the percentage caries in the three categories of surfaces.

Combining results *from both parts of the analysis*, van Eck (1987) concluded:

> The results of this study show that the use of fluoridated water until eruption only, has a greater effect than the use only between eruption and examination in

all categories of surfaces of the first molar. However, additional use of fluoridated water consumed continuously from birth, results in the greatest effect: pre- as well as post-eruptive consumption are both necessary to benefit most from water fluoridation.

Since the publication of the thesis of van Eck (1987), Groeneveld, van Eck and Backer Dirks (1990) have discussed his findings in relation to '*in vitro*' and previous epidemiological evidence. They present an important explanation for the disagreement between laboratory workers and epidemiologists on the relative importance of the pre-eruptive effect of fluoride. While laboratory workers have almost exclusively studied the enamel lesion, epidemiologists have usually concerned themselves with dentinal lesions (i.e. caries cavities). While the number of dentinal lesions in fluoridated Tiel was about 50% less than in Culemborg, the total number of lesions (dentinal and enamel) was the same, in 18-year-olds, in both towns. It can be concluded that there was no difference in the solubility of enamel in the two areas, but that progression of lesions from enamel only to dentine was slower in Tiel than in Culemborg. Hence, there is no pre- or post-eruptive effect of fluoride on the formation of enamel-only lesions.

Groeneveld and co-workers presented further analyses of the Tiel and Culemborg data, and graphically illustrated the relative effectiveness of pre- and post-eruptive fluoride exposure (Figures 12.4 and 12.5). It can be seen that the observed percentage reductions approximate to curve C in both figures, indicating the presence of both pre- and post-eruptive effects on those surfaces. They concluded that:

> It is evident that fluoride has an important pre-eruptive effect on caries experience in all permanent dentition predilection sites. The maximum DMFS reduction in a fluoridated area at age 15 was due about half to the pre-eruptive and about half to the post-eruptive effect of fluoride. The initiation of the caries lesion is hardly affected by fluoride from drinking water. The cariostatic effect occurs when the lesion has progressed to the dentine following cavitation. The best effect is achieved if fluoride is available from birth, but about 85% of the greatest reduction is obtained when fluoride consumption starts between 3 and 4.

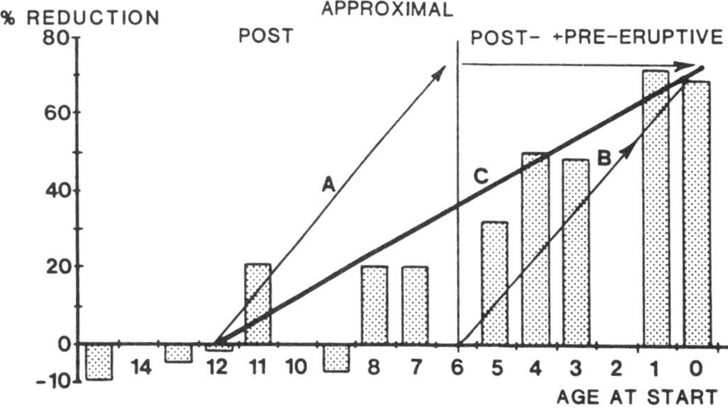

Figure 12.4 Observed percentage caries reductions (bars) in approximal surfaces of first permanent molars in 15-year-old children who were at different ages at the onset of water fluoridation. Lines A and B indicate the theoretical curves of pure post- and pre-eruptive effects, respectively. Line C indicates similar pre- and post-eruptive effects (Reproduced from Groeneveld *et al.*, 1990; reproduced by kind permission of the Editor, *Journal of Dental Research*)

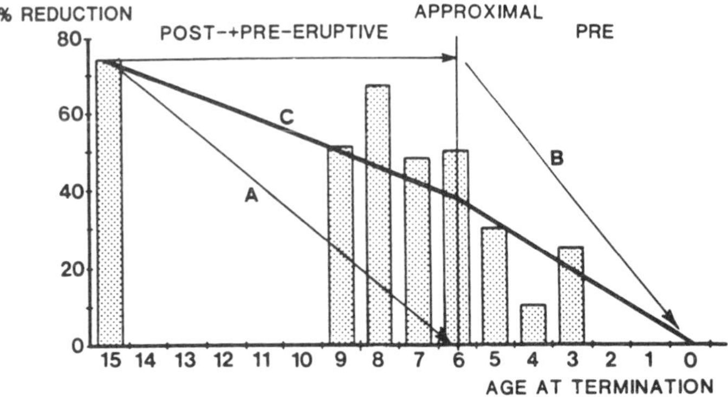

Figure 12.5 Observed percentage caries reductions (bars) in approximal surfaces of first permanent molars in 15-year-old children who were at different ages at the termination of water fluoridation. Lines A and B indicate the theoretical curves of pure post- and pre-eruptive effects, respectively. Line C indicates similar pre- and post-eruptive effects (Reproduced from Groeneveld *et al.*, 1990; reproduced by kind permission of the Editor, *Journal of Dental Research*)

In surfaces with high caries susceptibility, e.g. pits and fissures, the greater part of the reduction is derived from pre-eruptive fluoride, while in surfaces with low susceptibility, i.e. smooth surfaces, post-eruptive fluoride is more significant.

Because the pre-eruptive effect is less important in surfaces least susceptible to caries, it could be expected that the pre-eruptive effect will become less important overall as caries declines in a population. However, this argument is balanced somewhat by the fact that, as caries declines, a greater proportion of the remaining caries resides in fissure surfaces – the surfaces which gain most from pre-eruptive fluoride exposure.

Without a doubt, a pre-eruptive fluoride exposure prevents cavity formation. Reasons for this observed fact need to be clarified. Thylstrup (1990) put forward one possible explanation: that permanent teeth in fluoridated areas emerge into an oral environment with fewer carious deciduous teeth, with fewer plaque-retentive sites and a less cariogenic flora, than permanent teeth in fluoride-low areas. They, thus, 'get off to a better start' than teeth in children receiving insufficient fluoride. Further research would be welcomed.

References

Arnold, F. A. (1945) A discussion of the possibility of reducing dental caries by increasing fluoride ingestion. *J. Am. Coll. Dent.*, **12,** 61–62

Arnold, F. A., Dean, H. T., Jay, P. and Knutson, J. W. (1956) Effect of fluoridated public water supplies on dental caries prevalence. *Publ. Hlth Rep.*, **71,** 652–658

Arnold, F. A., Likens, R. C., Russell, A. L. and Scott, D. B. (1962) Fifteenth year of the Grand Rapids fluoridation study. *J. Am. Dent. Ass.*, **65**, 780–785

Beltran, E. D. and Burt, B. A. (1988) The pre- and post-eruptive effects of fluoride in the caries decline. *J. Publ. Hlth Dent.*, **48**, 233–240

Bibby, B. G. (1943) The effect of sodium fluoride application on dental caries. *J. Dent. Res.*, **22**, 207 (abstr.)

Bibby, B. G. (1945) Test of the effect of fluoride-containing dentifrices on dental caries. *J. Dent. Res.*, **24**, 297–303

Bibby, B. G., Zander, H. A., McKelleget, M. and Labunsky, B. (1946) Preliminary reports on the effect on dental caries of the use of sodium fluoride in a prophylactic cleaning mixture and in a mouthwash. *J. Dent. Res.*, **25**, 207–211

Deatherage, C. F. (1943a) Fluoride domestic waters and dental caries experience in 2026 white Illinois selective servicemen. *J. Dent. Res.*, **22,** 129–137

Deatherage, C. F. (1943b) A study of fluoride in domestic waters and dental caries experience in 263 white Illinois selective servicemen living in fluoride areas following the period of calcification of the permanent teeth. *J. Dent. Res.*, **22,** 173–180

van Eck, A. A. M. J. (1987) Pre- and post-eruptive effect of fluoridated drinking water on dental caries experience. *Thesis*, University of Utrecht, NIPG-TNO No. 87021

Ekstrand, J., Fejerskov, O. and Silverstone, L. M. (1988) *Fluoride in Dentistry*, Munksgaard, Copenhagen

Englander, H. R., Keyes, P. H., Gestwicki, M. and Sultz, H. A. (1967) Clinical anti-caries effect of repeated topical sodium fluoride applications by mouthpieces. *J. Am. Dent. Ass.*, **75**, 638–644

Fédération Dentaire Internationale (1985) Changing patterns of oral health and implications for oral health manpower. *Int. Dent. J.*, **35**, 235–251

Fejerskov, O., Manji, F., Baelum, V. and Moller, I. J. (1988) *Dental Fluorosis*, Munksgaard, Copenhagen

Forrest, J. R. (1956) Caries incidence and enamel defects in areas with different levels of fluoride in the drinking water. *Br. Dent. J.*, **100**, 195–200

Glass, R. L. (1982) The first international conference on the declining prevalence of dental caries. *J. Dent. Res.*, **61**, 1304–1383

Groeneveld, A., van Eck, A. A. M. J. and Backer Dirks, O. (1990) Fluoride in caries prevention; is the effect pre- or post-eruptive? *J. Dent. Res.*, **69** (spec. issue), 751–755

Gron, P., Spinelli, M., Trautz, O. and Brudevold, F. (1963) The effect of carbonate on the solubility of hydroxyapatite. *Arch. Oral Biol.*, **8**, 251–263

Hardwick, J. L., Teasdale, J. and Bloodworth, G. (1982) Caries increments over 4 years in children aged 12 years at the start of water fluoridation. *Br. Dent. J.*, **153,** 217–222

Healy, W. B. and Ludwig, T. G. (1966) Enamel solubility studies on New Zealand teeth. *N.Z. Dent. J.*, **62**, 276–278

Klein, H. (1945) Dental caries experience in relocated children exposed to drinking water containing fluorine, I. *Publ. Hlth Rep.*, **60**, 1462–1467

Klein, H. (1946) Dental caries (DMF) experience in relocated children exposed to water containing fluorine, II. *J. Am. Dent. Ass.*, **33**, 1136–1141

Klein, H. (1948) Dental effects of community water accidentally fluoridated for nineteen years, II. *Publ. Hlth Rep.*, **63**, 563–573

McKay, F. S. (1952) The study of mottled enamel (dental fluorosis). *J. Am. Dent. Ass.*, **44**, 133–137

Marthaler, T. M. (1979) Fluoride supplements for systemic effects in caries prevention. In *Continuing Evaluation of the Use of Fluorides* (eds E. Johansen, D. R. Taves and T. O. Olsen), AAAS, Washington, pp. 33–59

Ockerse, T. (1949) *Dental Caries; Clinical and Experimental Investigations*, Pretoria, South Africa, Department of Health

Russell, A. L. (1949) Dental effects of exposure to fluoride-bearing Dakota sandstone waters at various ages and for various lengths of time, II. *J. Dent. Res.*, **28,** 600–612

Thylstrup, A. (1990) Clinical evidence of the role of pre-eruptive fluoride in caries prevention. *J. Dent. Res.*, **69** (special issue), 742–750

Thylstrup, A., Bille, J. and Bruun, C. (1982) Caries prevalence in Danish children living in areas with low and optimal levels of natural water fluoride. *Caries Res.*, **16,** 413–420

Volker, J. F., Hodge, H. C., Wilson, H. J. and van Voorkis, S. N. (1940) The absorption of fluorides by enamel, dentine, bone and hydroxyapatite as shown by the use of the radioactive isotope. *J. Biol. Chem.*, **134**, 543–548

Weaver, R. (1944) Fluorine and dental caries; further investigations on Tyneside and in Sunderland. *Br. Dent. J.*, **57**, 185–193

Widenheim, J. (1985) On fluoride tablets; a retrospective study of intake pattern and the pre-eruptive effect on occurrence of caries, restorations and fluorosis in teeth. *Thesis*, University of Lund, Malmo

Widenheim, J., Birkhed, D., Granath, L. and Lindgren, G. (1986) Pre-eruptive effect of NaF tablets on caries in children from 12 to 17 years of age. *Community Dent. Oral Epidemiol.*, **14**, 1–4

Chapter 13

Epidemiology and measurement of dental fluorosis

Dental fluorosis is a hypoplasia or hypomaturation of tooth enamel or dentine produced by the chronic ingestion of excessive amounts of fluoride during the period when teeth are developing. The major cause of dental fluorosis is the consumption of water, containing high levels of fluoride, by infants and children during the first six years of life. Although both primary and permanent teeth may be affected by fluorosis, under uniform conditions of fluoride availability fluorosis tends to be greater in permanent teeth than primary teeth. This disparity may be due to the fact that much of the mineralization of primary teeth occurs before birth and the placenta serves as a barrier to the transfer of high concentrations of plasma fluoride from a pregnant mother to her developing fetus, thus controlling to a certain extent the delivery of fluoride to the developing primary dentition. Other reasons may be that the period of enamel formation for primary teeth is shorter than for permanent teeth and that the enamel of primary teeth is thinner than that of permanent teeth (Moller, 1982; Horowitz, 1986).

Interest in dental fluorosis has increased over the past 10 years or so, not only in areas like India and Kenya where there are communities with high levels of fluorosis, associated with high concentrations of fluoride in the water supply, but also in temperate climates with optimal or low fluoridated water supplies where fluoride uptake from other sources, in particular fluoride supplements and fluoride toothpaste in early infancy, have resulted in an increase in the prevalence of enamel mottling. With the decline in caries, following fluoride therapy, increasing attention is now being given to levels of dental fluorosis (Fejerskov *et al.*, 1985). In a sense history is turning full circle, because the history of water fluoridation really started with trying to ascertain the cause of 'Colorado stain' in the early 1900s. In this chapter, the development of the various indices advocated to measure dental fluorosis will be reviewed and the effect of fluoride ingestion from vehicles other than water will be considered.

Historical aspects

One of the first reports of what was probably dental fluorosis was made by Kuhns in 1888, who described teeth of persons in areas of Mexico that were opaque, discoloured and disfigured (Kuhns, 1888; Moller, 1982). An Assistant Surgeon of the US Marine Hospital Service reported the condition in Italians emigrating to the USA from Naples (Eager, 1901). He surmised that the aetiology:

> seems to be connected with volcanic fumes or the emanations of subterranean fires, either fouling the atmosphere or forming a solution in drinking water. In Naples it is more often attributable to water than the air and since the Serino water, brought in conduits from a distant mountain height, has been in use and local wells condemned, the incidence among infants has greatly diminished.

He described affected children as having 'characteristic black teeth (denti neri)' or teeth 'marred by a line of fine black markings crossing the incisor teeth in a horizontal direction'.

The next report in the literature came when McKay and Black (1916) published a series of articles in *Dental Cosmos* (see Chapter 2, pages 7–8). Black introduced the term 'mottled enamel' and described affected teeth in the following way: 'The teeth are of normal form, but not of normal colour. When not stained brown or yellow they are ghastly opaque white that comes prominently into notice whenever the lips are opened. . . . In many cases the teeth appear absolutely black. . . .'

Ainsworth (1933) gave a similar description of a 15-year-old girl from Maldon, Essex (see Chapter 2, page 13). Her teeth 'were curiously opaque and flecked with brownish black spots'.

Dean's index and subsequent modifications

After the discovery that the fluoride concentration in the drinking water was correlated with mottled enamel, Dean (1934) developed an index for assessing the presence and severity of mottled enamel. He used the following classification – normal, questionable, very mild, mild, moderate, moderately severe, severe, and commented:

> To the experienced investigator, 'very mild' presents separate and distinct characteristics. The classification of 'questionable' is often a baffling problem. There are areas where the causative factor in mottling of the enamel is apparently just between the maximum harmless amount and the minimum amount capable of producing the milder forms of mottling. In such areas, occasional minute flecks and small white spots on the enamel often show in an unusually high percentage of children.

Dean made it clear that under his classification all those showing 'hypoplasia, other than mottling of the enamel . . . (Hutchinsonianism, disorders caused by exanthematous disease and nutritional disturbances)' were placed in the 'normal category'. He also described the difficulty in deciding between 'normal' and 'very mild', even for the experienced investigator.

In Dean's method, each individual receives a score corresponding to the clinical appearance of the second most severely affected tooth in the mouth.

Examinations were made in good natural light with the child seated facing a window. All tooth surfaces were examined. Dean made it clear, particularly in his study on the minimal threshold of the dental sign of chronic endemic fluorosis (Dean and Elvove, 1935), that children who had not lived in a community continuously, or who had obtained their domestic water from other than the public water supply, were eliminated from further study. No specific information as to whether the teeth were cleaned or dried before examination is given, although mouth mirrors and new probes 'were utilized in making the examination'. Having completed the examination each child was then given a 'mouth classification' by summarizing the 'general impression of the degree of severity' (normal, questionable, very mild, mild, moderate, moderately severe, severe).

Dean, Dixon and Cohen (1935) then proposed that their classification should be used to determine a mottled enamel index of a community, deeming it necessary for 'epidemiological purposes and subsequent correlation with chemical and other studies':

Negative: less than 10% of the children show 'very mild' or more severe types of mottled enamel.
Borderline: 10% or more, but less than 35%, show 'very mild' mottled enamel or worse.
Slight: 35% or more show 'very mild' or worse, but less than 50% are mild or worse, and less than 35% 'moderate' or worse.
Medium: 50% or more are mild or worse, but less than 35% are 'moderate' or worse.
Rather marked: 35% or more, but less than 50% are 'moderate' or worse, but less than 35% are 'moderately severe' or worse.
Marked: 50% or more are 'moderate' or worse, but less than 35% are 'moderately severe' or worse.
Very marked: 35% or more are 'moderately severe' or worse.

In 1942, Dean modified his index by reducing the number of categories (Table 13.1) and developed a scoring system so as to derive a Community Fluorosis Index score (Dean, 1942). The scoring system ranged from 0 (normal enamel) to 4 (severe

Table 13.1 Criteria for Dean's classification system for dental fluorosis* (From Dean, 1942)

Classification (score)	*Criteria*
Normal (0)	The enamel represents the usual translucent semi-vitriform type of structure. The surface is smooth, glossy and usually of a pale, creamy white colour
Questionable (0.5)	The enamel discloses slight aberrations from the translucency of normal enamel, ranging from a few white flecks to occasional white spots. This classification is used in those instances where a definite diagnosis of the mildest form of fluorosis is not warranted and a classification of 'normal' not justified
Very mild (1)	Small, opaque, paper white areas scattered irregularly over the tooth, but not involving as much as approximately 25% of the tooth surface. Frequently included in this classification are teeth showing no more than about 1–2 mm of white opacity at the tip of the summit of the cusps of the bicuspids or second molars
Mild (2)	The white opaque areas in the enamel of the teeth are more extensive, but do not involve as much as 50% of the tooth
Moderate (3)	All enamel surfaces of the teeth are affected, and surfaces subject to attrition show wear. Brown stain is frequently a disfiguring feature
Severe (4)	All enamel surfaces are affected and hypoplasia is so marked that the general form of the tooth may be affected. The major diagnostic sign of this classification is discrete or confluent pitting. Brown stains are widespread and teeth often present a corroded-like appearance.

*See also Plates 1–6 (Driscoll *et al.*, 1983).

fluorosis) – see Plates 1–6. In a given population, the proportion in each category was multiplied by the weight given to derive a score for the community:

$$F_{ci} = \frac{(n \times w)}{N}$$

where F_{ci} is the community index of fluorosis, n the number of children in each category, w the weighting for each category, and N the total population. This gave an indication of the public health significance of the fluorosis (Table 13.2).

Table 13.2 Public health significance of Community Fluorosis Index scores, as defined by Dean (From Dean, 1946)

Range of scores for Community Fluorosis Index	*Public health significance*
0.0–0.4	Negative
0.4–0.6	Borderline
0.6–1.0	Slight
1.0–2.0	Medium
2.0–3.0	Marked
3.0–4.0	Very marked

In an attempt to make Dean's index more sensitive, Moller (1965) introduced three intermediate classifications and a variation in the weightings to be ascribed to each category (Table 13.3).

From his study in Denmark, Moller (1965) concluded that both the prevalence and the degree of severity of dental fluorosis are lower in Denmark than in the USA, with identical contents of fluorine in the drinking water. He felt this was due to quantitative differences in the consumption of drinking water, but also in part due to differences in diet and nutrition. He felt that the type of enamel classified as 'optimal' in his study was found to be most frequent with 1.2–1.6 ppm F in the drinking water. The enamel was of a creamy colour, looking somewhat like mother-of-pearl and was clinically deemed to be ideally mineralized, having no signs of dental fluorosis, enamel hypoplasia or other defects in enamel structure. He further concluded that 'the occurrence of localized interval enamel hypoplasia of unknown aetiology (non-fluoride enamel opacities) is inversely proportional to the fluorine ion concentration in the drinking water'.

These observations by Moller are most important. A non-fluoride opacity or hypoplasia can be just as unacceptable aesthetically as a case of dental fluorosis, and in terms of the dental health of a community the best outcome is minimal enamel defects, whether due to fluoride or non-fluoride factors.

Climate and dental fluorosis

Dean's Community Fluorosis Index was used by Galagan and Lamson (1953) in their investigation of climate and endemic dental fluorosis. They showed (Figure 13.1) that in water supplies of the Arizona communities studied with a mean annual temperature of 70°F (21°C), concentration of fluoride above 0.8 ppm resulted in

Table 13.3 Dental fluorosis index as described by Moller (From Moller, 1965)

Weighting	*Diagnosis*	*Clinical criteria*
0	Normal	The enamel shows the usual translucency. The surface is smooth, shiny and usually of a pale, creamy white to grey white colour. In this group are also opacities, which are not considered to be of fluoritic character
0	Optimal	The enamel is on clinical inspection completely homogeneously mineralized without hypomineralization of any sort. The enamel is smooth and mirror-like, and has a shiny, 'varnished' look. The colour is creamy white to yellowish white
¼	Questionable	In areas with relatively low fluoride content in drinking water, there are cases which even the most experienced researchers cannot classify as either normal or very mild. These cases show mainly labially in the upper front teeth as very narrow, opaque, paper-white, horizontal lines in the tooth's incisal third especially. In the back teeth are now and then seen small, opaque spots (about 0.5 mm in diameter) directly on the cusp tips, while the rest of the tooth is completely normally mineralized. The features of these opaque lines and spots are so fine that they are often confused with perichymata. This fine feature shows more clearly with drying the tooth, a procedure which should always be done while diagnosing
½–1	Very mild	Clearer opaque, paper-white, transversely oriented striations or spots, found spread especially on the upper incisors' labial surfaces and most concentrated in the incisal third. In the back teeth are seen opaque regions (<1 mm in diameter) directly on the cusp tips. Opaque, paper-white, narrow, transversely running lines reach down over the cusp, while the rest of the tooth is normal. The opaque regions cover at most a fourth of the surface of the tooth. When viewed from a distance, the tooth seems to have a slightly mother-of-pearl sheen. The lower grades of very mild dental fluorosis are rated ½ and the worse 1.

objectionable dental fluorosis, but concentrations below 0.6 ppm did not cause objectionable fluorosis. They surmised that because of several climatological influences, Arizona children drink more water than children living in more temperate climates and as a result there is increased ingestion of fluoride in relation to the concentration found in the water supply. From these findings, Galagan and Vermillion (1957) were able to establish an empirical relationship in the form of an equation which related ounces of water consumed per day, per pound of body weight, to the mean maximum temperature, which was found to apply over the temperature range 50–80°F (10–27°C).

Minoguchi (1970) refined the analysis of Galagan and Vermillion (1957) to take into account the total fluoride content from the diet by a community. Myers (1978) suggested a graphic method of obtaining optimal fluoride concentration by comparing the Community Fluorosis Index against water fluoride content, at different temperatures (Figure 13.2). He summarized the results from 14 countries (Table 13.4) and where possible computed the Community Fluorosis Index.

Weighting	*Diagnosis*	*Clinical criteria*
1½–2	Mild	The mainly transversely running opaque lines and spots are more clear and stretch further down over the tooth's surface towards the outer circumference. One can detect that the opaque lines begin to merge together into diffuse regions, so that the tooth seen at a distance (40–50 cm) seems whiter – more opaque – than a normally mineralized tooth. Seen close to, these opaque areas take up, however, at most half of the tooth's surface. Changes in the front teeth's lingual surfaces are considerably less obvious than on the labial. As far as the back teeth are concerned, the changes in labial and lingual surfaces are of more or less the same degree. On the cusps of canines, premolars and molars there are cases where the cusp tips are worn, so that the wear facets peripherally are bordered by a narrow, opaque ring (an expression of the fluoritic surface layer) surrounded by the clearer underlying enamel. In pronounced cases the development of pigment can be seen, especially in the upper incisors. Lower grades of mild dental fluorosis are scored 1½ and the worse degrees 2
2½–3	Moderate	The opaque regions take up practically all the tooth's surface. Tooth shape is normal, but a weak 'pit' development can be found, especially on premolar buccal and palatal surfaces, as well as upper incisor labial surfaces. Pigment where present can vary in colour from yellow to brown. The lower grades of moderate dental fluorosis are rated 2½ and the worse 3
3½–4	Severe	The shape of the tooth can be changed. The development of pits is pronounced. Merging of pits is often seen. Sometimes the outer layer of enamel is partly or completely missing, and the tooth has a corroded look. Pigmentation varies in colour from brown, to dark brown, to black. Lower degrees of severe dental fluorosis score 3½ and the worse degrees 4

Disadvantages of Dean's index

Dean's index has been the most widely used index to measure dental fluorosis. There is no doubt that its use helped to indicate the prevalence of moderate and severe fluorosis in various communities, as can be seen from Table 13.4, and the index was successful in monitoring the changes in Bauxite and other communities after the water supply had been changed (Dean, McKay and Elvove, 1938; Dean and McKay, 1939). The difficulty, which Dean himself recognized, was to differentiate between normal, questionable and very mild fluorosis. He said that 'to the experienced observer "very mild" presents separate and distinct characteristics. The classification of "questionable" is often a baffling problem' (Dean, 1934). In the 1950s, Forrest (1956) used Dean's index to assess the incidence of enamel defects in six areas in the south-east of England. Her results are summarized in Table 13.5 and include the footnote 'Not due to fluoride ingestion, but graded as if they were'. These results show that the low-fluoride areas (Surrey schools) gave a

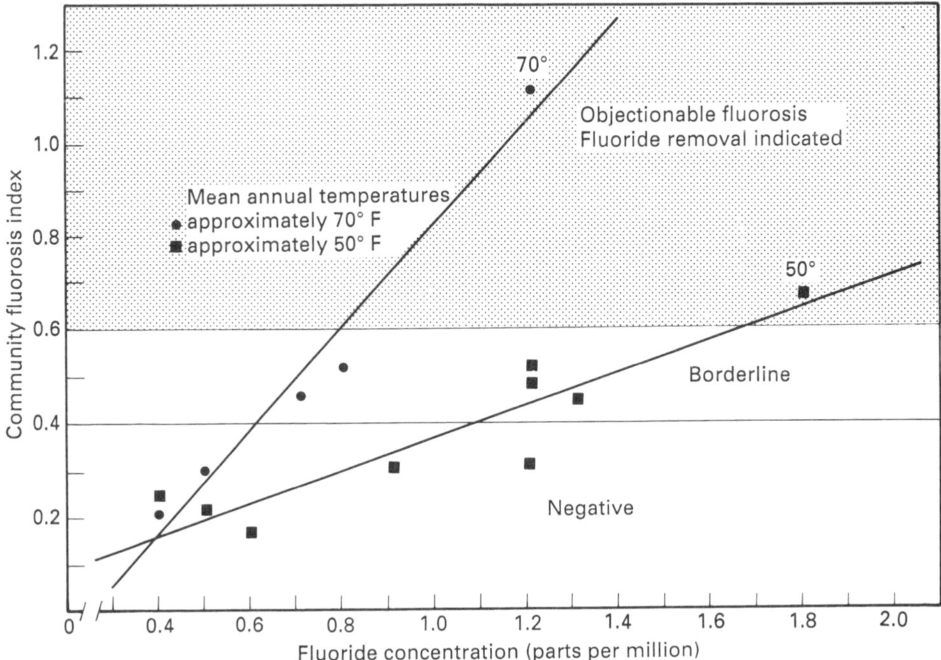

Figure 13.1 Relationship between fluoride concentration of municipal waters and fluorosis index for communities with mean annual temperatures of approximately 50°F (10°C), Midwest, and 70°F (21°C), Arizona (From Galagan and Lamson, 1953, by kind permission of the US Department of Health, Education and Welfare)

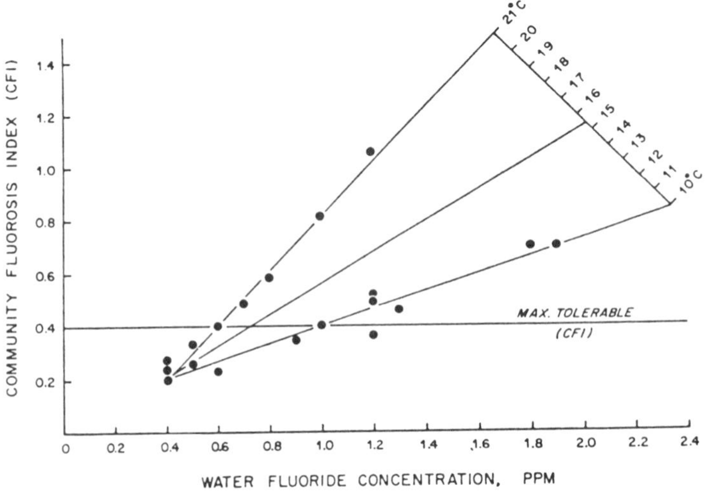

Figure 13.2 Graphic method of obtaining optimal fluoride concentration (From Myers, 1978, by kind permission of Karger, Basel)

Table 13.4 Incidence and severity of dental fluorosis as influenced by climate and drinking water concentration of fluoride (From Myers, 1978)

Location	*Average temperature* (°C)	H_2O (F ppm)	*CFI*	*Severity of fluorosis (percentage of total)*					*Percentage afflicted*	*Reference*
				Doubtful	*Very mild*	*Mild*	*Moderate*	*Severe*		
Sweden	6	1.0	–	36	23	41	0	0	64	Forsman (1974)
Sweden	6	5.0	–	8	0	65	5	20	90	Forsman (1974)
Sweden	6	10.0	–	0	0	0	35	65	100	Forsman (1974)
Austria	7	1.0	–	–	18	0	0	0	18	Binder (1973)
Austria	7	1.5	–	–	43	5	0	0	48	Binder (1973)
Austria	7	3.0			19	27	6	0	52	Binder (1973)
England	10.5	0.0	0.60	45	0	12	6	0	63	Forrest (1965)
England	10.5	0.0	–	–	4	1	2	0	47	Forrest (1965)
England	10.5	0.12	–	–	5	3	0.6	1.4	10	Goward (1976)
England	10.5	0.9	0.32	16	–	–	–	–	16	Forrest (1965)
England	10.5	1.0	–	9	3	0	0	0	12	Murray *et al.* (1956)
England	10.5	2.0	0.80	–	0	0	8	0	66	Forrest (1965)
England	10.5	3.5	1.9		–	–	–	11	92	Forrest (1965)
England	10.5	5.8	2.6	35	–	–	–	31	96	Forrest (1965)
USA	10	0.4	0.25	37	5	1	0	0	6	Galagan and Lamson (1953)
USA	10	0.5	0.22	35	4	1	0	0	5	Galagan and Lamson (1953)
USA	10	0.6	0.17	21	6	0.5	0	0	7	Galagan and Lamson (1953)
USA	10	0.7	–	3	2	0	0	0	2	Dean and Elvove (1937)
USA	10	0.9	0.31	35	10	2	0	0	12	Galagan and Lamson (1953)
USA	10	0.9	–	21	9	2	0	0	11	Dean and Elvove (1937)
USA	10	1.2	0.32	32	14	1	0	0	15	Galagan and Lamson (1953)
USA	10	1.2	0.49	32	30	2	0	0	32	Galagan and Lamson (1953)
USA	10	1.2	0.51	28	29	4	0	0	33	Galagan and Lamson (1953)
USA	10	1.3	0.46	34	22	3	0	0	25	Galagan and Lamson (1953)
USA	10	1.5	–	20	18	6	1	0	25	Dean and Elvove (1937)
USA	10	1.6	–	8	22	4	0	0	26	Dean and Elvove (1937)
USA	10	1.7	–	21	37	5	0	0	42	Dean and Elvove (1937)
USA	10	1.8	0.67	32	30	9	0	0	39	Galagan and Lamson (1953)
USA	10	1.9	0.69	27	40	6	1	0	47	Galagan and Lamson (1953)
USA	10	2.5	–	14	28	22	14	3	67	Dean and Elvove (1937)
Italy	16	1.3	1.2	–	23	17	10	8	58	Massler and Schour (1952)
Italy	16	3.5	2.5	–	5	38	53	4	100	Massler and Schour (1952)
Israel	20	2.0	0.80	–	–	–	–	–	57	Milgalter *et al.* (1974)

Table 13.4 continued

Location	Average temperature (°C)	H_2O (F ppm)	CFI	Severity of fluorosis (percentage of total)					Percentage afflicted	Reference
				Doubtful	Very mild	Mild	Moderate	Severe		
USA	20	0.4	0.21	32	2	1	0	0	3	Gallagan and Vermillion (1957)
USA	20	0.5	0.30	38	9	1	0	0	10	Gallagan and Vermillion (1957)
USA	21	0.6	–	–	+	+	0	0	–	Richards *et al*. (1967)
USA	20	0.7	0.46	45	12	3	2	0	17	Gallagan and Vermillion (1957)
USA	20	0.8	0.52	39	9	6	2	0	17	Gallagan and Vermillion (1957)
USA	20	1.0	0.85	38	30	18	0	0	48	Gallagan and Vermillion (1957)
USA	20	1.2	1.12	20	26	14	13	3	56	Gallagan and Vermillion (1957)
USA	18	1.2	–	–	+	+	0	0	–	Richards *et al*. (1967)
Morocco	20	0.4	2.2	6	20	29	29	13	91	Møller and Poulsen (1976)
Taiwan	24	0.0	0.10	–	11	4	0	0	15	Pu and Lilienthal (1961)
Taiwan	24	0.3	0.27	–	26	8	0	0	34	Pu and Lilienthal (1961)
Taiwan	24	0.7	0.44	–	40	14	5	0	54	Pu and Lilienthal (1961)
Taiwan	24	0.9	0.74	–	36	38	9	0	83	Pu and Lilienthal (1961)
Taiwan	24	1.6	1.02	–	21	37	24	2	84	Pu and Lilienthal (1961)
Pescadores	24	0.5	0.88	–	33	33	19	–	85	Pu and Lilienthal (1961)
Pescadores	24	0.5	0.51	–	35	22	5	1	63	Pu and Lilienthal (1961)
South Africa	25	2.4	–	–	15	27	41	–	83	Bischoff *et al*. (1976)
USA	27	0.3	–	–	+	+	0	0	–	Richards *et al*. (1967)
USA	27	0.6	–	–	+	+	+	0	–	Richards *et al*. (1967)
Australia	27	1.3	–	–	–	–	–	–	–	Kallis and Silva (1970)
Thailand	28	0.1	–	–	–	–	–	–	3	Leatherwood *et al*. (1965)
Thailand	28	0.1	–	–	–	–	–	–	42	Leatherwood *et al*. (1965)
Thailand	28	0.2	–	–	–	–	–	–	60	Leatherwood *et al*. (1965)
Thailand	28	0.6	–	–	–	–	–	–	56	Leatherwood *et al*. (1965)
Thailand	28	0.7	–	–	–	–	–	–	61	Leatherwood *et al*. (1965)
Uganda	29	0.2	0.04							Møller and Poulsen (1976)
Uganda	29	0.7	0.82							Møller and Poulsen (1976)
Uganda	29	2.5	1.74							Møller and Poulsen (1976)
India	32	0.2	–	–	11	1	0	0	12	Nanda *et al*. (1974)
India	32	0.6	–	–	18	5	1	0	24	Nanda *et al*. (1974)
India	32	1.0	–	–	18	16	7	0	34	Nanda *et al*. (1974)
India	32	>1.2	–	–	2.6	17	23	0	56	Nanda *et al*. (1974)

Plate Section

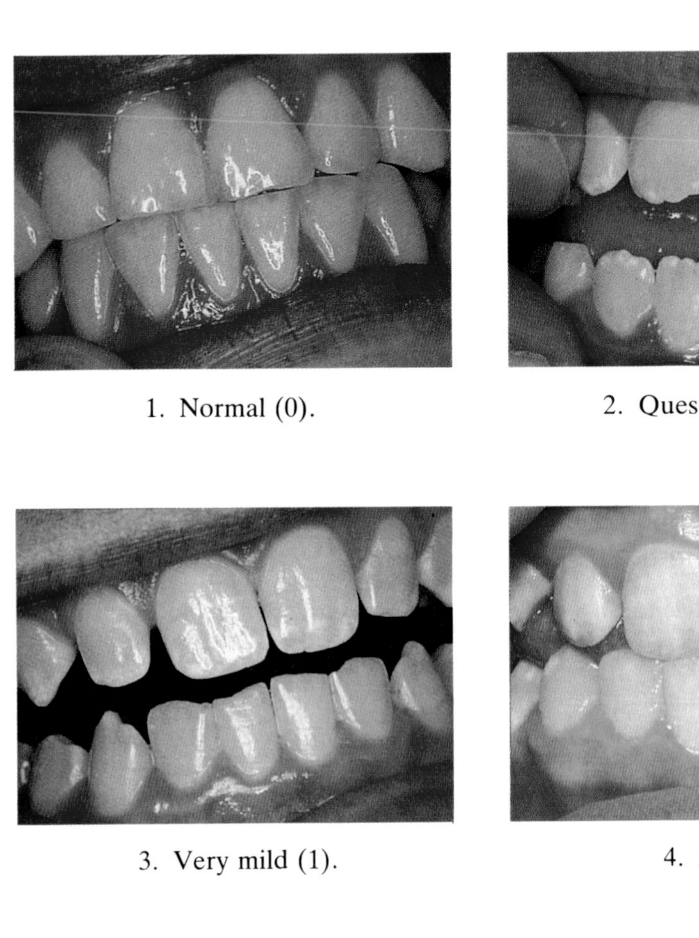

1. Normal (0).

2. Questionable (0.5).

3. Very mild (1).

4. Mild (2).

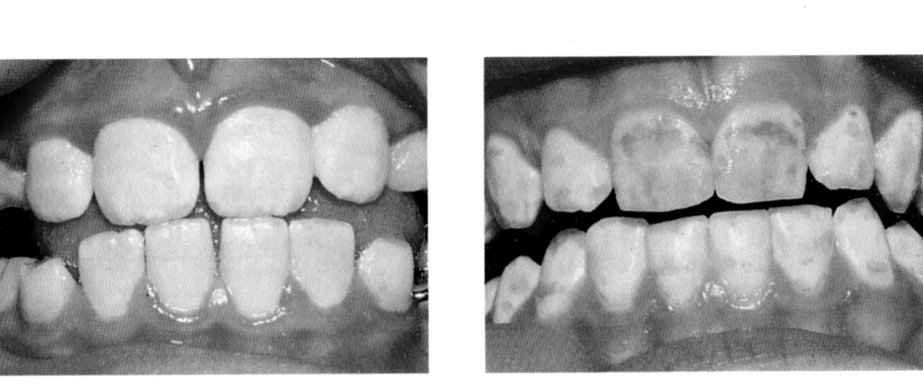

5. Moderate (3).

6. Severe (4).

Plates 1–6 Examples of Dean's classification system for dental fluorosis and assigned scores (From Driscoll *et al.*, 1983, by kind permission of the Authors and the *Journal of the American Dental Association*)

Erratum
Plate 7 and Plate 10 have been transposed in error.

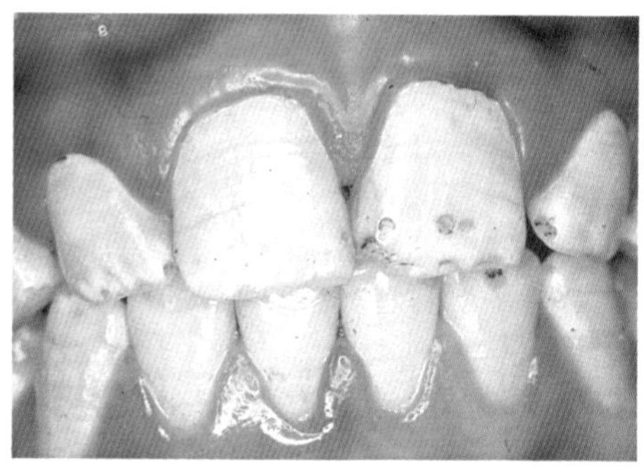

7. TF score 1.
Fine lines across the entire tooth surface.

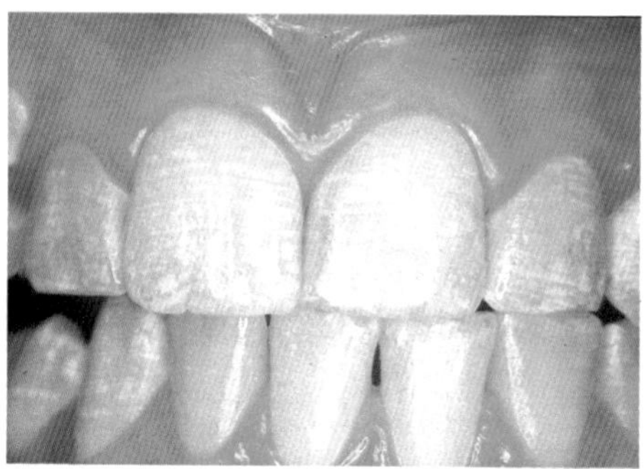

8. TF score 2.
Fine lines frequently merge.

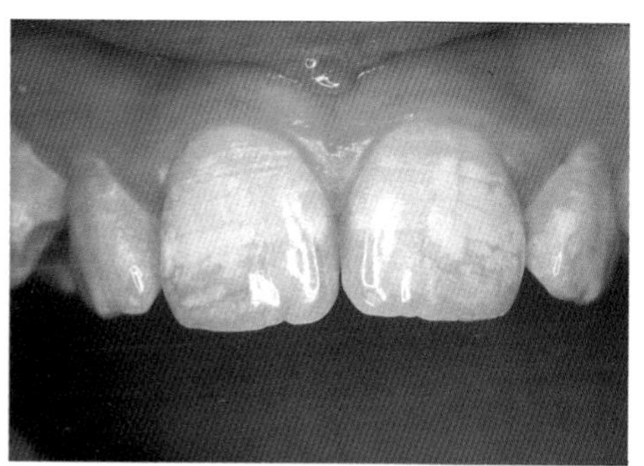

9. TF score 3.
Irregular cloudy white areas.

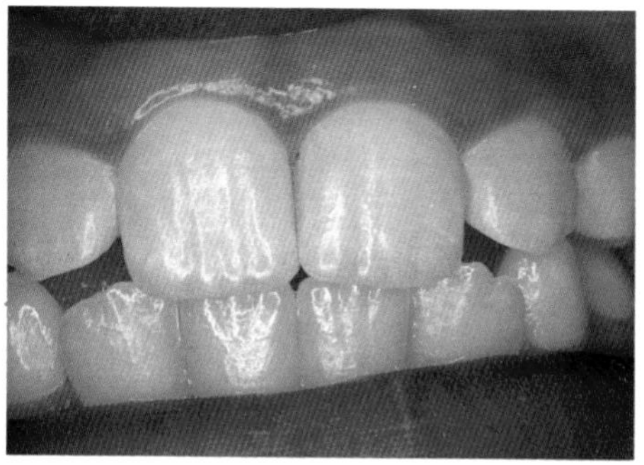

10. TF score 4 (right incisor) and score 5 (left incisor).

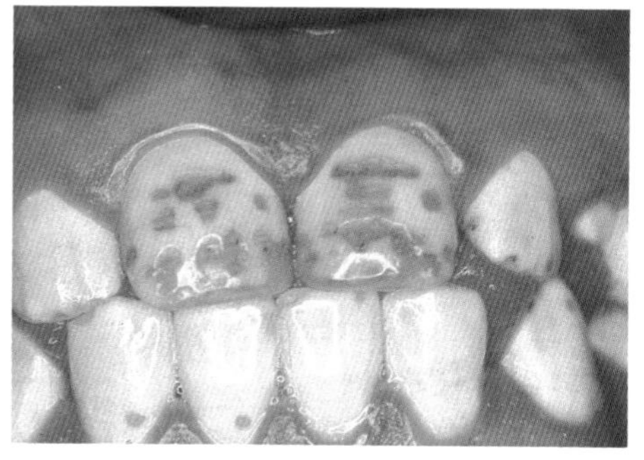

11. TF score 7.

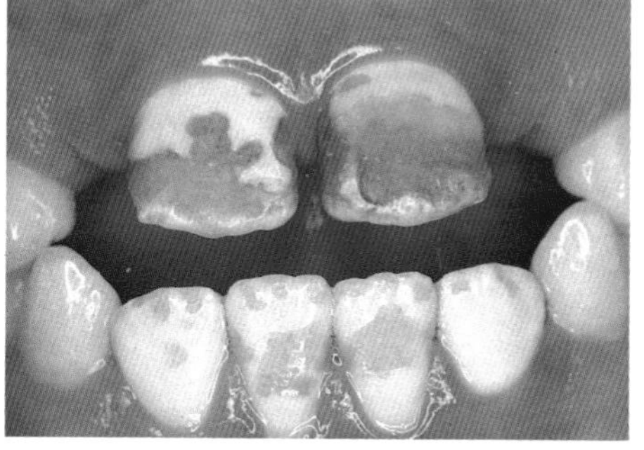

12. TF scores 8 and 9.

Plates 7–12 Examples of the Thylstrup–Fejerskov index (By kind permission of Professor O. Fejerskov and Munksgaard Publishers, Copenhagen)

Table 13.5 Prevalence of various types of enamel opacities in children aged 12–14 in fluoride and non-fluoride areas (From Forrest, 1956)

Area	*Fluoride content of water* (ppm)	*No. children examined*	*No opacities*	*Idiopathic spots only*	*Percentage of children with enamel opacities (degree of mottling)*					*Index of mottling*†	
					Not noticeable		*Noticeable*			*Excluding idiopathic spots*	*Including idiopathic spots*
					Questionable	*Very mild*	*Mild*	*Moderate*	*Moderately severe*		
West Mersea	5.8	51	0	4	16	12	2	25	31	2.5	2.6
Burnham-on-Crouch	3.5	62	5	3	10	29	16	26	11	1.88	1.9
Harwich	2.0	92	18	16	22	32	4	8	–	0.7	0.8
Slough	0.9	119	50	31	10	6	2	1	–	0.17	0.32
Saffron Walden and District	0.1	145	37	30	12*	9*	6*	6*	–	0.45*	0.6*
Surrey schools	0.1–0.2	114	40	30	14*	3*	2*	11*	–	0.45*	0.6*

* Not due to fluoride ingestion, but graded as if they were.
† By Dean's method of computation. The threshold of objectionable mottling lies between 0.4 and 0.6.

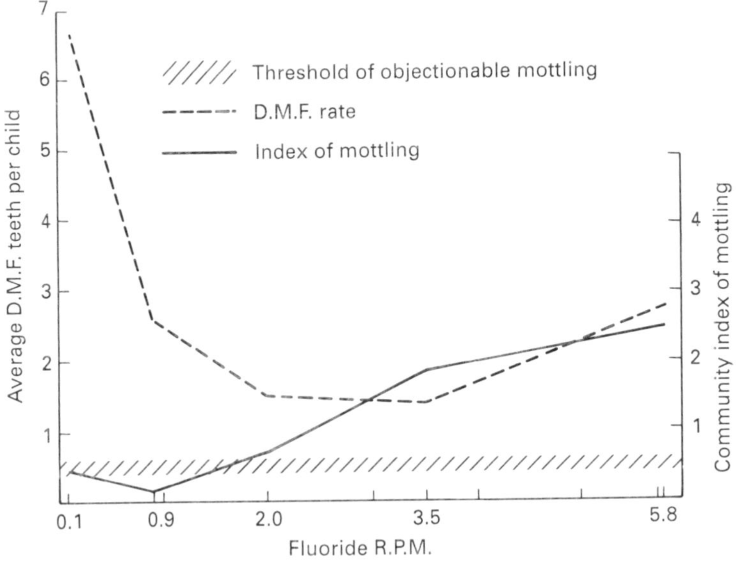

Figure 13.3 Fluoride content of water, caries experience and enamel mottling in children aged 12–14 years (From Forrest, 1956; reproduced by courtesy of the Editor, *British Dental Journal*)

Community Fluorosis Index of 0.45–0.6, on the threshold of objectionable mottling. The best score (CFC 0.17–0.32) was achieved in Slough, with 0.9 ppm F in drinking water (Figure 13.3).

Clarkson (1989) summarized the main criticisms of Dean's classification in the following way:

1. Since the index is based on the two most severely affected teeth, it does not allow for the measurement of the extent of defects on the remaining teeth.
2. It gives no indication of the location of the teeth or the tooth surfaces affected.
3. The use of the term 'questionable' is too vague.
4. The index appears to describe the milder forms of fluorosis accurately, but is not sensitive enough to distinguish between degrees of fluorosis in high-fluoride areas.
5. The statistical basis for using the arithmetic mean to calculate the CFI is questionable on the grounds that the classification is based on an ordinal and not an interval scale.
6. The Community Fluorosis Index, because of its method of calculation, may not give a true reflection of the severity of fluorosis within a community.

Descriptive classifications

Forrest (1956) was of the opinion that 'severe degrees of fluoride mottling were unmistakable but in milder cases the cause of enamel defects cannot always be stated with certainty' and referred to the high incidence of enamel defects reported by Parfitt (1955), Hurme (1949) and Zimmerman (1954) in areas with no fluoride in the water. She also pointed out the balance required between caries protection and the level of mottling and concluded that 'it is probably better to accept some degree of caries rather than risk the occurrence of enamel defects which are associated with excessive amounts of fluoride'.

A number of workers became concerned about the presumption in Dean's index concerning dental fluorosis, when many enamel defects are caused by other factors. Jackson in particular (Al-Alousi *et al.*, 1975; Jackson, James and Wolfe, 1975) argued that an index depends upon the principle that, when recording any conditions, once the criteria are defined, the results must depend on the definitions laid down and not be based on any presumed aetiology. The classification system used by Jackson and co-workers was based on the principle that investigators should record only what they see. Their index was also based on the principle that a simple descriptive index is preferable to a weighted one.

A summary of their definitions and the results of this approach are given in Tables 13.6 and 13.7. The idea was that the investigators should record what they saw, in both fluoride and low-fluoride areas, and make no decision on individual subjects, but rather compare the results for both fluoride and low-fluoride communities at the end of the study. On this basis, Al-Alousi *et al.* (1975) concluded that the prevalence of enamel opacities on anterior teeth was higher in low-fluoride Leeds than fluoridated Anglesey, and Murray *et al.* (1984) showed that, while the overall prevalence of enamel opacities was similar in fluoridated Newcastle compared with low-fluoride Northumberland, the prevalence of horizontal white lines was higher and the prevalence of hypoplasia was lower in Newcastle. The general thrust of this approach was to try to quantify whether fluoridation at 1 ppm had any public health implications in terms of an increasing prevalence of enamel defects, and followed the line of thinking articulated by Forrest in 1956.

The principal criticisms of descriptive indices were also summarized by Clarkson (1989): (a) the scores are not arranged in a well-ordered fashion; (b) the use of such criteria as 'areas greater or less than 2 mm' does not take into account the total area of a tooth surface which may be affected; (c) the criteria do not cover the full range of defects, and there is no attempt to differentiate between the configuration or demarcation of opacities; and (d) the criteria of diagnosis are not clearly stated, e.g. if two defects occur on the same surface, no indication is given as to which should be recorded.

In their paper, Al Alousi *et al.* (1975) make clear that the main purpose of their investigation was to measure the effect of fluoride in drinking water at 1 ppm F on the prevalence and distribution of mottled incisor teeth. Each child was seated on a portable dental examination chair fitted with a headrest. Natural lighting was used (as did Dean in his investigations). For each child there were two examiners: no charting was made unless both examiners agreed about the classification. There were only a few instances when food debris could have masked the possible diagnosis of mottling; in these instances debris was removed with a dental napkin. These studies were restricted to incisor teeth because the principal purpose of the investigations was to determine whether there was any aesthetic public health problem in fluoridating water at 1 ppm.

One possible complication in the diagnosis of enamel opacities is the presence of saliva which can reflect the light. Murray and Shaw (1979) and Murray *et al.* (1984) examined children in artificial light, in order to provide a uniform source of light, and dried the teeth gently with compressed air. This difference in methodology may explain in part the high values obtained by the latter investigators.

Table 13.6 Classifications used to quantify enamel opacities

Young (1973)	*Al Alousi* et al. *(1975)*	*Murray and Shaw (1979)*
Class 1 White fleck areas of enamel not greater than 2 mm in any direction	*Type A* White opaque spots <2 mm in diameter	*Type 1* White opaque spots (or flecks) <2 mm in diameter
Class 2 Coloured flecks same as white flecks but usually varying shades of yellow or brown	*Type B* White opaque spots >2 mm in diameter	*Type 2* White opaque spots (or patches) >2 mm when measured in any direction. Well demarcated from the surrounding area
Class 3 White patches – opaque white areas >2 mm when measured in any direction. Well demarcated from the surrounding enamel	*Type C* Coloured spots <2 mm in diameter	*Type 3* Coloured spots, flecks or patches
Class 4 Outline and form same as white patches, but also coloured. Usually varying shades of yellow or brown	*Type D* Coloured spots >2 mm in diameter	
Class 5 Spaced white lines. These are seen as fine opaque lines in the enamel. Ill-defined areas of chalky white appearance also seen occasionally	*Type E* Horizontal white lines irrespective of there being any white non-linear lines	*Type 4* Horizontal white lines, irrespective of there being any white non-linear lines. Not associated with deficiency of enamel substance (hypoplasia)
Class 6 As for Class 5, but associated with hypoplasia	*Type F* Coloured or white areas associated with roughened and badly shaped enamel	*Type 5* Hypoplasia, in association with any of categories 1–4
Class 7 A mixture of white lines, opaque and coloured areas. Lines often difficult to distinguish from the diffuse ill-defined areas		*Type 6* Possible early carious lesions
Class 8 As for Class 7, but associated with hypoplasia		

The FDI index: Developmental Defects of Enamel

The development of indices of a descriptive nature was considered by a Working Group of the FDI Commission in Oral Health, Research and Epidemiology in 1977. The Working Group concluded that:

1. Lack of a well-defined and internationally accepted classification of enamel defects has led to much confusion and lack of comparability of numerous studies of enamel defects.

Table 13.7 Distribution of teeth with specified types of mottling

Type of mottling	*Al-Alousi* et al. *(1975)*				*Jackson* et al. *(1975)*			
	Anglesey (n = 1312)		*Leeds (n = 1383)*		*Anglesey (n = 691)*		*Bangor/Caernarvon (n = 758)*	
	No. teeth affected	*%*	*No. teeth affected*	*%*	*No. teeth affected*	*%*	*No. teeth affected*	*%*
A	85	6.5	105	7.6	23	3.3	30	4.0
B	25	1.9	42	3.0	23	3.3	17	2.2
C	0	0	1	0.1	0	0	0	0
D	5	0.4	13	0.9	3	0.5	0	0
E	4	0.3	4	0.3	2	0.3	3	0.4
F	0	0	0	0	4	0.6	8	1.1
Total	119	9.1	165	11.9	55	8.0	58	7.7

2. Classifications based on aetiological considerations are premature because only a few defects can be assigned an aetiology.
3. A classification of defects based on descriptive criteria is the preferred basis of an epidemiological index.
4. A descriptive classification should have the flexibility for recording data on a person, tooth or tooth surface basis (Ainamo and Cutress, 1982).

They recommended the use of a descriptive index entitled Developmental Defects of Enamel (DDE) in which the type (opacity, hypoplasia, discoloration), number (single and multiple), demarcation (demarcated and diffuse) and location of defects on the buccal and lingual surfaces of teeth could be recorded (FDI, 1982; Clarkson and O'Mullane, 1989). Results from a number of studies (Suckling and Pearce, 1984; King and Brook, 1984; Cutress *et al.*, 1985; King and Wei, 1986; Dummer, Kingdon and Kingdon, 1986) have shown that the DDE index gives information on a wide range of defects, their distribution and location. However, the large amounts of data generated have caused difficulties in presenting results in a meaningful fashion. For example, Suckling and Pearce (1984) examined 243 children aged 12–14 years using the FDI index. The teeth were not cleaned or dried prior to examination and fibre-optic lighting was used. At least 1 tooth with defective enamel was seen in 60% of children, with a demarcated white opacity present in 44% of children. Defects were found most frequently in maxillary central incisors. The prevalence according to the FDI code is recorded in Table 13.8.

Table 13.8 Prevalence of enamel defects in 243 children according to type and number (From Suckling and Pearce, 1984)

FDI code	*Children*		*Teeth*	
	n	%	*n*	%
White opacities				
1.1 Demarcated single	108	44.4	247	4.2
(small, <2 mm diameter)	47	19.3	72	1.2
1.2 Demarcated multiple	24	9.9	30	0.5
1.3 Diffuse horizontal parallel lines	7	2.9	12	0.2
1.4 Diffuse patchy distribution	40	16.5	259	4.4
Yellow opacities				
2.1 Demarcated single	40	16.5	67	1.1
2.2 Demarcated multiple	4	1.7	4	0.1
Hypoplasia				
3 Pits	22	9.1	34	0.6
4 Grooves, horizontal	7	2.9	13	0.2
5 Grooves, vertical	1	0.4	3	0.1
6 Missing enamel	17	7.0	26	0.4
7 Discoloured enamel	1	0.4	8	0.1
8 Other	2	0.8	6	0.1
Combination of types				
9 Fillings	21	8.6	30	0.5
Extractions	5	2.1	20	–
Any defect	152	62.6	692	11.7

Table 13.9 Modified DDE index for use in general-purpose epidemiology studies (From Clarkson and O'Mullane, 1989)

Normal
Demarcated opacities
White/cream
Yellow/brown
Diffuse opacities
Diffuse – lines
Diffuse – patchy
Diffuse – confluent
Confluent/patchy + staining + loss of enamel
Hypoplasia
Pits
Missing enamel
Any other defects
Extent of defects
Normal
<1/3
At least 1/3 < 2/3
At least 2/3

Table 13.10 Modified DDE index for use in screening surveys (From Clarkson and O'Mullane, 1989)

Normal
Demarcated opacity
Diffuse opacity
Hypoplasia
Other defects

Clarkson and O'Mullane (1989) suggested that the DDE index needed to be simplified and proposed two modifications – one for general-purpose epidemiological studies (Table 13.9) and one for simple screening surveys (Table 13.10). The authors also recommended that the teeth be examined wet and that artificial light be used when teeth are examined on a full-mouth basis. The light source should not be so strong as to create a glare which might mask defects.

Approach by Thylstrup and Fejerskov (1978)
In contrast to the descriptive approach, Thylstrup and Fejerskov (1978) suggested a 10-point classification system (Table 13.11; see also Plates 7–12) designed to characterize the degree of dental fluorosis affecting buccal/lingual and occlusal surfaces.

An important feature of the system proposed by Thylstrup and Fejerskov (1978) is that it attempts to validate the visual appearance against the histological defect. Extracted teeth from the area were sampled, rinsed under tap water and stored in thymol-containing bottles. After drying with a cottonwool roll the surfaces were assigned to one of the 10 categories proposed, photographed and then ground sections prepared. The sections were approximately 80 μm thick and were examined in ordinary and polarized light. As far as score 1 was concerned, when the sections were examined dry in air, pseudo-isotopic areas were observed mainly along the striae of Rezius, giving rise to accentuated perichymata. As the clinical scores increased, the microscopic changes showed an ever-increasing width of the porous subsurface lesion. With the aid of polarized and ordinary light microscopy the histological features behind the individual scores were described. They applied their classification system to samples of children born in areas of 3.5, 6.0 and 21.0 ppm F and reported that the macroscopic appearance of increasing degrees of dental fluorosis were well correlated to the degree of subsurface porosity. For the clinical study, the children were examined in a portable chair by one investigator.

The examination was carried out in daylight using a plane mirror and probe. Prior to the examination the teeth were dried with cottonwool rolls. They reported that 'the present study has shown that the degree of fluorosis classically described as "severe" includes a wide range of clinical and histologic changes corresponding to our scores of 6–9. This explains why Dean's index was not sensitive enough to

Table 13.11 Classification of the clinical appearance of fluorotic enamel changes characterizing the single tooth surface* (From Thylstrup and Fejerskov, 1978)

Score	*Clinical appearance*
0	Normal translucency of enamel remains after prolonged air drying
1	Narrow white lines located corresponding to the perichymata
2	*Smooth surfaces* More pronounced lines of opacity which follow the perichymata. Occasionally confluence of adjacent lines *Occlusal surfaces* Scattered areas of opacity <2 mm in diameter and pronounced opacity of cuspal ridges
3	*Smooth surfaces* Merging and irregular cloudy areas of opacity. Accentuated drawing of perichymata often visible between opacities *Occlusal surfaces* Confluent areas of marked opacity. Worn areas appear almost normal but usually circumscribed by a rim of opaque enamel
4	*Smooth surfaces* The entire surface exhibits marked opacity or appears chalky white. Parts of surface exposed to attrition appear less affected *Occlusal surface* Entire surface exhibits marked opacity. Attrition is often pronounced shortly after eruption
5	*Smooth and occlusal surfaces* Entire surface displays marked opacity with focal loss of outermost enamel (pits) <2 mm in diameter
6	*Smooth surfaces* Pits are regularly arranged in horizontal bands <2 mm in vertical extension *Occlusal surfaces* Confluent areas <3 mm in diameter exhibit loss of enamel. Marked attrition
7	*Smooth surfaces* Loss of outermost enamel in irregular areas involving less than one-half of entire surface *Occlusal surfaces* Changes in the morphology caused by merging pits and marked attrition
8	*Smooth and occlusal surfaces* Loss of outermost enamel involving >½ of surface
9	*Smooth and occlusal surfaces* Loss of main part of enamel with change in anatomic appearance of surface. Cervical rim of almost unaffected enamel is often noted

*See also Plates 7–12.

distinguish between the severity of dental fluorosis in areas with 6.0 and 21.0 ppm F'.

Clarkson (1989) reported that Thylstrup and Fejerskov examined the teeth after a two-minute period of air drying, which creates an unnatural situation. He suggested that 'the changes described in scores 1 and 2 of their index are very minor, and the effect of drying the teeth tends to show these diffuse areas more clearly. The aesthetic significance of such changes is therefore questionable'.

The Tooth Surface Index of Fluorosis

The Tooth Surface Index of Fluorosis (TSIF) was developed by Horowitz *et al.* (1984). It was introduced to overcome some of the shortcomings of Dean's index. With the TSIF, a separate score is given for each tooth surface and contains no 'questionable' category. In this respect the TSIF index is similar to the TF index, because Horowitz (1986) maintained, as did Fejerskov and Thylstrup, that it was possible for trained and experienced examiners to make a definite diagnosis of dental fluorosis using differential diagnostic criteria for fluoride and non-fluoride opacities suggested by Russell (1961) (Table 13.12). The descriptive criteria for the TSIF are given in Table 13.13.

The index was used in communities grouped into four categories according to the relation of their water fluoride concentration to the recommended optimal fluoride

Table 13.12 Differential diagnosis: milder forms of dental fluorosis (questionable, very mild and mild) and non-fluoride opacities of enamel (From Russell, 1961)

Characteristic	*Milder forms of fluorosis*	*Non-fluoride enamel opacities*
Area affected	Usually seen on or near tips of cusps or incisal edges	Usually centred in smooth surface; may affect entire crown
Shape of lesions	Resembles line shading in pencil sketch; lines follow incremental lines in enamel, form irregular caps on cusps	Often round or oval
Demarcation	Shades off imperceptibly into surrounding normal enamel	Clearly differentiated from adjacent normal enamel
Colour	Slightly more opaque than normal enamel; 'paper white'. Incisal edges, tips of cusps may have frosted appearance. Does not show stain at time of eruption (in these milder degrees, rarely at any time)	Usually pigmented at time of eruption; often creamy-yellow to dark reddish-orange
Teeth affected	Most frequent on teeth that calcify slowly (cuspids, bicuspids, second and third molars). Rare on lower incisors. Usually seen on six or eight homologous teeth. Extremely rare in deciduous teeth	Any tooth may be affected. Frequent on labial surfaces of lower incisors. May occur singly. Usually 1–3 teeth affected. Common in deciduous teeth
Gross hypoplasia	None. Pitting of enamel does not occur in the milder forms. Enamel surface has glazed appearance, is smooth to point of explorer	Absent to severe. Enamel surface may seem etched, be rough to explorer
Detection	Often invisible under strong light; most easily detected by line of sight tangential to tooth crown	Seen most easily under strong light on line of sight perpendicular to tooth surface

Table 13.13 Descriptive criteria and scoring system for the Tooth Surface of Fluorosis (TSIF) (From Horowitz, 1986)

Numerical score	*Descriptive criteria*
0	Enamel shows no evidence of fluorosis
1	Enamel shows definite evidence of fluorosis, namely areas with parchment-white colour that total less than one-third of the visible enamel surface. This category includes fluorosis confined only to incisal edges of anterior teeth and cusp tips of posterior teeth ('snowcapping')
2	Parchment-white fluorosis totals at least one-third of the visible surface, but less than two-thirds
3	Parchment-white fluorosis totals at least two-thirds of the visible surface
4	Enamel shows staining in conjunction with any of the preceding levels of fluorosis. Staining is defined as an area of definite discoloration that may range from light to very dark brown
5	Discrete pitting of the enamel exists, unaccompanied by evidence of staining of intact enamel. A pit is defined as a definite physical defect in the enamel surface with a rough floor that is surrounded by a wall of intact enamel. The pitted area is usually stained or differs in colour from the surrounding enamel
6	Both discrete pitting and staining of the intact enamel exist
7	Confluent pitting of the enamel surface exists. Large areas of enamel may be missing and the anatomy of the tooth may be altered. Dark-brown stain is usually present

concentration for the area (one, two, three or four times optimal). Air was not used to dry the teeth. Horowitz (1986) commented that 'some investigators advocate the use of compressed air to dry the teeth thoroughly before examining for fluorosis, a procedure that accentuates any existing fluorosis. Because teeth are normally kept moist by saliva, they should be examined in their natural state to determine whether they display fluorosis under conditions that more closely approximate normal social interactions'.

The results (Table 13.14) showed that fluorosis was absent in 84.5% of all tooth surfaces examined in the optimal fluoride area. There was an obvious dose response pattern, with only 31.9% of surfaces said to be free of dental fluorosis in the 4 × optimal fluoride area. Horowitz (1986) further commented that 'because of its sensitivity, the TSIF index permitted special analyses of fluorosis that occurred

Table 13.14 Percentage distribution of TSIF scores for all permanent tooth surfaces according to water fluoride level, Illinois communities (From Horowitz, 1986)

Water fluoride level	*No. children*	*Percentage distribution of TSIF scores*							
		0	*1*	*2*	*3*	*4*	*5*	*6*	*7*
Optimal	336	84.5	12.4	2.0	1.1	0.0	0.0	0.0	0.0
2 × optimal	143	58.1	28.4	7.6	5.6	0.1	0.1	0.0	0.0
3 × optimal	192	50.4	25.7	13.2	9.3	0.4	0.8	0.0	0.2
4 × optimal	136	31.9	27.0	17.1	20.5	0.4	2.1	0.1	0.8

in the labial surfaces of maxillary anterior teeth, those surfaces of greatest aesthetic concern'. This is the very point Jackson made in 1975.

Horowitz (1986) concluded by reiterating the balance to be struck between fluorosis and dental decay, which is a disease that may cause a cosmetic problem greater than fluorosis. The data from Illinois showed that as the level of fluoride in water increased to two and three times the optimal level, there was a trend of less dental caries than in the community with an optimal fluoride concentration.

Photographic methods of assessment

Al-Alousi *et al.* (1975) took colour transparencies of each child examined to show them to professional and lay observers. Neither group reported an enhanced level of mottling in Anglesey. Levine, Beal and Fleming (1989) measured the prevalence of enamel hypoplasia in children from Birmingham (1.0 ppm F) and Leeds (low fluoride). They used a photographic technique to eliminate possible observer bias. Scoring was done using the Jackson–Al-Alousi (J–A) index, and the Tooth Surface Index of Fluorosis (TSIF). Both were compared with the results from conventional clinical recordings using the J–A index. Results (Table 13.15) showed that, using the J–A index, photographically, in Leeds 38.2% of upper central incisors were defect free, compared with 68.3% when the same observer viewed the teeth clinically. The corresponding figures for Birmingham were 16.6% and 59.2%. The difference was largely accounted for by the increase in Grade E scores – horizontal white striations with photographic recording.

Distribution of enamel opacities by tooth type and surface

It is evident that between 1934 and 1984 a variety of different methods were used to measure dental fluorosis/enamel opacities and hardly any of the studies are strictly comparable. One major difference is whether all teeth should be examined or whether the investigation should be restricted to incisor teeth only. Although the illustrations in Dean's studies show only incisor teeth, it appears from his papers that all surfaces of all teeth were examined and that the person was categorized according to the second worst surface.

Moller (1965) recorded the distribution of dental fluorosis in children for seven areas of Denmark where the fluoride concentration in the drinking water varied from 0.34 ppm to 3.4 ppm. He reported that premolars are the teeth most severely affected by dental fluorosis, followed by the upper incisors, canines, first molars and, lastly, lower incisors. He concluded that this general pattern occurred in all seven areas and was independent of the degree of fluorosis observed in the individual, and of the fluoride concentration in the drinking water.

Larsen *et al.* (1986) examined 106 children, aged 14–16 years, from five fluoride areas in Denmark with 1.0–2.1 ppm F in the drinking water. Half the children were 'new arrivals' into the fluoride areas; they were compared with children who had lived continuously in one of the five areas since birth. The distribution of dental fluorosis, using the T–F index, in individual tooth types, confirmed Moller's observation that premolars were the teeth most frequently affected (Table 13.16) (Larsen *et al.*, 1986; Fejerskov *et al.*, 1988).

Jackson and co-workers restricted their observations to the labial surfaces of incisor teeth because they felt that these surfaces were of greatest public health

Table 13.15 Comparison of clinical and photographic methods of assessment of enamel hypoplasia (From Levine, Beal and Fleming, 1989)

	Clinical assessment (Jackson–Al-Alousi index)					*Photographic assessment (Jackson–Al-Alousi index)*					*Photographic assessment (TSIF index)*			
Grade	*Central incisors*				*Grade*	*Central incisors*				*Grade*	*Central incisors*			
	Leeds		*Birmingham*			*Leeds*		*Birmingham*			*Leeds*		*Birmingham*	
	n	%	*n*	%		*n*	%	*n*	%		*n*	%	*n*	%
0	422	68.3	293	59.2	0	229	38.2	80	16.6	0	233	38.8	80	16.6
A	74	12.0	51	10.3	A	95	15.8	48	10.0	1	304	50.7	291	60.4
B	74	12.0	63	12.7	B	88	14.7	66	13.7	2	37	6.2	66	13.7
C	0	0.0	1	0.2	C	0	0	0	0	3	7	1.2	22	4.6
D	2	0.3	5	1.0	D	10	1.7	10	2.1	4	11	1.8	13	2.7
E	42	6.8	80	16.2	E	170	28.3	268	55.6	5	3	0.5	5	1.0
F	4	0.6	2	0.4		8	1.3	10	2.1	6	3	0.5	2	0.4
										7	2	0.3	3	0.6
Total	618		495			600		482			600		482	

Table 13.16 Percentage affected by dental fluorosis in 53 Danish children from 5 areas (F = 1.2–2.1 ppm) (From Larsen *et al.*, 1986)

	Central incisor	*Lateral incisor*	*Canine*	*First premolar*	*Second premolar*	*First molar*	*Second molar*
Maxilla	48	45	55	77	80	60	70
Mandible	5	7	15	62	76	48	72

significance, whereas a discoloured occlusal surface of a first permanent molar was of little consequence. Very different values can be obtained if the score is computed for *mouth* prevalence (one or more teeth affected) or *tooth* prevalence (the percentage of total teeth present in the mouth which are affected). These issues were considered by Murray and Shaw (1979) in a study of two populations, both from low-fluoride areas. In the first study, 303 6-year-old children were involved; in the second, 1214 13-year-olds were examined. In both studies the teeth were dried with compressed air and examined under artificial light. The occlusal, buccal and lingual surfaces of each tooth were examined and scored separately, using the criteria previously described (see page 234). The differences between values for *mouth* prevalence or *tooth* prevalence for primary teeth are compared in Table 13.17. Although almost one-third of children had at least one affected tooth, 95% of teeth were unaffected.

Table 13.17 Enamel opacities in primary teeth of 6-year-olds (From Murray and Shaw, 1979)

Classification	*Mouth prevalence of opacities*		*Tooth prevalence of opacities*	
	No.	*%*	*No.*	*%*
No opacities	204	67.3	4674	95.4
Flecks	23	7.6	73	1.5
White patches	1	0.3	2	0.04
Coloured flecks/patches	62	20.5	121	2.5
Horizontal lines	0	0	0	0
Hypoplasia with or without 1–4	13	4.3	27	0.6

The prevalence of enamel opacities in each tooth type and in specified surfaces is summarized in Tables 13.18 and 13.19. Mandibular second molars and maxillary central incisors were the teeth most commonly affected, with almost 10% having some enamel opacity. Buccal surfaces were by far the most commonly affected surface.

Table 13.18 Percentage of each tooth type (primary dentition) affected by enamel opacities in 6-year-olds (From Murray and Shaw, 1979)

	Central incisor	*Lateral incisor*	*Canine*	*First molar*	*Second molar*
Maxilla	10	1	5	4	6
Mandible	2	1	2	5	10

Table 13.19 Prevalence of enamel opacities in specified surfaces of primary teeth in 6-year-old children (From Murray and Shaw, 1979)

	No. surfaces	*No. affected*	*Percentage affected*
Occlusal	2267	37	1.6
Buccal	4887	187	3.8
Lingual	4887	7	0.1

Similar information for the permanent dentition is given in Tables 13.20–13.22. Eighty-two per cent of children had at least one tooth surface affected. Overall, 14% of surfaces had some enamel opacity. In contrast to the primary dentition where mottling was equally prevalent in maxillary and mandibular teeth, enamel opacities in the permanent dentition were twice as prevalent in the maxilla. The most commonly affected tooth was the maxillary central incisor. A similar pattern

Table 13.20 Enamel opacities in permanent teeth of 13–14-year-old children (From Murray and Shaw, 1979)

Classification	*Mouth prevalence of opacities*		*Tooth prevalence of opacities*	
	No.	*%*	*No.*	*%*
No opacities	219	18	27 089	86
Flecks	158	13	1 423	4.5
White patches	460	38	2 264	7.2
Coloured flecks/patches	240	20	474	1.5
Horizontal lines	29	2	92	0.3
Hypoplasia with or without 1–4	108	9	159	0.5

Table 13.21 Percentage of each permanent tooth type with enamel opacities in 13–14-year-old children (From Murray and Shaw, 1979)

	Central incisor	*Lateral incisor*	*Canine*	*First premolar*	*Second premolar*	*First molar*	*Second molar*
Maxilla	30	20	9	12	13	28	15
Mandible	5	4	5	10	8	23	16

Table 13.22 Prevalence of enamel opacities in specified surfaces of permanent teeth in 13–14-year-olds (From Murray and Shaw, 1979)

	No. surfaces	*No. affected*	*Percentage affected*
Occlusal	17 216	900	5.2
Buccal	31 501	3 563	11.3
Lingual	31 501	515	1.6

Table 13.23 Percentage of each tooth type affected by some enamel defect (From Suckling and Pearce, 1984)

	Central incisor	*Lateral incisor*	*Canine*	*First premolar*	*Second premolar*	*First molar*	*Second molar*
Maxilla	24	13	11	9	12	18	10
Mandible	6	5	7	9	10	17	7

of surface involvement was observed in both primary and permanent dentitions, with the buccal surface being the most commonly affected surface. Thus if a partial recording system is to be used, particularly in the permanent dentition, the most at-risk surfaces are the labial surfaces of maxillary central and lateral incisors.

Suckling and Pearce (1984) used the FDI index to assess developmental defects of enamel in 243 children aged 12–14 years in a low-fluoride area of New Zealand. Sixty-three per cent of the children had at least one tooth with defective enamel; 11.7% of teeth were affected. They also looked at the distribution of defects in each tooth type (Table 13.23). This pattern for individual tooth types is similar to that found by Murray and Shaw (1979), also in a low-fluoride area, but different from that found by Moller (1965) and Larsen *et al.* (1986), in seven predominantly high-fluoride areas. A comparison of the pattern of enamel defects by tooth type is shown in Figure 13.4.

Effect of fluoride ingestion from vehicles other than water

The vast majority of the literature is concerned with fluorosis due to the consumption of water containing high levels of fluoride. Some workers have, however, been concerned with fluoride ingestion from other sources and its possible effect on tooth enamel. The clinical and photographic study by Levine, Beal and Fleming (1989), referred to in the previous section, considered the effect of fluoride toothpaste and concluded that its use by young children in fluoridated areas is unlikely to produce aesthetically unacceptable levels of fluorosis.

Effect of fluoride supplements

Aasenden and Peebles (1974) were probably the first investigators to measure dental fluorosis in children receiving fluoride supplements. Their subjects received 0.5 mg F/day from shortly after birth to the age of 3 years and 1 mg/day thereafter. Enamel fluorosis was classified according to Moller's modification (Moller, 1965) of Dean's index (Dean, 1942). Each tooth was classified and the individual's index was determined by the *most* pronounced type found in two teeth (this is rather different from Dean's method.) Their results (Table 13.24) showed that fluorosis was twice as high in the fluoride supplementation group compared with children who were lifelong residents of a fluoride community.

In the majority of cases the individual index was determined by the scores of the maxillary central incisors. Fluorosis in deciduous teeth was found in only four cases; it was classified as the very mild type. The group index of enamel fluorosis for the children given fluoride supplements was 0.88. The appearance of 4–5

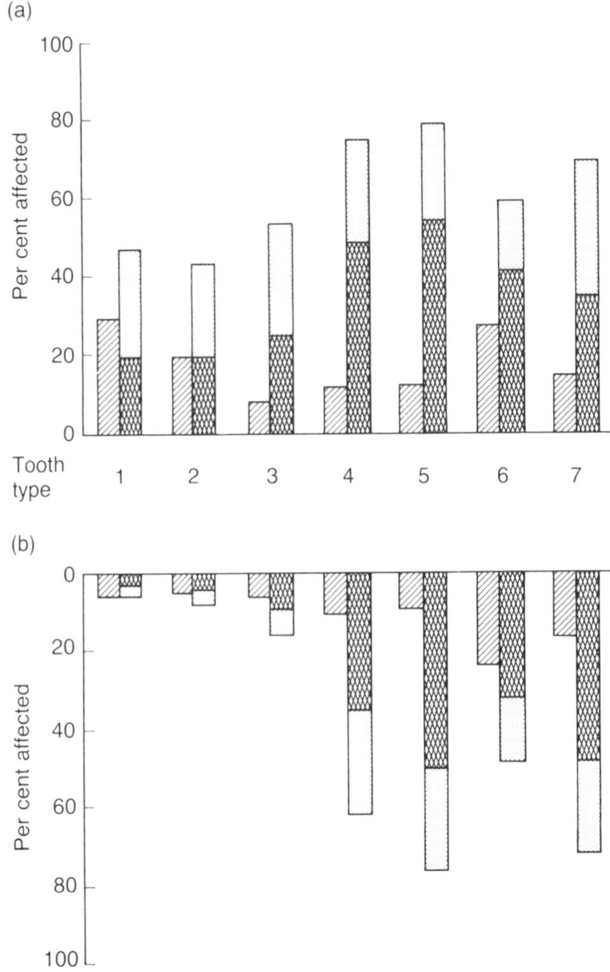

Figure 13.4 Comparison of pattern of enamel defects by tooth type: (a) upper jaw; (b) lower jaw (hatching, enamel opacities in a low-fluoride area; stippling, TF score 1 – dental fluorosis, 1.2–2.1 ppm; cross-hatching, TF score 2 – dental fluorosis, 1.2–2.1 ppm)

Table 13.24 Index of enamel fluorosis in percentage distribution by degree of severity (From Aasenden and Peebles, 1974)

	*Percentage distribution**					
	Mean index	*Normal*	*Questionable*	*Very mild*	*Mild*	*Moderate*
I. F supplement	0.88 ± 0.08†	16.0	17.0	34.0	19.0	14.0
II. No F supplement	0.07 ± 0.02	82.8	12.9	3.2	1.1	0
III. F water	0.40 ± 0.06	37.0	30.4	21.7	8.7	2.2

* No severe fluorosis was observed.
† Standard error.

children was considered undesirable, although there was no colouring or pitting of the enamel. The authors concluded that the fluoride dose given during the first years of life in their study were at the very borderline of the tolerable limit. The same authors re-examined available subjects (35 in the fluoride supplement group and 16 in the control group) at the age of 12–17 years (Aasenden and Peebles, 1978). The mean caries score of the fluoride supplement group was lower at the second than at the first examination, suggesting that enamel fluorosis of the very mild and mild degrees may fade to some extent with time, possibly due to continued mineralization or to abrasion.

Hennon, Stookey and Beiswanger (1977) came to a different conclusion concerning the effect of vitamin fluoride supplements on fluorosis. Using Dean's index they reported (Table 13.25) no clinically significant fluorosis in any group.

Table 13.25 Distribution of fluorosis severity (From Hennon, Stookey and Beiswanger, 1977)

Group (mg F dosage)	*No. participants*	*Normal*	*Questionable*	*Very mild*	*Mild*	*Index*
A (0.5/1.0)	32	21	8	2	1	0.250
C (0.5)	32	21	10	1	0	0.188
B (0.0)	30	28	2	0	0	0.033

Andersson and Grahnen (1976) carried out an investigation to determine whether the use of fluoride tablets (approximately 0.55 mg F/day) had any obvious effect on the frequency of clinically demonstrable enamel mineralization defects. Enamel fluorosis was classified according to the criteria of Dean (1934) and Moller (1965). Examinations were carried out for 127 children who had consumed fluoride tablets up to the age of 5 years, and 129 control children who had received no fluoride supplementation. Their results (Table 13.26) showed that the tooth prevalence of enamel mineralization defects was of the same order in the experimental as well as the control group.

The authors considered in detail the possible reasons for scoring 'enamel fluorosis' in the control group, who lived in an area with 0.2–0.28 ppm F in the

Table 13.26 Prevalence of enamel mineralization defects in permanent incisors and/or six-year molars (From Andersson and Grahnen, 1977)

Group	*No. children*	*Children with enamel fluorosis according to Dean's classification*					*Children with enamel hypoplasia and/or opacities, not fluorosis*		*Grand total (%)*
		0.5	*1*	*2*	*3*	*total (%)*	*No.*	*%*	
Experimental									
Children	127	6	4	4	1	12	39	31	43
Control									
Children	129	5	7	2	1	12	44	34	46

drinking water. In one child of the control group, the cause may be attributed to the consumption of Ramlösa mineral water, which contains more than 4 mg F/litre. In a further three controls it was suggested that the defects may be ascribed to an increased intake of fluoride with the drinking water during the summer holidays. Nevertheless there remained 11 children with diagnosed enamel fluorosis without any known exposure to fluoride, except that in a fluoride toothpaste. Of these 11 children, 5 had not been exposed to fluoride toothpaste at an early age. The authors commented: 'It is true that the information we received about exposure to fluoride was anamnestic, but it is most probable that the recorded frequency of enamel fluorosis is too high.'

Bagramian, Narendran and Ward (1989) reported the results of the relationship of fluorosis to fluoride supplement history in a sample of 206 Michigan children living in an area with low fluoride levels in the water supply. Fluorosis was assessed by the TSIF index; 20% of the sample were said to have fluorosis of the mild type, with most occurrence on posterior teeth. No significant relation was revealed with evidence of fluorosis and the use of fluoride supplements (Table 13.27). The

Table 13.27 Percentage distribution of TSIF scores for all permanent tooth surfaces by reported use of dietary fluoride supplements (n = 159) (From Bagramian, Narendran and Ward, 1989)

Supplement use	*TSIF score*		
	0	*1*	*2*
Daily	86.7	13.0	1.0
Not daily	89.9	10.1	0.0
Never	91.5	8.5	0.0

authors concluded that, based on this study, 'it appears that reported use of dietary fluoride supplements does not have a significant effect on the prevalence of dental fluorosis for this population from a fluoride deficient area'. This poses the question as to what caused the fluorosis. Was it due to consumption of fluoride from other sources, for example toothpaste, or was the diagnosis of fluorosis correct?

Effects of fluoride toothpaste

Hargreaves and Chester (1973) reported the results of a 3-year clinical trial of a fluoride dentifrice containing 2% MFP (2400 ppm F), in the Island of Lewis, Scotland – a low-fluoride area. The children at the start of the trial were aged 11 years, but sufficient supplies of toothpaste were provided for the whole family, including younger siblings. Houwink and Wagg (1979) carried out a follow-up study of 133 of the younger siblings of the original trial participants, the criterion for inclusion in the study being that they were aged 1–4 years at the commencement of the dentifrice trial. Sixty-six children belonged to families who received the active paste and 67 came from families receiving the placebo (non-fluoride) paste. A clinical examination was carried out in 1974 and intra-oral colour transparencies taken in 1976. The authors realized the difficulties involved in measuring enamel defects in these types of studies: 'Whenever data are derived from sensory impressions rather than instrumental measurements, there is a danger of confusing observation and interpretation, so that the observer subconsciously ignores observations which he does not consciously recognise as relevant to the hypothesis he is attempting to test.' In order to try to overcome this problem the authors scored the teeth twice. The first score was made on the prevalence of enamel defects, irrespective of how they might be caused. The second score was made by assigning to each of the defects identified in the first round a 'most probable aetiology'. In making these judgements, reliance was placed on Dean's published descriptions of enamel fluorosis.

The frequency of distribution of the number of teeth with mottling of enamel is given in Table 13.28. Children receiving the fluoride dentifrice had significantly fewer affected teeth. The results of the photographic examination (Table 13.29) found no difference between the test and control groups in terms of enamel defects.

Table 13.28 Developmental defects of enamel; frequency distributions of the number of affected teeth per child in the two groups* (From Houwink and Wagg, 1979)

Group	*n*	*No. affected teeth per child*								
		0	*1*	*2*	*3*	*4*	*5*	*6*	*7*	*8*
Test	66	22	18	13	8	1	3	0	0	1
Placebo	67	12	13	18	10	5	2	1	2	2

* Difference between groups significant ($P = 0.0178$).

Table 13.29 Prevalence of developmental defects as assessed from intra-oral colour transparencies (From Houwink and Wagg, 1979)

Group	*No. children*		*No. affected teeth*		
	Total	*Without enamel defects*	*F related*	*Non-F related*	*Doubt as to cause*
Test	76	69	0	11	7
Placebo	70	63	0	11	8

The photographic technique gave slightly lower numbers of opacities in both groups, probably because it considered the buccal surfaces only and the total number of teeth examined was smaller. The authors concluded that, in a low-fluoride area, no association could be found between enamel mottling and the use of a toothpaste containing 2% MFP by young children during the period of amelogenesis of their permanent teeth.

Topical fluoride application

Larsen *et al.* (1985) investigated the prevalence of dental fluorosis among children who, from the age of 6 years, have received routine fluoride gel treatments twice or more per year. They were examined for dental fluorosis at 14–16 years of age.

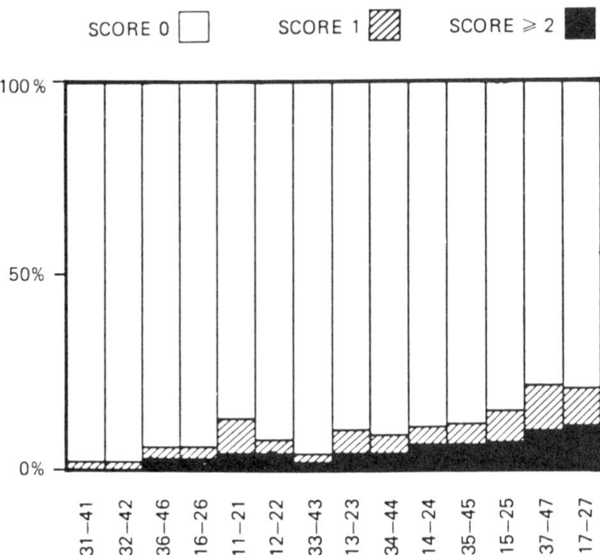

Figure 13.5 Percentage prevalence of dental fluorosis scores within the single tooth types. The tooth types are ranked in order of mineralization (From Larsen *et al.*, 1985; reproduced by courtesy of the Editor, *Journal of Dental Research*)

Dental fluorosis was recorded for each tooth using the scoring system developed by Thylstrup and Fejerskov (1978). An increased prevalence of dental fluorosis was not observed, even after up to five twice-yearly treatments were given during the tooth formation periods. The authors therefore assumed that the 'fluorosis' they observed originated from background fluoride intake. The percentage prevalence of dental fluorosis for each tooth type was illustrated diagrammatically (Figure 13.5) and showed an increase in the prevalence of dental fluorosis with tooth age, indicating that from birth to the maturation of the second molars, the population of children may be subjected to increasing fluoride exposure.

Effect of airborne fluoride

The effect of airborne fluoride on dental fluorosis was reported by Haikel *et al.* (1989), who carried out a study in the partially fluoridated area of Khouribga and the non-fluoridated area of Beni Mellal in Morocco. In Khouribga, the fluoride content of the drinking water was 0.17 ppm in the urban centre and 0.7 ppm in the rural area, whereas in Beni Mellal the fluoride content was 0.07 ppm. Dean's index was used to measure fluorosis. Over 90% of subjects of Khouribga were affected by fluorosis, of which approximately one-third had moderate fluorosis and 12% severe fluorosis. In contrast, in Beni Mellal, only 4% of subjects exhibited signs of dental fluorosis. It was suggested that the cause of fluorosis in Khouribga was due to the chronic exposure to fluoride-containing phosphate particles, because 167 metric tonnes of these particles were ejected daily into the atmosphere.

Effect of consumption of powdered milk or cow's milk

In a relatively small study, the prevalence of dental fluorosis in two locations was measured – one in which powdered milk had been consumed during tooth mineralization, and one in which natural cow's milk had been used. During the 1960s and 1970s, condensed milk powder for suspension in tap water was the milk product of choice for families with children in Greenland. In 1981, dental fluorosis was recorded in 127 children from Narssaq, Greenland (1.1 ppm F in drinking water). In Vordingborg, Denmark (1.4–1.6 ppm F in drinking water), 149 children were examined. Dental fluorosis in each tooth type was recorded using Thylstrup and Fejerskov's (1978) classification system.

More dental fluorosis was observed in Greenland in the primary dentition, where powdered milk had been consumed, but the prevalence of fluorosis in premolars was higher in Vordingborg than Narssaq, suggesting a pattern of slowly increasing intake of fluoride over the years, reflecting an increasing background fluoride intake from drinking water. This study must be viewed with some caution. The samples were relatively small and the two communities were examined 6 years apart. The authors said that the consumption of fluoride from food, toothpaste and other fluoride-containing preventive methods 'may be supposed to be similar in both populations'. The importance of the study is that it draws attention to aspects of food and drink intake that might provide vehicles for increased fluoride uptake.

Risk factors in the prevalence of dental fluorosis

Concern has been expressed that with an increase in the range of fluoride preparation there is a possibility of increasing amounts of fluoride in the food chain for infants and young children, raising the risk of dental fluorosis. Forsman (1977) studied enamel fluorosis in 1094 children from areas with a water fluoride content of from 0.2 ppm F to 2.75 ppm F, with and without supplementary fluoride. She concluded that fluorosis was correlated with different infant diets and also with the calculated supply per kilo body weight: 0.1 mg F/kg body weight appeared to cause fluorosis. Enamel fluorosis can be avoided or minimized in areas with up to at least 1.2 ppm F if water-diluted gruel and/or supplementary fluoride is not commenced until 6 months of age.

Osuji *et al.* (1988) conducted a case control study to determine the sources of fluoride which are particular risk factors to dental fluorosis. A total of 633 children, aged 8–10 years, living in the fluoridated community of East York, Canada, were involved. Their parents were interviewed about the child's first 5 years of residence and about diet and caries-preventive practices. The prevalence of mild fluorosis (1–4 on the Thylstrup and Fejerskov index) was 13%. Those who brushed their teeth before the age of 25 months had 11 times the odds of fluorosis compared with those toothbrushing later. Prolonged use of infant formulas (greater than 13 months) was associated with 3.5 times the risk of fluorosis, compared with none on shorter duration of formula use. They estimated that these two factors were responsible for 72% and 22%, respectively, of the cases of dental fluorosis occurring in the population studied and concluded that parents should be advised to supervise toothbrushing by children under 2 years of age.

In the USA, in particular, because more food and beverages are being processed in fluoridated communities and the use of various fluoride vehicles for caries prevention has become widespread, there is concern that the ingestion of fluoride

Table 13.30 Percentage distribution of TSIF scores for all permanent tooth surfaces of 8–10-year-olds by water fluoride level in 1980 and 1985 (From Heifetz *et al.*, 1988)

Water fluoride level	*No. children*	*Percentage distribution of TSIF scores*							
		0	*1*	*2*	*3*	*4*	*5*	*6*	*7*
1980									
Optimal	113	81.2	14.8	2.3	1.6	0.0	0.1	0.0	0.0
2× optimal	61	53.0	33.0	6.9	6.8	0.2	0.2	0.0	0.0
3× optimal	82	48.5	30.6	10.9	8,1	0.5	1.0	0.1	0.3
4× optimal	59	30.3	28.5	17.1	19.7	0.3	2.8	0.1	1.2
1985									
Optimal	156	72.0	20.6	5.6	1.8	0.0	0.1	0.0	0.0
2× optimal	102	48.0	30.4	11.6	8.7	0.0	1.3	0.0	0.0
3× optimal	112	48.0	29.4	12.3	8.2	0.2	1.5	0.0	0.4
4× optimal	62	24.2	32.2	18.7	19.7	0.6	3.1	0.1	1.4

Table 13.31 Percentage distribution of TSIF scores for all permanent tooth surfaces of 13–15-year-olds by water fluoride level in 1980 and 1985 (From Heifetz *et al.*, 1988)

Water fluoride level	*No. children*	*Percentage distribution of TSIF scores*							
		0	*1*	*2*	*3*	*4*	*5*	*6*	*7*
1980									
Optimal	111	88.6	9.1	1.5	0.8	0.0	0.0	0.0	0.0
2× optimal	39	61.7	25.4	7.8	5.0	0.0	0.1	0.0	0.0
3× optimal	50	54.0	21.6	13.7	9.6	0.2	0.7	0.0	0.1
4× optimal	34	36.9	25.6	16.7	18.6	0.3	1.3	0.1	0.5
1985									
Optimal	94	70.7	21.6	4.9	2.8	0.1	0.0	0.0	0.0
2× optimal	23	33.5	32.5	18.6	13.8	0.3	1.3	0.0	0.0
3× optimal	47	30.8	34.9	18.2	13.6	0.3	1.2	0.1	0.9
4× optimal	29	22.5	30.8	18.8	22.1	0.5	3.9	0.0	1.5

Table 13.32 Percentage distribution of TSIF scores for labial surfaces of maxillary incisors in 8–10-year-olds in 1980 and 1985 by water fluoride level (From Heifetz *et al.*, 1988)

Water fluoride level	*Percentage distribution of TSIF scores*					
	1980			*1985*		
	0	*1–3*	*4–7*	*0*	*1–3*	*4–7*
Optimal	67.0	33.0	0.0	59.7	40.3	0.0
2× optimal	29.1	70.0	1.4	32.2	66.9	0.8
3× optimal	26.4	67.9	5.7	28.8	68.0	3.3
4× optimal	9.4	80.8	9.8	8.3	79.6	12.0

has significantly increased with a concomitant rise in dental fluorosis (Heifetz *et al.*, 1988). The prevalence of dental caries and fluorosis among lifetime residents in four areas of Illinois, with water fluoride concentrations of 1×, 2×, 3× and 4× above the optimal level, were measured in 1980 and 1985. The distributions of TSIF scores for each fluorosis category (Tables 13.30 and 13.31) showed little difference for 8–10-year-olds between 1980 and 1985, but for 13–15-year-olds there was a greater prevalence and severity of fluorosis in 1985 compared with 1980. The TSIF scores were then grouped by combining scores 1, 2 and 3 (whitish discolorations of intact enamel) and 4, 5, 6 and 7 (more severe forms of fluorosis, involving staining, pitting or both). Results for 8–10-year-olds, for labial surfaces of maxillary incisors (Table 13.32) showed little difference between 1980 and 1985, but in the older group the intensity of fluorosis had increased over the 5-year period (Table 13.33) especially in the areas with 3× and 4× optimal fluoride.

Table 13.33 Percentage distribution of TSIF scores for labial surfaces of maxillary incisors and canines in 13–15-year-olds in 1980 and 1985 by water fluoride level (From Heifetz *et al.*, 1988)

Water fluoride level	*Percentage distribution of TSIF scores*					
	1980			*1985*		
	0	*1–3*	*4–7*	*0*	*1–3*	*4–7*
Optimal	87.5	12.5	0.0	66.6	33.0	0.4
2× optimal	56.3	43.7	0.0	15.3	77.1	7.6
3× optimal	43.9	53.3	2.8	17.1	76.4	6.6
4× optimal	24.2	69.0	6.8	6.7	81.7	11.6

However, in the optimal area no labial surfaces of the younger children received TSIF scores of 4–7 and for the 13–15-year-olds only 0.4% were placed in this category. The authors concluded that there was no need to modify the recommended optimal fluoride concentration, but that at twice the optimal, the additional intake of fluoride from extraneous sources could be approaching a critical threshold for producing the higher grades of fluorosis.

The trend in the prevalence of dental fluorosis in the USA was reviewed by Szpunar and Burt (1987). In an excellent paper, which compared recent published evidence with Dean's pioneering work, they concluded that there was a slight trend towards more fluorosis today than would be expected based upon findings in the later 1930s and early 1940s. This suggested increase in fluorosis is not as clear cut or as widely accepted as the recent decline in the prevalence of caries. Data for 50 communities from studies quoted by Szpunar and Burt (Dean *et al.*, 1941, 1942; Galagan and Lamson, 1953; Driscoll *et al.* 1983, 1986; Segreto *et al.*, 1984; Leverett, 1986) have been gathered together, in descending order of water fluoride concentration, and show clearly the relationship between fluoride concentration and the prevalence of fluorosis. Of greater importance from a public health point of view is not so much the CFI score, but the percentage in a given community with moderate or severe fluorosis (Table 13.34).

Pendrys and Stamm (1990) advocated the use of multivariate analysis in studies concerning the relationship of total fluoride intake to beneficial effects and enamel fluorosis. They concluded:

Table 13.34 Percentage distribution of children by fluorosis index score, the CFI score and overall percentage prevalence of fluorosis

Authors	*US city*	*ppm F*	*N*	*Fluorosis index category*						*CFI*	*Prevalence (%)*
				Normal	*Questionable*	*Very mild*	*Mild*	*Moderate*	*Severe*		
Segreto *et al*. (1984)	Taylor	4.3	190	0.5	4.7	32.6	30.5	31.1	0.5	1.91	94.7
Driscoll *et al*. (1983)	Bushnell and Table Grove	4.0	136	12.5	15.4	16.9	25.0	7.4	22.8	1.88	72.1
Segreto *et al*. (1984)	Gatesville	3.1	113	12.4	10.6	44.2	28.3	4.4	0.0	1.19	76.9
Driscoll *et al*. (1983)	Abingdon, Elmwood and Ipava	3.0	192	22.9	26.0	15.1	19.8	7.8	8.3	1.25	51.0
Segreto *et al*. (1984)	Abernathy	2.9	67	4.5	1.5	19.4	41.8	32.8	0.0	2.02	94.0
Segreto *et al*. (1984)	Perryton	2.7	90	8.9	8.9	42.2	33.3	6.7	0.0	1.33	82.2
Segreto *et al*. (1984)	Monahans	2.7	170	20.0	4.1	32.4	30.0	13.5	0.0	1.35	75.9
Segreto *et al*. (1984)	Hillsboro	2.7	200	2.5	7.0	52.0	34.5	4.0	0.0	1.37	90.5
Dean *et al*. (1941)	C. Springs, CO	2.6	404	6.4	19.8	42.1	21.3	8.9	1.5	1.27	73.8
Segreto *et al*. (1984)	Ft. Stockton	2.5	301	20.9	13.3	38.2	24.2	3.3	0.0	1.03	65.7
Segreto *et al*. (1984)	Littlefield	2.3	109	17.4	4.6	37.6	25.7	14.7	0.0	1.35	78.0
Segreto *et al*. (1984)	Alpine	2.3	23	21.7	4.3	21.7	39.1	13.0	0.0	1.41	73.8
Driscoll *et al*. (1983)	Monmouth	2.0	143	18.2	28.7	23.1	16.8	8.4	4.9	1.16	53.2
Dean *et al*. (1941)	Galesburg, IL	1.9	273	25.3	27.1	40.3	6.2	1.1	0.0	0.69	48.0
Dean *et al*. (1941)	Elmhurst, IL	1.8	170	28.2	31.8	30.0	8.8	1.2	0.0	0.67	40.0
Segreto *et al*. (1984)	Kerrville	1.4	128	52.3	32.0	14.8	0.8	0.0	0.0	0.32	15.6
Segreto *et al*. (1984)	Angleton	1.3	187	39.0	28.3	21.4	10.2	1.1	0.0	0.59	32.7
Segreto *et al*. (1984)	Alvin	1.3	211	49.8	21.3	22.3	5.7	0.9	0.0	0.47	28.9
Dean *et al*. (1941)	Joliet, IL	1.3	447	40.5	34.2	22.2	3.2	0.0	0.0	0.46	25.3

Dean *et al*. (1941)	Maywood, IL	1.2	171	39.2	27.5	29.2	4.1	0.0	0.0	0.51	33.3
Dean *et al*. (1941)	Aurora, IL	1.2	633	53.2	31.8	13.9	1.1	0.0	0.0	0.32	15.0
Dean *et al*. (1941)	E. Moline, IL	1.2	152	36.8	31.6	29.6	2.0	0.0	0.0	0.49	32.0
Dean *et al*. (1941)	Kewanee	1.0	336	56.0	29.5	7.4	4.8	1.8	0.6	0.39	14.6
Segreto *et al*. (1984)	Kingsville	1.0	361	39.6	21.1	36.6	2.5	0.3	0.0	0.53	39.4
Leverett *et al*. (1986)	New York State (F)	1.0	729	73.1	–	22.6	3.2	1.1	–	–	26.9
Dean *et al*. (1941)	Kewanee, IL	0.9	123	52.8	35.0	10.6	1.6	0.0	0.0	0.31	12.2
Dean *et al*. (1941)	Pueblo, CO	0.6	614	72.3	21.2	6.2	0.3	0.0	0.0	0.17	6.5
Dean *et al*. (1941)	Elgin, IL	0.5	403	60.5	35.3	3.5	0.7	0.0	0.0	0.22	4.2
Dean *et al*. (1941)	Marion, OH	0.4	263	57.4	36.5	5.3	0.8	0.0	0.0	0.25	6.1
Segreto *et al*. (1984)	San Antonio	0.4	126	92.1	5.6	2.4	0.0	0.0	0.0	0.05	2.4
Segreto *et al*. (1984)	San Marcos	0.3	223	81.2	10.3	8.5	0.0	0.0	0.0	0.14	8.5
Segreto *et al*. (1984)	N. Braunfels	0.3	103	60.2	31.1	6.8	1.9	0.0	0.0	0.26	8.7
Dean *et al*. (1941)	Lima, OH	0.3	454	84.1	13.7	2.2	0.0	0.0	0.0	0.09	2.2
Dean *et al*. (1941)	Middletown, OH	0.2	370	84.3	14.6	1.1	0.0	0.0	0.0	0.08	1.1
Dean *et al*. (1941)	Zanesville, OH	0.2	459	85.4	13.1	1.5	0.0	0.0	0.0	0.08	1.5
Dean *et al*. (1941)	Quincy, IL	0.1	330	93.0	6.7	0.3	0.0	0.0	0.0	0.04	0.3
Dean *et al*. (1941)	Elkhart , IN	0.1	278	91.3	8.3	0.4	0.0	0.0	0.0	0.04	0.4
Dean *et al*. (1941)	Portsmouth, OH	0.1	469	88.9	9.8	1.3	0.0	0.0	0.0	0.06	1.3
Dean *et al*. (1941)	Mi. City, IN	0.1	236	97.5	2.5	0.0	0.0	0.0	0.0	0.02	0.0
Leverett *et al*. (1986)	New York State (Non-F)	0.1	564	95.6	–	2.7	1.1	0.6	–	–	4.4
Dean *et al*. (1941)	Evanston, IL	0.0	256	91.8	6.6	1.6	0.0	0.0	0.0	0.5	1.6
Dean *et al*. (1941)	Oak Park, IL	0.0	329	90.6	8.8	0.6	0.0	0.0	0.0	0.05	0.6
Dean *et al*. (1941)	Waukegan, IL	0.0	423	97.9	1.9	0.2	0.0	0.0	0.0	0.1	0.2
Driscoll *et al*. (1986)	Bella Plain and 3 others, IA	0.0	316	93.0	4.1	1.9	1.0	0.0	0.0	0.06	2.9

> Recent North American studies suggest that in contrast to an increase of about 33% in the prevalence of enamel fluorosis in fluoridated areas, there has been more than a 10-fold increase in the prevalence of enamel fluorosis in non-fluoridated communities. It is important to note that fluorosis prevalence reports from fluoridated areas assess the effects not just of the 1-ppm-fluoride in the drinking water, but also of that exposure combined with additional exposure to other common fluoride sources, such as diet and dentifrices. For this reason, the relatively small increase in fluorosis prevalence that has been observed in optimally fluoridated areas since the time of Dean's studies is not unexpected. On the contrary, it is difficult to explain why the prevalence of dental fluorosis in these communities has not increased more markedly, given the suggested association of these other sources with fluorosis.

They felt that

> a body of evidence is clearly developing to indicate that there remains a strong risk of mild to moderate enamel fluorosis associated with the ingestion of fluoride supplements. Further this evidence suggests that reductions in dosage for the first two years of life alone may not be sufficient to prevent fluorosis in children being supplemented under the existing protocol in the United States.

They suggested that

> A prime obstacle facing all serious studies of dental fluorosis and potentially associated risk factors is the disparity in the diagnosis of clinical fluorosis. This arises for at least two reasons. First, the scientific community has not reached a consensus as to which diagnostic systems or indices are most appropriate to use. What is more, the best index for use in a prevalence study may not be the best index for use in an analytical study investigating specific risk factors. Second, there remains variability in the application of clinical procedures and the interpretation of clinical observations even within a given diagnostic system.

Conclusions

Over the years a certain polarization of views concerning the measurement of dental fluorosis has occurred. Some workers, for example Jackson, James and Wolfe (1975) and the FDI Technical Report (1982), argued that an index should be based on what a clinical examiner could see, without consideration being given to the aetiology of the lesion. Horowitz (1986) considered that although this concept sounded intellectually correct it seemed 'rather schizophrenic to use an index based on a premise that it is inappropriate to ascribe etiological considerations to observations, and then to actually make such attributions'. Fejerskov *et al.* (1988) went further and said that this concept arose out of ignorance of, or lack of experience in, the nature of fluoride-induced enamel changes: 'Implicitly these indices dismiss the results of the meticulous, methodical and extensive studies of Dean and his co-workers which established the very distinctive features of dental fluorosis.' They claimed that if the criteria of the TF index are applied meticulously, the earliest sign of dental fluorosis should not be confused with any of the non-fluoride-induced lesions. They gave criteria for differential diagnosis between non-fluoride-induced opacities and the milder forms of dental fluorosis (Table 13.35) which make similar points to those given by Russell (1961).

Table 13.35 Differential diagnosis: milder forms of dental fluorosis (TF scores 1–3) and enamel opacities of non-fluoride origin (From Fejerskov *et al.*, 1988)

Characteristics	*Dental fluorosis*	*Enamel opacities*
Area affected	The entire tooth surfaces (all surfaces) often enhanced on or near tips of cusps/incisal edges	Usually centred in smooth surface of limited extent
Lesion shape	Resemble line shading in pencil sketch which follows incremental lines in enamel (perichymata). Lines merging, and in score 3, a cloudy appearance. At cusps/incisal edges formation of irregular white caps ('snow cap')	Round or oval
Demarcation	Diffuse distribution over the surface of varying intensity	Clearly differentiated from adjacent normal enamel
Colour	Opaque white lines or clouds; even a chalky appearance! 'Snow caps' at cusps/incisal edges. Score 3 may become brownish discoloured at mesio-incisal part of central upper incisors after eruption	White opaque or creamy-yellow to dark reddish-orange at time of eruption
Teeth affected	Always on homologous teeth. Early erupting teeth (incisors/1st molars) least affected. Premolars and second molars (and third molars) most severely affected	Most common on labial surfaces of single or occasionally homologous teeth. Any tooth may be affected but mostly incisors

Notwithstanding these views, in part derived from studies in communities with high concentrations of fluoride in the drinking water, there is a consistent thread running through the literature of difficulties in diagnosing the prevalence of dental fluorosis in communities with 0.5–1.2 ppm F in drinking water.

The concern was, from a public health point of view, that the aesthetic problems of mild dental fluorosis should be no worse than the problems of enamel opacities in low-fluoride areas. Indeed, Moller (1965) pointed out that the occurrence of non-fluoride opacities is universely proportional to the fluoride ion concentration in the drinking water.

Pendrys and Stamm (1990) concluded that

> . . . there is a pressing need for additional analytical epidemiological studies to confirm existing findings, specifically related to the role of fluoride supplementation and fluoride dentifrice use in the pathogenesis of enamel fluorosis, and to determine whether any other fluoride sources may be associated with enamel fluorosis. These investigations are necessary in both fluoridated and non-fluoridated communities.

Summary

In this chapter the main indices used to measure dental fluorosis have been reviewed and results from the various studies have been summarized. Attention has been drawn to a number of difficulties and variations in approach that are apparent from the literature. These include:

1. There is little need to be concerned about the weighted values Dean ascribed to the various forms of mottled enamel. Quoting the proportion of the population with mild, moderate and severe fluorosis allows one to compare communities with one another.
2. Differences in method, particularly with respect to the type of lighting used and whether the teeth were dried, can have a bearing on results produced. Dean used natural lighting – most observers now use artificial light. Some workers remove plaque and debris only if it obscures the tooth surface; others use compressed air to remove excessive saliva and loose debris (Thylstrup and Fejerskov were said to dry the teeth with air for two minutes before examining the tooth surface).
3. It is important to appreciate the reasoning behind the development of certain indices. Moderate and severe fluorosis can be identified easily and none of the indices has made substantial improvements on Dean's original observations for the moderate and severe forms of the condition. The greatest difficulty arises in trying to differentiate between 'normal' and 'questionable'.
4. Some of the indices have been developed in communities with relatively high fluoride concentrations in the drinking water (Thylstrup and Fejerskov – up to 21 ppm F; Horowitz and co-workers – up to four times optimal fluoride concentration; Dean – up to 4 ppm F). The specific work of Jackson and co-workers was concerned with making comparisons between communities with 0.1–1.0 ppm F.
5. Ideally an index should be simple to use and be reproducible. The original DDE index was complex and produced considerable data that was not appropriate for screening purposes.
6. Maxillary central incisors are probably the tooth type most affected by enamel defects and are also the most important from an aesthetic standpoint. If a partial scoring system is to be used, there is some justification for concentrating on maxillary incisors.
7. Some investigators have used photographs as a means of producing a permanent record and reducing the possibility of examiner bias. Photographs can be complicated by highlights from the flashlight and are best used for anterior teeth only. There is a suggestion that scoring is higher using photographs compared with clinical examination.
8. In view of the multitude of fluoride sources available today, there is a need to monitor the prevalence and severity of dental fluorosis in fluoridated and non-fluoridated communities.

References

Aasenden, R. and Peebles, T. C. (1974) Effects of fluoride supplementation from birth on human deciduous and permanent teeth. *Archs Oral Biol.*, **19**, 321–326

Aasenden, R. and Peebles, T. C. (1978) Effects of fluoride supplementation from birth on dental caries and fluorosis in teenaged children. *Archs Oral Biol.*, **23**, 111–115

Ainamo, J. and Cutress, T. W. (1982) An epidemiological index of developmental defects of dental enamel (DDE index). Commission on Oral Health, Research and Epidemiology. *Br. Dent. J.*, **32**(2), 159–167

Ainsworth, N. J. (1933) Mottled teeth. *Br. Dent. J.*, **55**, 233

Al-Alousi, W., Jackson, D., Compton, G. and Jenkins, O. C. (1975) Enamel mottling in a fluoride and in a non-fluoride community. *Br. Dent. J.*, **138**, 9–15, 56–60

Andersson, R. and Grahnen, H. (1976) Fluoride tablets in pre-school age – effect on primary and permanent teeth. *Swed. Dent. J.*, **69**, 137–143

Bagramian, R. A., Narendran, S. and Ward, M. (1989) Relationship of dental caries and fluorosis to fluoride supplement history in a non-fluoridated sample of schoolchildren. *Adv. Dent. Res.*, **3**(2), 161–167

Binder, K. (1973) Comparison of the effects of fluoride drinking water on caries frequency and mottled enamel in three similar regions of Austria over a ten year period. *Caries Res.*, **7**, 179–183

Bischoff, J. I., Van der Merwe, E. H. M., Rettef, D. H., Barbakow, F. H. and Cleaton-Jones, P. E. (1976) Relationship between fluoride concentration in enamel, DMFT index and degree of fluorosis in a community residing in an area with a high level of fluoride. *J. Dent. Res.*, **55**, 37–42

Clarkson, J. (1989) Review of terminology, classifications, and indices of developmental defects of enamel. *Adv. Dent. Res.*, **3**(2), 104–109

Clarkson, J. and O'Mullane, D. (1989) A modified DDE index for use in epidemiological studies of enamel defects. *J. Dent. Res.*, **68**(3), 445–450

Cutress, T. W., Suckling, G. W., Pearce, E. I. F. and Ball, M. E. (1985) Defects of tooth enamel in children in fluoridated and non-fluoridated water areas of the Auckland Region. *N.Z. Dent. J.*, **81**(363), 12–19

Dean, H. T. (1934) Classification of mottled enamel diagnosis. *J. Am. Dent. Ass.*, **21**, 1421

Dean, H. T. (1938a) Chronic endemic dental fluorosis (mottled enamel). In *Dental Science and Dental Art* (ed. S. M. Gordon), Henry Kimpton, London

Dean, H. T. (1938b) Endemic fluorosis and its relation to dental caries. *Publ. Hlth Rep.* (*Wash.*), **53**, 1443

Dean, H. T. (1942) The investigation of physiological effects by the epidemiological method. In *Fluorine and Dental Health* (ed. F. R. Moulton), Publ. No. 19, American Association for the Advancement of Science, Washington, pp. 23–31

Dean, H. T. (1946) Epidemiological studies in the United States. In *Dental Caries and Fluorine* (ed. F. R. Moulton), American Association for the Advancement of Science/Science Press, Lancaster, pp. 5–31

Dean, H. T., Dixon, R. M. and Cohen, C. (1935) Mottled enamel in Texas. *Publ. Hlth Rep.* (*Wash.*), **50**, 424–442

Dean, H. T. and Elvove, E. (1935) Studies on the minimal threshold of the dental sign of chronic endemic fluorosis (mottled enamel). *Publ. Hlth Rep.* (*Wash.*), **50**, 1719–1729

Dean, H. T. and Elvove, E. (1937) Further studies on the minimal threshold of chronic endemic dental fluorosis. *Publ. Hlth Rep.* (*Wash.*), **52**, 1249–1264

Dean, H. T., Jay, P., Arnold, F. A. and Elvove, E. (1941) Domestic waters and dental caries. II. A study of 2832 white children ages 12–14 years of eight suburban Chicago communities, including *Lactobacillus acidophilus* studies of 1761 children. *Publ. Hlth Rep.* (*Wash.*), **56**, 761–792

Dean, H. T., Jay, P., Arnold, F. A., McClure, F. J. and Elvove, E. (1939) Domestic waters and dental caries including certain epidemiological aspects of oral *Lactobacillus acidophilus*. *Publ. Hlth Rep.* (*Wash.*), **54**, 862–888

Dean, H. T. and McKay, F. S. (1939) Production of mottled enamel halted by a change in common water supply. *Am. J. Pub. Hlth*, **29**, 590–596

Dean, H. T., McKay, F. S. and Elvove, E. (1938) Mottled enamel survey of Bauxite, Ark., ten years after a change in the common water supply. *Pub. Hlth Rep.* (*Wash.*), **53**, 1736–1748

Driscoll, W. S., Horowitz, H. S., Meyers, R. J., Heifetz, S. B., Kingman, A. and Zimmerman, E. R. (1983) Prevalence of dental caries and dental fluorosis in areas with optimal and above-optimal water fluoride concentrations. *J. Am. Dent. Ass.*, **107**, 42–47

Driscoll, W. S., Horowitz, H. S., Meyers, R. J., Heifetz, S. B., Kingman, A. and Zimmerman, E. R. (1986) Prevalence of dental caries and dental fluorosis in areas with negligible, optimal, and above-optimal fluoride concentrations in drinking water. *J. Am. Dent. Ass.*, **113**, 29–33

Dummer, P. M., Kingdon, A. and Kingdon, R. (1986) Prevalence of enamel developmental defects in a group of 11 and 12 year old children in South Wales. *Community Dent. Oral Epidemiol.*, **14**, 119–122

Eager, J. M. (1901) Denti di chiaie (chiaie teeth). *Publ. Hlth Rep.* (*Wash.*), **16**, 2576

FDI (1982) An epidemiological index of developmental defects of dental enamel (DDE index). Technical Report No. 15. *Int. Dent. J.*, **32**, 159–167

Fejerskov, O., Baelum, V., Manji, F. and Moller, I. J. (1988) *Dental Fluorosis – A Handbook for Health Workers,* Munksgaard, Copenhagen

Forrest, J. R. (1956) Caries incidence and enamel defects in areas with different levels of fluoride in the drinking water. *Br. Dent. J.,* **100**(8), 195–200

Forrest, J. R. (1965) Mottled enamel. *Br. Dent. J.,* **119**, 316–319

Forsman, B. (1974) Dental fluorosis and caries in high fluoride districts in Sweden. *Community Dent. Oral. Epidemiol.,* **2**, 132–148

Forsman, B. (1977) Early supply of fluoride and enamel fluorosis. *Scand. J. Dent. Res.,* **85**, 22–30

Galagan, D. J. and Lamson, G. G. (1953) Climate and endemic dental fluorosis. *Publ. Hlth Rep. (Wash.),* **68**, 497

Galagan, D. J. and Vermillion, J. R. (1957) Determining the optimum fluoride concentrations. *Publ. Hlth Rep. (Wash.),* **72**, 491–493

Goward, P. E. (1976) Enamel mottling in a non-fluoride community in England. *Community Dent. Oral. Epidemiol.,* **4**, 111–114

Haikel, Y., Cahen, P. M., Turlot, J. C. and Frank, R. M. (1989) The effects of airborne fluorides on oral conditions in Morocco. *J. Dent. Res.,* **68**(8), 1238–1241

Hargreaves, J. A. and Chester, C. G. (1973) Clinical trial among Scottish children of an anticaries dentifrice containing 2 per cent sodium monofluorophosphate. *Community Dent. Oral Epidemiol.,* **1**, 41–46

Hargreaves, J. A., Chester, C. G. and Wagg, B. J. (1975) An assessment of children in active and placebo groups, one year after termination of a clinical trial of a 2 per cent sodium monofluorophosphate dentifrice. *Caries Res.,* **9**, 291 (abstr.)

Heifetz, S. B., Driscoll, W. S., Horowitz, H. S. and Kingman, A. (1988) Prevalence of dental caries and dental fluorosis in areas with optimal and above optimal water-fluoride concentrations: a 5-year follow-up survey. *J. Am. Dent. Ass.,* **116,** 490–493

Hennon, D. K., Stookey, G. K. and Beiswanger, B. B. (1977) Fluoride-vitamin supplements: effects on dental caries and fluorosis when used in areas with suboptimum fluoride in the water supply. *J. Am. Dent. Ass.,* **95**, 965–971

Horowitz, H. S. (1986) Indexes for measuring dental fluorosis. *J. Pub. Dent. Hlth,* **46**(4), 179–183

Horowitz, H. S., Driscoll, W. S., Meyers, R. J., Heifetz, S. B. and Kingman, A. (1984) A new method for assessing the prevalence of dental fluorosis – the Tooth Surface Index of Fluorosis. *J. Am. Dent. Ass.,* **109**, 37–41

Houwink, B. and Wagg, B. J. (1979) Effect of fluoride dentifrice usage during infancy upon enamel mottling of the permanent teeth. *Caries Res.,* **13,** 231–237

Hurme, V. O. (1949) Developmental opacities of teeth in a New England community. *Am. J. Dis. Child.,* **77**, 61

Jackson, D., James, P. M. C. and Wolfe, W. B. (1975) Fluoridation in Anglesey: a clinical study. *Br. Dent. J.,* **138**, 165–171

Kallis, D. G. and Silva, D. G. (1970) Carnarvon studies. III. Detailed investigations related to endemic fluorosis present in children in Carnavon, Western Australia (Aug. 1963). *Aust. Dent. J.,* **15**, 35–43

King, N. M. and Brook, A. H. (1984) A prevalence study of enamel defects among young adults in Hong Kong: use of the FDI index. *N.Z. Dent. J.,* **80**(360), 47–49

King, N. M. and Wei, S. H. (1986) Developmental defects of enamel; a study of 12 year olds in Hong Kong. *J. Am. Dent. Ass.,* **112**, 835–839

Kuhns, C. (1888) *Dtsch. Monattschr. Zahnheilkd,* **6**, 446

Larsen, M. J., Kirkegaard, E., Fejerskov, O. and Poulsen, S. (1985) Prevalence of dental fluorosis after fluoride-gel treatments in a low-fluoride area. *J. Dent. Res.,* **64**(8), 1076–1079

Larsen, M. J., Kirkegaard, E., Poulsen, S. and Fejerskov, O. (1986) Enamel fluoride, dental fluorosis and dental caries among immigrants to and permanent residents of five Danish fluoride areas. *Caries Res.,* **20**, 349–355

Leatherwood, E. C., Burnett, G. W., Chandravejjsmarn, R. and Sirikaya, R. (1965) Dental caries and dental fluorosis in Thailand. *Am. J. Publ. Hlth,* **55**, 1792–1799

Leverett, D. H. (1986) Prevalence of dental fluorosis in fluoridated and non-fluoridated communities, a preliminary investigation. *J. Publ. Hlth Dent.,* **46**, 184–187

Levine, R. S., Beal, J. F. and Fleming, C. M. (1989) A photographically recorded assessment of enamel hypoplasia in fluoridated and non-fluoridated areas in England. *Br. Dent. J.*, **166**, 249–252

McKay, F. S. and Black, G. V. (1916) An investigation of mottled teeth: an endemic development imperfection of the enamel of the teeth, heretofore unknown in the literature of dentistry. *Dent. Cosmos,* **477**, 627, 781, 894

Massler, M. and Schour, I. (1952) Relation of endemic fluorosis to malnutrition. *J. Am. Dent. Ass.*, **44**, 156–169

Milgalter, N., Zadik, D., Gedalia, I. and Kelman, M. (1974) Fluorosis and dental caries in the region of Jotvata Israel. *J. Dent. Med.,* **23**, 104–109

Minoguchi, G. (1970) Japanese studies on water and food fluoride and general dental health. In *Fluorides and Human Health*, WHO, Geneva, pp. 294–304

Møller, I. J. (1965) *Dental Fluorosis of Caries*, Rhodos Publ., Copenhagen

Møller, I. J. (1982) Fluorides and dental fluorosis. *Int. Dent. J.*, **32**, 134–137

Møller, I. J. and Poulsen, S. (1976) A study of dental mottling in children in Khouribga, Morocco. *Archs Oral Biol.,* **20**, 601–607

Murray, J. J., Gordon, P. H., Carmichael, C. L., French, A. D. and Furness, J. A. (1984) Dental caries and enamel opacities in 10-year-old children in Newcastle and Northumberland. *Br. Dent. J.,* **156**, 255–258

Murray, J. J. and Shaw, L. (1979) Classification and prevalence of enamel opacities in the human deciduous and permanent dentitions. *Archs Oral Biol.,* **24**, 7–13

Murray, M. M., Forrest, J. R., Griffith, G. W. and Longwell, J. (1956) Iodine and fluorine nutrition. *Nature, Lond.,* **177,** 912–914

Myers, H. M. (1978) Fluorides and dental fluorosis, Monogr. Oral. Sci., No. 7, Karger, Basel

Osuji, O. O., Leake, J. L., Chipman, M. L., Nikiforuk, G., Locker, D. and Levine, N. (1988) Risk factors for dental fluorosis in a fluoridated community. *J. Dent. Res.,* **67**(12), 1488–1492

Parfitt, G. J. (1955) Report of the bone and tooth society. *Br. Dent. J.,* **98**, 177–178

Pendrys, D. G. and Stamm, J. W. (1990) Relationship of total fluoride intake to beneficial effects and enamel fluorosis. *J. Dent. Res.,* **69** (spec. iss.), 529–538

Pu, M. Y. and Lilienthal, B. (1961) Dental caries and mottled enamel among Formosan children. *Archs Oral Biol.,* **5**, 125–136

Richards, L. F., Westmoreland, W. W., Tashiro, M., McKay, C. H. and Morrison, J. T. (1967) Determining optimum fluoride levels for community water supplies in relation to temperature. *J. Am. Dent. Ass.,* **74**, 389–397

Russell, A. L. (1961) The differential diagnosis of fluoride and non-fluoride enamel opacities. *Publ. Hlth Rep.,* **21**, 143–146

Segreto, V. A., Collins, E. M., Camann, D. and Smith, C. T. (1984) A current study of mottled enamel in Texas. *J. Am. Dent. Ass.,* **113**, 29–33

Suckling, G. W. and Pearce, E. I. F. (1984) Developmental defects of enamel in a group of New Zealand children: their prevalence and some associated etiological factors. *Community Dent. Oral Epidemiol.,* **12**, 177–184

Szpunar, S. M. and Burt, B. A. (1987) Trends in the prevalence of dental fluorosis in the United States: a review. *J. Publ. Hlth Dent.,* **47**(2), 71–79

Thylstrup, A. and Fejerskov, O. (1978) Clinical appearance of dental fluorosis in permanent teeth in relation to histologic changes. *Community Dent. Oral Epidemiol.,* **6**, 315–328

Young, M. A. (1973) An epidemiological study of enamel opacities and other dental conditions in children in temperate and sub-tropical climates. *Ph.D. thesis*, University of London

Zimmerman, E. R. (1954) Fluoride and nonfluoride enamel opacities. *Publ. Hlth Rep.* (*Wash.*), **69**, 1115

Chapter 14

Physiology of fluoride

Availability of fluoride

Fluorine is the most electronegative of all chemical elements. It has an atomic weight of 19.0 and an atomic number of 9. Combined chemically in the form of fluorides, chiefly as fluorspar (CaF_2), fluorapatite ($Ca_{10}[PO_4]_6F_2$) or cryolite (Na_3AlF_6), it is seventeenth in the order of abundance of elements in the earth's crust (Fleischer, 1953). Barth (1947) estimated that the earth's crust contained 880 ppm. The F concentration in soils varies enormously from place to place, the published figures ranging from 10 to 1070 ppm, with average values between 200 and 300 ppm (Vinogradov, 1954; Largent, 1960). When different levels have been studied, it has usually been found that the fluoride concentration is lowest on the surface. Fluoride also occurs in sea water, in concentrations ranging from 0.8 to 1.4 ppm (Thompson and Taylor, 1933; Wattenberg, 1943; Kappana *et al.*, 1962). It is present in nearly all fresh ground waters, although the concentration in some water supplies may be too low to be detectable by routine methods. The range of fluoride levels in drinking water varies in different parts of the world. In Africa, areas have been reported with as much as 95 ppm in the drinking water (Tanganyika Government Chemist, 1955); the range in the USA is given as 0–16 ppm (WHO, 1970), whereas in England most supplies are well below 1 ppm: the highest concentrations found naturally (2.5 and 5.8 ppm) have now been reduced to below 2 ppm (Heasman and Martin, 1962).

Additional fluorides are widely distributed in the atmosphere, originating from the dusts of fluoride-containing soils (Williamson, 1953), from gaseous industrial wastes (MacIntire, Harden and Lester, 1952), from the burning of coal fires in populated areas (Cholak, 1959), and from gases emitted in areas of volcanic activity (Noguchi *et al.*, 1963). Thus fluoride, in varying concentrations, is freely available in nature. It is difficult to understand how any form of life, in land, sea or air, evolved and survived unless it was fully able to cope with continuous uptake of fluoride from its environment. The fluoride content of plants remains remarkably constant whether they are grown in soil with much or little fluoride (McClure, 1949a). There is no consistent difference in the fluoride content of the soft tissues of fresh-water and salt-water fish: very little fluoride appears in cow's milk and the amount is increased only slightly, if at all, by the addition of large amounts of fluoride to the drinking water or grain ration (McClure, 1949a). Negligible amounts of fluoride are stored in human soft tissues and these concentrations do not rise with increased levels of fluoride in the individual's drinking water (Smith *et al.*,

(1960). It is clear that no serious imbalance can or does exist between the life processes and ordinary amounts of fluoride acquired from the environment.

Intake of fluoride

The only comprehensive survey of the fluoride concentration in foods was reported by McClure in 1949 based on the analytical methods then available that are of doubtful reliability for estimating low levels in complex mixtures like foods. However, his main conclusion that with two exceptions most foods contain very low concentrations, usually below 1 ppm (wet weight), has been confirmed by more recent work with improved methods (Marier and Rose, 1966; Taves, 1983; Walters *et al.*, 1983). Taves compared the fluoride content of 93 foods before and after ashing and found very little difference, indicating that the fluoride is present in an unbound form except for three foods (two dried cereals and pepper) in which the fluoride was significantly higher after ashing (the nature of the bound fluoride is not known). The only two common dietary constituents high in fluoride are fish and tea. The importance of fish as a source of fluoride has been exaggerated, since McClure published high figures but did not make clear which parts of the fish were included in his samples. Later analyses have shown that only the skin and bones are especially high, 8 and 500 ppm respectively being typical (Jenkins and Edgar, 1973), so that unless these are edible, as, for example, in tinned sardines or tinned salmon, which may contain 1–2 mg of fluoride in a typical helping (but absorption from this source is poor, see later), the contribution from fish is no greater than from other foods. For unknown reasons, the tea plant takes up exceptionally high concentrations from the soil which eventually reach the leaves and, when purchased in dried form, may contain between 50 and 350 ppm, depending on the brand. The fluoride in tea is readily soluble in water, mostly as fluoride ions, although about 20% is complexed with aluminium, manganese and unidentified substances (Speirs, 1983), and tea infusion as drunk may contain 1–3 ppm (Duckworth and Duckworth, 1978). Most of the fluoride is extracted from tea quite quickly and, if water is added to the tea after the first infusion has been poured out, the second infusion contains much less fluoride (Harrison, 1949).

In view of the small contribution made by foods, fluoride is unusual in that its intake is dominated by the concentration in the drinking water and by the amount of tea consumed. This is illustrated by estimates of the total fluoride intake, by residents of American cities with or without fluoride in their drinking water, based on direct analysis of their foods. Singer, Ophaug and Harland (1980) estimated that the mean fluoride intake for young American men in unfluoridated Kansas City was 0.91 mg/day compared with 1.72 mg/day (75% from the water) in fluoridated Atlanta. In Britain, with its much heavier tea consumption, intakes by adults of 3 mg/day are quite common in unfluoridated areas, as are 4–5 mg/day in areas with fluoridation. A heavy tea drinker may even reach intakes of 8–10 mg/day (Jenkins and Edgar, 1973; Walters *et al.*, 1983).

It has been pointed out that in fluoridated areas not only do drinks contain more fluoride but some fluoride may enter the food during cooking or industrial processing (Martin, 1951; Marier and Rose, 1966). Although this must occur to some extent, no significant increase in fluoride intake from food has been revealed since extensive fluoridation was introduced in the USA (Rao, 1984; Singer, Ophaug and Harland, 1985).

The fluoride of milk

There is still some uncertainty about the fluoride of milk and the forms in which it is present, as the concentration of one of the fractions is near or below that which can be readily estimated. Most of the published figures suggest that the free ionic fluoride is below 0.01 ppm, but that if the milk is ashed or treated with strong acid the fluoride detected (total fluoride) is about six times greater (Backer Dirks *et al.*, 1974; Hargreaves, 1989). It is assumed that the bound fluoride is probably associated with the calcium salts of the milk and is released during digestion. The fluoride of human milk is increased only very slightly by 1 ppm in the drinking water, although high doses of 25 mg NaF (as given in the treatment of osteoporosis) did increase it by about 4-fold (Ekstrand *et al.*, 1984). The concentration in cow's milk has usually been found to be somewhat higher than in human milk, but the proportion of free and bound fluoride is about the same (Backer Dirks *et al.*, 1974; Duff, 1981).

The fluoride in fluoridated milk has been shown to be well absorbed, although more slowly than from water (Ericsson, 1958). Presumably the fluoride has to be released from the bound form by digestions before it can be absorbed. Another suggested explanation for that slower absorption is that milk will raise the pH of the gastric juice by its powerful buffering action, so that at the higher pH a smaller proportion of the fluoride will form the readily absorbed HF (Spak, Ekstrand and Zylberstein, 1982).

Ekstrand *et al.* (1984) stated that breast-fed infants are in negative balance, i.e. their urinary excretion is higher than their intake. This conclusion is based on the concentrations they reported for milk, 0.004–0.008 ppm; they made no attempt to estimate the bound fluoride whose existence this group of workers seems to doubt (Spak, Ekstrand and Zylberstein, 1982). These concentrations are close to those found by others for free ionic fluoride. If the ionic fluoride is taken to be 15% of the total, as Backer Dirks and colleagues and Duff reported, then the total intake would be about 0.024 and 0.048 mg – very near to their urinary output, indicating an approximate balance.

Ekstrand *et al.* (1984) point out that breast-fed infants receive a lower fluoride intake after birth (from the low concentration in milk if the existence of bound fluoride is ignored) than before birth via the placenta. When babies are fed on dried milk preparations diluted with fluoridated water, their fluoride intake may be as much as 150 times that of a breast-fed infant. Two surveys have shown that bottle-fed babies have a higher fluorosis index than do breast-fed babies, although the opacities were within the aesthetically acceptable level. This may arise because the absorption of fluoride from baby foods made up with fluoridated water was found in one experiment to be only about 70% (Spak, Ekstrand and Zylberstein, 1982).

Non-dietary source of fluoride

In addition to dietary sources, most people in developed countries have in the past few years been exposed daily to extremely high concentrations of fluoride as tablets, toothpastes, mouthrinses and, less frequently, to topical applications as solutions or gels. With adults and older children little of the fluoride from these sources is swallowed, but children younger than 4 years are often unable to clear their mouths by rinsing and spitting and much of the fluoride is swallowed (Hargreaves, Ingram and Wagg, 1970, 1972; Naylor *et al.*, 1971). The fluoride of dentifrices containing NaF and Na_2PO_3F is in a form in which all is absorbed (Ekstrand and Ehrnebo, 1980). Provided that the amount is not too large this is probably beneficial, because it allows the fluoride to exert a systemic effect on the developing teeth in addition to the topical effects in the mouth. This may explain why the fall in caries which has occurred since the early 1970s (widely thought to be caused in Britain by the use of fluoride toothpastes and involving children who have used them from an early age) is in general larger (about 50%) than the average reduction found in clinical trials (25%), carried out mostly on 12–15-year-old children. However, there is danger of over-dosing, leading to some fluorosis, especially if toothpastes are used along with other measures such as tablets or fluoridated water. It is strongly recommended that young children should use either toothpastes low in fluoride (500 ppm instead of the more usual 1000 ppm) and/or use a smear of toothpaste 'no larger than a pea' (Ericsson and Forsman, 1969).

Airborne fluoride (see page 262) is not an important source, but has been detected in the vicinity of some industrial plants, such as aluminium smelters, at average levels no higher than 8 μg/m^3; even if this air were breathed all day it would result in the inhalation of only 0.16 mg – negligible in comparison with the intake from other sources (see page 250 for an exception to this).

Absorption of fluoride

Fluoride can be readily absorbed into the body, although many factors may delay or reduce this process. Experiments on rats and the cheek pouch of hamsters have shown a slow absorption of fluoride in the mouth for up to 2.5 h (Gabler, 1968; Whitford, Callan and Wang, 1982). Although it is unlikely that significant absorption could occur from foods and drinks during the short time they are in the mouth, some absorption is probable when fluoride tablets are slowly sucked. Absorption from the mouth, as elsewhere, is greatly accelerated when the pH is reduced, because it is non-ionized HF, and not fluoride ions, that can permeate cell walls. This explains why fluoride, unlike most nutrients, is absorbed largely from the stomach, where the HCl of the gastric juice will lead to the formation of HF and may in favourable circumstances, such as an empty stomach, convert almost all the fluoride into HF. Absorption is rapid as plasma fluoride reaches a peak within 1 h of ingesting NaF, and in the absence of calcium absorption is almost complete, less than 10% of the intake being in the faeces.

In the presence of calcium, as in experiments with calcium fluoride or dietary bone meal, absorption is greatly reduced as the calcium salts have a very low solubility and, even if dissolved in the stomach, would probably precipitate in the intestine as the pH rises. In experiments with rats, addition of calcium to a diet containing soluble fluoride reduced its absorption, and addition of calcium and phosphate together reduced it still further (Wagner and Muhler, 1952). These experiments explain the low availability of the fluoride in bone meal or tinned fish and the delay in absorption of fluoride added to milk. Presumably the calcium phosphate that would form binds the fluoride in several ways, making it less available even than the only slightly soluble calcium fluoride that would form when calcium was added alone. Ingestion of aluminium also reduces fluoride absorption, probably by forming complexes that make less fluoride available for converting into HF. Other factors also influence absorption, e.g. 2 mg of sodium fluoride taken with 80 g of sucrose was absorbed more slowly than when taken alone – probably the sucrose stimulated the secretion of digestive juices and diluted the fluoride.

Fluoride absorption occurs by simple diffusion of HF, its rate depending on the concentration gradient of HF, and does not involve any metabolic activity (Ekstrand and Whitford, 1988).

Fluoride in blood

The results of fluoride analyses of complicated biological materials low in fluoride, such as blood and saliva, carried out by the methods available before the mid-1960s are now known to be much too high. The results on mineralized tissues and urines that are relatively high in fluoride and require little or no pretreatment, such as ashing, are acceptable. When the specific ion electrode was introduced (Frant and Ross, 1966), it became possible to estimate accurately much smaller quantities of fluoride, although even with this method great care is needed especially at the lower end of its sensitivity.

It is now agreed that in areas with water containing less than 0.25 ppm F, the mean concentration of fluoride ions in blood is about 0.5 μmol/l (0.01 ppm). Ekstrand (1978) published data on the fluoride of plasma at intervals over 36 h in 15 subjects of varied ages on three different levels of fluoride in water. The results detected a difference in plasma fluoride between subjects with water 0.25 and 1.2 ppm F (0.01 and 0.02 ppm, respectively), and showed that plasma fluoride increased with age over the range 10–38 years. With older subjects on 9.6 ppm, there was clear evidence of a diurnal rhythm – values in the afternoon being double those at 8 a.m. There were signs of it even with 1.2 ppm F. A diurnal rhythm has also been found in dogs under a laboratory regimen, but their plasma fluoride was highest in the morning (Whitford, 1990). Earlier values published before the use of the electrode had failed to show any difference in plasma fluoride in subjects consuming water containing 2.4 ppm or less, and it had been concluded that plasma fluoride was controlled within narrow limits so that 1 ppm in the water did not affect it. This conclusion was clearly wrong and arose simply because of the insensitivity of the analyses.

When ^{18}F is added to blood, about one-quarter of it enters the red cells. When the CO_2 tension of the blood is raised, an 'F shift' from the plasma into the cells occurs similar to the chloride shift but with a different explanation: a rise in CO_2 tension lowers the pH of the plasma thus increasing the formation of HF, the form which can permeate cell walls.

Although the plasma fluoride is not nearly as static as was once thought, the rapid rise after ingesting a few mg of fluoride lasts only for an hour or so, even if the basal value is not reached for several hours. A mechanism must exist therefore for the rapid elimination of most of an absorbed dose. One mechanism is uptake by the skeleton – especially the young, growing skeleton which, being low in fluoride, has a greater capacity for taking it up. In older people, the bone fluoride is higher and the plasma approaches equilibrium with it; hence the rise in plasma fluoride with advancing years. Another mechanism for lowering the plasma fluoride is the rapid excretion by the kidney (see later).

Whitford and Pashley (1982) showed that blood drawn from different sites may differ in its fluoride concentration. Fluoride was infused into adult dogs and young puppies over 20 min and samples were collected from the femoral artery and the femoral and jugular veins. The fluoride of the arterial samples was consistently 20–25% higher than that of the venous blood in the adults and 75% higher in the puppies. This could be explained by an uptake by the skeleton of the infused fluoride in the arterial blood, especially by the young bone. After stopping the infusion, arterial levels of fluoride fell and venous levels rose, in some cases exceeding the arterial values. This implies that the skeleton takes up fluoride when the blood level is rising and is the most direct evidence that fluoride can be released from the skeleton into the venous blood when the blood levels are falling. This work also suggests a possible source of error in metabolic studies if the site of collection is not taken into account.

The F concentration of ashed blood (i.e. blood dried and heated strongly to remove all organic matter, with precautions taken to avoid loss of fluoride during the heating) has been found to imply a concentration of about 0.1 ppm in the original blood – 10 times the value found with the electrode (Taves, 1966, 1968). This was thought at first to indicate that about 90% of the fluoride in blood was bound to plasma proteins. Later, Guy, Taves and Brey (1977) fractionated 20 litres of plasma and identified the non-ionic fraction as perfluoro-octanoic acid, a surfactant widely used in modern products and entering the body as a pollutant. This work does not seem to have been repeated and remains unconfirmed. Bound fluoride was stated by Taves (1971) to be absent from the sera of several animal species (perhaps because they breathe an atmosphere unpolluted with surfactants!). Other workers have found, however, that when large doses of fluoride (3 mg/kg of body weight) were injected into sheep, rabbits and rats a considerable proportion of the fluoride in the sera was in a bound form (Patterson, Kruger and Dales, 1977). Apparently, blood is capable of binding high concentration of fluorides but whether blood normally contains bound fluoride (other than in fluoride-containing pollutants) is still uncertain.

Fluoride in saliva

Fluoride is secreted into saliva at concentrations related to, but lower than, those of plasma – some of the reported figures are near or below the limits of accurate estimation and must be accepted with caution. Unstimulated saliva contains a higher fluoride concentration than stimulated (e.g. 0.018 ppm unstimulated and 0.013 ppm stimulated), but once stimulated there is no consistent relation between concentration and flow rate (Shannon, Suddick and Edmonds, 1973). The fluoride of whole saliva collected from the mouth (i.e. after contact with the oral tissues) is higher than in saliva collected from the ducts. After centrifuging, the concentration of whole saliva is lower, presumably because some of the fluoride is bound to precipitates of calcium phosphate that form in saliva after secretion (Birkeland, 1973): there is no evidence of significant binding with the soluble constituents. Saliva collected simultaneously from the parotid and submandibular ducts have similar concentrations.

In one experiment, 1 mg of fluoride (as NaF) in a gelatin capsule was swallowed by 5 subjects and the fluoride concentration in plasma and parotid saliva at two different rates of flow was estimated over 2 h. The fluoride of the saliva at both rates of flow rose from a mean baseline of about 0.2 μmol (0.004 ppm) to a maximum of 1.5 μmol (0.03 ppm) 30 min after the dose, remained at this level for a further 30 min, then steadily fell but did not reach baseline within 2 h. There was no significant difference between the saliva at the two rates of flow (0.25 and 0.5 ml per min) (Oliveby *et al.*, 1989). The saliva/plasma ratio was about 0.6 at the maximum rate.

Effect of fluoridated water on saliva fluoride

The mean concentration in stimulated mouth saliva from residents of 1 ppm fluoridation areas was significantly higher than in those from unfluoridated areas (0.033 compared with 0.011 ppm), but the difference in parotid saliva (0.009 and 0.007) was not significant (Yao and Gron, 1970).

Most of these differences must arise therefore from direct contact of the soft tissue and plaque (including plaque-like deposits on the tongue) and with the drinking water, rather than systemically. This was confirmed by Bruun and Thylstrup (1984) who measured the fluoride concentration of mouth saliva before and 15 min after a 30 g rinse with 10 ml fluoridated tap water (F = 2.3). The saliva fluoride rose from 0.028 to 0.092 ppm: even a rinse with water containing only 0.36 ppm raised the saliva from 0.018 to 0.032 ppm. The salivary fluoride is probably an important source of fluoride in plaque which may be crucial in the action against caries (see Chapter 15). After 30 s use of toothpastes containing 500, 1000 or 1500 ppm of F as NaF or MFP, the concentration in the salivary toothpaste slurry immediately after brushing varied between 60 and 250 ppm, depending on the concentration in the toothpaste. Within 3 min, the concentrations had fallen to between 3 and 11 ppm and fell exponentially to 0.1–0.3 ppm after 30 min and were still detectably above baseline (0.016 ppm in these experiments) after 60 min. With MFP, the figures for total fluoride were similar, but free fluoride was only about 4% in the slurries, 40% in 3 min and 65% in the later samples (Bruun *et al.*, 1984). Fluoride is released from MFP fairly rapidly by salivary enzymes (Pearce and Jenkins, 1977).

Saliva movements within the mouth are quite rapid but unilateral (Jenkins and Krebsbach, 1985). One effect of this is that when fluoride tablets are placed in one side of the mouth and allowed to dissolve slowly, the fluoride concentration in the mouth can vary very widely from levels (2600 ppm in one experiment) potentially toxic to the soft tissues on one side of the mouth to less than 4 ppm on the other side (Weatherell *et al.*, 1984). Even after rinsing with 1000 ppm F solution, the rate of clearance in different parts of the mouth varied greatly, e.g. the lower central mandibular area cleared much more quickly than the central upper labial vestibule (Weatherell *et al.*, 1986).

Excretion of fluoride

Fluoride is excreted in the urine, lost through sweat and excreted in the faeces. The principal route of fluoride excretion is via the urine and the urinary fluoride level is widely regarded as one of the best indices of fluoride intake.

In the USA, a country in which tea drinking is not very common, it was shown many years ago that the urinary fluoride concentration depended on that of the drinking water (McClure and Kinser, 1944) (Figure 14.1). There have been few data published on this since the introduction of fluoride-containing toothpastes, so it is uncertain whether this relation still holds. In tea-drinking communities, it would be expected that urinary fluoride would be dominated by the amount of tea drunk, but as the strength of tea and therefore its fluoride concentration is so variable, the relationship is not likely to be clear-cut.

The clearance of fluoride by the kidney is less than that of inulin, which indicates that some of the fluoride filtered through the glomerulus is reabsorbed by the tubules (Chen *et al.*, 1956; Carlson *et al.*, 1960a). Between 35% and 45% of the

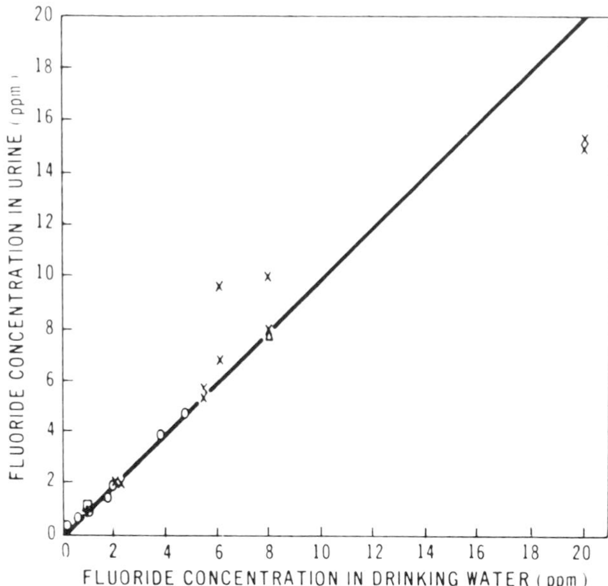

Figure 14.1 Relation between fluoride concentration in human urine and that in the water supplies used (Reproduced from *Fluorides and Human Health* (WHO Monograph Series No. 59), by courtesy of the World Health Organisation)

fluoride is reabsorbed in the proximal tubule, but if the pH of the fluid in the distal tubule falls, more reabsorption occurs as the fluoride ions are converted into HF, the form in which fluoride is diffusible into cells.

There is no evidence for fluoride secretion by the kidney tubules (Whitford, 1990).

Fluoride is rapidly excreted from the body. Even small amounts, for example 1.5 mg (Hodge and Smith, 1965) or 5 mg (Zipkin and Leone, 1957) taken in a glass of water are absorbed and excreted so rapidly that 20% of the fluoride can be found in the urine after 3 h (Figure 14.2). Using ^{18}F, Carlson, Armstrong and Singer (1960b) and Ericsson (1958) found that up to 30% of a 1 mg dose was detectable in the urine in 4 h. The very rapid rate of excretion is one of the most protective factors in severe fluoride poisoning: usually either death occurs within 4 h or the individual recovers. The critical period is short because fluoride is rapidly removed from the blood stream and extracellular fluid via the kidney and because skeletal deposition is extremely rapid.

In an individual relatively unexposed to fluoride, about half a single dose of fluoride is excreted in the urine in the following 24 h and about half is deposited in the skeleton. Largent (1960) collected samples of everything he ate and drank and of everything he excreted, over a period of several months, so that he was able to make definitive measurements of the retention of fluoride when daily doses of 1–18 mg were ingested. This fluoride balance study showed that fluoride retention followed closely a simple straight line, indicating storage of 50% of the absorbed fluoride (Figure 14.3).

Younger individuals, who have a greater proportion of their skeleton available to the circulation and who are actively laying down bone mineral, excrete a lower percentage of a given dose of fluoride than do adults. Infants excrete 40% of the fluoride ingested daily (Ham and Smith, 1954). Longwell (1957) reported that children in the London area aged 5–6 years excreted half as much fluoride in the urine as did those aged 10–12 years (0.16 mg per 24 h compared with 0.35 mg per 24 h).

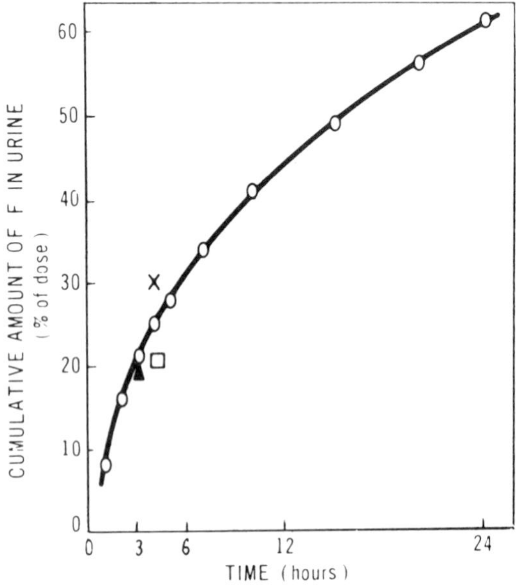

Figure 14.2 Cumulative secretion of fluoride in the human urine following the oral administration of sodium fluoride (Reproduced from *Fluorides and Human Health* (WHO Monograph Series No. 59), by courtesy of the World Health Organisation)

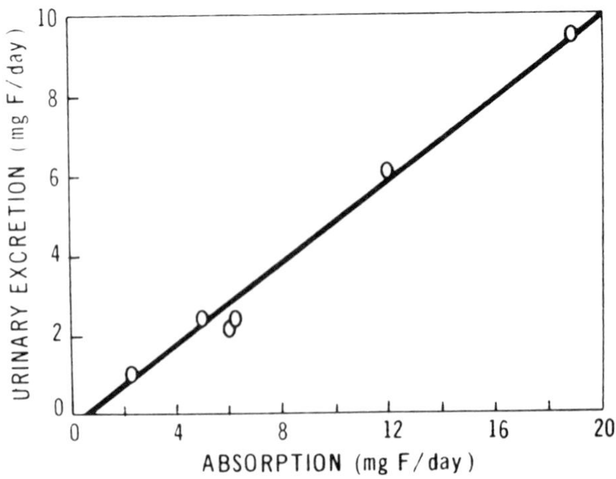

Figure 14.3 Relation between absorption and urinary excretion of fluoride (After Machle and Largent, 1943; reproduced from *Fluorides and Human Health* (WHO Monograph Series No. 59), by courtesy of the World Health Organisation)

Fluoride in sweat

The fluoride concentration of sweat and the role it plays in metabolism is still somewhat uncertain, as there have been very few studies on sweat with the fluoride electrode. Early work (McClure *et al.*, 1945; Crosby and Shepherd, 1957) had suggested that sweat contained sufficiently high concentrations of fluoride (0.3–0.7 ppm was a typical range) to indicate that the skin was a significant route of excretion, especially when sweating was profuse. This seemed to be authenticated by reports that the proportion of fluoride eliminated in the urine in 'comfortable' conditions was higher (77%) than in 'hot–moist' conditions (44%) when the corresponding figures for the sweat were stated to rise from 24% to 49%. A fall in the average fluoride content of urine collected first thing in the morning in summer from Australian 5-year-old children was attributed to a greater output via the sweat in summer, although several other possible influences were not controlled (Dooland and Carr, 1985).

Analyses with the electrode have failed to confirm a high concentration of fluoride in sweat. Even after ingesting 10 mg F, which raised plasma levels to 0.24 ppm, sweat was reported to contain only about 0.05 ppm (Henschler, Buttner and Patz, 1975). G. M. Whitford (pers. comm.) found a similar concentration after vigorous exercise (about 0.06 ppm). Although more work is required, recent results suggest that fluoride excretion in sweat is negligible – even with hard manual labour under hot conditions (where 4–6 litres of sweat may be excreted daily) fluoride elimination would not appear to exceed 0.2–0.3 mg. There is no explanation for the earlier results in which the analytical methods used gave quite acceptable values for the urine fluoride but apparently grossly overestimated the fluoride of sweat. If a fall in urine fluoride did occur under hot conditions, it would seem more likely to arise from some unrecognized effect on kidney function rather than a rise in loss of fluoride through the sweat.

Storage of fluoride in soft tissues

The mineralized tissues are the main site of storage of fluoride and contain about 99% of the total. Analysis of healthy soft tissues invariably gives low values for fluoride and their validity is confirmed by study of the ratio between the concentrations in the tissues and the plasma (the T/P ratio) after the injection of ^{18}F. This ratio was found to be less than 1.0 in all tissues except two – the kidney (with its concentrate of glomerular fluid) and bone with T/P ratios of 4.16 and 7.5, respectively (Whitford, Pashley and Reynolds, 1979). The lowest was brain (0.084), suggesting that fluoride does not readily cross the blood–brain barrier, followed by adipose tissue (0.112), presumably low from its poor vascularity. A high fluoride concentration in a soft tissue suggests that it is undergoing pathological mineralization (Mohamedally, 1984).

The fluoride of nails and hair is related to the fluoride intake. The mean fluoride concentrations reported for nails from groups of about 35 residents of areas with 0.1, 0.8 and 1.9 ppm in their water were 0.79, 1.31 and 2.31 ppm, respectively (Schamschula *et al.*, 1985). The fluoride of nails might be used as a means of identifying subjects suspected of receiving excessive fluoride, although nail parings would be indicative of fluoride intake some months previously, when the nails were forming. The fluoride concentration in hair is too low (0.2–0.4 ppm) for accurate routine estimation and too variable to be diagnostic of fluoride intake.

Interaction of fluoride and apatite crystals

The principal mineral of skeletal tissues is the particular crystallized form of calcium phosphate known as apatite: $Ca_{10}(PO_4)_6X_2$. When X is OH, the crystal is known as hydroxyapatite (HA) and impure HA is the main constituent of the mineralized tissues.

An important property of apatite is that several different ions can occupy positions in the crystal with only minor changes in its dimensions and without significant change in its form; for example, calcium ions can be replaced by strontium ions and phosphate by carbonate ions (heteroionic exchange). Experiments with radioactive isotopes show that one ion (e.g. Ca) may leave the crystal and be replaced by another Ca ion (isoionic exchange). In addition, some ions, too large to enter the crystal, may become adsorbed onto the crystal surfaces or enter the 'hydration shell' (the layer of adsorbed water that normally surrounds the crystal).

Neuman and Neuman (1958) proposed a three-stage mechanism to describe the entry of ions into the apatite crystal lattice. The first stage is that fluoride ions exchange with one of the ions or polarized molecules present in the loosely integrated hydration shell. The second stage involved the exchange of fluoride in the hydration shell with an ion group at the surface of the apatite crystal. The ionic exchange would occur between fluoride ions and hydroxyl and bicarbonate groups and also with fluoride ions already present in the crystal. Finally, ions present in the crystal surface might migrate slowly into vacant space in the crystal interior during recrystallization.

Pure HA interacts with concentrations of fluoride ions up to about 100 ppm by exchanging with the OH ions forming a fluorohydroxyapatite (FHA) or, if it goes to completion, fluorapatite (FA) with no hydroxyl ions left but a fluoride content of 3.8% (38 000 ppm). Some fluoride is always present in the calcified tissues, so its mineral is FHA.

Because HA is a complicated crystal (each unit containing 18 ions), when it crystallizes it tends to contain imperfections and occasional ions are absent forming 'vacancies' or 'voids' in the crystal. Studies by X-ray and neutron diffraction suggest that this is specially likely to occur in the hydroxyl groups which form a column running through the middle of each crystal (Figure 14.4). The orientation of the OHs is reversed at various places within the crystal, some OH ions pointing 'downwards' and others pointing 'upwards'. Where this reversal occurs, two adjacent OH ions cannot point in opposite directions (OH HO) because the H atoms would be too close together and would not fit into the lattice. A vacancy must therefore occur between two OH ions pointing in opposite directions and this vacancy introduces an instability into the crystal that increases its solubility. The dimensions of fluoride and OH ions are similar, so that a fluoride ion can fill the vacancy and be also attached to the neighbouring OH ions by hydrogen bonds, thus making the crystal more stable, i.e. dissolve less readily (Kay, Young and Posner, 1964).

With concentrations of fluoride higher than 100 ppm, another reaction occurs with apatite resulting in the formation of CaF_2:

$$Ca_{10}(PO_4)(OH)_2 + 20F^- = 10CaF_2 + 6(PO_4)^{3+} + 2(OH)^-$$

The concentrations of fluoride applied topically in solutions, gels or toothpastes are sufficiently high for CaF_2 to form, and its spherical crystals can be seen in SEMs of

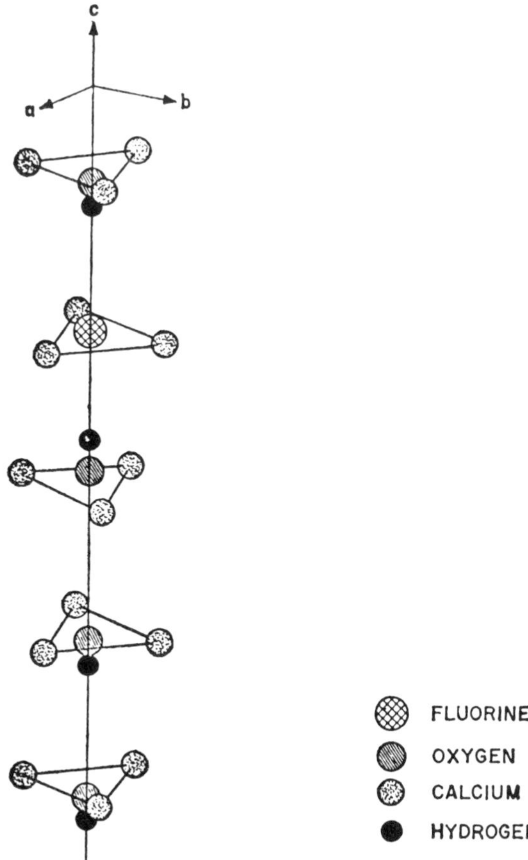

Figure 14.4 Perspective drawing of the inner part of the apatite crystal (the 'calcium triangles'). When the H of the OH ions (in the centre of the triangles) face each other they cannot occupy adjacent triangles because there is insufficient room to accommodate them. Consequently, an OH is missing from the triangle between the two H atoms facing each other and this 'void' makes the crystal less stable and more soluble. Fluoride ions can enter this void and remove the instability and reduce the solubility of the crystal (From Young and Elliott, 1966, with kind permission of the Editor, *Archives of Oral Biology*)

the enamel surface after the treatments. The CaF_2 gradually dissolves and acts as a reservoir of fluoride ions that can enter plaque and also diffuse into the enamel in concentrations that lead to the filling of voids or to ionic exchange with hydroxyl ions. Calcium fluoride is soluble in KOH, so that estimations of the fluoride soluble and insoluble in a KOH solution differentiates between apatite CaF_2 and F (Caslavska, Moreno and Brudevold, 1975).

Although CaF_2 has a low solubility in water (reported at about 16 ppm), its retention on the teeth after formation following topical applications of fluoride is longer than would be predicted in view of the fairly large throughput of water in the mouth as drinking fluid and saliva. Rolla and Ogaard (1986) have shown that CaF_2 is less soluble in saliva than in water and they suggest that, in the mouth, crystals of CaF_2 become coated with some salivary constituents identified as protein, phosphate or apatite derived from it which make them less soluble.

Reactions of enamel with fluoride in topical application or toothpastes

In the belief, now seriously questioned, that the effectiveness of topical application of fluoride depends on the extent to which fluoride is introduced into the apatite of enamel, methods for increasing the uptake have been intensively studied.

The uptake of fluoride by HA is greatly favoured by an acid medium, and two explanations have been suggested for this effect. First, the acid will dissolve some HA, releasing calcium and phosphate ions (making the enamel more porous) and when these ions meet fluoride ions they will form FA (or FHA: partially fluoridated hydroxyapatite) which, being less soluble than HA, will precipitate leading to its incorporation in the enamel. Secondly, in an acid medium, the concentration of OH is extremely low which reduces the probability of isoionic exchange of OH ions in apatite, thereby increasing the probability of heteroionic exchange of hydroxyl with fluoride. However, acidity also converts phosphate ions (PO_4^{3-}) to the protonated forms: HPO_4^{2-} and $H_2PO_4^{1-}$. The higher the concentration of acid, the lower the concentration of PO_4 and hence the lower the common ion effect preventing the PO_4^{3-} of the apatite from being released and preventing the crystal from dissolving. Brudevold *et al.* (1963) realized that if an acidified solution of fluoride also contained phosphate, the fluoride uptake would be favoured (by the acid) and the dissolution of the enamel would be disfavoured (by the common ion effect of the phosphate). Phosphate also favours the entry of fluoride into the apatite rather than the formation of CaF_2 (Gron, 1977). A solution of 1.23% of fluoride as NaF in 0.1 M H_3PO_4 at pH of about 3, which came to be called APF (acidulated phosphate fluoride), has been widely used for topical application in gels and was shown *in vivo* to increase about 4-fold the concentration of fluoride in enamel, mostly as CaF_2 which, as mentioned above, gradually dissolves to form very dilute solutions in plaque and saliva (which are unsaturated with CaF_2) and some of the fluoride eventually becomes firmly bound in the apatite crystal.

In the first clinical trial of APF, two topical applications at yearly intervals on 115 children with 113 controls produced a 70% reduction in caries increments (Wellock and Brudevold, 1963). This was a much greater reduction than obtained by any other workers and it should be noted that the APF solution was made up somewhat differently from that used subsequently. It consisted of 2% NaF in 0.1 M H_3PO_4, the fluoride being made up to 1.23% by the dropwise addition of HF. Later workers have used 1.23% F (as NaF) in 0.15 M H_3PO_4 (i.e. excluding HF). There seems no obvious theoretical reason for expecting these two solutions to differ in caries-preventing action and the difference may be quite irrelevant but should be borne in mind.

Other fluoride salts have been shown to increase the concentration and retention of fluoride by enamel more than APF, e.g. acidified solution (pH 4.4) of ammonium fluoride and fluoride bound to certain long-chain aliphatic amines (Baijot-Stroobants and Vreven, 1980), but in both cases considerable loss eventually occurred. Other procedures for increasing the effectiveness of topical application is to etch the enamel with phosphoric acid followed by APF or other F solutions. The pretreatment with acid may act either by dissolving some apatite, thus increasing the diffusion pathways enabling more fluoride to enter, or by increasing the reformation (as FA) of the apatite dissolved by the acid – it is known that fluoride favours FA formation from saturated solutions of Ca and P rather than other crystalline forms of calcium phosphate. This pretreatment has been shown to be more effective clinically than APF alone (although of borderline significance), and the fluoride of biopsy samples from the upper central incisors were still significantly higher than controls after 1 year (DePaula, Aasenden and Brudevold, 1971). However, Wei and Scholtz (1975) found a very high uptake from APF and from ammonium fluoride preceded by acid, but after 3 months the surface fluoride was *lower* than before the treatment – possibly the increased diffusion pathways increased the access of oral fluids which washed away the deposited fluoride. Pretreatment of the teeth with acid solution of 'dical' (calcium acid phosphate dihydrate $CaHPO_4 \cdot 2H_2O$) also favours fluoride uptake (Chow, 1990).

In one respect these biopsies on the intact enamel usually of upper incisors, upon which the above conclusions were based, may be misleading because fluoride accumulates preferentially in the more permeable enamel of early white spot lesions and there are no estimations of uptake and retention *in vivo* from topical fluoride in these sites. The etching used before some of the topicals presumably affects the enamel in a way similar, but not identical, to that of early caries. When fluoride uptake and retention by bovine enamel were compared after treatment with APF and KF, with or without previous etching, followed by washing in running water for 8 weeks, the APF + etch gave the highest uptake and retention. This treated enamel was also the least acid-soluble, i.e. the retained fluoride did exert an effect on the enamel solubility (Valk *et al.*, 1985).

Effect of stannous fluoride on enamel

Studies by the electron microprobe of enamel treated with 10% SnF_2 for 4 min show that the surface becomes irregular and that tin is deposited on the irregular surface. SEMs confirm the roughening of the surface which, especially after prolonged exposure (24 h), suggests that the original surface is dissolved (SnF_2 solution is very acid) and that new material is deposited on the exposed inner enamel (Wei, 1974). The deposits, after prolonged exposure, show the same infra-red spectra as a previously unknown substance, tin fluoride phosphate $Sn_3F_3PO_4$ (Krutchkoff *et al.*, 1972), along with some spherical crystals of CaF_2. These changes seem to be too slow to occur on an intact enamel surface with 4 min exposure to 10% SnF_2, but may take place in early carious lesions when the increased surface area might be expected to increase its reactivity (Krutchkoff *et al.*, 1972).

The interaction of tin, as well as fluoride, with enamel treated with SnF_2 may explain why this substance alters the wettability of the enamel surface (Glantz, 1969) that, in turn, may account for the finding that SnF_2 has a greater effect than NaF in reducing plaque formation.

Effect of fluoride on apatite formation

This is a convenient place to describe the important effects that fluoride ions have on supersaturated solutions of calcium and phosphate (Brudevold, McCann and Gron, 1965). Among the several salts that might precipitate, octacalcium phosphate [$Ca_8H_2(PO_4)_6$] is the form kinetically favoured but, in the presence of traces of fluoride, apatite crystallizes, especially if a crystal of apatite is added to act as a 'seed'. The higher the concentration of fluoride, the larger are the crystals and the fewer imperfections they contain, i.e. the higher is their 'crystallinity'. The importance of this effect is that apatites are the least soluble and most stable of all the calcium phosphates and this may be of significance in the protection of enamel. It is known that many metallic ions (Zn, Pb, Sn and Cd) do, like fluoride, reduce the solubility of apatite but do not reduce caries, nor favour the precipitation of apatite from saturated solutions, suggesting that this property is apparently unique to fluoride, and may play a part in its anti-caries action.

Metabolism and role in caries prevention of monofluorophosphate

Physiology

Most of the *in vivo* effects of monofluorophosphate (MFP) are identical with those of NaF or other soluble fluorides with the same fluoride content, because the MFP ion is rapidly broken down before absorption, probably by non-specific phosphatases. The main differences occur in the gut before the breakdown takes place. Saliva has little effect on ingested MFP because its contact is so brief, but MFP remaining in the mouth after the use of a toothpaste is rapidly broken down by bacterial enzymes. MFP is quite stable in the stomach as the pH is too low to allow enzymic breakdown, but usually not low enough for acid hydrolysis which occurs only below pH 2.5. Unlike fluoride, MFP is not absorbed from the stomach, so immediately after swallowing, absorption of fluoride is more rapid, but shortly after entering the intestine its breakdown and absorption are rapid. It is unlikely that any intact MFP enters the blood, but if it did it would be immediately hydrolysed by enzymes in the blood and liver. One important difference between fluoride and MFP is that the latter is not precipitated by Ca and therefore its absorption is not delayed, should it be ingested with it. After absorption, the metabolism of fluoride from MFP is the same as that of NaF.

Effects of MFP in the mouth that influence caries

There is no evidence that MFP itself inhibits enzymes, but it is broken down quite rapidly by plaque (Pearce and Jenkins, 1977; Jackson, 1982) and, after toothbrushing with an MFP toothpaste, concentration of fluoride ions released may be sufficient to reduce plaque acid production. *In vivo*, the ions released by the plaque enzymes can be expected to play the same part as fluoride from any source, i.e. to exchange with hydroxyls in the enamel apatite and favour remineralization during episodes of acid production. In view of the rapidity of the hydrolysis of MFP by plaque, discussions of interaction with apatite are somewhat academic. Nevertheless, there has been considerable discussion about mechanisms whereby MFP may react with enamel. One suggestion is that MFP exchanges with PO_4 or HPO_4 ions in the apatite crystal (Ingram, 1972, 1973), the main alternative view being that after a preliminary hydrolysis, perhaps brought about by contact with the apatite as well as by enzymes, the fluoride ions then exchange with OH ions (Ericsson, 1967; Gron, Brudevold and Aasenden, 1971). In both cases, PO_4 would be released – on the first hypothesis from the apatite and on the second from the MFP. Most of the evidence supports the first hypothesis, e.g. when apatite and MFP interact, PO_4 is released but there is no rise in free fluoride ions (Duff, 1983), and if apatite is treated with a mixture of both PO_4 and MFP, less fluoride from MFP enters the apatite than with MFP alone because it has to compete with the PO_4 for the ionic exchange.

Uptake of fluoride in hard tissue

Fluoride content of bone

Because fluoride ions can enter the hydroxyapatite lattice, the concentration in human bone builds up slowly with age, its concentration depending on the fluoride intake (Blayney, Bowers and Zimmerman, 1962). The data collected by Jackson and Weidmann (1958) suggested that the fluoride concentration in the skeleton reached a plateau by middle age, but this did not agree with the findings of either Smith, Gardner and Hodge (1960) or of Weatherell (1969) that showed a continued rise with age (Figure 14.5).

Although the number of analyses over the age of 80 is limited, the rise in fluoride seems to be more rapid after this age than before, a result also obtained by Mohamedally (1984). Although this may be a misleading result arising from few data, it is possible that as the mass of bone diminishes in later life the bone that remains is the oldest and contains the highest fluoride concentration. Also, as some bone is removed, the fluoride it releases might be taken up by the surviving bone in the neighbourhood (Zipkin, 1972).

The incorporation of fluoride slightly alters the chemical composition of bone and tooth mineral; the carbonate and citrate contents are lowered and the magnesium level increased. The Ca/P ratio, however, remains unchanged (Weidmann and Weatherell, 1970).

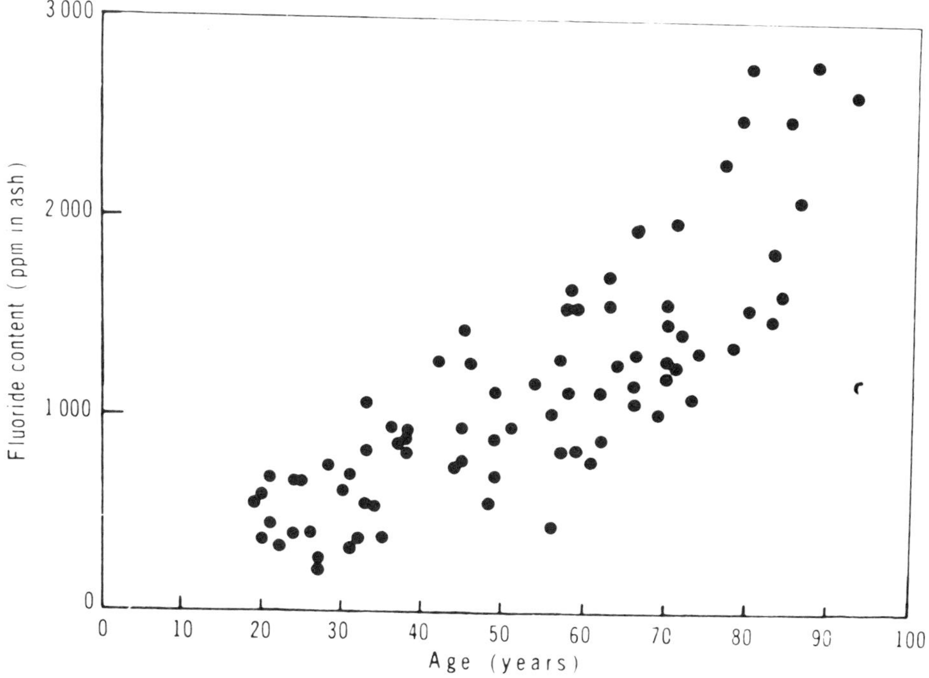

Figure 14.5 Fluoride content of femoral compacta from humans of different ages living in low-fluoride areas (From Weatherell, 1969; reproduced from *Mineral Metabolism in Paediatrics*, edited by Barltrop, D. and Burland, W. L., by kind permission of Blackwell Scientific Publications, 1969)

If the intake of fluoride is markedly reduced, some of the fluoride accumulated by bone is gradually lost. For example, when the fluoride in the water supply in Bartlett, Texas, was reduced from the excessive 8 ppm to approximately 1 ppm, urinary fluoride excretion was over 4 ppm for about 20 weeks after defluoridation and continued to fall, although more slowly, so that even 2 years after it was still more than 2 ppm (Likins, McClure and Steere, 1956). It was suggested that the rapid initial drop occurred as the fluoride in superficial parts of the fluoride-rich bone exchanged with hydroxyl ions and approached a new equilibrium. The later slower loss probably occurred from the replacement of old bone by new, low in fluoride, in the course of remodelling (Likins, McClure and Steere, 1956).

The distribution of fluoride within bone is not uniform. It is highest in those areas of most active growth; for example, endosteal and periosteal surfaces usually have a higher fluoride content than the central parts of compact bone (Weidmann and Weatherell, 1959). This makes the sampling of bone for analysis very difficult: most workers now take all their samples from one location, such as rib cortex. In addition to age, the main factor controlling the fluoride of bone is the fluoride intake, which means in practice the fluoride concentration of the drinking water and the amount of tea consumed. The average fluoride of bone samples from American residents is lower than in comparable samples from tea-drinking Britain (Zipkin *et al.*, 1958).

Fluoride content of teeth

Enamel

As in bone, the distribution of fluoride in the dental tissues as formed is not uniform. When the fluoride concentrations are estimated in sequential layers of enamel, either ground off or dissolved with acid, from a tooth of a young person, the outer 5 μm of permanent teeth are found to contain typically between 1000 and 3000 ppm depending on the fluoride of the drinking water (for a summary of the data up to 1974, see Mellberg and Singer, 1977). The concentration falls off to about one-tenth of these figures at a depth of about 50 μm (Jenkins and Speirs, 1954; Brudevold, Gardner and Smith, 1956; Weatherell and Hargreaves, 1966) and remains fairly constant until the amelodentinal junction is approached where there is a small rise (Figures 14.6 and 14.7). The absolute values obtained for the outer layers depend very much on the thickness of each layer removed – the thicker the layer the more of the inner enamel, relatively low in fluoride it will include. This is illustrated by the higher values found by the secondary ion micro-analyser (the 'ion probe'). In this method, the sample is bombarded with mono-energetic ions focused onto a small area of enamel and the ions sputtered off the surface are analysed by mass spectrometry. Fluoride concentrations of 3650 and 5500 ppm were found in 2 teeth from 12-year-old children in a low-fluoride area, in layers only 0.04 μm thick (Petersson *et al.*, 1976).

Another example is the fluoride analyses of exfoliated deciduous teeth from children in Japan after exposure to 0.5 M perchloric acid for only 5 s which dissolved a layer less than 1 μm thick. Values of 14 380 and 1600 ppm were found in teeth from areas with 1.74 and 0.1 ppm F, respectively, in their water and 1000 and 300 ppm at depths of 30 μm (Iijima and Katayama, 1985). The latter figures are in reasonable agreement with previous findings for deciduous teeth in Britain at a

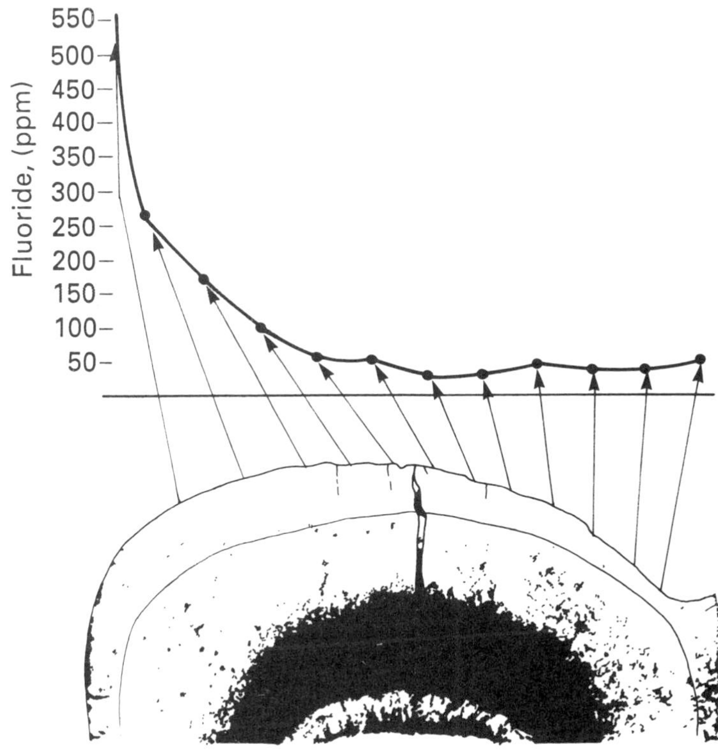

Figure 14.6 Distribution of fluoride in enamel of a permanent incisor (From Weatherell and Hargreaves, 1965; reproduced from *Archives of Oral Biology*, by kind permission of the Editor and Pergamon Press)

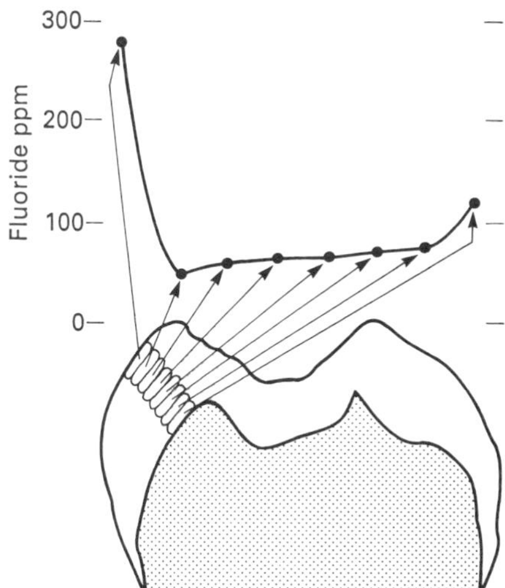

Figure 14.7 Distribution of fluoride across the cuspal enamel of an unerupted mandibular third molar from a female aged 51 years (From Hallsworth and Weatherell, 1969; reproduced by courtesy of the Editor, *Caries Research*)

depth of 30 µm – about 1000 and 400 ppm, respectively, from towns with 2 and 0.1 ppm F (Hargreaves, 1967). The influence of fluoridated drinking water on the fluoride of surface enamel has been well established by several groups of workers (Isaac *et al.*, 1958; Jackson and Weidmann, 1959; Iijima and Katayama, 1985).

Estimation of enamel fluoride in vivo

Three procedures have been used in living subjects for collecting biopsy samples and estimating their fluoride concentration. The most accurate method is by placing a drop of 0.5 M perchloric acid for a few seconds on a 'window' of known area, cut out of a piece of sticking plaster previously placed on the enamel, followed by a drop of washing water (Munksgaard and Bruun, 1973). The F, Ca and/or P of the combined drops are then analysed, from which the weight of enamel removed can be estimated (on the basis that the composition of enamel is 36% Ca and 17% P). From the weight and the area, the depth can be calculated. An alternative method is to place a circle of filter paper soaked in acid on the enamel and wash out and analyse the acid for F and Ca or P (Aasenden, Moreno and Brudevold, 1972). Although measurements showed that the enamel became thinner with increasing age as a result of abrasion (but significantly only for the occlusal surfaces of molars and the incisal and palatal surfaces of canines), the individual variation was so great that there was no consistent difference in fluoride with age in deciduous teeth (Hargreaves, 1967). In the third method (Brudevold, McCann and Gron, 1968), a sample of enamel is ground off and the powder collected, but it is more difficult to get a uniform layer and to estimate its depth than with dissolving off the layer. These procedures usually have no detectable effect on the appearance of the enamel, but if a slight chalkiness is visible it rapidly disappears within a few days.

Acquisition of fluoride by the enamel

The gradients are present in unerupted teeth and presumably arise because after the full thickness of the enamel is formed it remains in contact with tissue fluid for, in some teeth, several years before eruption. During this time it would be expected that fluoride would be taken up by the apatite even from the low concentrations in the tissue fluid. The fact that the interval between formation and eruption is much shorter with the deciduous teeth would explain the lower values reached.

The capacity for apatite to bind fluoride is so great that it was at first assumed that fluoride entered enamel and other calcified tissue because it became bound to the high concentration of apatite that they contain. It was therefore surprising to find that the fluoride concentration of fetal enamel, measured as the F/P ratio in the rat and cow (Deutsch, Weatherell and Hallsworth, 1972; Deutsch, Weatherell and Robinson, 1974), pig (Speirs, 1975, 1978) and human (Deutsch and Gedalia, 1982), was at its highest *before* mineralization was complete and that it actually fell in the later stages of maturation (Figure 14.8). This suggested that the fluoride of inner enamel was deposited with the protein during the secretory stage and was either diluted by the influx of more mineral or partly removed, along with the protein, during maturation. In the very last stage of post-eruptive development, the fluoride of the enamel rose slightly, probably because the surface layer was already highly mineralized and could take up fluoride from the tissue fluid. This is shown in Figure 14.8, in the oldest stage of human fetal teeth (later, post-natal teeth were not available in this study). The rise has been shown more convincingly in animal experiments in which older teeth were available (Speirs, 1978).

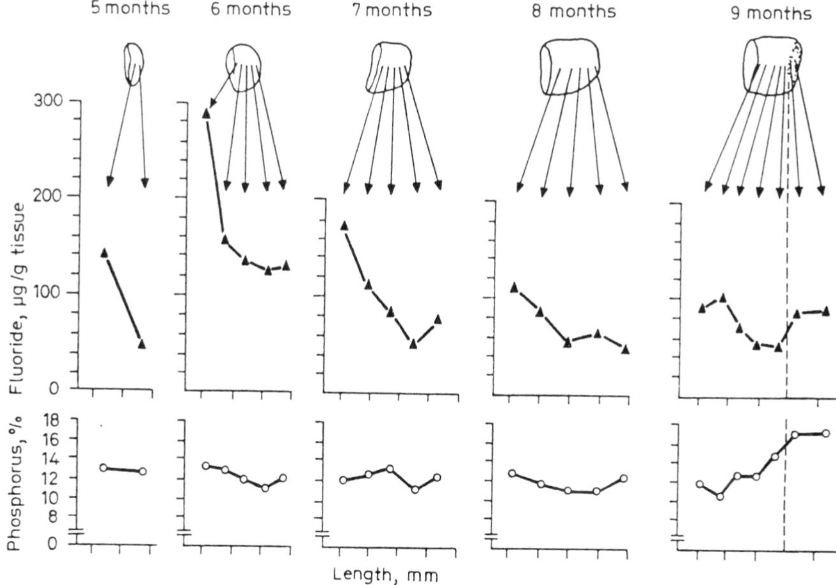

Figure 14.8 Fluoride and phosphorus distribution along the developing enamel of maxillary incisors taken from human fetuses aged 5–9 months. The teeth from the 5- to 8-month-old fetuses contain forming enamel only and show a steady fall in fluoride concentration, whereas the tooth from the 9-month-old fetus contains both forming and mature enamel (From Deutsch and Gedalia, 1982, by kind permission of Karger, Basel)

As mentioned elsewhere, the soft tissues contain very low concentrations of fluoride and it had been assumed that fluoride did not readily combine with tissue proteins. An alternative explanation is that the pH of most tissues is never sufficiently low to convert many fluoride ions into HF – the non-ionized form to which cell walls are permeable. When enamel matrix proteins were equilibrated with ^{18}F, by Crenshaw, Wennburg and Bawden (1978), they reported that considerable binding did occur, thus supporting the concept of protein-bound fluoride in developing enamel, but they were unable to confirm this in later experiments (Bawden, Deaton and Crenshaw, 1987; Lussi *et al.*, 1988). They suggested that the fluoride uptake in the early stages of enamel development occurs because the apatite crystals are small and have a large surface area that favours uptake and that the fall in fluoride concentration (on a weight basis), which had been interpreted as a removal of fluoride coinciding with the removal of protein, occurs because, as more mineral enters, it dilutes the concentration (but does not change the absolute amount) of fluoride present. This could be tested by estimating the fluoride on a volume basis (a fall in fluoride concentration per mm^3 would represent a removal of fluoride), but there are no reports of this experiment being carried out.

Fluoride of the outer surface of different types of teeth

Estimations of the fluoride of the outer surfaces of central and lateral incisors and canines in groups of about 100 12–16-year-old children, reported by Aasenden, Moreno and Brudevold (1973), showed (a) that contralateral teeth from children with the same exposure to fluoride have very similar concentrations, and (b) that the central incisors have significantly lower fluoride than lateral incisors (a similar trend was reported by Wei and Schultz, 1975) that in turn have lower concentrations than the canines, except in areas with 5–7 ppm F in the water. These differences are explicable on the assumption that the fluoride of the outer enamel is acquired mostly in the intervals between the completion of enamel formation and eruption, which are approximately 3, 4 and 5 years for the central and lateral incisors and canines, respectively (Aasenden, Moreno and Brudevold, 1973).

The fluoride control of surface enamel of boys was reported to be significantly ($P = 0.05$) higher than in girls of the same age in a fluoride area, with a non-significant trend in a non-fluoride area (Aasenden *et al.*, 1971). There are several possible explanations: (a) the interval between the completion of tooth formation and eruption during which the enamel is taking up fluoride is several months longer in boys than in girls; (b) girls are known to be more conscientious in toothbrushing and would therefore tend to remove more of the fluoride surface than boys; (c) the greater body size and activity of boys may lead to a higher water intake. This difference in fluoride may account for the slightly higher caries prevalence in girls, in spite of their more thorough oral hygiene.

Effect of age on the fluoride of enamel

Early studies based on the exposure to acid of the crowns of whole teeth or of powdered enamel ground off the crowns, and estimation of the fluoride removed, suggested that the concentration of fluoride rose with increasing age at a rate that depended on the fluoride of the drinking water (Brudevold, Gardner and Smith, 1956; Jenkins and Speirs, 1953). Jackson and Weidmann (1959) reported that the fluoride concentration reached a plateau at the age of 40–50, the height of the plateau again depending on the fluoride ingested.

When the fluoride concentration of very small areas of enamel, less than 1 mm across, etched off with 4 μl of acid were measured by meticulous micro-techniques, the picture that emerged showed that over most of the enamel, at least of the anterior teeth, the trend was for the concentration to fall with increasing age (Figure 14.9) (Weatherell, Hallsworth and Robinson, 1973). A rise in the fluoride concentration was found in only two groups of sites: the cervical areas of the anterior teeth, and early white spot lesions. A significant fall in fluoride concentration was detectable when enamel from children aged 7–10 was compared with that of children aged 15–19 and, in high-fluoride towns, even between children with ages as close as 11–13.5 and 13.5–15 (Aasenden, 1975).

These results strongly suggested that the outer layer was being removed and the lower fluoride concentrations of the inner layer became exposed. This loss of surface enamel had been demonstrated previously by microscopy of teeth at different ages (Scott, Kaplan and Wyckoff, 1949). Several factors might lead to this abrasion: toothbrushing, and contact with tough, fibrous foods. A similar distribution of fluoride was reported in cervical and non-cervical areas of enamel in mediaeval teeth which it could be presumed had not been subjected to any form of toothbrushing (Richards, Larsen and Fejerskov, 1979). It would seem that abrasion from food is the most likely cause.

There is good evidence that for some time (how long is not known) after eruption, fluoride and other constituents can be taken up by enamel. It has been found, by several groups conducting clinical trials of fluoride-containing toothpastes, that the caries reduction is about twice as great in teeth erupting

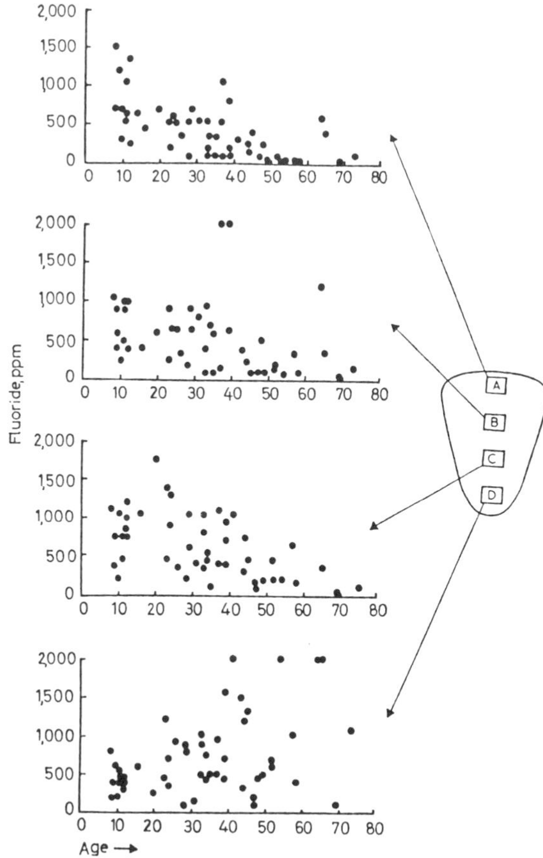

Figure 14.9 Variation of fluoride concentration with age in different regions of the labial or buccal tooth surfaces. Note that the fluoride concentration falls with age except in the cervical region (From Weatherell, Hallsworth and Robinson, 1972, by kind permission of Karger, Basel)

during the trial as in the teeth already erupted when the trial began (Naylor and Emslie, 1967). Newly-erupted teeth are incompletely mineralized (Crabb, 1976) and take up further minerals (Sakae and Hirai, 1982) and fluoride from saliva and food shortly after eruption, which increases their caries resistance. The data of Weatherell, Hallsworth and Robinson (1972) (Figure 14.10), on groups of 10 teeth of individuals varying in age from 11 to 65, do show a tendency for a higher mean fluoride concentration at age 12 than at age 11 – a possible indication of post-eruptive maturation. Animal experiments have also shown that rats receiving a cariogenic diet at weaning develop higher caries scores than a matched group put onto the cariogenic diet for the same duration but 3 weeks after weaning, i.e. their caries resistance increased during the 3 weeks (Fanning, Shaw and Sognnaes, 1953) presumably from mineral uptake.

The high fluoride concentration in the cervical area might occur either by reduced abrasion in this relatively sheltered area or by uptake from the gingival fluid (with a fluoride concentration similar to that of plasma – about 0.01 ppm) and

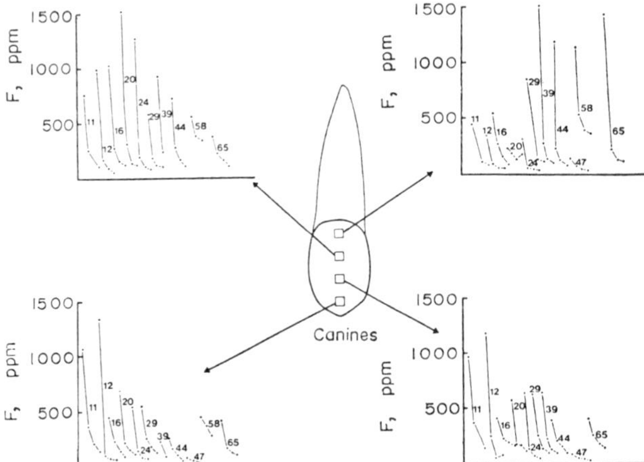

Figure 14.10 Fluoride distribution curves in four regions of the buccal surfaces of 10 canines. The ages of the individuals from whom the teeth had been obtained are shown against the curves (From Weatherell, Hallsworth and Robinson, 1972, by kind permission of Karger, Basel)

from the plaque that readily builds up on this site. The plaque contains a surprisingly high fluoride concentration (see page 306) and its pH frequently falls to about 5, a value that favours the uptake of fluoride by apatite as well as releasing fluoride ions in plaque from bound forms. The concentration was often higher than in younger teeth, strongly suggesting an uptake rather than reduced abrasions.

Another area where fluoride accumulates is in early carious lesions (Dowse and Jenkins, 1957). Enamel ground out from 'white spots' contained over twice the fluoride concentration of similar borings from intact enamel from the same teeth and it was pointed out that this suggests that under normal physiological conditions fluoride might accumulate in early cavities and exert its effect just where it could be most beneficial (see page 300 for further discussion). The acidity that causes the lesion would favour fluoride uptake and the increased permeability would allow the fluoride from plaque and saliva to diffuse throughout the lesion.

The question arises as to why the earlier work (carried out in the 1950s) suggested an uptake with ageing rather than the fall so convincingly shown by the more recent data. There is no certain answer, but it may be relevant that the older work was carried out largely on the entire enamel surface of unselected teeth as they became available, and included molars (not yet studied by the newer methods), some of the older teeth having been erupted as long ago as the last century when toothbrushing might have been less thorough with less abrasion than in recent years. Also, when these teeth were analysed it was not known that white spots were high in fluoride and their presence was ignored.

The abrasion in old teeth may be sufficient to reduce the thickness of the enamel, e.g. in two groups studied by Kidd *et al.* (1984) the mean width of enamel from 10 teeth from subjects over 65 was $915 \pm 213\,\mu m$ compared with that from a group of teenagers ($1416 \pm 160\,\mu m$; $P < 0.001$). Surprisingly, even the heavily abraded 'old' teeth showed a gradient in fluoride from the outside to inside of 450 ppm at 10 μm, to slightly more than 100 ppm at 80 μm. In view of the loss of about 500 μm, none of the original high fluoride could have survived; thus the exposed inner enamel must take up fluoride, presumably from toothpastes.

The fluoride of dentine and cementum

The fluoride concentrations in dentine are two to three times higher than those of enamel and its distribution is the reverse: the inner dentine close to the vascularized pulp contains higher concentrations than the outer layers near the amelodentine junction (Yoon *et al.*, 1960). The concentration increases steadily with age, presumably because fluoride in tissue fluid diffuses along the dentinal tubules and is taken up by the apatite.

The fluoride concentration in cementum has been estimated by grinding successive layers off sections of the roots of extracted teeth and dissolving the powder in perchloric acid and estimating fluoride and phosphate (*P* is 12.2% of cementum). The outer layer usually has the higher concentration with a steep fall in the inner layers, but in a few teeth the highest concentration is some distance in from the outer layer. There is usually a sharp fall in the boundary between the outer acellular cementum (which forms slowly) and the inner cellular tissue which forms more quickly. Complete fluoride profiles through all three of the tissues of 20 teeth from subjects ranging in age from 13 to 75 years (Figure 14.11) illustrate many of the above points. The total fluoride content of the tissues at different ages was calculated and the results are shown in Figure 14.12, which emphasize the lack of consistent effect in enamel and the clear rise in dentine and especially cementum.

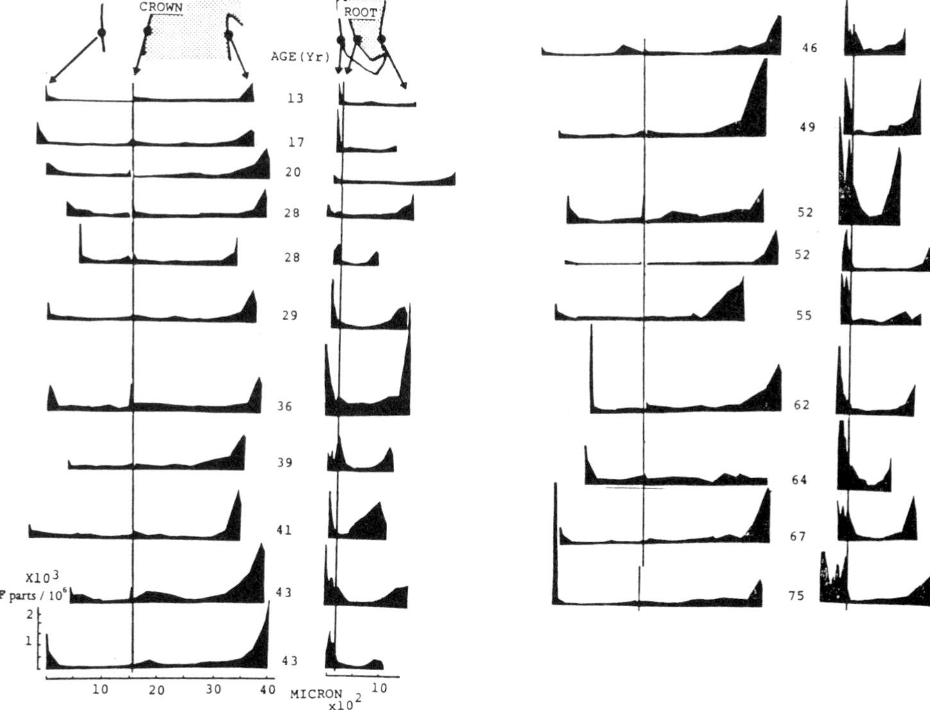

Figure 14.11 Fluoride concentrations in each of 20 teeth of ages ranging from 13 years (top left) to 75 years (lower right) expressed as black silhouettes (scale at bottom left). As indicated on the top left-hand side of the figure, the wide silhouettes represent the crowns of the teeth and the narrow silhouettes the apical regions of the roots. The vertical lines in the crowns indicate the amelodentinal junction and, in the roots, the cementodentinal junction. Note the sharp rise in fluoride near the enamel surface (left of each crown silhouette) and the larger but more gradual rise in the dentine of both crowns and roots (right side of all silhouettes) as the pulp is approached (From Nakagaki *et al.*, 1987, with kind permission of Pergamon Press)

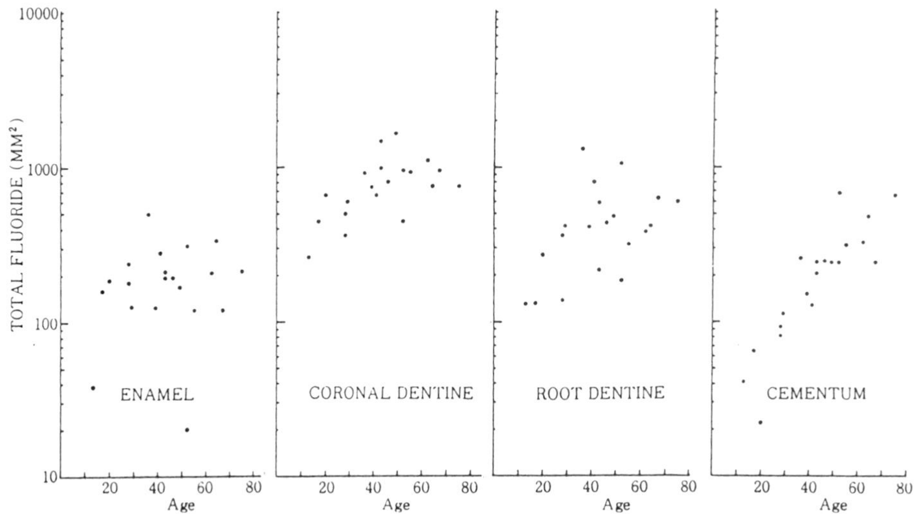

Figure 14.12 Total fluoride in the various dental tissues in relation to age (From Nakagaki *et al.*, 1987, by kind permission of Pergamon Press)

Fluoride in placenta and fetus

Early attempts to study the placental transfer of fluoride compared the fluoride concentration in fetal and maternal blood with those in the placenta in women receiving additional fluoride either in water (Gardner *et al.*, 1952) or in tablets (Feltman and Kosel, 1955). The results indicated higher values for the placenta, suggesting that it was at least a partial barrier to fluoride, but the methods of analysis available at the time were inadequate for estimating blood levels accurately or distinguishing between total and ionic fluoride.

Ericsson and Malmnas (1962) studied the transfer of ^{18}F across the placenta of patients undergoing therapeutic abortions. The ^{18}F content of fetal blood was found to be very low 5–30 min after intravenous injection – always less than one-third of the simultaneous concentration in the maternal blood. The concentration in the placenta was between that in the fetal and maternal blood, again suggesting a partial barrier. This was confirmed by Ericsson and Ullberg (1958) who injected pregnant mice with ^{18}F, killed them at intervals after the injection and made autoradiographs from rapidly prepared sections of the whole animals (Figure 14.13). The results showed uptake in the maternal skeleton within 2 min and some accumulation in the placenta (perhaps in areas of mineralization), but none was detectable in the fetus at this time. Thirty minutes later, the fetal skeleton was clearly labelled, showing that the barrier at 2 min was eventually overcome. The radiographs also show, incidentally, the very low uptake by the soft tissues except for the kidney.

Gedalia *et al.* (1964) analysed bone and teeth from fetuses varying in age from 4 to 9 months in a low-fluoride area (F = 0.05–0.10 ppm) and a moderate-fluoride area (F = 0.5–0.6 ppm) in Israel. The results clearly showed a rise in fluoride concentration of the fetal bones in the moderate-fluoride area, and it was detectable but smaller and less consistent in the low-fluoride area.

There is therefore no doubt that some fluoride can cross the placenta and that the fetal uptake depends on that of the mother. Whether fluoride supplements during pregnancy can provide sufficient fluoride to the fetus to increase its caries resistance is still controversial (see page 113).

Chemical and X-ray diffraction analysis and SEMs of the enamel from 10 children who had received 1 mg of prenatal fluoride daily were compared with similar samples from 7 controls without prenatal fluoride, but 3 of whom had received postnatal tablets, in what was described as a 'preliminary' double-blind study (Legeros *et al.*, 1985). The results did show some differences: the mineral density was higher and the fluoride concentration significantly higher and the CO_2

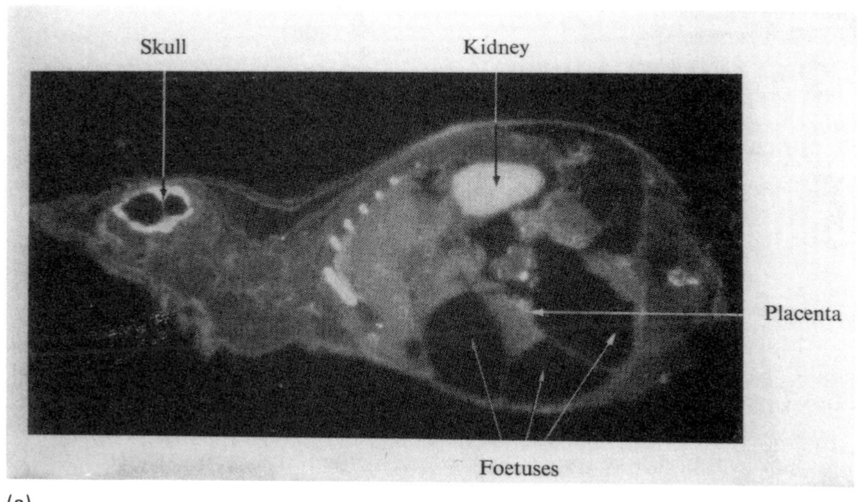

(a)

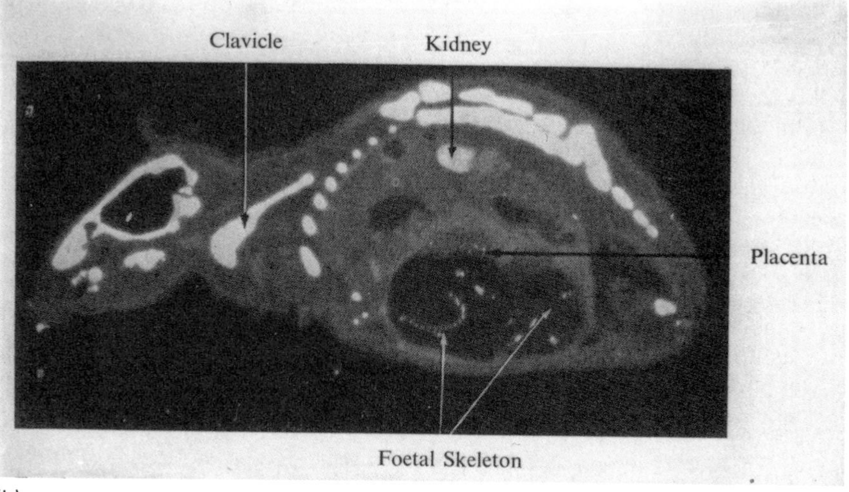

(b)

Figure 14.13 (a) Autoradiogram of section through a mouse 2 min after intravenous injection of ^{18}F. (b) As (a) but 30 min after injection (From Ericsson and Ullberg, 1958; reproduced with kind permission of the Editor, *Acta Odontologica Scandinavica*)

lower in the fluoride group. The lattice parameters of the apatite also showed differences consistent with a high fluoride content. The prenatal fluoride teeth showed less severe etching when exposed to acid. Although very little enamel is formed during fetal life, it is possible that the prenatal fluoride entered the fetal bones and was released later in concentrations sufficient to have some effect on the developing enamel.

Fluorine: an essential mineral nutrient?

Fluorine occurs naturally in a great number of foods and drinking water supplies and is universally present in the bodies of all higher animal species. The question has been raised as to whether fluorine plays a physiological role, or whether it is present in the tissues as an accidental constituent because it is ingested from food (Sharpless and McCollum, 1933). No human diet is free from fluoride, and it is extremely difficult to prepare a diet for experimental animals which is very low in fluoride

Studies carried out between 1933 and 1957 on the effect of minimal fluoride intake in rats failed to show that fluorine was an essential nutrient (Sharpless and McCollum, 1933; Muhler, 1954; Maurer and Day, 1957), although in some cases the minimal diets employed contained fluoride, as judged by carcass fluoride analyses, and in others the purified diets employed were inadequate for support of normal reproductive performance. Doberenz *et al.* (1964) fed a minimal fluoride (<0.005 ppm F) diet for a 10-week period to weanling rats and demonstrated significantly lower levels of bone fluoride in the study animals compared with a control group receiving the minimal diet plus 2 ppm F. Messer and co-workers have shown marked effects on haematocrit values and litter production in mice fed on a diet based on milk and cereals which had a very low fluoride content. Messer *et al.* (1972) reported that the low fluoride intake did not influence the haematocrit values of non-pregnant adult female mice or of newborn pups. However, the stresses of pregnancy and rapid growth in the newborn period produced a severe anaemia in mice on the low fluoride intake. They suggested that fluoride may play a hitherto unidentified role in haemopoiesis which is manifested only during stress on the haemopoietic system. In another study, Messer, Armstrong and Singer (1972) demonstrated that fluorine satisfies the major criteria for an essential trace element in the mouse. They reported that female mice maintained on a low-fluoride diet over two generations showed a progressive decline in litter production, whereas mice receiving the same diet supplemented with fluoride reproduced normally and at constant intervals. Furthermore, this impaired reproductive capacity was prevented and cured by the addition of fluoride alone to the diet.

References

Aasenden, R. (1975) Post-eruptive changes in the fluoride concentrations of human tooth surface enamel. *Arch. Oral Biol.*, **20**, 359–363

Aasenden, R., Allukian, M., Brudevold, F. and Wellock, W. D. (1971) An *in vivo* study of enamel fluoride in children living in a fluoridated and non-fluoridated area. *Arch. Oral Biol.*, **16**, 1399–1411

Aasenden, R., Moreno, E. C. and Brudevold, F. (1972) Control of sampling areas for human tooth enamel biopsies. *Arch. Oral Biol.*, **17**, 355–358

Aasenden, R., Moreno, E. C. and Brudevold, F. (1973) Fluoride levels in the surface enamel of different types of human teeth. *Arch. Oral Biol.*, **18**, 1403–1410

Backer Dirks, O., Jongeling-Eijndhoven, J. M. P. A., Flisselbaalje, T. D. and Gedalia, I. (1974) Total and free ionic fluoride in human and cow's milk as determined by gas–liquid chromatography and the fluoride electrode. *Caries Res.*, **8**, 181–186

Baijot-Stroobants, J. and Vreven, J. (1980) *In-vivo* uptake of topically applied fluoride by human dental enamel. *Arch. Oral Biol.*, **25**, 617–621

Barth, T. F. W. (1947) The geochemical cycle of fluoride. *J. Geol.*, **55**, 420–426

Bawden, J. W., Deaton, T. G. and Crenshaw, M. A. (1987) Uptake and retention of fluoride in developing enamel and bone. *J. Dent. Res.*, **66**, 1587–1590

Birdsong-Whitford, N. L., Dickinson, A. and Whitford, G. M. (1986) Effect of haematocrit on plasma F concentrations. *J. Dent. Res.*, **65** (special issue), Abs. 129, p. 184

Birkeland, J. M. (1973) The effect of pH on the interaction of fluoride and salivary ions. *Caries Res.*, **7**, 11–18

Blayney, J. R., Bowers, R. C. and Zimmerman, M. (1962) Evanston dental caries study, II. A study of fluoride deposition in bone. *J. Dent. Res.*, **41**, 1037–1044

Brudevold, F., Gardner, D. E. and Smith, F. A. (1956) The distribution of fluorine in human enamel. *J. Dent. Res.*, **35**, 420–429

Brudevold, F., McCann, H. G. and Gron, P. (1965) Caries resistance as related to the chemistry of enamel. In *Caries Resistant Teeth* (eds W. E. G. Wolstenholme and M. O'Connor), Churchill, London

Brudevold, F., McCann, H. G. and Gron, P. (1968) An enamel biopsy method for determination of fluoride in human teeth. *Arch. Oral Biol.*, **13**, 377–385

Brudevold, F., Savory, A., Gardner, D. E., Spinelli, M. and Speirs, R. (1963) A study of acidulated fluoride solutions: *in vitro* effects on enamel. *Arch. Oral Biol.*, **8**, 167–177

Bruun, C., Givskow, H. and Thylstrup, A. (1984) Whole saliva fluoride after toothbrushing with NaF and MFP dentifrices with different F concentrations. *Caries Res.*, **18**, 282–288

Bruun, C. and Thylstrup, A. (1984) Fluoride in whole saliva and dental caries experience in areas with high or low concentrations of fluoride in the drinking water. *Caries Res.*, **18**, 450–456

Carlson, C. H., Armstrong, W. D. and Singer, L. (1960a) Distribution and excretion of radio fluoride in the human. *Proc. Soc. Exp. Biol. Med.*, **104**, 235–239

Carlson, C. H., Armstrong, W. D. and Singer, L. (1960b) Distribution, migration and binding of whole blood fluoride evaluated with radio fluoride. *Am. J. Physiol.*, **199**, 187–189

Caslavska, V., Moreno, E. C. and Brudevold, F. (1975) Determination of calcium fluoride formed from *in vitro* exposure of human enamel to fluoride solutions. *Arch. Oral Biol.*, **20**, 333–339

Cholak, J. (1959) Fluorides: a critical review, I. The occurrence of fluoride in air, food and water. *J. Occup. Med.*, **1**, 501–511

Chow, L. C. (1990) Tooth-bound fluoride and dental caries. *J. Dent. Res.*, **69**, 595–600

Crenshaw, M. A., Wennburg, A. and Bawden, J. W. (1978) Fluoride-binding by the organic matrix of developing bovine enamel. *Arch. Oral Biol.*, **23**, 285–287

Crosby, N. D. and Shepherd, P. A. (1957) Studies on patterns of fluid intake, water balance and fluoride retention. *Med. J. Aust.*, **ii**, 341–346

DePaula, P. F., Aasenden, R. and Brudevold, F. (1971) The use of topically applied acidulated phosphate–fluoride preceded by mild etching of the enamel: a one-year clinical trial. *Arch. Oral Biol.*, **16**, 1155–1163

Deutsch, D. and Gedalia, I. (1982) Fluoride concentration in human fetal enamel. *Caries Res.*, **16**, 428–432

Deutsch, D., Weatherell, J. A. and Hallsworth, A. S. (1972) Uptake and distribution of fluoride in developing enamel. *J. Dent. Res.*, **51**, 1278 (Abstract)

Deutsch, D., Weatherell, J. A. and Robinson, C. A. (1974) Distribution of fluoride in developing bovine enamel. *J. Dent. Res.*, **53**, 1053 (Abstract)

Doberenz, A. R., Kurnick, A. A., Kurtz, E. B., Kemmerer, A. R. and Reid, B. L. (1964) Effect of a minimal fluoride diet on rats. *Proc. Soc. Exp. Biol. Med.*, **117**, 689–693

Dooland, M. B. and Carr, S. M. (1985) Urinary fluoride levels in South Australian pre-school children in summer and winter. *Aust. Dent. J.*, **30**, 410–413

Dowse, C. M. and Jenkins, G. N. (1957) Fluoride uptake *in vivo* in enamel defects and its significance. *J. Dent. Res.,* **36**, 816 (Abstract)

Duckworth, C. S. and Duckworth, R. (1978) The ingestion of fluoride in tea. *Br. Dent. J.,* **145**, 368–370

Duff, E. J. (1981) Total and ionic fluoride in milk. *Caries Res.,* **15,** 406–408

Duff, E. J. (1983) Reaction of monofluorophosphate with apatitic substances. *Caries Res.,* **17** (Suppl. 1), 77–87

Ekstrand, J. (1978) Relationship between fluoride in the drinking water and the plasma fluoride in man. *Caries Res.,* **12**, 123–127

Ekstrand, J. and Ehrnebo, M. (1980) Absorption of fluoride from fluoride dentifrices. *Caries Res.,* **14**, 96–102

Ekstrand, J., Hardell, L. I. and Spak, C.-J. (1984) Fluoride balance studies in a 1 ppm-water-fluoride area. *Caries Res.,* **18**, 87–92

Ekstrand, J., Spak, C.-J., Falch, J., Afseth, J. and Ulverstad, H. (1984) Distribution of fluoride to human breast milk. *Caries Res.,* **18**, 93–95

Ekstrand, J. and Whitford, G. M. (1988) Fluoride metabolism. In *Fluoride in Dentistry* (eds J. Ekstrand, O., Fejerskov and L. M. Silverstone), Munksgaard, Copenhagen, pp. 150–170

Ericsson, Y. (1958) The state of fluorine in milk and its absorption and retention when administered in milk: investigations with radioactive fluorine. *Acta Odontol. Scand.,* **16,** 51–77

Ericsson, Y. (1967) Biological splitting of PO_3F ions. *Caries Res.,* **1**, 144–152

Ericsson, Y. and Forsman, B. (1969) Fluoride retained from mouthwashes and dentifrices in preschool children. *Caries Res.,* **3**, 290–299

Ericsson, Y. and Malmnas, C. L. (1962) Placental transfer of fluorine, investigated with F18 in man and rabbit. *Acta Obstet. Gynecol. Scand.,* **41**, 144–158

Ericsson, Y. and Ullberg, S. (1958) An autoradiographic investigation of the distribution of ^{18}F in mice and rats. *Acta Odont. Scand.,* **16,** 263–282

Fanning, R. J., Shaw, J. H. and Sognnaes, R. F. (1954) Salivary contribution to enamel maturation and caries resistance. *J. Am. Dent. Ass.,* **49**, 668–671

Feltman, R. and Kosel, G. (1955) Prenatal ingestion of fluorides and their transfer to the fetus. *Science,* **122**, 560–561

Fleischer, M. (1953) Recent estimates of the abundance of the elements in the earth's crust. U.S. Geological Survey Circular No. 285, Washington, DC

Frant, M. S. and Ross, J. W. Jr (1966) Electrode for sensing fluoride ion activity in solution. *Science,* **134**, 1553–1555

Gabler, W. L. (1968) Absorption of fluoride through the oral mucosa of rats. *Arch. Oral Biol.,* **13**, 619–623

Gardner, D. W., Smith, F. A., Hodge, H. C. and Overton, D. E. (1952) The fluoride content of placental tissue as related to the fluoride content of drinking water. *Science,* **115**, 208–209

Gedalia, I., Brzezinski, A., Bercovici, B. and Lazarov, E. (1961) Placental transfer of fluorine in human fetus. *Proc. Soc. Exp. Biol. Med.,* **106**, 147–149

Glantz, P.-O. (1969) On wettability and adhesiveness. *Odont. Revy,* **20**, Suppl. 17

Gron, P. (1977) Chemistry of topical fluorides. *Caries Res.,* **11** (Suppl. 1), 172–204

Gron, P., Brudevold, F. and Aasenden, R. (1971) Monofluorophosphate interaction with hydroxyapatite and intact enamel. *Caries Res.,* **5**, 202–214

Guy, W. S. (1979) Inorganic and organic fluoride in human blood. In *Continuing Evaluation of the Use of Fluorides*, AAAS Selected Symposium, 11 (eds E. Johansen, D. R. Taves and T. O. Olsen), Westview Press, Boulder, Colorado, pp. 124–147

Guy, W. S., Taves, D. R. and Brey, W. S. Jr (1977) Organic fluorocompounds in human plasma: prevalence and characteristics in filler; biochemistry involving carbon–fluorine bonds. *Am. Chem. Soc. Symp.,* ser. 28, 117

Hallsworth, A. S. and Weatherell, J. A. (1969) The microdistribution, uptake and loss of fluoride in human enamel. *Caries Res.,* **3**, 109–118

Ham, M. P. and Smith, M. D. (1954) Fluorine balance studies on four infants. *J. Nutr.,* **53**, 215–223

Hargreaves, J. A. (1967) Enamel wear in deciduous teeth with age, related to surface fluoride content. *Caries Res.,* **1**, 32–41

Hargreaves, J. A. (1989) Daily variation of ionic and total fluoride in human milk. *J. Dent. Res.*, **68** (Abstract 1767), p. 402

Hargreaves, J. A., Ingram, G. S. and Wagg, B. J. (1970) Excretion studies on the ingestion of a monofluorophosphate toothpaste by children. *Caries Res.*, **4**, 256–268

Hargreaves, J. A., Ingram, G. S. and Wagg, B. J. (1972) A gravimetric study of the ingestion of toothpaste by children. *Caries Res.*, **6**, 237–243

Harrison, M. F. (1949) Fluorine content of teas consumed in New Zealand. *Br. J. Nutr.*, **3**, 162–166

Heasman, M. A. and Martin, A. E. (1962) Mortality in areas containing natural fluoride in their water supplies. *Monthly Bull. Minist. Hlth*, **21**, 150–160

Henschler, D., Buttner, W. and Patz, J. (1975) Absorption, distribution in body fluid and bioavailability of fluoride. In *Calcium Metabolism, Bone and Metabolic Disease* (eds F. Kuhlencordt and H. P. Kruse), Springer-Verlag, Berlin, pp. 111–121

Hodge, H. C. and Smith, F. A. (1965) Fluoride absorption: metabolism of inorganic fluorides. In *Fluorine Chemistry*, Vol. 4 (ed. J. H. Simons), Academic Press, New York, pp. 137–176

Iijima, Y. and Katayama, T. (1985) Fluoride concentrations in deciduous teeth in high- and low-fluoride areas. *Caries Res.*, **19**, 262–265

Ingram, G. S. (1972) Reaction of monofluorophosphate with apatite. *Caries Res.*, **6**, 1–15

Ingram, G. S. (1973) Some factors affecting the interaction of hydroxyapatite with sodium monofluorophosphate. *Caries Res.*, **7**, 315–323

Isaac, S., Brudevold, F., Smith, F. A. and Gardner, D. E. (1958) Solubility rate and natural fluoride content of surface and subgingival enamel. *J. Dent. Res.*, **37**, 254–263

Jackson, L. R. (1982) *In vitro* hydrolysis of monofluorophosphate by dental plaque microorganisms. *J. Dent. Res.*, **61**, 953–956

Jackson, D. and Weidmann, S. M. (1958) Fluorine in human bone related to age and the water supply of different regions. *J. Pathol. Bacteriol.*, **76**, 451–459

Jackson, D. and Weidmann, S. M. (1959) The relationship between age and the fluoride content of human dentine and enamel: a regional survey. *Br. Dent. J.*, **107**, 303–306

Jenkins, G. N. and Edgar, W. M. (1973) Some observations on fluoride metabolism in Britain. *J. Dent. Res.*, **52**, 984 (Abstract)

Jenkins, G. N. and Krebsbach, P. H. (1985) Experimental study of the migration of charcoal particles in the human mouth. *Arch. Oral Biol.*, **30**, 697–700

Jenkins, G. N. and Speirs, R. L. (1953) Distribution of fluoride in human enamel. *J. Physiol.*, **121**, 21–22P (Abstract)

Kappana, A. N., Gadre, G. T., Bhavnagary, H. M. and Joshi, J. M. (1962) Minor constituents of Indian sea-water. *Curr. Sci.*, **31**, 273–274

Kay, M. I., Young, R. A. and Posner, A. S. (1964) Crystal structure of hydroxyapatite. *Nature* (*Lond.*), **204**, 1050–1052

Kidd, E. A. M., Richards, A., Thylstrup, A. and Fejerskov, O. (1984) The susceptibility of 'young' and 'old' human enamel to artificial caries *in vitro*. *Caries Res.*, **18**, 226–230

Krutchkoff, D. J., Jordan, T. H., Wei, S. H. Y. and Nordquist, W. D. (1972) Surface characteristics of the stannous fluoride–enamel interaction. *Arch. Oral Biol.*, **17**, 923–930

Largent, E. J. (1960) Excretion of fluorine. In *Fluorine and Dental Health: the Pharmacology and Toxicology of Fluorine* (eds J. C. Muhler and M. K. Hine), Indiana University Press, Bloomington, p. 132

Legeros, L. Z., Glenn, F. B., Lee, D. D. and Glenn, W. D. (1985) Some physicochemical properties of deciduous enamel with and without prenatal fluoride supplementation (PNF). *J. Dent. Res.*, **64**, 465–469

Likins, R. C., McClure, J. F. and Steere, A. C. (1956) Urinary excretion of fluoride following defluoridation of water supply. *Pub. Hlth Rep.*, **71**, 217–220

Longwell, J. (1957) Symposium on the fluoridation of public water supplies. (d) Chemical and technical aspects. *R. Soc. Hlth J.*, **77**, 361–370

Lussi, A., Fridell, R. A., Crenshaw, M. A. and Bawden, J. W. (1988) Absence of *in vitro* fluoride-binding by the organic matrix of developing bovine enamel. *Arch. Oral Biol.*, **33**, 531–533

Machoy, Z. (1989) Effects of environment upon fluoride content in nails of children. *Fluoride*, **22**, 169–173

McClure, F. J. (1949) Fluorine in foods. *Publ. Hlth Rep. (Wash.)*, **64**, 1061–1074

McClure, F. J. and Kinser, L. A. (1944) Fluoride domestic waters and systemic effects: fluoride content of urine in relation to fluorine in drinking water. *Publ. Hlth Rep. (Wash.)*, **59**, 1575–1591

McClure, F. J., Mitchell, H. H., Hamilton, T. S. and Kinser, A. C. (1945) Balance of fluorine ingested from various sources in food and water by five young men. Excretion of fluorine thru the skin. *J. Ind. Hygiene Toxicol.*, **27**, 159–170

MacIntire, W. H., Harden, L. J. and Lester, W. (1952) Measurement of atmospheric fluorine: analyses of rainwater and Spanish moss exposures. *Engng Chem.*, **44**, 1365–1370

Marier, J. R. and Rose, D. (1966) Fluoride content of some foods and beverages – a brief survey using a modified Zr-SPADNS method. *J. Food Sci.*, **31**, 941–946

Martin, D. J. (1951) The Evanston dental caries study VIII. Fluorine content vegetables cooked in fluorine containing water. *J. Dent. Res.*, **30**, 676–681

Maurer, R. J. and Day, H. G. (1957) The non-essentiality of fluorine in nutrition. *J. Nutr.*, **62**, 561–573

Mellberg, J. R. and Singer, L. (1977) Discussion of paper by Weatherell, J. A. *et al. Caries Res.*, **11** (Suppl. 1), 101–115

Messer, H. H., Armstrong, W. D. and Singer, L. (1972) Fertility impairment in mice on a low fluoride intake. *Science*, **177**, 893–894

Messer, H. H., Wong, K., Wegner, M., Singer, L. and Armstrong, W. D. (1972) Effect of reduced fluoride intake by mice on haematocrit values. *Nature (New Biol.)*, **240**, 218–219

Mohamedally, S. M. (1984) Studies on the relative fluoride content of normal and pathologically mineralized human tissues. *Fluoride*, **17**, 246–251

Muhler, J. C. (1954) Retention of fluorine in the skeleton of the rat receiving different levels of fluorine in the diet. *J. Nutr.*, **54**, 481–490

Munksgaard, E. C. and Bruun, C. (1973) Determination of fluoride in superficial enamel biopsies from human teeth by means of gas chromatography. *Arch. Oral Biol.*, **18**, 735–743

Nakagaki, H., Koyama, Y., Sakakibara, Y., Weatherell, J. A. and Robinson, C. (1987) Distribution of fluoride across human dental enamel, dentine and cementum. *Arch. Oral Biol.*, **32**, 651–654

Naylor, M. N. and Emslie, R. D. (1967) Clinical testing of stannous fluoride and sodium monofluorophosphate dentifrices in London schoolchildren. *Br. Dent. J.*, **126**, 17–23

Naylor, N. M., Melville, M., Wilson, R. F., Ingram, G. and Wagg, B. J. (1971) Ingestion of dentifrice by young children: a pilot study using a fecal marker. *J. Dent. Res.*, **50**, 687 (Abstract)

Neuman, W. F. and Neuman, M. W. (1958) *The Chemical Dynamics of Bone Mineral*. University of Chicago Press, Chicago

Noguchi, K., Ueno, S., Kanuiya, H. and Nishiido, T. (1963) Chemical composition of the volatile matters emitted by the eruptions of Miyake Island in 1962. *Proc. Jpn Acad.*, **39**, 364–369

Oliveby, A., Lagerlof, F., Ekstrand, J. and Dawes, C. (1989) Studies on fluoride excretion in human whole saliva in relation to flow rate and plasma fluoride levels. *Caries Res.*, **23**, 243–246

Patterson, C. M., Krugher, B. J. and Dales, J. J. (1977) Differences in fluoride levels in the blood between sheep, rabbit and rat. *Arch. Oral Biol.*, **22**, 419–423

Pearce, E. I. F. and Jenkins, G. N. (1977) The decomposition of monofluorophosphate by enzymes in whole human saliva. *Arch Oral Biol.*, **22**, 405–407

Petersson, L. G., Odelius, H., Loddings, A., Larson, S. J. and Frostell, G. (1976) Ion probe study of fluoride gradients in outermost layers of human enamel. *J. Dent. Res.*, **55**, 980–990

Rao, S. G. (1984) Dietary intake and bioavailability of fluoride. *Ann. Rev. Nutr.*, **4**, 115–136

Richards, A., Larsen, M. J. and Fejerskov, O. (1979) Fluoride content of buccal surface enamel from caries-free mediaeval subjects. *Arch. Oral Biol.*, **24**, 83–84

Rolla, G. and Ogaard, B. (1986) Studies on the solubility of calcium fluoride in human saliva. In *Factors Relating to Demineralization and Remineralization of the Teeth* (ed. S. A. Leach), IRL Press, Washington, pp. 45–50

Sakae, T. and Hirai, G. (1982) Calcification and crystallisation in bovine enamel. *J. Dent. Res.*, **61**, 57–59

Schamschula, R. G., Sugar, E., Un, P. S. H., Toth, K., Barmes, D. E. and Adkins, B. L. (1985) Physiological indicators of fluoride exposure and utilisation: an epidemiological study. *Commun. Dent. Oral Epidemiol.*, **13**, 104–107

Scott, D. B., Kaplan, H. and Wyckoff, R. W. G. (1949) Replica studies of changes in tooth surface with age. *J. Dent. Res.*, **28**, 31–47

Shannon, I. L., Suddick, R. P. and Edmonds, E. (1973) Effect of rate of gland function on parotid saliva fluoride concentrations in the human. *Caries Res.*, **7**, 1–10

Sharpless, G. R. and McCollum, E. V. (1933) Is fluorine an indispensable element in the diet? *J. Nutr.*, **6**, 163–178

Singer, L., Ophaug, R. H. and Harland, B. F. (1980) Fluoride intake among young male adults in the United States. *Am. J. Clin. Nutr.*, **33**, 328–332

Singer, L., Ophaug, R. H. and Harland, B. F. (1985) Dietary fluoride intake of 15–19-year-old male adults residing in the United States. *J. Dent. Res.*, **64**, 1302–1305

Smith, F. A., Gardner, D. E. and Hodge, H. C. (1953) Age increase in fluoride content in human bone. *Fed. Proc.*, **12**, 368

Smith, F. A., Gardner, D. E., Leone, N. C. and Hodge, H. C. (1960) The effects of the absorption of fluoride, V. The chemical determination of fluoride in human soft tissues following prolonged ingestion of fluoride at various levels. *Arch. Indust. Health*, **21**, 330–332

Spak, C.-J., Ekstrand, J. and Hardell, L. I. (1983) Fluoride in human breast milk. *Caries Res.*, **17**, 161 (Abstract)

Spak, C.-J., Ekstrand, J. and Zylberstein, D. (1982) Bioavailability of fluoride added to baby formula and milk. *Caries Res.*, **16**, 249–256

Speirs, R. L. (1975) Fluoride incorporation into developing enamel of permanent teeth in the domestic pig. *Arch. Oral Biol.*, **20**, 877–883

Speirs, R. L. (1978) Fluoride concentrations in tooth germs of permanent teeth of the domestic pig. *Arch. Oral Biol.*, **23**, 1019–1027

Speirs, R. L. (1983) Correlations between the concentration of fluoride and some other constituents of tea infusions and their possible dental caries-preventive effect. *Arch. Oral Biol.*, **28**, 471–475

Tanganyika Government Chemist (1955) *Annual Report of the Government Chemist*, 1954. Government Printer, Dar es Salaam

Taves, D. R. (1966) Normal human serum fluoride concentrations. *Nature, Lond.*, **211**, 192–193

Taves, D. R. (1968) Evidence that there are two forms of fluoride in human serum. *Nature, Lond.*, **217**, 1050–1051

Taves, D. R. (1971) Comparison of 'organic' fluoride in human and non-human species. *J. Dent. Res.*, **50**, 783

Taves, D. R. (1983) Dietary intake of fluoride ashed (total fluoride) v. unashed (inorganic fluoride) analysis of individual foods. *Br. J. Nutr.*, **49**, 295–301

Thompson, T. G. and Taylor, H. J. (1933) Determination and occurrence of fluorides in sea water. *Indust. Engng Chem. Analyt. Edn.*, **5**, 87–89

Valk, J. W. P., Duijsters, P. P. E., ten Cate, J. M. and Davidson, C. L. (1985) Long-term retention and effectiveness of APF and neutral KF fluoridation agents on sound and etched bovine enamel. *Caries Res.*, **19**, 46–52

Vinogradov, A. P. (1954) *Geochemie seltener und nur in Spuren vorhandener chemischer Elemente in Boden*, Akademie Verlag, Berlin. Cited in *Fluorides and Human Health* (1970), WHO Monogr. Ser. No. 59, WHO, Geneva, p. 21

Wagner, M. J. and Muhler, J. C. (1952) The effect of calcium and phosphate on fluoride absorption. *J. Dent. Res.*, **39**, 49–52

Walters, C. B., Sherlock, J. C., Evans, W. H. and Read, I. (1983) Dietary intake of fluoride in the United Kingdom and fluoride content of some foodstuffs. *J. Sci. Food Agric.*, **34**, 523–528

Wattenberg, H. (1943) Zur chemie des Meerwassers: uber die in Spuren vorkommenden Alimente. *Z. Anorg. Allg. Chem.*, **251**, 86–91

Weatherell, J. A. (1969) Fluoride in bones and teeth and the development of fluorosis. In *Mineral Metabolism in Paediatrics* (eds D. Barltrop and W. L. Burland), Blackwell Scientific Publications, Oxford, pp. 53–69

Weatherell, J. A., Hallsworth, A. S. and Robinson, C. (1972) Changes in the labial enamel surface with age. *Caries Res.*, **6**, 312–324

Weatherell, J. A., Hallsworth, A. S. and Robinson, C. (1973) The effect of tooth wear on the distribution of fluoride in the enamel surface of human teeth. *Arch. Oral Biol.*, **18**, 1175–1189

Weatherell, J. A. and Hargreaves, J. A. (1965) The micro-sampling of enamel. *Arch. Oral Biol.,* **10**, 139–142

Weatherell, J. A. and Hargreaves, J. A. (1966) Effect of resorption on the fluoride content of human deciduous teeth. *Arch. Oral Biol.,* **11**, 749–756

Weatherell, J. A., Robinson, C., Ralph, J. P. and Best, J. S. (1984) Migration of fluoride in the mouth. *Caries Res.,* **18**, 343–353

Weatherell, J. A., Strong, M., Robinson, C. and Ralph, J. P. (1986) Fluoride distribution in the mouth after fluoride rinsing. *Caries Res.,* **20**, 111–119

Wei, S. H. Y. (1974) Scanning electron microscope study of stannous fluoride-treated enamel surfaces. *J. Dent. Res.,* **53**, 57–63

Wei, S. H. Y. and Schultz, E. M. Jnr (1975) *In vivo* micro-sampling of enamel fluoride concentrations after topical treatments. *Caries Res.,* **9**, 50–58

Weidmann, S. M. and Weatherell, J. A. (1959) The uptake and distribution of fluorine in bones. *J. Pathol. Bacteriol.,* **78**, 243–255

Weidmann, S. M. and Weatherell, J. A. (1970) Distribution in hard tissues. In *Fluoride and Human Health (1970)*, WHO Monogr. Ser. No. 59, WHO, Geneva, pp. 104–128

Wellock, W. D. and Brudevold, F. (1963) A study of acidulated fluoride solution. The caries-inhibitory effect of single annual topical applications of acidic fluoride and phosphate solutions. A two-year experience. *Arch. Oral Biol.,* **8**, 179–182

Whitford, G. M. (1990) *The Metabolism and Toxicity of Fluoride*, Monographs in Oral Science, Vol. 13, Karger, Basle

Whitford, G. M., Callan, R. S. and Wang, H. S. (1982) Fluoride absorption through the hamster cheek pouch: a pH-dependent event. *J. Appl. Toxicol.,* **2**, 303–306

Whitford, G. M. and Pashley, D. H. (1982) Plasma fluoride levels: influence of sampling site. *J. Dent. Res.,* **61**, 291 (Abstract 1019)

Whitford, G. M., Pashley, D. H. and Reynolds, K. E. (1979) Fluoride tissue distribution: short-term kinetics. *Am. J. Physiol.,* **236**, F141–F148

Williamson, M. M. (1953) Endemic dental fluorosis in Kenya: a preliminary report. *E. Afr. Med. J.,* **30**, 217–233

World Health Organisation (1970) *Fluorides and Human Health*, WHO Monogr. Ser. No. 59, WHO, Geneva

Yao, K. and Gron, P. (1970) Fluoride concentration in duct saliva and whole saliva. *Caries Res.,* **4**, 321–331

Yoon, S. H., Brudevold, F., Gardner, D. E. and Smith, F. A. (1960) Distribution of fluoride in teeth from areas with different levels of fluoride in the water supply. *J. Dent. Res.,* **39**, 845–856

Young, R. A. and Elliott, J. C. (1966) Atomic-scale bases for several properties of apatites. *Arch. Oral Biol.,* **11**, 699–707

Zipkin, I. (1972) Mobilization of fluoride from the bones and teeth of growing and mature rats. *Arch. Oral Biol.,* **17**, 479–494

Zipkin, I. and Leone, N. C. (1957) Rate of urinary fluoride output in normal adults. *Am. J. Public Hlth,* **47**, 848–851

Zipkin, I., McClure, F. J., Leone, N. C. and Lee, W. A. (1958) Fluoride deposition in human bones after prolonged ingestion of fluoride in drinking water. *Publ. Hlth Rep. Wash.,* **73**, 732–740

Chapter 15

Modes of action of fluoride in reducing caries

The mechanism of the effect of fluoride in reducing caries is a very controversial subject and although a consensus has emerged in recent years about the most important mechanism, there is still doubt about several possible subsidiary effects. There is wide agreement that the final result probably arises from the combined effect of several different actions. Although the same basic mechanisms may operate at both the low concentrations in fluoridated water and the much higher concentrations involved in the various methods of topical application, their relative importance may differ with those contrasting concentrations. It may be of interest to point out that it is virtually impossible to measure the full effect of fluoride in human subjects because the 'low F controls' with which the 'high F' material is compared all contain some fluoride whether they be teeth, saliva or plaque. It is possible only to study the effect of the additional fluoride received from water, toothpastes or other topicals.

The facts that have to be explained by hypotheses on the mode of action may be summarized as follows: (a) that fluoridated water taken during tooth development and before eruption reduces caries; (b) that for the full effect, exposure to fluoride must continue after eruption (and people receiving fluoridated water only after their teeth have erupted also gain some benefit); (c) that the benefit lasts well into adulthood and, at least with 2 ppm, is still detectable in the elderly; (d) that applications of high concentrations of fluoride daily as toothpastes, every few days as a rinse or once or twice a year in a gel, are effective; (e) that the effects of fluoride in the water and in toothpastes supplement each other.

Three main hypotheses have been proposed to account for the anti-caries effect of fluoride. One suggestion is that fluoride affects the morphology of the teeth in ways that makes them more self-cleansing. The hypothesis that has received most attention is based on the observation that fluoride makes apatite less soluble and therefore more resistant to the acids formed by the plaque bacteria. A more recent development is the finding that fluoride favours the precipitation of crystals of apatite, or the growth of pre-existing crystals, from saturated or supersaturated solutions, i.e. it favours remineralization. Clearly, de- and remineralization are closely linked and may in some circumstances be difficult to distinguish. The third hypothesis emphasizes that fluoride is a well-known enzyme inhibitor and might be expected to reduce bacterial acid production.

In this chapter, the evidence for and against these hypotheses is presented in some detail.

Effects on the morphology of teeth

Forrest (1956) and Ockerse (1949) commented on the 'well-rounded cusps and shallow fissures' of teeth from fluoridated areas in Great Britain and South Africa, respectively, but presented no statistical data. Wallenius (1959) reported, from the results of 10 000 measurements of plaster casts of the teeth from 419 children, that those on water containing 0.5–1.0 ppm F were 1.7% wider than those receiving less than 0.5 ppm F. The importance of this observation was doubtful, however, as the difference, although significant, was mostly in the boys' mandibular teeth; the girls' teeth and the boys' maxillary teeth differed by only about 1%. Simpson and Castaldi (1969) also reported that the teeth in a fluoride area (1.2 ppm in Canada) were larger than in a low-fluoride control area and had shallower fissures (the differences in mandibular molars were highly significant) and more obtuse inter-cuspal angles. Cooper and Ludwig (1965) found that the mesial–distal diameters of models of the lower first molars in children from fluoridated areas of New Zealand were 2% *smaller* than in fluoride-free controls, but with significantly lower cusp heights and highly significant reductions in buccal convexity. Lovius and Goose (1969) measured cusps of teeth from groups of 100 children from the fluoride and non-fluoride areas of Anglesey and concluded that, overall, the results suggested that the molars were slightly smaller and with lower cusp heights, although results with each dimension separately failed to reach significance. Aasenden and Peebles (1974) reported, without giving actual measurements, that 47% of their 100 subjects on 0.5–1.0 mg F supplements had 'atypically shallow' pits and fissures compared with 24% of a similar sized group on fluoridated water and 4.3% without fluoride from either source.

The results on tooth size are contradictory and were probably caused by variations unrelated to fluoride, but there is a consensus that occlusal surfaces are more rounded under the influence of fluoride. This might be expected to make the teeth more self-cleansing, but the effect is generally considered to be too small to be of much practical importance. This is one effect of fluoride that obviously occurs during tooth development.

Possible mechanisms of the morphological effects of fluoride

Animal experiments have suggested some possible mechanisms for these morphological effects.

When female rats were fed 6 ppm of fluoride in their food during pregnancy and lactation, the teeth of the offspring were smaller and the fissures more rounded than in controls (Paynter and Grainger, 1956). Kruger (1966) found that injecting high doses of fluoride (0.1 mg/day) into newborn rats reduced the thickness of the enamel and dentine resulting in smaller teeth with wider, but not deeper, fissures.

Kruger (1968) followed up these observations and attempted to elucidate their mechanism by injecting a range of doses of fluoride into newborn rats and found changes in the ultrastructure of the ameloblasts. With the highest dose used (7 mg/kg of body weight daily, equivalent to about 24 mg for a newborn baby), large vacuoles appeared in the rough endoplasmic reticulum (the organelle concerned with protein synthesis), visible within 30 min of the injection. With a dose more comparable with what a newborn child would receive on formula milk made up with fluoridated water (0.1 mg/kg body weight), the change was qualitatively similar but very much smaller and not detectable until 90 min after the injection. This change would be expected to affect the synthesis of protein and later work showed that even the lowest dose used reduced the uptake by ameloblasts of labelled proline for up to 90 min (Kruger, 1970). Reductions in the amount of matrix protein would be expected to reduce the thickness of the enamel and thus change the shape of the fissures.

The solubility hypothesis

Some of the earliest studies on the mode of action of fluoride showed that if whole teeth or powdered enamel were exposed to fluoride solutions (even in concentration lower than 1 ppm), washed to remove excess fluoride solution and then shaken with acid buffers, their rate of dissolution in acid was reduced (Volker, 1939). It was assumed that fluoride was entering the apatite and producing a crystal that was less soluble, suggesting that fluoride reduces caries by solubility effects on the enamel. This hypothesis was tested by measurements of the solubility rate of teeth extracted from residents of towns with different levels of fluoride in their water supplies.

Three methods have been mainly used to compare enamel solubilities. One is to grind off successive layers of enamel, shake weighed amounts of the enamel powder in an acid buffer for standard times and measure the weight loss (which is equal to the amount dissolving). Another technique is to cover the enamel of intact teeth with wax or nail varnish, except for a 'window', usually of 4 mm diameter, shake the teeth in an acid buffer for a standard time and estimate the Ca, P or both that dissolved in the buffer. This method measures the solubility *rate* of thin layers of the outer enamel and not the true solubility at equilibrium. Usually, the window was exposed to acid several times and it was found that, in general, the solubility rate of each succeeding layer was higher which was readily explained from the high concentration of fluoride and the low concentration of carbonate (carbonate raises the solubility of apatite) known to be on the outer enamel surface. More recently, factors influencing solubility rate (such as the concentration of fluoride and Ca in the solvent) have been measured by the third technique, the 'rotating disc method'. Synthetic apatites of known composition are compressed into pellets, embedded in Araldite and mounted on a shaft that is rapidly rotated in an acid buffer, samples of which are withdrawn periodically and analysed for Ca or P to monitor the rate of dissolution (Foreward, 1977; Nelson *et al.*, 1983) (this method is not suitable for comparing the solubility of teeth).

The results with teeth all agree in giving some limited support to the concept that enamel formed in high-fluoride areas has a lower solubility rate than enamel from low-fluoride areas (Isaac *et al.*, 1958; Jenkins, 1963; Healy and Ludwig, 1966; Cutress, 1972). The differences were small and not always statistically significant (Table 15.1) and some anomalous results were found. For example, Isaac *et al.* (1958) reported that two layers of enamel with fluoride containing 460 and 1080 ppm differed in solubility by only 1.9%, whereas in two sets of inner enamel with almost identical fluoride concentration (198 and 219 ppm) the solubilities differed by 5.5%. Results with the window method also showed a higher mean solubility rate in teeth from a low-fluoride area compared with that from two high-fluoride areas, but the differences did not reach significance in deciduous teeth from an area with 1 ppm F or from the sound enamel of permanent teeth with 2 ppm (Table 15.1).

Table 15.1 Effect of fluoride in drinking water on the solubility rate of outer enamel

A: μg/ml P dissolved during exposure of 4 mm windows of enamel to acetate buffer pH 4.0 for 10 min; *n* in parentheses

F in water (ppm)	*0*	*1*	*1.8*	*% dif.*	*Sig. of dif.*
Deciduous teeth	10.4 (77)	9.2 (79)	–	12	not sig.
Deciduous teeth	12.0 (108)		9.5 (109)	21	$P < 0.05$
Permanent teeth, non-carious surfaces	12.7 (108)		12.1 (112)	5	not sig.
Early carious surfaces of same permanent teeth	8.2 (108)		6.7 (112)	18	$P < 0.05$

Data from Jenkins (1963).

B: Weight loss in mg of batches of 50 mg pooled powdered outer enamel shaken with acetate buffer pH 4.0 for 1 h

F in water (ppm)	*0*	*1*	*5*	*% dif.*	*Sig. of dif.*
Young permanent	32.5		26.8	17.6	sig. not stated
Old permanent	35.7	32.8		8.1	

Data from Isaac *et al.* (1958).

Tyler *et al.* (1986) studied the fluoride concentration and solubility of enamel in three groups of deciduous teeth from English children: two from Bristol – one collected before 1960 and the other after 1975 – and the third from Birmingham, collected 10 years after that city was fluoridated. Both the later groups had higher surface fluoride than the pre-1960 samples: in Bristol the fluoride was 1.3 times higher, presumably from fluoride toothpastes, and in Birmingham 3.4 times higher from the combined effect of toothpastes and fluoridated water. Only the Birmingham teeth showed increased resistance to acid and they differed from the other groups only by 10%. These workers compared the solubilities by measuring the depth of the lesions produced when the teeth were exposed to acid gels. This method is a standard technique for producing *in vitro* lesions closely resembling natural caries and is widely used to study factors that influence caries, but has seldom been used to compare the solubilities of clinical specimens. It is apparently insufficiently sensitive to detect the effect of the comparatively small increase in fluoride which occurred in Bristol.

A serious difficulty in comparing solubilities of teeth is the great individual variation from tooth to tooth and even between parts of the same tooth, presumably arising from the irregular distribution of the fluoride and other constituents on the enamel surface. Consequently, large numbers of teeth (preferably caries-free and of comparable morphological type) are needed to obtain statistically significant results and these are rarely available. However, all the investigations mentioned above showed the same trend towards lower solubility in teeth from the high-fluoride areas, although they were widely distributed geographically and the solubility was measured by different methods. It may be concluded that this evidence on clinical material suggests that reduced solubility plays a part in the protective effect of fluoride.

Difficulties in the solubility hypothesis

In vitro studies of the effect of fluoride contained in apatite on its solubility are contradictory. Moreno, Kresok and Zahradnik (1977) reported that they had synthesized a number of apatites with fluoride concentrations varying, in 0.5% increments, between 0% and 3.8% (pure FA) from which impurities, such as carbonate, had been rigorously excluded and had compared their solubilities at equilibrium after exposure to acid for 30 days. They found (and Larsen and Jensen, 1989, confirmed) that the inclusion of fluoride up to 10% of the maximum possible has very little effect on solubility. Typical figures for the fluoride concentration of the outer surfaces of enamel from high- and low-fluoride areas are 3000 and 2000, respectively, i.e. about 7.9% and 5.3% of the maximum, and the difference of 2.6% would, from the results of Moreno and colleagues, have a negligible effect on solubility, so this hypothesis tended to be discredited. Okazaki *et al.* (1981), on the other hand, studying powdered apatites that did contain carbonate, found that the solubility was proportional to the log of the fluoride concentration and that with a concentration of 0.1 mmol/g (1900 ppm) fluoride, solubility was reduced by about 25%. In both of these studies true solubility at equilibrium was measured after prolonged exposure to acid, whereas the studies on teeth have measured solubility rate sometimes over periods as short as 10 min. It is uncertain whether equilibrium conditions are reached during a caries attack *in vivo* and therefore difficult to decide which set of data is most relevant to caries.

Enamel does contain carbonate, suggesting that the quite large effects of fluoride on solubility found by Okazaki and co-workers might be applicable to the caries situation, in which case the solubility idea would be supported. However, Larsen and Jensen (1989) treated enamel samples (which, of course, contained carbonate) with fluoride and produced a range of surface fluoride from 2000 to 3000 ppm and also found that the effect of the fluoride on solubility was small. A similar result was obtained by Nelson *et al.* (1983) who compared the solubilities of pelleted apatites containing carbonate and 0, 76 and 713 ppm F and found that they were virtually identical. These fluoride concentrations were smaller than would occur on enamel surfaces, but the difference (713 minus 76) is comparable with that on the enamel surfaces of teeth from fluoride or non-fluoride areas. The presence of carbonate does not, therefore, seem to explain the difference between the results of Moreno and colleagues and Okazaki and colleagues.

A further contribution was made by Wong, Cutress and Duncan (1987) who measured the solubilities of synthetic apatites containing one of three levels of fluoride (44, 602 or 30 476 ppm) incorporated into the crystals or two levels (60 and 706 ppm) adsorbed onto preformed HA. They were tested as powders and also as compressed pellets to resemble teeth. The apatites were shaken in acid buffer and samples were taken periodically over 6 h for powders or 30 h for pellets (which, of course, dissolve more slowly). The results showed that the powders for all three fluoridated apatites were less soluble than HA, but with the pellets only the sample with the highest fluoride was affected (30 476 ppm), very much higher than occurs in human enamel. The solubility of pellets (and of intact enamel) is affected not only by their composition, but by factors influencing the permeability inwards of acid and outwards of Ca and P. Both levels of adsorbed fluoride reduced the solubility of the powder and the pellets. The various apatites were also tested in buffers containing fluoride and as little as 0.1 ppm reduced the solubility of all the powders and the pellets with the highest levels of fluoride incorporated (see later for more evidence that low concentrations of fluoride in an acid solvent are more effective in reducing solubility than much higher concentrations in or on the apatite crystals). With the apatites containing the higher levels of fluoride, much less than the theoretical quantity of fluoride was released into the buffer as the apatite dissolved, the implication being that either the fluoride was recombining with apatite newly exposed by the dissolution of the surface layers or, as the buffer approached saturation, precipitation of FHA occurred (i.e. remineralization). The extra fluoride acquired in these ways could have accounted for some of the reductions in solubility that were found and illustrates another complication in studying the effect of fluoride on solubility.

How can we reconcile the observation that enamel from high-fluoride areas is less soluble, with the laboratory evidence mostly suggesting that the fluoride levels on the outer enamel are too low too exert this effect? One possibility is that the concentrations on extremely thin layers of outer enamel are, as mentioned on page 278, much higher than the usually accepted figures based on layers many microns thick and may be within the range that would be expected to affect solubility even on the findings of Moreno and co-workers (Margolis, Murphy and Moreno, 1990).

These concentrations of fluoride in outer enamel might account for a lower solubility in teeth shortly after eruption but, as Weatherell's group have shown (page 282), much of the fluoride in the outer enamel is removed by abrasion a few years after eruption, and could not protect the enamel as a whole for long periods and certainly not in adults. Alternatively, it is suggested that the fluoride may be distributed unevenly throughout the enamel rods and that the outer part of each rod may be richer in fluoride than the cores and thus protect it from acid attack. Studies with the SEM do show that the core of the rods, and even of some individual crystals, dissolve first, leaving hollow shells which eventually disintegrate (Johnson, 1967; Simmelink and Nygaard, 1982; Frank, 1990).

Another hypothesis to explain how low levels of fluoride may reduce enamel solubility is that fluoride may fill the vacancies in the columns of hydroxyl ions running through the middle of the apatite crystal (see Figure 14.4, page 273) and very small additions in this situation (well within the differences found in high- and low-fluoride areas) could stabilize the crystal and exert considerable effect on its solubility (Young and Elliott, 1966).

Effect of early caries on the fluoride and solubility of enamel

Myers, Hamilton and Becks (1952) showed that when teeth were exposed to solutions of $Na^{18}F$, the ^{18}F attached itself to the whole enamel as a thin layer but collected in higher concentrations and to a greater depth in early white spot lesions and other defects in the enamel. This suggested that fluoride might enter early carious lesions *in vivo*. Analysis of enamel ground out from the early lesions in teeth from both high- and low-fluoride areas was found to contain 2–3 times the fluoride concentration in sound enamel ground to a similar depth from the same teeth (Table 15.2) (Dowse and Jenkins, 1957) and the high fluoride of early caries has been fully confirmed by others (e.g. Little and Steadman, 1966; Hallsworth and Weatherell, 1969). 'Windows' over white spot enamel were found to dissolve much

Table 15.2 Fluoride content of normal and carious enamel from towns with 0 ppm F and 2 ppm F in the water supply (After Jenkins, 1963)

	Non-carious enamel		*Carious enamel*	
	0 ppm	2 ppm	0 ppm	2 ppm
F ppm	250	440	640	850
No. of teeth	108	112	108	112

more slowly than adjacent areas of sound enamel (see Table 15.1). This suggested that, even if fluoride had only a small effect on the solubility of intact enamel, the fluoride accumulated in the lesion is at a site where it can be most effective in reducing the inward extension of caries. This is a natural version of the idea of treating enamel with an acid before topical application (see page 274) and of the concept of Koulourides *et al.* (1980) that the uptake of fluoride after exposure to acid ('priming') represents an adaptation to the cariogenic challenge.

There are several possible explanations for this rise in the fluoride concentration of slightly carious enamel. One is that the dissolution of some of the apatite crystals makes the affected enamel more porous and may allow fluoride from saliva and plaque to permeate and bind with the inner enamel, as the results with ^{18}F suggest. Another possibility which may contribute is that the more soluble crystals, low in fluoride, dissolve first leaving behind a higher proportion of less soluble apatite high in fluoride. The most widely held view is that, in the intervals between acid attacks, remineralization occurs and the newly deposited apatite takes up more fluoride from the environment of the tooth, which contains higher concentration of fluoride (at least 0.05 ppm, see page 304) than is present in tissue fluid (0.01 ppm) from which the original crystals were formed.

The role of carbonate

An alternative explanation for the effect of fluoride on solubility is based on data suggesting that there is a reciprocity between the concentrations of carbonate and fluoride in enamel, as there is in bone (see page 277). Carbonate has been described as the Achilles heel of the enamel because the mineral lost in the first stages of caries contains a much higher proportion of carbonate (and Mg) than is contained in intact enamel (Hallsworth, Weatherell and Robinson, 1973), showing that these ions are the ones most readily dissolved from the enamel. When HA is formed *in vivo* in a low-fluoride area, carbonate ions tend to attach to the growing crystals and block the accretion of phosphate, thereby reducing the growth of the crystals and introducing imperfections; they will be more soluble on account of their small size and poor crystallinity (Ingram, 1973). A higher concentration of fluoride reverses this tendency by accelerating the growth of the crystals and reducing their carbonate content. Nikiforuk *et al.* (1962) showed that enamel high in fluoride was lower in carbonate, especially in caries-resistant teeth (Table 15.3). The ratio carbonate/F was very significantly different in high-fluoride, non-carious enamel compared with that from other groups. On this hypothesis, it is not the fluoride itself that protects the enamel, but the indirect effect of fluoride in reducing the carbonate concentration with its attendant effects on solubility and crystal form.

Table 15.3 Relationship between F and CO_3 of enamel to the fluoride of drinking water in carious and non-carious teeth (each figure is the mean of 3 groups of 20 teeth) (Data from Nikiforuk, 1961)

	F of water	*% CO_3*	*ppm F*	*Ratio ×100*
Non-carious teeth	None	2.07 ± 0.06	136 ± 21	1.52
	1 ppm	1.90 ± 0.08	357 ± 94	0.53
Sound enamel from carious teeth	None	2.03 ± 0.01	83 ± 13	2.45
	1 ppm	2.13 ± 0.05	229 ± 50	0.93

Cutress (1972) supported this hypothesis when he found, among groups of teeth from many geographical areas, a low positive correlation (P between 0.1 and 0.05) between solubility and the fluoride of outer enamel, a more significant one for carbonate concentration and a highly significant correlation ($P < 0.001$) between solubility and the carbonate/F ratio (Figure 15.1). More data are desirable on the

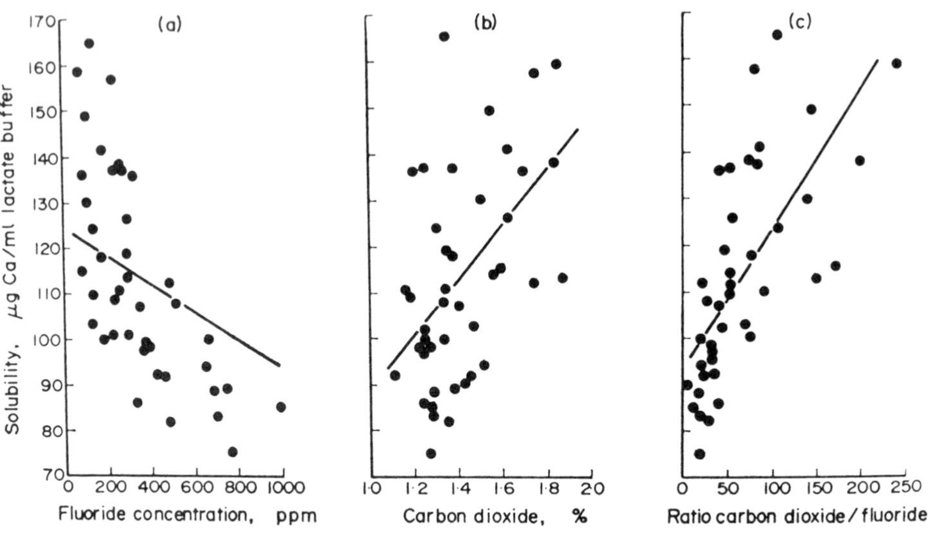

Figure 15.1 Scatter diagrams and regression lines of 42 enamel samples (6 teeth each) according to their solubility and (a) fluoride concentration; (b) CO_2 concentration; and (c) the ratio of CO_2 to F (From Cutress, 1972, with kind permission of the Editor, *Archives of Oral Biology*)

relation between the carbonate and fluoride concentrations entering enamel during its formation and its solubility and caries resistance, but this would be almost impossible to obtain now as, in most communities, the fluoride of enamel is influenced erratically by the fluoride of toothpastes and other topicals.

Fluoride of the enamel surface in relation to caries activity

If the fluoride concentration of outer enamel reduces its solubility and if the solubility is a factor in caries, then it would be predicted that the enamel fluoride of individuals who are caries-resistant would be higher than in those who are caries-prone. The data on this are contradictory, but the majority of surveys fail to show a correlation or show a correlation so weak as to preclude any clinical importance. For example, Spector and Curzon (1979) found $r = -0.16$ ($P < 0.01$), indicating that only 4% of the variability in DMFT was accounted for by the enamel fluoride. The study of DePaola *et al.* (1975) on 1447 subjects from 7 areas with waters varying in fluoride from 0.06 to between 5 and 7 ppm did show a significant correlation of 0.4, but this probably arose from the wide range of fluoride. It is not surprising that the caries was low and the enamel fluoride high with a water containing 5–7 ppm F and the reverse with 0.06 ppm. The correlation within each individual town was not significant.

There are several reasons why this correlation is difficult to investigate. First, biopsy estimations of fluoride are usually made on very small areas of the buccal surface of the premolars or upper incisors which are not typically caries-prone. Secondly, the surface fluoride is known to fall steadily with increasing age, so that the fluoride at the time of the survey could be very different from what it was when much of the caries developed years before and, thirdly, there are now wide short-term fluctuations in surface fluoride from the use of toothpastes and other topical sources of fluoride. Also, in some communities, children especially prone to caries may be encouraged to have more frequent topical applications of fluoride which would tend to reverse a negative correlation between enamel fluoride and caries. In view of these factors affecting the outer surface of enamel, Schamschula *et al.* (1979) calculated the correlation of DMFT with the fluoride in the deeper layers (4 μm from the surface) and found them to be highly significant. Keene, Mellberg and Pederson (1980) found the reverse: on small groups of subjects, they found (contrary to most other workers) a significant correlation in outer enamel ($P < 0.05$) but not in the deeper layers ($P = 0.63$).

Another possible reason for the failure to establish a significant relation between surface fluoride and the caries score is that the comparisons were made on intact non-carious surfaces. In view of the accumulation of fluoride in early lesions, where it may exert a major effect, it would be of interest to know whether the fluoride concentration in these areas correlated with caries activity.

Role of fluoride ions in reducing solubility rate and favouring remineralization

So far we have discussed mainly the effect of fluoride incorporated in the enamel on solubility rate, but many workers have shown that concentrations of fluoride as low as 0.05 ppm in an acid buffer reduce the amount of enamel that will dissolve in it (Manly and Harrington, 1959; ten Cate and Duijsters, 1983; Featherstone *et al.*, 1990). The reduced solubility is accompanied by a rise in fluoride concentration of the undissolved solid which may occur in several ways (Spinelli, Brudevold and Moreno, 1971). In these experiments, if the solvent becomes saturated with HA, then precipitation of FHA (i.e. remineralization) will occur (see later). If the solvent does not become saturated (as in some short-term experiments), the fluoride may be adsorbed onto the HA and gradually penetrate the crystal and form FHA or it may form FHA by immediate exchange with hydroxyl ions.

In the production of experimental carious lesions in acidified gels, the effect of fluoride in the gel is to reduce the depth of the lesion and to favour the formation of the well-mineralized layer on the surface of the lesion. Borsboom, Mei and Arendt (1985) showed that as little as 0.12 ppm F determined whether or not a well-mineralized layer formed.

The fluid environment of the teeth, saliva and the fluid phase of plaque ('plaque fluid') contain fluoride, and as the pH falls during a caries attack the concentration of free fluoride ions increases as they are released from bound sources in the plaque (Birkeland and Charlton, 1976). Experiments by Larsen, von der Fehr and Birkeland (1976), by Margolis, Moreno and Murphy (1986) and by Margolis and Moreno (1990), although using different procedures and materials, have led to a similar hypothesis on the role of fluoride in the acid solvent on the solubility of enamel. The basic principle of these two groups of experiments was the same, but Larsen and colleagues worked with synthetic apatite and enamel powder, whereas Margolis and colleagues used windowed surfaces of wax-covered human teeth. The powders were shaken with a pH 5.0 buffer for 1 or 2 weeks until it was almost saturated with HA or enamel (it was not quite saturated even after this time). Fluoride (0.5 or 1.0 ppm) was then added, making the solution highly supersaturated with FA (see page 275) which precipitated out, and the consequent removal of Ca and P from the solution made it unsaturated with HA which continued to dissolve. Margolis and co-workers exposed groups of windowed teeth to demineralizing solutions containing a range of fluoride concentrations up to 1 ppm and measured, by polarized light microscopy of sections of the teeth, the depth of the lesion and the thickness of the surface layer with each level of fluoride. They found that with increasing fluoride (i.e. with increasing degrees of saturation with FA) the depth of the lesion was decreased and the thickness of the outer layer increased. In separate experiments, the uptake of fluoride by the enamel was found to be negligible from neutral solutions containing fluoride in which, of course, no enamel dissolved, but was quite large from acid demineralizing solutions unsaturated with HA but saturated with FA, confirming that some HA had to dissolve before the fluoride of the enamel could increase by the precipitation of FA.

Applying these results to the caries situation, it is suggested that when apatite dissolves in the acidified saliva and plaque fluid, the Ca, P and F released, added to those already present before the environment became acidified, form a saturated solution of a fluoridated apatite which then precipitates to an extent depending on the fluoride concentration. As mentioned above, this removes Ca and P from the liquid environment and reduces the degree of saturation with HA, so that more dissolves, but this loss of enamel is partly compensated for by the precipitate. The effect of fluoride, on this hypothesis, is to reduce the apparent (net) solubility rate by favouring the reverse process – the precipitation of a more heavily fluoridated apatite, i.e. remineralization. A requirement for this process is that the rate of precipitation exceeds the rate of outward diffusion of Ca and P, otherwise there would be too few ions available to form the precipitate. Diffusion is reduced by protective pellicles on the enamel surface and by concentrations of Ca and P in the plaque fluid.

The practical issue arising is that, to exert this effect, fluoride ions must be present during the acid attack on the enamel. This can be achieved by building up the fluoride in the plaque and on the enamel surface as FHA or CaF_2; the latter acts as a reservoir slowly dissolving into plaque and saliva. When CaF_2 is formed in saliva *in vitro*, the solid deposits become surrounded by phosphate, pyrophosphate and proteins from the saliva which reduces their solubility. This might be expected to occur *in vivo* (although it has not been shown experimentally) and, if so, it would greatly extend the time during which CaF_2 releases fluoride (Lagerlof *et al.*, 1987). When enamel dissolves, it will also release its fluoride into its environment, but the majority of the fluoride ions in this location probably comes from plaque and saliva which in turn comes from drinks and toothpastes. This is probably why, to achieve its full effect, a source of fluoride is needed throughout life. It also suggests an explanation of how caries is reduced even if fluoride is received only after the teeth are fully erupted. Naturally, any other factor that increases the level of saturation of the plaque fluid with apatite (such as raising the concentration of Ca or P ions or reducing the intensity of the acid attack) will reinforce this effect of fluoride.

This hypothesis suggests that both fluoride in FHA of the enamel and fluoride ions outside the tooth contribute to the protective effect and this agrees with the results of an experiment in rats (Larsen, von der Fehr and Birkeland, 1976). Five groups of rats 22–25 days old were fed a non-cariogenic diet for 7 days, during which their drinking water contained different levels up to 150 ppm of fluoride which led to the incorporation of fluoride into their enamel. All the rats were then put on to a cariogenic diet for 56 days, one-half of each group having 10 ppm of fluoride in their water while the other half received fluoride-free water. The results showed that the fluoride built into the enamel had the greater effect on caries in the fissures, but the fluoride provided in the water was most effective on the smooth surfaces and had a greater overall effect.

Clinical evidence for remineralization

The first suggestion that enamel could be remineralized by saliva was made as long ago as 1912 by Head, but was not followed up. Backer Dirks (1966) drew attention to this possibility when he reported that many 'white spot' lesions in the teeth of 8-year-old children had either not progressed into cavities or had even disappeared by the age of 15. A similar observation has been made in experimental caries in human subjects (von der Fehr, Loe and Theilade, 1970; Edgar *et al.*, 1978). When the subjects abstained from toothbrushing for 23 days (von der Fehr and co-workers) or even for 9 days (Edgar *et al.*, 1978) during which they took 6 daily rinses of 10% sucrose, white spots, presumed to be similar to early caries, were detectable microscopically (with a magnification of 15). When oral hygiene was resumed and the mouth rinsed with fluoride solutions for some weeks, the white spots disappeared. The relative importance of the saliva and fluoride in this remineralization is not known as, for ethical reasons, the effect of saliva alone has not been tested in case it was ineffective.

Two further examples of remineralization may be mentioned. The well-mineralized outer layer of an early carious lesion is now thought to be formed by the precipitation of mineral as the Ca and P ions diffuse out from the body of the lesion. The earlier view, that this layer occurred because the outermost enamel was less soluble (from its high fluoride and low carbonate concentration), was shown to be incorrect because exposure to acid of enamel with its outer layer removed resulted in the formation of a well-mineralized outer layer (Sperber and Buonocore, 1963). Also, Ogaard *et al.* (1986) have shown that this layer is not present during the first 4 weeks of experimental lesions produced by applying orthodontic bands on teeth scheduled for extraction: evidently it takes some time to develop, but if it were caused by the fluoride-rich outer layer it would be present from the beginning of the lesion.

It is also suggested that the lower score of idiopathic opacities in areas with 1 ppm F than in non-fluoride areas (Forrest, 1956) may occur because they are mineralized and become less conspicuous under the influences of fluoride. Also, the score of mild enamel fluororis in 7–12-year-old children has been reported to fall during the following 5 years (Aasenden and Peebles, 1978). Mineralization is a likely explanation, although loss of superficial blemishes from abrasion is another possibility.

To summarize this confusing data on solubility – the evidence is contradictory on whether the concentration of fluoride in sound enamel is sufficient to reduce its solubility but, even if it is too low, the fluoride could reduce caries in three other ways: (a) it reduces the carbonate of enamel, an ion that increases its solubility; (b) after dissolution by acid it provides fluoride ions which, along with those from plaque and saliva, would favour remineralization; (c) it accumulates in early lesions to concentrations that are often sufficiently high to reduce solubility.

This group of effects is now widely believed to be the most important mechanism of anti-caries action of fluoride. It might also be said that fluoride built into the enamel has a sort of 'fail-safe' effect on caries. If its concentration is high enough, the evidence suggests that its solubility is reduced but if the concentration is too low to do this, then more enamel will dissolve during each cariogenic episode and the released fluoride will contribute to the pool arising also from plaque and saliva which brings about remineralization. The earlier belief that the fluoride incorporated into the apatite of enamel exerted the greatest cariostatic effect has now been replaced by the view that it is a constant supply of soluble, ionic fluoride that is most effective.

Effect of fluoride on bacterial acid production

Fluoride has been known as an enzyme inhibitor for many years, and among the early attempts to explain the effect of fluoride on caries was the possibility that it inhibited acid production by the plaque bacteria. Two questions must be answered before the validity of this hypothesis can be decided: (a) what concentrations of fluoride are needed to inhibit acid production significantly, and (b) do the concentrations in saliva or plaque reach the inhibitory levels? Bibby and Van Kesteren (1940) began the search for an answer to the first question. They showed that 1–2 ppm F had a detectable effect on acid production by pure cultures of various oral acidogenic bacteria, but 10 ppm were needed for a decisive inhibition (Figure 15.2) and about 100 ppm for reducing growth. Similar results were found with mixed salivary organisms (Wright and Jenkins, 1954). The fluoride concentration in saliva was reported to be about 0.1 ppm – not nearly enough to inhibit bacteria – so the idea was virtually abandoned. It was assumed up to the 1950s that the fluoride concentration of plaque was similar to that of saliva, although no estimations were attempted as pooled samples from 1000 people were thought to have been needed to measure it by the insensitive methods then available! Two developments in the late 1950s renewed interest in this hypothesis. The first was the finding that the sensitivity of bacteria to fluoride greatly increased as the pH fell (Shiota, 1956; Jenkins, 1959). When saliva is adjusted to pH 5.0 and incubated with sugar and more than 6 ppm F, acid production is completely inhibited and the pH *rises* because base production (formation of amines and ammonia from amino acids) continues unopposed (Figure 15.3). The second development was improvements in the methods of fluoride analysis, so that Hardwick and Leach (1963) were able to estimate the concentration in plaque and obtained the astonishing result that it was more than 100 times higher than that of saliva, mean values of 25 and 47 ppm being recorded in plaques from towns low and high in fluoride, respectively. By the 1960s, there seemed good evidence that the fluoride concentration in plaque was adequate to support the inhibitory hypothesis.

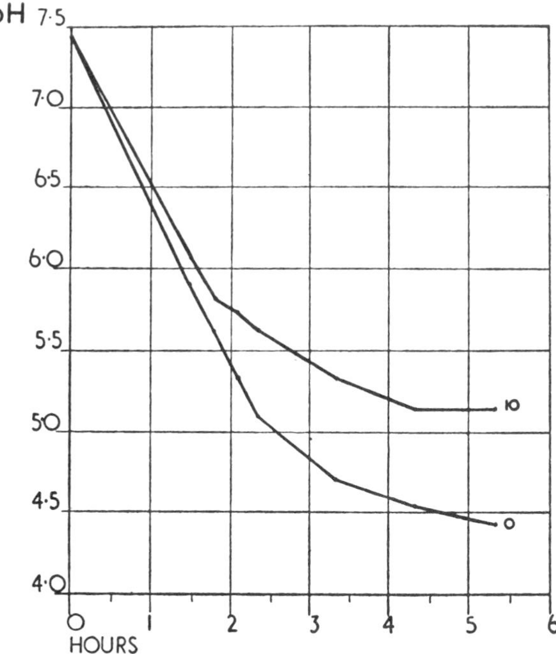

Figure 15.2 The pH changes during the incubation of saliva and glucose with 10 ppm F (upper curve) and without F (lower curve). Note that the inhibition is negligible until the pH falls below 6.0 (From Jenkins, 1959, with kind permission of the Editor, *Archives of Oral Biology*)

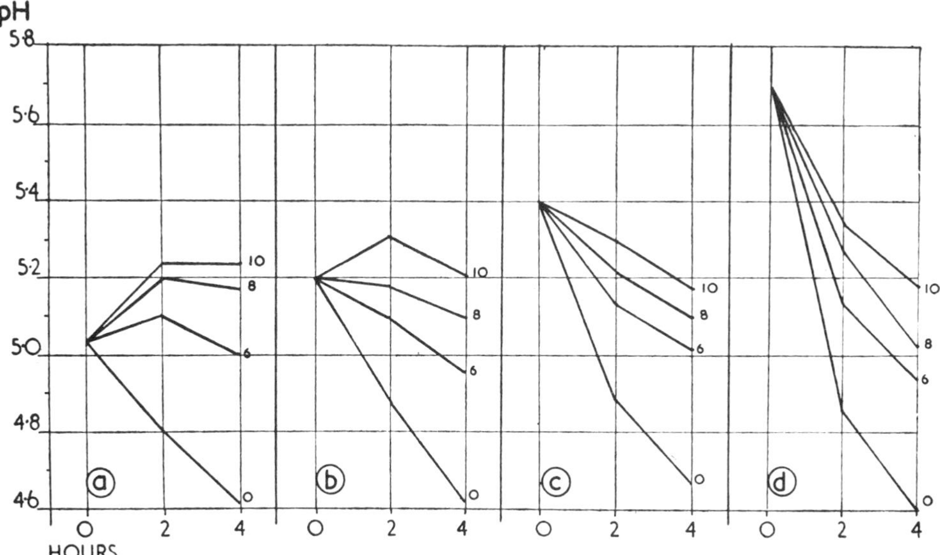

Figure 15.3 Effect of 0, 6, 8 and 10 ppm of F on the pH changes of incubated saliva–glucose mixtures adjusted to pH values (a) 5.04, (b) 5.2, (c) 5.4, (d) 5.7. When adjusted to 5.05 (a), acid production is completely inhibited for 2 h by 8 and 10 ppm and the pH rises (From Jenkins, 1959, with kind permission of the Editor, *Archives of Oral Biology*)

Later results for plaque fluoride with the specific ion electrode, introduced in the 1960s (Frant and Ross, 1966), have shown that the early figures were too high, up to 5 ppm being typical but with great variability from subject to subject (for summary of later results see Tatevossian, 1990). The electrode also revealed that the early figure of 0.1 ppm F for the concentration in saliva was too high, the true figure being about 0.01–0.02 ppm, confirming that plaque fluoride is over 100 times higher.

Source of plaque fluoride

The fluoride of plaque in low-fluoride areas probably arises from the saliva and gingival fluid: the importance of the latter has been shown in dogs injected with ^{18}F. Within 30 min of the injection, the ^{18}F concentration of gingival fluid equalled that of plasma but, in agreement with previous results, saliva concentrations never reached those of plasma (MacFadyen *et al.*, 1979). In some experiments with injected ^{18}F, saliva secretion was suppressed by atropine and in others it was stimulated by pilocarpine. The plaque ^{18}F rose in both experiments, but was higher and reached its peak earlier when saliva was stimulated, suggesting that both saliva and gingival fluid are the sources of plaque fluoride in unfluoridated areas. The higher level of plaque fluoride in fluoridated areas may come partly from the slightly raised levels in plasma (and therefore presumably in gingival fluid as well) and in saliva. It is probably also supplemented by direct contact with drinking water: rinsing with 10 ml of water containing 2.3 ppm F raised plaque fluoride (see page 268). The absolute amount of fluoride in an individual's plaque is, of course, extremely small. The daily production of plaque averages about 10 mg so, assuming a concentration of 5 ppm, the absolute weight is 0.05 μg of fluoride, equal to the amount contained in 0.05 ml of fluoridated water or about 5–10 ml of saliva.

The binding of plaque fluoride

It is obvious that these concentrations could not remain in plaque unless they were bound in some way, and the nature of the binding clearly influences the ability of plaque fluoride to inhibit acid production. Three constituents of plaque might bind F: (a) the protein and polysaccharide matrix; (b) the high concentrations of Ca and P which, if present as apatite, would bind it tightly at neutrality as FHA; and (c) the bacteria. Tests failed to show any binding by matrix, and various solvents showed that the Ca and P of plaque could be dissolved without releasing fluoride, which implies that at least some of the fluoride is not in apatite (Edgar and Jenkins, 1972). X-ray diffraction has been reported to detect apatite crystals in plaque (Kaufman and Kleinberg, 1973), but this process involves the drying of the plaque which would encourage the formation of apatite not present in the original wet plaque. Although the form of the Ca and P of plaque and whether it binds any fluoride is still uncertain, there is much evidence suggesting that at least a large part of plaque fluoride is present within the bacteria. When bacteria are grown in cultures containing fluoride, many species take it up, especially under acid conditions reaching concentrations many times higher than the medium (Jenkins, Edgar and Ferguson, 1969; Kashket and Rodriguez, 1976; Yotis *et al.*, 1979; Edgar, Cockburn and Jenkins, 1981).

There are at least two types of binding of fluoride by oral bacteria and there has been confusion in naming them. Kashket and Bunick (1978) found that some fluoride was readily washed out with buffers ('loosely bound'), whereas the remainder required 0.5 M perchloric acid to extract it ('tightly bound'). Jenkins and Edgar (1977) also described a fraction as 'tightly bound' which they found could be extracted only by the complete destruction of the proteins by 11 M perchloric acid, but the existence of this fraction has not been confirmed (Gallagher and Bruton, 1982; Ophaug *et al.*, 1987).

When fluoride was added to the cytoplasmic contents released by ultrasonication from several species of oral bacteria which were then separated by chromatography, it was found that at least 11 constituents bound fluoride, including the enzyme enolase (Kashket and Bunick, 1978), and similar results were reported by Psarros, Feige and Duschner (1990). The amount of fluoride binding by enolase differed in different species and correlated with the sensitivity of that species to inhibition by fluoride, e.g. *Streptococcus mutans* is much less sensitive to fluoride than is *S. salivarius* and its enolase has a lower affinity for fluoride. Kashket and Rodriguez (1976) found that changing the external pH of a culture of *S. sanguis* from 7 to 5.5 raised the total fluoride of the bacteria by only 25%, but the loosely bound fluoride rose six-fold, from 0.3 to about 2 ppm. They suggested that the pH of the medium not only controls the uptake of fluoride but has an even larger effect on the distribution of fluoride within the cell. The sensitivity of enolase itself to fluoride has been shown not to increase at lower pH values; it is in fact more sensitive at neutrality than at pH 5 and 6 (Bunick and Kashket, 1981; Edgar, Cockburn and Jenkins, 1981).

There are contradictory opinions on the importance of the different fractions of fluoride as inhibitors. Hamilton (1969), Weiss *et al.* (1965) and Jenkins, Edgar and Ferguson (1969) found that the bacterial inhibition by fluoride was still present after the cells had been washed and the loosely bound fluoride presumably removed, implying that the tightly bound fraction contained the inhibitor. Agus *et al.* (1980) came to a similar conclusion in their finding of a much more significant correlation between DMFS and bound fluoride ($P < 0.005$) than with ionic fluoride ($P < 0.05$). Edgar, Cockburn and Jenkins (1981), on the other hand, found that several strains and species of oral bacteria took up fluoride, but when transferred to a fluoride-free medium showed little inhibition but were quite sensitive to free ionic fluoride added to the medium. It is likely that these differences arose from variations in the metabolic state and stage of growth of the organisms tested and of species differences: it is still unclear which results apply to the situation *in vivo*.

Control of the entry of fluoride into bacteria and its consequences

The pH inside bacterial cells is usually considerably higher than that of the external environment; for example at neutrality, a difference in pH (ΔpH) of 0.6 has been reported between the inside and outside of the cells of *S. salivarius*, rising to 0.9 when the medium pH was 5.0 (Kashket and Kashket, 1985). If the pH of a medium containing fluoride falls (i.e. the concentration of H^+ rises), some of the fluoride ions are converted into the non-ionized HF molecule which diffuses into the cells because the cell walls are permeable to it (but not to free fluoride ions). This is one explanation of the greater sensitivity of bacteria to fluoride at low pH values; another explanation is discussed later (see page 312). When the HF reaches the higher pH inside the cell it ionizes again into H^+ and F^+. This has three consequences: (a) it lowers the concentration of HF in the cell, thus maintaining a gradient between the inside and the outside and encouraging more diffusion into the cell; (b) it increases the intracellular concentration of fluoride ions which are usually thought to be the active enzyme inhibitor; and (c) it increases the H^+ concentration (i.e. lowers the pH) in the cell and this may reach a level so far removed from the optimum pH of the enzymes that acid production is reduced or may even cease (Eisenberg and Marquis, 1980). On this hypothesis, the inhibition is not caused directly by fluoride ions, but the fluoride (as HF) is simply a vehicle for increasing the intracellular H^+. Evidence for this is that with 10 ppm F in the medium at 5.5, the ΔpH in *S. salivarius* cells fell from 0.9 to 0.17 (Kashket and Kashket, 1985).

The two factors controlling the entry of F into cells are therefore the fluoride concentration outside the cell and the ΔpH (Whitford *et al.*, 1977). The uptake is independent of metabolic activity, e.g. it occurs in the absence of sugar (although if sugar is present it will indirectly increase uptake by lowering the pH) and is hardly affected by temperature changes over the range 22–37°C (Kashket and Rodriguez, 1976).

The concentration of fluoride ions in neutral plaque is extremely low, averaging 0.05 ppm, but increases (e.g. to 0.27 ppm) when the pH falls, and fluoride ions are released from bound forms (Birkeland and Charlton, 1976; Agus *et al.*, 1980). Most experiments on the uptake of fluoride by bacteria have studied concentrations such as 1–10 ppm, but the limited data on uptake from levels similar to those in plaque fluid do suggest that some species can take it up even from these low concentrations (Edgar, Cockburn and Jenkins, 1981 and unpublished; Psarros, Feige and Duschner, 1990). However, more work is desirable on a variety of bacterial species before this can be fully accepted and its clinical importance assessed. The fact that ionic fluoride increases when plaque is acidified suggests that some fluoride is bound to an acid-soluble substance and some workers suggest that this is a fluoridated apatite, although evidence against this (at least as the only binder) has already been mentioned. Some critics dismiss the possibility of bacterial uptake of fluoride in plaque and the resulting inhibition on the grounds that the concentration of ionic fluoride released even in an acidified plaque is too low (Tatevossian, 1990). Although there is some evidence, not yet confirmed, that certain bacteria can take up fluoride even from concentrations similar to those in plaque fluid, it is also possible, in an environment as heterogeneous as plaque, that the fluoride concentration may build up to much higher values in the immediate vicinity in which it is released from bound forms and thus facilitate bacterial uptake locally. Following topical applications, the fluoride concentrations would for a short time be quite high and, if CaF_2 is formed, its gradual dissolution would probably maintain for longer periods a level adequate for bacterial uptake. If the bacteria can take up fluoride from the concentrations in plaque fluid, then the release from bound forms is not only unnecessary for inhibition but is undesirable because if the fluoride were released as free ions it would no longer be combined with the enzymes that are inhibited.

The nature of fluoride inhibition

The main site of fluoride inhibition in the Emden–Myerhof pathway of acid production has long been known to be enolase, the enzyme that converts phosphoglyceric acid (PG) to phosphoenolpyruvic acid (PEP). When this reaction is blocked, PG accumulates and later products such as PEP and lactic acid are not formed (Figure 15.4). This has several consequences when it occurs in plaque:

1. The reduced production of lactate obviously impairs the ability of the bacterial plaque to cause caries.
2. In many bacteria, the uptake of glucose requires the presence of PEP (the PEP–phosphotransferase system), so uptake is reduced by fluoride (Hamilton, 1977).
3. Some bacteria, including *S. mutans*, also take up glucose (and some other nutrients) by 'proton motive force' (Hamilton, 1990) (Figure 15.4). The uptake by this mechanism depends on the ability of the organism to expel protons which in turn is controlled by fluoride-sensitive enzymes, the 'proton-translocating ATPases' (Konings *et al.*, 1987) which Psarros, Feige and Duschner (1990) have reported are inhibited by concentrations of fluoride as low as those in plaque fluid. Thus, by reducing PEP production and by inhibiting proton extrusion, fluoride interferes with the uptake of glucose by two independent mechanisms.

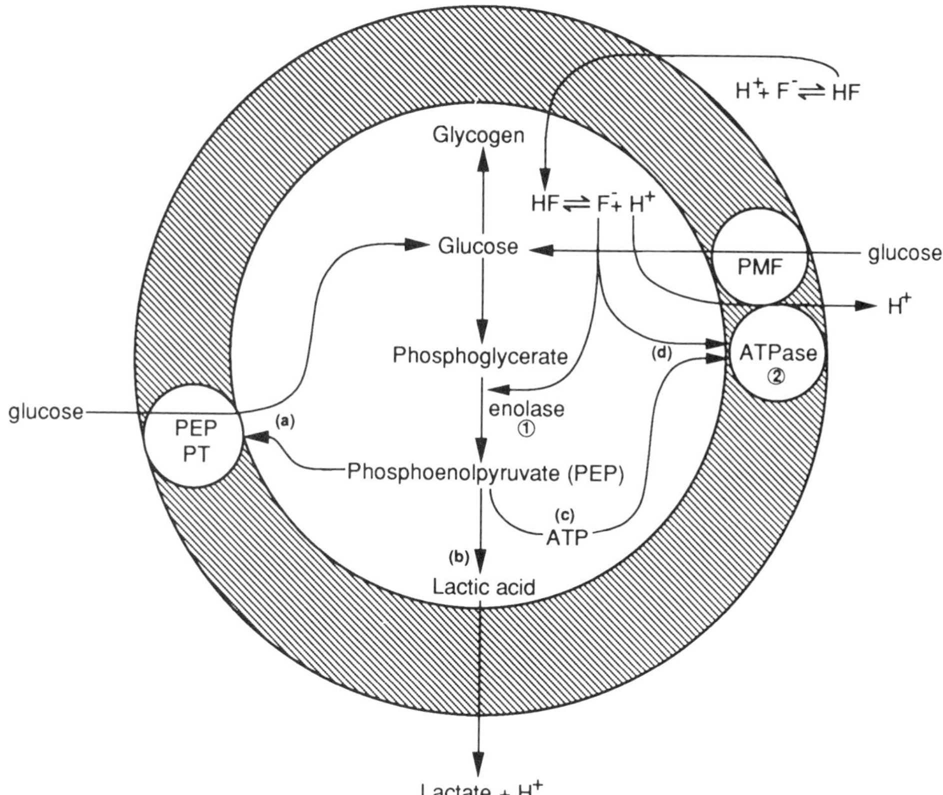

Figure 15.4 Simplified scheme for the uptake of glucose by bacteria and the sites of inhibition by F. Fluoride inhibits enolase reducing the formation of PEP and consequently (a) reducing the uptake of glucose by the PEP phosphotransferase system (PEP PT), thus (b) reducing lactic acid production and (c) reducing ATP synthesis required by the proton motive force system (PMF). F also inhibits the ATPase required for (d), the uptake of glucose by the PMF system

4. The reduced glucose uptake also prevents the synthesis of glycogen, the intracellular polysaccharide that acts as a store of carbohydrate and makes it possible for oral bacteria to continue to produce acid after the dietary sugar has been washed away by saliva.
5. The effect of fluoride in reducing the pH within the bacteria from the ionization of diffused HF has already been mentioned.

The second hypothesis to explain the pH sensitivity of fluoride inhibition

The last point above also suggests the second possible explanation for the greater sensitivity of many bacteria to fluoride at low pH values. An important characteristic of cariogenic bacteria is their aciduricity (their ability to produce acid at pH values even as low as 4.0). The suggestion is that fluoride reduces their aciduricity, e.g. *S. mutans* ceases to produce acid at about pH 5 in the presence of 10 ppm fluoride but in fluoride-free controls it continues, although more slowly, down to pH 4 (Eisenberg, Bender and Marquis, 1980). The aciduricity of bacteria depends on their power to extrude H^+ from their cytoplasm, a process that requires the membrane-bound proton-translocating ATPase mentioned above. This enzyme is very sensitive to fluoride in *S. mutans*. Marquis (1990) suggested that fluoride in plaque may inhibit this ATPase, thus reducing the extrusion of H^+ by the bacteria, leading to a build-up of acid which in turn inhibits enolase and other enzymes. A striking piece of circumstantial evidence for this hypothesis is that the acid tolerance of several species of bacteria is directly related to the concentration of ATPase in their membranes (Marquis, 1989).

Effect of fluoride on the synthesis of extracellular polymers

The synthesis of extracellular polymers (dextrans and fructans) has generally been found not to be inhibited by fluoride, although one piece of unconfirmed work suggests the contrary (Broukal and Zajicek, 1974). Several reports show that fluoride, in concentrations similar to those in plaque, *increases* dramatically the synthesis of these polymers *in vitro* (Zameck and Tinanoff, 1987). This may be an effect secondary to the inhibition of sugar intake making more substrate available for extracellular synthesis or, by inhibiting acid production, it may provide a more favourable pH. If these explanations are correct, it is unlikely that this increased synthesis of polymers would occur *in vivo* because the uptake of sugar by plaque bacteria is very small in absolute terms (a few milligrams of plaque would use very little of a mouthful of 10% sugar). Also, the effect of plaque fluoride on pH, although perhaps enough to affect de- and remineralization, would be too small to influence enzyme action (see later). As mentioned above, plaque fluoride inhibits the intracellular synthesis of glycogen as this depends on the fluoride-sensitive uptake of sugars by the bacteria (Wegman *et al.*, 1984).

Clinical evidence on the effect of fluoride on acid production

Although the effect of fluoride in reducing bacterial acid production *in vitro* has been thoroughly studied and is well established, there have been surprisingly few attempts to test whether the fluoride entering plaque from fluoridated water influences acid production *in vivo*.

The only work known to us in which DMFS was correlated with plaque fluoride and with acid production was carried out by Agus *et al.* (1980) on 75 children in a low-fluoride area in Australia. These workers collected plaque from every alternate tooth for the measurements of pH and fluoride concentration of 'resting' plaque. The plaque from the remaining teeth was collected 1 min after two supervised sugar rinses, each of 45 s duration. Acid production would occur while the samples were being prepared for analysis, so that the results of the second samples indicated the composition of 'fermented' plaque. Among the more important findings were: (a) the ionic fluoride increased during the fermentation (confirming the results of others); (b) there were significant correlations between DMFS and acid production ($P < 0.01$), fluoride ions in fermented plaque ($P < 0.05$) and very highly significant correlation with bound fluoride ($P < 0.0005$). Although a correlation is not a proof of a causal relationship, the strong implication is that plaque fluoride, especially in the bound form (i.e. probably mostly in the bacteria), even in a low-fluoride area influences acid production and DMFS.

In the first of two other studies, plaque acid production *in vitro* was compared in samples collected from residents of towns with different levels of fluoride in their water (Table 15.4). Plaques were collected simultaneously from children in the two areas and transported to the laboratory; plaques from children with similar DMF scores were pooled (the reason for this is explained later), incubated with sugar and their pH measured (Jenkins, Edgar and Ferguson, 1969). In the second study, on university students, the pH changes during incubation were compared in plaques from Newcastle upon Tyne before, and 2 months after, that city was fluoridated, with plaques from Durham City which was non-fluoridated on both occasions

Table 15.4*

A: *In vitro* pH changes during incubation of plaques with sugar from low- and high-fluoride towns (20 mg of plaque incubated with 20 μl 20% sucrose solution)

F of water (ppm)	*pH after incubation*	*Difference*	*n*	*P*
0 1.8	4.89 5.04	0.15 ± 0.12	34	<0.001
0 1.0	4.88 4.93	0.05 ± 0.09	13	between 0.1 and 0.05

B: Plaque pH changes with subjects from town with 1.8 ppm F classified on the basis of DMF

DMF	*No F in water*		*1.8 ppm in water*	
	pH	*n*	*pH*	*n*
<2	4.82	6	5.00	29
2–8	4.56	37	4.76	28
>8	4.67	16	4.60	7

* In addition to showing the significant difference in pH between the plaques from the high- and low-fluoride areas, the results indicate also (a) that (except for one group) the pH after incubation is lower in subjects with a high DMF, (b) the effect of fluoride on the DMF (there are more subjects with a low DMF in the high-fluoride town and vice versa).

(Edgar, Jenkins and Tatevossian, 1970). The results of both studies were consistent in showing significantly smaller pH drops in the high-fluoride towns (Table 15.5), although some workers think that the differences were too small to be of practical importance. It is now accepted that demineralization of enamel occurs only if the

Table 15.5 Mean pH after incubation with sugar of plaques from Newcastle, before and after fluoridation, and from Durham City (no fluoride) (Data from Edgar, Jenkins and Tatevossian, 1970)

	*Before fluoridation**	*After fluoridation**
Newcastle	5.21 ± 0.44 (17)	5.07 ± 0.20 (22)
Durham city	5.21 ± 0.26 (17)	4.94 ± 0.24 (32)
Difference	0.0	0.13 ($P = 0.01$)

* Number of observations in parentheses.

pH of plaque falls below some critical figure, usually between 5 and 6 (Fosdick and Starke, 1939), but varies in different plaques depending on their Ca and P content (Margolis, Murphy and Moreno, 1985). It must be emphasized that the relevant factor for demineralization is the degree of saturation with FHA which is influenced by the Ca, P and F concentration as well as the pH; hence the great variability in the critical pH in different plaques. If the critical pH of a particular plaque is, say, 5.5 and that without fluoridated water it would go down to 5.4 after sugar, but with fluoridated water it fell to only 5.5, then this difference of 0.1 pH would change a small degree of demineralization to none at all!

A difficulty in correlating plaque pH drops with fluoride is that, in fluoride areas, there is a higher proportion of individuals who are caries-free or have low caries scores. It is known that plaques from such individuals show smaller pH drops than those who are more caries-prone (Stephan, 1944; Englander, Carter and Fosdick, 1956). A difference in pH drop between the plaques from towns high and low in fluoride might therefore merely be a reflection of the smaller pH drops of the more numerous caries-free individuals. It was to avoid the risk of this spurious result that, in the study of Jenkins and colleagues, mentioned above, the plaques from children with similar caries activities were pooled: comparison of their pH drops still shows an effect of fluoride (Table 15.4b). Comparison of the figures in the various caries groups also confirms that plaque pH drop is related to caries and even with these small numbers the distribution of the subjects in the groups demonstrates the effect of fluoride (more with a low DMF in the fluoride area).

A similar point arises when the fluoride concentrations of saliva are compared in high- and low-fluoride areas in subjects subdivided into caries-free and caries-prone. In one survey, saliva fluoride in caries-free and caries-prone subjects were 0.041 and 0.020 ppm, respectively, in the high-fluoride area and 0.034 and 0.024 ppm in the low-fluoride area. When adjusted for caries experience, salivary fluoride levels were not significantly different in the two areas (Leverett *et al.*, 1987).

In another investigation on plaque fluoride in relation to acid production, samples of plaque were collected from schoolchildren, weighed, and their fluoride concentration estimated along with their pH drop when incubated with sugar (Rugg-Gunn *et al.*, 1981). A significant correlation was found between the fluoride and the final pH, but it was also found that the final pH and fluoride were inversely related to the weight of the plaque. In other words, the heavier the plaque sample, the lower was the fluoride concentration and the more acid it produced: the correlation of plaque weight with its fluoride concentration had been reported previously by Hardwick and Leach (1963), Birkeland, Jorkjend and von der Fehr (1971) and Agus *et al.* (1976). The explanation for these correlations is still speculative (see Rugg-Gunn *et al.*, 1981), but could lead to the false conclusion that the low fluoride concentrations were the cause of the higher acid production and vice versa. However, there is no evidence that fluoridated water influences plaque weight, so probably this complication does not cast doubt on the validity of the finding that plaques from high-fluoride areas produced smaller pH drops *in vitro* than those from low-fluoride areas.

Antibacterial effects of topical fluoride and fluoride in toothpastes

In contrast to the borderline effects of fluoridated water on plaque pH, there is no doubt that the various forms of topical fluoride do have a marked action on plaque acid production and may even alter the bacterial composition of plaque (see page 317). Effects on acid production are illustrated in the following description of three contrasting experiments. Woolley and Rickles (1971) applied a 2% solution of NaF daily for 1 week to half of the maxillary teeth of 63 girls and 2% NaCl to the other half. Plaque pH changes after a sugar rinse were measured with an antimony electrode on both halves of the mouth 8 h, 3–4 days and 1, 2 and 4 weeks after the end of the fluoride application. The inhibitory effect of fluoride was highly significant at 8 h and was detectable at 3–4 days and 1 week but was not significant, clearly indicating that topical application must be frequent to have an effect on acid production. Geddes and McNee (1982) studied the effect of daily mouthrinses with 0.2% NaF on 40 subjects for 1–2 months on plaque fluoride and Stephan curves. Mean plaque fluoride was raised 12-fold and the pH minimum was raised by an average of 0.11 (P between 0.025 and 0.01). The difference was larger (0.20) among the 27 subjects with the largest pH drops (probably because fluoride is more effective as a bacterial inhibitor at low pH values). Plaque fluoride and the pH drops returned to the baseline values within 4–10 days after the end of the rinsing.

Brown *et al.* (1981) tested the effect of a daily application of 1% NaF gels for up to 5 years on bacterial counts and acid production (measured as the concentrations of lactic and acetic acids) in plaques of xerostomic patients, in whom the clearance of the applied fluoride would be delayed due to their lack of saliva and the bacteria would be exposed to fluoride for much longer times than would occur in subjects with a normal saliva flow. Plaque fluoride rose and acid production decreased. After 1 year it was found that an increasingly high proportion of the *S. mutans* cells were fluoride-resistant, although enough of them must have remained sensitive to fluoride because the reduction in acid production continued. The development of fluoride-resistant bacteria had been reported previously *in vitro* by Williams (1964) and in animal experiments (van der Hoevan and Franken, 1984). The mechanism is not known, but it has been shown that it is not due to inability of the cells to take up fluoride or to changes in the sensitivity of enolase (Kashket and Preman, 1985). In some species, the resistance is lost when they are grown in a fluoride-free medium for a few generations, but in others the effect remains after exposure to fluoride ceases and is presumably genetic. There have been few studies on the adaptation of oral bacteria to the concentrations of fluoride present in plaque exposed to fluoridated water, but the limited data suggest that this does not occur. One report showed that plaque from users of fluoride toothpastes was still sensitive to 5 ppm F (Eisenberg *et al.*, 1985), suggesting that frequent exposure even to 1000 ppm had not induced significant resistance.

Effect of fluoride toothpastes and mouthrinses on fluoride of saliva and plaque

Bruun, Givskov and Thylstrup (1984) studied the fluoride concentration in saliva at intervals after one single brushing with toothpastes containing either 500 or 1500 ppm F as NaF or MFP, followed by a water rinse that was expectorated. Although there were differences between the fluoride concentrations in saliva from NaF and MFP during the first 10 min, the later values were similar – it had already been shown that MFP is rapidly broken down by enzymes in the saliva and plaque (Pearce and Jenkins, 1977). Immediately after brushing, the fluoride concentration varied between 60 and 220 ppm in different subjects, falling to between 3 and 11 ppm by 3 min, and then fell exponentially reaching baseline values after about 60 min. In a study by Ogaard *et al.* (1986) with a mouthrinse containing 0.2% (2000 ppm) fluoride, the saliva did not reach baseline till 4 h after the rinse (and in one subject remained at about 20 ppm from 2 to 5 h after the rinse).

Duckworth, Morgan and Murray (1987) found that after daily rinsing for 5–6 weeks with solutions containing NaF providing 100, 250 and 1000 ppm F, plaque and saliva collected 18 h after the last rinse showed marked increases in fluoride proportional to the concentration in the rinse. There was a significant correlation between the levels in plaque and saliva. After the rinsing finished, it took 2–3 weeks before the saliva reached baseline fluoride levels, presumably from the slow release of fluoride from deposits of CaF_2 on the enamel. This slow release suggests that with daily use of fluoride either as a toothpaste or rinse, the concentrations remain at physiologically active levels throughout the day. Although with toothpastes much of the plaque would be removed, the CaF_2 known to be formed on the enamel would slowly dissolve into the plaque formed during the day. Somewhat similar studies on toothpastes containing 1000, 1500 and 2500 ppm F as MFP were reported by Duckworth, Morgan and Burchell (1989). They confirmed that plaque uptake was related to the concentration in the toothpaste, but did not correlate with the amount of toothpaste used, and that two brushings per day were more effective than one, only with the toothpaste containing 1000 ppm. Mean plaque fluoride of the groups was significantly inversely related to the 3-year caries increment, but there was no correlation in the data for individual subjects.

Sidi (1989) collected approximal plaque from 22 students after they had used for periods of 1 week, on a cross-over basis, toothpastes with or without 1000 ppm of fluoride either as NaF or MFP. The plaque was collected 1 h after the last toothbrushing of each week and it is surprising that the reported weight of plaque (over 3 mg dry weight) was available so soon after brushing the teeth! The plaque fluoride was approximately doubled by the NaF toothpaste (from 1.79 in the fluoride-free control to 3.61 ppm dry weight), with a somewhat smaller increase with MFP to 3.19 ppm ($P < 0.01$). This work confirms the general conclusion that fluoride toothpastes can increase plaque fluoride, although the concentrations are very much lower than those reported by other workers.

Effect of fluoride on plaque formation and its bacterial composition

There is no evidence that fluoridated water reduces plaque formation, but some data show that APF may do this (see below). Stannous fluoride, however, has a much more powerful antibacterial effect than NaF (Andres, Shaffer and Windeler, 1974; Tinanoff *et al.*, 1983) and has been shown to reduce plaque accumulation. Leverett, McHugh and Jensen (1984) found in tests over 28 months, with mouthrinses containing either 0.05% NaF or 0.1% SnF_2, no effect on plaque with the NaF but a small reduction with the SnF_2 at 4 months, but it was not apparent at 16 or 28 months. As this is an effect of Sn and not fluoride it will not be discussed further (for references and suggested mechanisms see Camosci and Tinanoff, 1984, and Leverett, McHugh and Jensen, 1984).

Loesche, Murray and Mellberg (1973) reported a reduction in the percentage of *S. mutans* (but not of *S. sanguis*) in approximal plaques after 5–10 daily applications of APF gels which was still detectable 6 weeks after the end of the treatment. The suggested explanation for the selective inhibition of *S. mutans* was that this organism is found only in plaque or on the enamel surface, and if it is suppressed by the APF there is no surviving reservoir on the tongue or gingivae that could recolonize the plaque. *Streptococcus sanguis*, on the other hand, exists on many oral surfaces and can rapidly recolonize cleaned enamel. In a similar experiment (Loesche *et al.*, 1975), a 75% reduction in the proportion of *S. mutans* occurred in occlusal, but not approximal, plaque and remained significantly lower 12 weeks after the treatment ended. In both experiments, the plaque scores were reduced by the APF: for up to 6 days after the rinses in the first experiment and for as long as 12 weeks in the second. The prolonged effect was probably caused by the slow release of fluoride from CaF_2 formed by the interaction of the APF with the enamel. Two experiments provide further evidence that topical fluoride influences acid production as well as reducing solubility. Zahradnik, Propas and Moreno (1978) took extracted human teeth, split them in halves and treated one set of the halves with APF, leaving the other halves as controls. Some of the teeth were exposed to lactic acid, others to *S. mutans* (1B1600) and 2% sucrose for some days: the protection against demineralization of the fluoride-treated halves was much greater in the *S. mutans* groups than in the lactic acid group. This implied that fluoride released from that acquired from the topical application has a greater effect in inhibiting acid production than it had on the solubility of the enamel. The protective effect was absent after the treated teeth were exposed to KOH, showing that it was CaF_2 on the enamel that had brought about the inhibition. SEMs showed that fewer *S. mutans* were attached to the enamel of the treated teeth than the untreated controls.

The other experiment supporting the importance of antibacterial effects from topical fluoride was reported by van Loveren, Fielmich and Ten Brink (1987). The principle of the experiment was to compare the microradiographic profiles and the amount of Ca dissolving from enamel during demineralization *in vitro* by *S. mutans* in the presence of either fluoride or the bacterial inhibitors nigericin and in controls without either additive. Nigericin acts like fluoride in reducing the difference between the pH inside and outside the cell (see pages 312–313), but has no effect on apatite solubility. Concentrations of fluoride and nigericin were chosen that had similar inhibitory effects on acid production, so that any difference in demineralization by fluoride would represent an additional effect on solubility. The results indicated that, with this procedure, 75% of the effect of fluoride was related to reduced acid production.

The effect of two common constituents of fluoride toothpastes, a flavouring agent and the detergent sodium lauryl sulphate, on the availability of fluoride in saliva was studied on 13 subjects by Bruun, Qvist and Thylstrup (1987). The flavouring agent increased saliva flow which diluted the fluoride and led to a more rapid clearance. The detergent delayed the fall in salivary fluoride concentration which Bruun and colleagues assumed arose because the increased wetting capacity facilitated the uptake of CaF_2 by the enamel, thus slowing its release into saliva. This explanation is probably incorrect: Barkvoll, Rolla and Lagerlof (1988) showed very clearly from SEMs that sodium lauryl sulphate greatly reduces the deposition of CaF_2 on enamel probably because it complexes Ca and thus makes CaF_2 more soluble. The detergent also inhibits the enzymes that break down MFP resulting in the concentration of free fluoride ions in saliva being much less from the MFP toothpaste than from one containing NaF.

Conclusions

Fluoride must be regarded as a multi-factorial method of reducing caries, as many of its properties may contribute to this action. The question is not what is the mode of action, but rather what is the relative importance of the different effects. The current opinion is that the solubility–remineralization concept, with its emphasis on a constant flow of ionic fluoride, is the major effect. Bacterial inhibition probably plays a part in the high concentrations produced by topical applications and toothpastes, but there is still no agreement as to whether sufficiently high concentrations of fluoride, in an inhibitory form, can build up from fluoridated water.

References

Aasenden, R. and Peebles, T. C. (1974) Effects of fluoride supplementation from birth on human deciduous and permanent teeth. *Arch. Oral Biol.,* **19**, 321–326

Aasenden, R. and Peebles, T. C. (1978) Effects of fluoride supplementation from birth on dental caries and fluorosis in teenaged children. *Arch. Oral Biol.,* **23,** 111–115

Agus, H. M., Schamschula, R. G., Barmes, D. E. and Brunzel, M. (1976) Associations between the total fluoride content of dental plaque and individual caries experience in Australian children. *Commun. Dent. Oral Epidemiol.,* **4**, 210–214

Agus, H. M., Un, P. S. H., Cooper, M. H. and Schamschula, R. G. (1980) Ionized and bound fluoride in resting and fermenting dental plaques and individual caries experience. *Arch. Oral Biol.,* **25**, 517–522

Andres, C. J., Shaffer, J. C. and Windeler, A. S. Jr. (1974) Comparison of antibacterial properties of stannous fluoride and sodium fluoride mouth-washes. *J. Dent. Res.,* **53**, 457–460

Backer Dirks, O. (1966) Posteruptive changes in dental enamel. *J. Dent. Res.,* **45**, 503–511

Barkvoll, P., Rolla, G. and Lagerlof, F. (1988) Effect of sodium laurylsulphate on the deposition of alkali-soluble fluoride on enamel *in vitro. Caries Res.,* **22**, 139–144

Bibby, B. G. and Van Kesteren, M. (1940) The effect of fluoride on mouth bacteria. *J. Dent. Res.,* **19**, 391–402

Birkeland, J. M. and Charlton, G. (1976) Effect of pH on the fluoride ion activity of plaque. *Caries Res.,* **10**, 72–80

Birkeland, J. M., Jorkjend, L. and von der Fehr, F. R. (1971) The influence of fluoride rinses on the fluoride content of dental plaque in children. *Caries Res.,* **5**, 169–179

Borsboom, P. C. F., Mei, H. C. and Arends, J. (1985) Enamel lesion formation with and without 0.12 ppm F in solution. *Caries Res.,* **19**, 396–402

Briner, W. W. and Francis, M. D. (1962) The effect of enamel fluoride on acid production by *Lactobacillus casei*. *Arch. Oral Biol.*, **7**, 541–550

Broukal, Z. and Zajicek, O. (1974) Amount and distribution of extracellular polysaccharide in dental microbial plaque. *Caries Res.*, **8**, 97–104

Brown, L. R., White, J. O., Horton, I. M., Perkins, D. H., Strekfuss, J. L. and Driezen, S. (1981) Effects of a single application of sodium fluoride gel on dental plaque acidogenesis. *J. Dent. Res.*, **60**, 1396–1402

Bruun, C., Givskov, H. and Thylstrup, A. (1984) Whole saliva fluoride after toothbrushing with NaF and MFP dentifrices with different F concentration. *Caries Res.*, **18**, 282–288

Bruun, C., Qvist, V. and Thylstrup, A. (1987) Effect of flavour and detergent on fluoride availability in whole saliva after use of NaF and MFP dentifrices. *Caries Res.*, **21**, 427–434

Bunick, F. J. and Kashket, S. (1981) Enolases from fluoride-sensitive and fluoride-resistant Streptococci. *Infect. Immun.*, **34**, 856–863

Camosci, D. A. and Tinanoff, N. (1984) Anti-bacterial determinants of stannous fluoride. *J. Dent. Res.*, **63**, 1121–1125

Cooper, V. K. and Ludwig, T. G. (1965) Effect of fluoride and of soil trace elements on the morphology of the permanent molars in man. *N.Z. Dent. J.*, **61**, 33–40

Cutress, T. W. (1972) The inorganic composition and solubility of dental enamel from several specified population groups. *Arch. Oral Biol.*, **17**, 93–109

Dawes, C., Jenkins, G. N., Hardwick, L. J. and Leach, S. A. (1965) The relation between the fluoride concentration in the dental plaque and in the drinking water. *Br. Dent. J.*, **119**, 164–167

DePaola, P. F., Brudevold, F., Aasenden, R., Moreno, E. C., Englander, H., Bakhos, Y., Bookstein, F. and Warram, J. (1975) A pilot study of the relationship between caries experience and surface enamel fluoride in man. *Arch. Oral Biol.*, **20**, 859–864

Dowse, C. M. and Jenkins, G. N. (1957) Fluoride uptake *in vivo* in enamel defects and its significance. *J. Dent. Res.*, **36**, 816 (Abstract)

Duckworth, R. M., Morgan, S. N. and Burchell, C. K. (1989) Fluoride in plaque following use of dentifrices containing sodium monofluorophosphate. *J. Dent. Res.*, **68**, 130–133

Duckworth, R. M., Morgan, S. N. and Murray, A. M. (1987) Fluoride in saliva and plaque following use of fluoride-containing mouthwashes. *J. Dent. Res.*, **66**, 1730–1734

Edgar, W. M., Cockburn, M. A. and Jenkins, G. N. (1981) Uptake of fluoride and its inhibitory effects in oral microorganisms in culture. *Arch. Oral Biol.*, **26**, 615–623

Edgar, W. M., Geddes, D. A. M., Jenkins, G. N., Rugg-Gunn, A. J. and Howell, R. (1978) Effects of calcium glycerophosphate and sodium fluoride on the induction *in vivo* of caries-like changes in human dental enamel. *Arch. Oral Biol.*, **23**, 655–661

Edgar, W. M. and Jenkins, G. N. (1972) The ionisable F of plaque. Proc. 50th Gen. Session IADR. Program and Abstract 173, p. 91

Edgar, W. M., Jenkins, G. N. and Tatevossian, A. (1970) The inhibitory action of fluoride on plaque bacteria. *Br. Dent. J.*, **128**, 129–132

Eisenberg, A. D., Bender, G. R. and Marquis, R. E. (1980) Reduction in the aciduric properties of the oral bacterium *Streptococci mutans* GS5 by fluoride. *Arch. Oral Biol.*, **25**, 133–136

Eisenberg, A. D. and Marquis, R. W. (1980) Uptake of fluoride by cells of *Streptococcus mutans* in dense suspensions. *J. Dent. Res.*, **59**, 1187–1191

Eisenberg, A. D., Wegman, M. R., Oldershaw, M. D. and Curzon, M. E. J. (1985) Effect of fluoride, lithium or strontium on acid production by pelleted human dental plaque. *Caries Res.*, **19**, 454–457

Englander, H. R., Carter, W. J. and Fosdick, L. S. (1956) The formation of lactic acid in dental plaques. III Caries-immune individuals. *J. Dent. Res.*, **35**, 792–799

Featherstone, J. D. B., Glena, R., Shariati, M. and Shields, C. P. (1990) Dependence of *in vitro* demineralization of apatite and remineralization of dental enamel on fluoride concentration. *J. Dent. Res.*, **69**, 620–625

von de Fehr, F. R., Loe, H. and Theilade, E. (1970) Experimental caries in man. *Caries Res.*, **4**, 131–148

Foreward, G. C. (1977) A new method of measuring hydroxyapatite dissolution rate. *Caries Res.*, **11**, 9–15

Forrest, J. R. (1956) Caries incidence and enamel defects in areas with different levels of fluoride in the drinking water. *Br. Dent. J.*, **100**, 195–200

Fosdick, L. S. and Starke, A. C. (1939) Solubility of tooth enamel in saliva at various pH levels. *J. Dent. Res.*, **18**, 417–430

Frank, R. M. (1990) Structural events in the caries process in enamel, cementum, and dentine. *J. Dent. Res.*, **69**, 558–566

Frant, M. S. and Ross, J. W. Jr. (1966) Electrode for sensing fluoride ion activity in solution. *Science*, **134**, 1553–1555

Gallagher, R. W. and Bruton, W. F. (1982) Fluoride concentration in dental plaque of naval recruits with and without caries. *Arch. Oral Biol.*, **27**, 269–272

Geddes, D. A. M. and McNee, S. G. (1982) The effect of 0.2 per cent (48 mM) NaF rinses daily on human plaque acidogenicity *in situ* (Stephan curve) and fluoride content. *Arch. Oral Biol.*, **27**, 765–770

Hallsworth, A. S. and Weatherell, J. A. (1969) The microdistribution, uptake and loss of fluoride in human enamel. *Caries Res.*, **3**, 109–118

Hallsworth, A. S., Weatherell, J. A. and Robinson, C. (1973) Loss of carbonate during the first stages of enamel caries. *Caries Res.*, **7**, 345–348

Hamilton, I. R. (1969) Studies with fluoride-sensitive and fluoride-resistant strains of *Streptococcus salivarius*. *Can. J. Microbiol.*, **15**, 1013–1020, 1021–1027

Hamilton, I. R. (1977) Effects of fluoride on enzymatic regulation of bacterial carbohydrate metabolism. *Caries Res.*, **11** (Suppl. 1), 262–291

Hamilton, I. R. (1990) Biochemical effects of fluoride on oral bacteria. *J. Dent. Res.*, **69**, 660–667

Hardwick, J. L. and Leach, S. A. (1963) The fluoride content of the dental plaque. *Arch. Oral Biol.*, Spec. Suppl.: Proc 9th ORCA Congress, 151–158

Harper, D. S. and Loesche, W. J. (1986) Inhibition of acid production from oral bacteria by fluorapatite-derived fluorine. *J. Dent. Res.*, **65**, 30–33

Head, J. A. (1912) A study of saliva and its action on tooth enamel in reference to its hardening and softening. *J. Clin. Med. Ass.*, **59**, 2118–2122

Healey, W. B. and Ludwig, T. G. (1966) Enamel solubility studied on New Zealand teeth. *N.Z. Dent. J.*, **62**, 276–278

van der Hoevan, J. S. and Franken, H. E. M. (1984) Effect of fluoride on growth and acid production by *Streptococcus mutans* in dental plaque. *Infect. Immun.*, **45**, 356–359

Ingram, G. S. (1973) The role of carbonate in dental mineral. *Caries Res.*, **7**, 217–230

Isaac, S., Brudevold, F., Smith, F. A. and Gardner, D. W. (1958) Solubility rate and natural fluoride content of surface and subsurface enamel. *J. Dent. Res.*, **37**, 254–263

Jenkins, G. N. (1959) The effect of pH on the inhibition of salivary acid production. *Arch. Oral Biol.*, **1**, 33–41

Jenkins, G. N. (1963) Theories on the mode of action of fluoride in reducing dental decay. *J. Dent. Res.*, **42**, 444–452

Jenkins, G. N. and Edgar, W. W. (1977) Distribution and forms of F in saliva and plaque. *Arch. Oral Biol.*, **11** (Suppl. 1), 226–242

Jenkins, G. N., Edgar, W. M. and Ferguson, D. B. (1969) The distribution and metabolic effects of human plaque fluorine. *Arch. Oral Biol.*, **14**, 105–119

Johnson, N. W. (1967) Some aspects of the ultrastructure of early human enamel caries seen with the electron microscope. *Arch. Oral Biol.*, **12**, 1515–1521

Kashket, S. and Bunick, F. J. (1978) Binding of fluoride in oral streptococci. *Arch. Oral Biol.*, **23**, 993–996

Kashket, S. and Kashket, E. R. (1985) Dissipation of proton motive force in oral streptococci by fluoride. *Infect. Immun.*, **48**, 19–22

Kashket, S. and Preman, R. J. (1985) Fluoride uptake and fluoride resistance in oral streptococci. *J. Dent. Res.*, **64**, 1290–1292

Kashket, S. and Rodriguez, V. M. (1976) Fluoride accumulates by a strain of human oral *Streptococcus sanguis*. *Arch. Oral Biol.*, **21**, 459–464

Kaufman, H. W. and Kleinberg, I. (1973) X-ray diffraction of calcium phosphate in dental plaque. *Calc. Tiss. Res.*, **11**, 97

Keene, H. J., Mellberg, J. R. and Pederson, E. D. (1980) Relationship between dental caries experience and surface enamel fluoride concentrations in young men from three optimally fluoridated cities. *J. Dent. Res.*, **59**, 1941–1945

Konings, W. H., De Vrij, W., Driessens, A. J. M. and Poolman, B. (1987) Primary and secondary transport in Gram-positive bacteria. In *Sugar Transport and Metabolism by Gram-positive Bacteria* (eds J. Reiger and A. Peterkovsky), Ellis Horwood, Chichester, UK, pp. 270–294

Koulourides, T., Keller, S. E., Mansson-Hing, L. and Lilley, V. (1980) Enhancement of fluoride effectiveness by experimental cariogenic priming of human enamel. *Caries Res.*, **14**, 32–39

Kruger, B. J. (1966) Interaction of fluoride and molybdenum on dental morphology in the rat. *J. Dent. Res.*, **45**, 714–725

Kruger, B. J. (1968) Ultrastructural changes in ameloblasts from fluoride treated rats. *Arch. Oral Biol.*, **13**, 967–977

Kruger, B. J. (1970) An autoradiographic assessment of the effect of fluoride on the uptake of ^{3}H-proline by ameloblasts in the rat. *Arch. Oral Biol.*, **15**, 103–108

Lagerlof, F., Oliveby, A. and Ekstrand, J. (1987) Physiological factors influencing salivary clearance of sugar and fluoride. *J. Dent. Res.*, **66**, 430–435

Larsen, M. J., von der Fehr, F. R. and Birkeland, J. M. (1976) Effect of fluoride on the saturation of an acetate buffer with respect to hydroxyapatite. *Arch. Oral Biol.*, **21**, 723–728

Larsen, M. J. and Jensen, S. J. (1989) Solubility unit cell dimensions and crystallinity of fluoridated human dental enamel. *Arch. Oral Biol.*, **34**, 969–973

Larson, R. H., Mellberg, J. R., Englander, H. R. and Senning, R. (1976) Caries inhibition in the rat by water-borne and enamel bound fluoride. *Caries Res.*, **10**, 321–331

Leverett, D. H., Adair, S. M., Shields, C. P. and Fu, J. (1987) Relationship between salivary and plaque fluoride levels and dental caries experience in fluoridated and non-fluoridated communities. *Caries Res.*, **21**, 179–180

Leverett, D. H., McHugh, W. D. and Jensen, D. E. (1984) Effect of daily rinsing with stannous fluoride on plaque and gingivitis: final report. *J. Dent. Res.*, **63**, 1083–1086

Little, M. F. and Steadman, L. T. (1966) Chemical and physical properties of altered and sound enamel IV. *Arch. Oral Biol.*, **11**, 273–278

Loesche, W. J., Murray, R. J. and Mellberg, J. (1973) The effect of topical acidulated fluoride on percentage of *Streptococcus mutans* and *Streptococcus sanguis* in interproximal plaque samples. *Caries Res.*, **7**, 283–296

Loesche, W. J., Syed, S. A., Murray, R. J. and Mellberg, J. (1975) The effect of topical acidulated fluoride on percentage of *Streptococcus mutans* and *Streptococcus sanguis* in plaque II. Pooled occlusal approximal plaque. *Caries Res.*, **9**, 139–155

van Loveren, C., Fielmich, A. M. and Ten Brink, B. (1987) Comparison of the effect of fluoride and the ionophone nigericin on acid production by *Streptococcus mutans* and the resultant enamel demineralization. *J. Dent. Res.*, **66**, 1658–1662

Lovius, B. B. J. and Goose, D. A. (1969) The effect of fluoridation of water on tooth morphology. *Br. Dent. J.*, **127**, 322–324

McFadyen, E. E., Hilditch, T. E., Stephen, K. W., Horton, P. W. and Campbell, J. R. (1979) Distribution of fluoride in gingival fluid and dental plaque of dogs. *Arch. Oral Biol.*, **24**, 427–431

Manly, R. S. and Harrington, D. P. (1959) Solution rate of tooth enamel in an acetate buffer. *J. Dent. Res.*, **38**, 910–919

Margolis, H. C. and Moreno, E. C. (1990) Physicochemical perspectives on the cariostatic mechanisms of systemic and topical fluorides. *J. Dent. Res.*, **69**, 606–613

Margolis, H. C., Moreno, E. C. and Murphy, B. J. (1986) Effect of low levels of fluoride in solution on enamel demineralization *in vitro*. *J. Dent. Res.*, **65**, 23–29

Margolis, H. C., Murphy, B. J. and Moreno, E. C. (1985) Development of caries-like lesions in partially saturated lactate buffer. *Caries Res.*, **19**, 36–45

Marquis, R. E. (1989) Physiology of fluoride inhibition of oral bacteria. *J. Dent. Res.*, **68**, 1694–1695

Marquis, R. E. (1990) Diminished acid tolerance of plaque bacteria caused by fluoride. *J. Dent. Res.*, **69**, 672–675

Moreno, E. C., Kresok, M. and Zahradnik, R. T. (1977) Physicochemical aspects of fluoride apatite systems relevant to the study of dental caries. *Caries Res.*, **11** (Suppl. 1), 142–160

Myers, H. M., Hamilton, J. G. and Becks, H. (1952) A tracer study of the transfer of F^{18} to teeth by topical application. *J. Dent. Res.*, **31**, 743–750

Nelson, D. G. A., Featherstone, J. D. B., Duncan, J. F. and Cutress, T. W. (1983) Effect of carbonate and fluoride on the dissolution behaviour of synthetic apatites. *Caries Res.*, **17**, 200–211

Nikiforuk, G. (1961) Carbonates and fluorides as chemical determinants of tooth susceptibility to caries. In *Caries Symposium, Zurich* (eds H. R. Muhlemann and K. G. Konig), Hans Huber, Berne

Nikiforuk, G., McLeod, I. M., Burgess, R. C., Grainger, R. M. and Brown, H. K. (1962) Fluoride–carbonate relationship in dental enamel. *J. Dent. Res.*, **41**, 1477

Ockerse, T. (1949) *Clinical and Experimental Investigations*, Department of Public Health, Union of South Africa

Ogaard, B., Arends, J., Schuthof, J., Rolla, G., Ekstrand, J. and Oliveby, A. (1986) Action of fluoride on initiation of early enamel caries *in vivo*. A microradiographical investigation. *Caries Res.*, **20**, 270–277

Okazaki, M., Aoba, T., Doi, Y., Takahashi, J. and Moriwaki, Y. (1981) Solubility and crystallinity in relation to fluoride content of fluoridated hydroxyapatite. *J. Dent. Res.*, **60**, 845–848

Ophaug, R. H., Jenkins, G. N., Singer, L. and Kresbach, P. H. (1987) Acid diffusion of different forms of fluoride in dental plaque. *Arch. Oral Biol.*, **32**, 459–461

Paynter, K. J. and Grainger, R. M. (1956) The relation of nutrition to the morphology and size of rat molar tooth. *J. Can. Dent. Ass.*, **22**, 529–531

Pearce, E. I. F. and Jenkins, G. N. (1977) The inhibition of acid production in human saliva by monofluorophosphate. *Arch. Oral Biol.*, **21**, 617–621

Psarros, N., Feige, V. and Duschner, H. (1990) Interactions of micromolar concentrations of fluoride with *Streptococcus rattus* FA1. *Caries Res.*, **24,** 189–192

Retief, D. H., Harris, B. E. and Bradley, E. L. (1987) Relationship between enamel fluoride concentration and dental caries experience. *Caries Res.*, **21**, 68–78

Rugg-Gunn, A. J., Edgar, W. M., Cockburn, M. A. and Jenkins, G. N. (1981) Correlations between fluoride concentration, sample weight and acid production in dental plaque from children. *Arch. Oral Biol.*, **26**, 61–63

Schamschula, R. G., Agus, H., Charlton, G., Dupenthala, J. L. and Un, P. (1979) Association between fluoride concentrations in successive layers of human enamel and individual dental caries experiences. *Arch. Oral Biol.*, **24**, 847–852

Shiota, T. (1956) Effect of sodium fluoride on oral lactobacilli isolated from the rat. *J. Dent. Res.*, **35**, 939–946

Sidi, A. D. (1989) Effect of brushing with fluoride toothpastes on the fluoride calcium and inorganic phosphate concentrations in approximal plaque in young adults. *Caries Res.*, **23**, 268–271

Simmelink, J. W. and Nygaard, V. K. (1982) Ultrastructure of striations in carious human enamel. *Caries Res.*, **16**, 179–188

Simpson, W. J. and Castaldi, C. R. (1969) A study in crown morphology of newly-erupted first permanent molars in Wetaskiwin, Alberta (optimum fluoride) and Camrose, Alberta (low-fluoride). *Odont. Revy*, **20**, 1–14

Spector, P. C. and Curzon, M. E. J. (1979) Surface enamel fluoride and strontium in relation to caries prevalence in man. *Caries Res.*, **13**, 227–230

Sperber, G. H. and Buonocore, M. G. (1963) Enamel surface in white-spot formation. *J. Dent. Res.*, **42**, 724–731

Spinelli, M. A., Brudevold, F. and Moreno, E. (1971) Mechanism of fluoride uptake by hydroxyapatite. *Arch. Oral Biol.*, **161**, 187–203

Stephan, R. M. (1944) Intra-oral hydrogen-ion concentration associated with dental caries activity. *J. Dent. Res.*, **23**, 257–266

Tatevossian, A. (1990) Fluoride in dental plaque and its effects. *J. Dent. Res.*, **69**, 645–652

ten Cate, J. M. and Duijsters, P. P. E. (1983) The influence of fluoride in solution on tooth demineralization. *Caries Res.*, **17**, 193–199, 513–519

Tinanoff, N., Klock, B., Camoschi, D. A. and Manwell, M. A. (1983) Microbiologic effects of SnF_2 and NaF mouthrinses in subjects with high caries activity: results after one year. *J. Dent. Res.*, **62**, 907–911

Tyler, J. E., Poole, D. F. G., Stack, M. V. and Dowell, T. B. (1986) Superficial fluoride levels and response to *in vitro* caries-like lesion induction of enamel from Bristol (U.K.) and Birmingham (U.K.) human deciduous teeth. *Arch. Oral Biol.,* **31**, 201–204

Volker, J. F. (1939) The effect of fluorine on solubility of enamel and dentine. *Proc. Soc. Exp. Biol. Med.,* **42**, 725–727

Wallenius, B. (1959) The mesiodistal width of the tooth in relation to the fluoride content in drinking waters. *Odont. Revy,* **10**, 76–81

Wegman, M. R., Eisenberg, A. D., Curzon, M. E. J. and Handelman, S. L. (1984) Effects of fluoride and of strontium on intracellular polysaccharide accumulation in *S. mutans* and *A. viscosis. J. Dent. Res.,* **63**, 1126–1129

Weiss, S., King, W. L., Kestenbaum, R. C. and Donohue, J. J. (1965) Influence of various factors on polysaccharide synthesis by *S. mitis. Ann. N.Y. Acad. Sci.,* **131**, 839–850

Whitford, G. M., Schuster, G. S., Pashley, D. H. and Venkateswarla, P. (1977) Fluoride uptake by *Streptococcus mutans* 6715. *Infect. Immun.,* **18,** 680–687

Williams, R. A. D. (1964) Biochemical aspects of the adaptation to fluoride by a micro-organism isolated from dental plaque. *J. Dent. Res.,* **43**, 946–947 (Abstract)

Williams, R. A. D. (1967) The growth of Lancefield group D streptococci in the presence of sodium fluoride. *Arch. Oral Biol.,* **12**, 109–117

Wong, L., Cutress, T. W. and Duncan, J. F. (1987) The influence of incorporated and absorbed fluoride on the dissolution of powdered and pelleted hydroxyapatite in fluoridated and non-fluoridated buffers. *J. Dent. Res.,* **66**, 1735–1741

Woolley, L. and Rickles, N. H. (1971) Inhibition of acidogenesis in human dental plaque following the use of topical sodium fluoride. *Arch. Oral Biol.,* **16**, 1187–1194

Wright, D. E. and Jenkins, G. N. (1954) The effect of fluoride on the acid production of saliva-glucose mixtures. *Br. Dent. J.,* **96**, 30–33

Yates, W. W. and Brennan, P. C. (1983) Binding of fluoride by oral bacteria. *Caries Res.,* **17**, 444–454

Yotis, W. W., Mante, S., Brennan, P. C., Kirchner, F. R. and Glendenin, L. E. (1979) Binding of fluorine-18 by the oral bacterium, *Streptococcus mutans. Arch. Oral Biol.,* **24**, 853–860

Young, R. A. and Elliott, J. C. (1966) Atomic-scale bases for several properties of apatites. *Arch. Oral Biol.,* **11**, 699–707

Zahradnik, R. T., Propas, D. and Moreno, E. C. (1978) Effect of fluoride topical solution on enamel demineralization by lactate buffers and by *Streptococcus mutans in vitro. J. Dent. Res.,* **57**, 940–946

Zamek, R. L. and Tinanoff, N. (1987) Effects of NaF and SnF_2 on growth acid and glucan production of several oral bacteria. *Arch. Oral Biol.,* **32**, 807–810

Chapter 16

Toxicity of fluoride

Fluoride intoxication – effect on bone

The manifestations of chronic fluoride intoxication depend upon the rate of ingestion, the duration of exposure and the age of the subject. The bone fluoride is roughly proportional to the fluoride intake from water which, through the fluoride of plasma and tissue fluid, may (a) be incorporated into newly formed bone and (b) exchange with the hydroxyl ions in bone already formed.

At water fluoride levels over 8 ppm, for example in South Africa (Ockerse, 1946) and India (Srikantia and Siddiqui, 1965), skeletal fluorosis may develop. This is characterized by an increase in the X-ray density of trabecular bone in the lumbar spine, pelvis and elsewhere, and an increase in the thickness of long bone cortices due to endosteal and periosteal apposition. In more advanced cases, calcification of ligaments occurs, especially in the spine, and a clinical picture is observed which bears some resemblance to ankylosing spondylitis (Steinberg *et al.*, 1955).

Histologically, fluorotic bone presents a very mixed picture. There may be a great increase in new bone formation, as well as increase in the width and number of areas of unmineralized osteoid (Weatherell and Weidmann, 1959). This apparent resemblance to osteomalacia has never been adequately explained, but one hypothesis is that fluoride stimulates the osteoblasts to produce more matrix but the supply of Ca and P may be too low to mineralize it. However, the plasma calcium is invariably normal and the plasma phosphate is believed to be the same. In addition, there are numerous resorption spaces with fibrous tissue replacement, which Faccini (1969) attributed to secondary hyperparathyroidism. He postulated that bone which has taken up fluoride becomes resistant to resorption which results in parathyroid overactivity and excessive turnover in less affected parts of the skeleton (see page 326). If this secondary hyperparathyroidism led to hypophosphataemia, the osteomalacic features of fluorotic bone would be explained, but such plasma phosphate values that are available do not suggest that this is the case. Although fluorotic bone is sclerotic, in the sense that there is more of it than normal, it is not as strong, weight for weight, as normal bone, nor as highly mineralized, and spontaneous fractures are common (Nordin, 1973).

Cases of severe chronic toxicity have occurred among cryolite workers studied by Roholm (1937). These men and women were absorbing 14–68 mg/day for a period of 20–30 years. A number of toxic effects were observed, principally gastric complaints, osteosclerosis, exostoses of long bones, vertebrae, jaws bones and other flat bones. Singh *et al.* (1962) studied the skeleton of a person living in an area where the fluoride content of the drinking water was 9.5 ppm. All the bones were heavy and irregular and were of a dull colour due to irregular deposition of fluoride. Irregular bone was laid down along the attachment of muscles and tendons and multiple exostoses developed. Continuous exposure to 20–80 mg of fluoride for 20–30 years results in deformities (Singh *et al.*, 1962). The crippling deformities are partly due to mechanical factors and partly to the immobilization necessitated by pain and paraplegia.

The radiological changes of skeletal fluorosis were described by Roholm (1937) In stage 1, the spinal column and the pelvis show roughening and blurring of the trabeculae. In stage 2, the trabeculae merge together and the bone has a diffuse structureless appearance. In stage 3, the bone appears as marble white shadows; the configuration is woolly. The cortex of long bones is thick and dense and the medullary cavity is diminished.

The effects of exposure to fluoride at the level of 8 ppm in drinking water has been studied in detail, in America, by Leone *et al.* (1954) in a survey of 116 persons in Bartlett (8 ppm) and 121 persons in Cameron (0.5 ppm). The study began in 1943, when each participant received a medical and dental examination and X-rays, blood and urine studies were performed. These were repeated 10 years later in 1953. No significant differences between the two towns were observed in the following characteristics measured: arthritic changes, blood pressure, bone changes, cataract and/or lens opacity, thyroid, hearing, tumours and/or cysts, fractures, urinary tract calculi and gall-stones. There was a slightly higher rate of cardiovascular abnormalities in Cameron and a marked predominance of dental fluorosis in Bartlett.

The effect of consuming drinking water containing up to 4.0 ppm F on bone has been investigated histologically, roentgenographically and chemically. Weidmann, Weatherell and Jackson (1963) examined histologically the ribs of individuals who had lived in areas containing 0.5, 0.8 and 1.9 ppm F in the drinking water, for width of cortex and number and thickening of the cortical trabeculae. No differences were seen in resorption areas of the trabeculae or of the compacta among the three groups.

Schlesinger *et al.* (1956) examined children drinking water containing 1.2 ppm F in Newburgh, over a period of 10 years. Roentgenograms of the right hand, both knees and the lumbar spine were taken and bone density and bone age were estimated. No difference of any significance could be found in any of the roentgenographic studies.

Increased bone density or osteosclerosis was not apparent roentgenographically when the concentration of fluoride in the drinking water was less than 4 ppm (Stevenson and Watson, 1957; Geever *et al.*, 1958a, b; Morris, 1965), when the urinary fluoride concentration was less than 10 ppm (Largent, Bovard and Heyroth, 1951) or when the bone contained less than about 5000 ppm F on a dry, fat-free basis (Weidmann, Weatherell and Jackson, 1963).

The possible effect of fluoride on the chemical constituents of bone has been studied by Zipkin, McClure and Lees (1960), using post-mortem specimens of the iliac crest, rib and vertebra of individuals exposed to drinking water containing up to 4.0 ppm F. Calcium, phosphorus and potassium in the bone ash were unaffected by mean concentrations of bone fluoride as high as 0.8%. The carbonate content decreased by about 10%, the citrate content decreased by about 30% whereas the magnesium content increased by about 15% when the fluoride showed an 8-fold increase. An increase in bone fluoride is associated with an increase in the crystallinity of bone apatite (Posner *et al.*, 1963).

Mechanisms of the toxic effect of fluoride on bone

Experiments on rats receiving 100 ppm F in their water have shown that the effect of this very large dose consists of three actions directly on bone cells. The first is an increase in the number of osteoblasts and in their activity in secreting bone matrix accompanied by a rise in serum alkaline phosphatase, probably derived from the osteoblasts (Baylink *et al.*, 1970). Fluoride is also found to increase the incorporation of ^{3}H thymidine into the DNA of osteoblasts in cultures of bone cells from chick calvaria: this is, at least partly, specific to osteoblasts as it does not have this effect on cells from the liver or kidney. The mechanism of this stimulation is uncertain and may seem surprising in view of the well-known effect of fluoride as an inhibitor. However, fluoride does stimulate some enzymes, including adenyl cyclase, and a 2–3-fold increase in the activity of this enzyme has been reported in the bones of rabbits on high doses of fluoride with smaller increases in the liver and kidney (Singh and Susheela, 1982). These workers also found non-significant indications of a rise in plasma cAMP (the product of adenyl cyclase) in three fluorosed patients in India. It seems likely therefore that stimulation of adenyl cyclase may play a part in bone fluorosis.

The second effect of fluoride on bone is to delay mineralization, but this delay is smaller than the increase in osteoid formation so the net effect is an increase in bone tissue but with a greater width of unmineralized osteoid than in normal bone. This can probably be explained by several changes in the composition of bone matrix that have been reported in rabbits receiving, in most experiments, 10 mg F/kg body weight (unfortunately, an excessive dose, much higher than is ever received by human patients). The amino acid composition of collagen was changed (proline was higher and hydroxyproline was lower than normal, indicating a defect in the hydroxylation of proline) and the number of cross-links between the three chains was fewer. The non-collagenous constituents were also affected by fluoride. Normally bone contains two forms of chondroitin sulphate (A and C), but in the fluorosed rabbits a third form (B or dermatan sulphate) was present (Susheela and Sharma, 1982).

A third effect was an increase in resorption on the endosteal surfaces, producing a larger marrow cavity, but again this effect was smaller than the increase in periosteal deposition. One hypothesis to explain these effects is that fluoride stimulates the parathyroid causing increased resorption and a compensatory bone deposition elsewhere. However, the stimulus to PTH secretion is a fall in ionic Ca in the plasma, but this has not been found even in the severe fluorosis induced in experimental animals. This hypothesis was completely disproved by the finding that the effect of 90 ppm F in the water of rats was substantially unchanged by parathyroidectomy (Liu and Baylink, 1977). Another suggested explanation for the effect of fluoride on increasing the bone mass is that the fluorotic bone is less soluble than normal and that this disturbs the usual balance between deposition and resorption in favour of deposition. The acid solubility *in vitro* of bones from rats given 100 ppm F for 100 days was very much less than of bone from the controls (Zipkin and McClure, 1952), but fluorotic bone cultured with PTH was not resorbed less quickly than controls (Raisz and Taves, 1967) and *in vivo* experiments have failed to support this hypothesis.

Use of sodium fluoride in bone disorders

The discovery that fluoride increased the bone mass suggested that it might be effective in treating osteoporosis. The early experiments confirmed those in animals in showing that fluoride in large doses did increase the bone mass in human subjects and that the bone laid down under its influence was under-mineralized. This led to the use of combinations of fluoride with substances that seemed likely to increase mineralization – vitamin D, calcium salts and oestrogens (which oppose the resorption of bone) (Jowsey *et al.*, 1972). A detailed study on 165 patients was reported by Riggs *et al.* (1982) in which various combinations of these substances were tested over 4 years. They found that calcium alone reduced the fracture rate (the most useful criterion for success) to half, but when combined with 40–60 mg NaF daily and oestrogens it fell to 10%, although fluoride had no effect in some patients. About one-third of the patients receiving fluoride had side-effects (nausea and vomiting or painful joints), which were so severe in 5 that they discontinued the treatment.

In a later 4-year trial (Riggs, Hodgson and O'Fallon, 1990), 202 post-menopausal women with vertebral fractures all received 1500 mg Ca daily and half of them had, in addition, 75 mg NaF. The mineral density of the lumbar spine (mostly cancellous bone) increased in the fluoride group by 35%, of the femur neck and trochanter (mixed cancellous and cortical bone) by 12% and 10%, respectively, and in the shaft of the radius (cortical bone) density *decreased* by 4%. The number of vertebral fractures was similar in both the fluoride and placebo groups, but the fluoride group incurred significantly more non-vertebral fractures. As in the earlier trial, many patients had side-effects necessitating a reduction in dose. Overall, this survey, along with others quoted by Riggs, Hodgson and O'Fallon (1990), does not support the clinical efficacy of a combination of F and Ca as a treatment for osteoporosis.

In cases of myelomatosis, once the myelomatosis is controlled by melphalan and corticosteroids (which correct the hypercalcaemia), sodium fluoride (30–60 mg/day) has been used to produce recalcification of the myeloma bone lesions without, as far as can be judged, affecting the underlying cellular abnormality (Carbone *et al.*, 1968).

Sodium fluoride (30–60 mg/day) was reported by Rich and Ensinck (1961) to reduce bone resorption and improve calcium balance in one case of Paget's disease. This was confirmed by Bernstein *et al.* (1963), but later denied by Higgins *et al.* (1965) on the basis of balance studies in three cases.

Sodium fluoride (4–6 mg/day) was said to reduce the fracture rate in one 20-month-old girl (Kuzemko, 1970) suffering from osteogenesis imperfecta, but so little is known of the real nature of this disease that no rational therapy can be recommended.

Fluoride intoxication: effect on teeth

Dental fluorosis is a specific disturbance of tooth formation caused by excessive fluoride intake. The clinical features of dental fluorosis are extremely variable. It is characterized clinically by lustreless, opaque white patches in the enamel which may be mottled, striated and/or pitted. The mottled areas may become stained yellow or brown. The affected teeth may show a pronounced accentuation of the perikymata, or have multiple pits. Hypoplastic areas may also be present to such an extent in severe cases that the normal tooth form is lost (Pindborg, 1970) (see Chapter 13).

Histology of fluorosed enamel

The histology of fluorosed enamel has been studied by the diffusion of stains such as silver nitrate, by chemical analysis, microradiography and measurements of birefringence with polarized light. The information from these methods suggests that the general arrangement of enamel into rods (prisms) is unchanged in fluorosis and that the underlying defect is hypomineralization accompanied by a higher proportion of protein than normal. The main features are well-mineralized outer layers and patchy areas of hypomineralization within the enamel extending, in mild cases, to about one-third of the thickness of the enamel; in severe cases (with water containing F >4 ppm) it may reach one-half to three-quarters the thickness. The rod cores seem relatively normal, but the intra-rod regions are wider and radiolucent and contain more protein. Polarized light studies show that in severe cases as much as between 10% and 25% of the mineral matter may be missing. The smaller degree of mineralization between the rods explains the greater permeability of fluoridated enamel and the ability of pigments or substances forming pigments to diffuse into the enamel and cause the yellow to brown stains.

Sensitivity of ameloblasts

The finding that enamel fluorosis is the first known toxic effect of fluoride has been interpreted as evidence that ameloblasts are the most sensitive cells in the body to fluoride. This is possibly true, although opponents of fluoridation point out that other cells may be equally or even more sensitive but changes in the tissues they produce are not so readily observed as in the enamel. An alternative explanation for the sensitivity of ameloblasts is that they are exposed to higher concentrations of fluoride than other cells (except perhaps osteoblasts), as fluoride accumulates and is released in the vicinity of the Ca taking part in mineralization and remodelling of bone.

Histopathology of dental fluorosis

The way in which fluoride might exert its effect has been studied principally using chemical and histopathological techniques. Bowes and Murray (1936) demonstrated a higher protein content in fluorosed enamel than in non-mottled enamel. This finding was confirmed by Bhussry (1959) and by later workers (reviewed by Richards, 1990).

An observation of great theoretical interest is that although the outermost layer of shark's teeth contains more than 100 times the fluoride content of human mottled enamel, there are no signs of disturbance in its mineralization. Using biophysical and chemical methods, Glas (1962) demonstrated that the size and orientation of the apatite crystallites in the shark 'enamel' and its degree of mineralization were the same as in human enamel. In contrast to the hydroxyapatite occurring in human enamel, the inorganic phase of shark 'enamel' consists of an almost pure fluorapatite, which is formed during normal mineralization (Buttner, 1966). Unlike human enamel, which is of epithelial origin, the shark 'enamel' develops from mesodermal tissues (Kvam, 1950) and has been referred to as 'durodentin' and 'petrodentin' (Lison, 1941; Schmidt and Keil, 1958).

Experimental dental fluorosis

Experimental dental fluorosis has been studied by peritoneal injections of fluoride (causing acute fluorosis) or by adding fluorides to drinking water or diet (causing chronic fluorosis). Acute fluorosis produces horizontal bands of pigment-free areas of the rat incisor enamel corresponding to the timing of injections. It is possible to detect histologic changes in the ameloblasts of the rat incisor as early as 1 h after the injection of fluoride. Injections of high concentrations of fluoride at intervals of a few days cause an accentuation of the incremental lines in enamel and dentine, changes which may be utilized in determining the amount of dentine formed during a given period (Schour and Smith, 1934).

As a result of dosages of fluoride much higher than those normally received by human subjects, four abnormalities may be seen in dentine: striations, hypoplastic defects, hypomineralized interglobular spaces, and gross deformations of the external outline of the dentine (Yaeger, 1966). Such changes have not been described in human fluorosed teeth (Pindborg, 1970).

Experimental production of fluorosis

Angmar-Mansson and Whitford (1982, 1984, 1985) have administered fluoride to rats in different ways and on different time schedules and have related the plasma fluoride to histological or radiological changes in the enamel.

The experiments have shown that doses for 1 week producing daily peaks in the plasma fluoride of 10 μmol (0.19 ppm) lead to disturbances in enamel mineralization but peaks of 5 μmol did not, even when produced twice a day. When maintained at steady levels, by subcutaneous constant infusions, plasma levels of 3.3 μmol (0.06 ppm) produced an increased incidence of defective enamel and at 4.7 μmol (0.09 ppm) the changes consistently occurred (Angmar-Mansson and Whitford, 1982). In a similar later experiment but carried on for 56 days, this general conclusion was confirmed, but in addition it was found that constant plasma concentration as low as 1.5 μmol (0.028 ppm) caused slight but definite interference with enamel formation, visible in those parts of the incisor incompletely mineralized. When the fully mineralized parts of the incisors were examined, it was found that only plasma levels of 7 μmol, and 12.5 μmol produced by 25 and 60 ppm F in the drinking water, had affected the enamel: with the lower concentration the effects visible in the earlier stage of mineralization had disappeared by the time mineralization was completed (Angmar-Mansson and Whitford, 1984). It was noted that at the plasma fluoride levels that produced impaired enamel, the plasma Ca was normal – evidence that dental fluorosis is caused by some mechanism other than lack of minerals.

In a further experiment, single doses of fluoride ranging from 0.75 to 14.0 mg were injected, the animals were killed and the teeth were examined microradiographically 15, 35 or 70 days after the injections which had caused a rise in plasma fluoride (and with the higher doses, a fall in plasma Ca) only for 24 h (Angmar-Mansson and Whitford, 1985). Estimations of the F and P of the enamel 15 days (but not at 35 or 70 days) after the doses showed, in spite of a plasma returned to normal, under-mineralization and increased fluoride concentration measurable even with the lowest dose, but marked with the higher doses. Slight disturbances in the parts of the enamel still only partially mineralized were found microradiographically, with the higher doses in animals killed 35 and 70 days after dosing.

The authors suggested that the most reasonable explanation for changes occurring so long after the dose and with normal plasma composition is that the fluoride became attached to the bone adjacent to the enamel organ and is slowly released in concentrations sufficient to affect the metabolism of the ameloblast. Another possibility not mentioned by Angmar-Mansson and Whitford is that the dose caused a prolonged damage to ameloblasts. It is clear that the injury was not caused by lack of Ca.

This work incidentally throws light on the previously unexplained fact that most experiments have shown that 10 ppm F in drinking water was needed by rats to have an anti-caries effect similar to 1 ppm F in human subjects. However, the plasma concentrations producing fluorosis in humans and rats are very similar: evidently the need for higher intake to produce fluorosis and prevent caries involves the control of plasma levels and does not arise from different sensitivities of the ameloblasts.

Stages of enamel formation

In what is called the secretory stage, the ameloblasts synthesize and secrete the enamel matrix – a mixture of two unusual proteins, amelogenins and enamelins – along with a mineral concentration about one-third that of the final enamel. When the full thickness of the enamel matrix has been formed and the shape of the crown determined by the position of the ameloblasts, the 'maturation stage' begins. Proteolytic enzymes break down the amelogenins and the breakdown products are removed, along with water, while simultaneously additional minerals enter so that the enamelins become fully mineralized, the inner layers next to the dentine being mineralized first. In rodents with continuously growing incisors, all stages are present even in adult animals.

Site of fluoride activity in fluorosis

As already mentioned, fluorosed enamel is under-mineralized and contains a higher percentage of protein than normal enamel. There are three ways in which this defect might arise: (a) there might be excessive secretion of proteins or there might be differences in their amino acid composition so that they resisted the later removal; (b) the proteolysis of amelogenins which precedes their removal might be inhibited; or (c) the removal of the amelogenins might be reduced and this would prevent the entry of the normal amount of mineral. Experiments with very high unphysiological doses of fluoride have shown that all three effects may occur, but evidence is accumulating that it is at the maturation stage that the levels of fluoride most comparable with those present in human plasma exert their effect. For example, in an experiment on pigs, 2 mg F/kg body weight was fed for 8 months and only those teeth receiving fluoride at the maturation stage were fluorosed (Richards *et al.*, 1986). The plasma fluoride in the experimental group showed peaks of as high as 70 μmol immediately after dosing, with pre-dose levels varying from 5 μmol at the beginning of the experiment to 12 μmol at the end. The rise during the experiment would occur because the bone fluoride would increase from the fairly high dosage and plasma fluoride reaches an equilibrium with that of bone.

Clinical data on the occurrence of mild fluorosis in 110 children in Umanak, Greenland, in relation to the time at which they had received 0.5 mg fluoride tablets also showed that the fluoride given only at the late secretion or early maturation stage caused fluorosis (Larsen, Richards and Fejerskov, 1985). The evidence cannot be regarded as final because the number of children in this experiment was small and there was still uncertainty about the ages at which the various types of teeth go through the stages of enamel development.

Biochemical experiments also suggest that two-dimensional gel electrophoresis of secretory proteins of rats, with and without fluoride in their drinking water for 5 weeks, failed to show any difference in the composition of the matrix even with the highest of the range of dosage used (100 ppm). This implies that fluoride did not affect the composition of secretory enamel. Gel chromatography of the early maturation proteins, however, showed that, even with the lowest fluoride intakes of 25 ppm, there were much greater quantities of the higher molecular weight amelogenins than in the control, clearly supporting the conclusion that it was at the maturation stage (probably by reduced removal of amelogenins) and not during secretion that fluorosis is caused (DenBesten, 1986).

Patterson, Basford and Kruger (1976) found that the absolute amount of protein secreted by ameloblasts was reduced and its amino acid composition changed in rats given 50 ppm in the drinking water for 10 days. This may be due to a reduction in the amount of enamel matrix formed (as found by DenBesten) and to changes in the proportion of amelogenins to enamelins secreted, as suggested by Eastoe (1979), rather than to changes in the composition of the proteins (DenBesten and Crenshaw, 1984). As mentioned on page 297, Kruger (1970) reported that protein synthesis by ameloblasts was reduced by fluoride.

Effect of high altitude on fluoride metabolism

Exposure to high altitudes leads to alkalosis, as the oxygen lack stimulates respiration and more CO_2 is expelled than the body is producing. This would be expected to increase urinary excretion of fluoride and lead to lower tissue levels. Whitford *et al.* (1983) found the reverse in rats exposed to low atmospheric pressure. This fits in with the finding that fluorosis is more severe at high altitudes than at sea level, but the explanation is still uncertain.

In further experiments on rats, Angmar-Mansson *et al.* (1984) discovered that exposure to low atmospheric pressure, simulating residence at 18 000 ft (5500 m), enhanced the effect of fluoride on the bones and teeth and led to disordered mineralization of the enamel even when fluoride supplements were absent. It seems likely that this disorder among human populations living at high altitudes has been sometimes mistaken for fluorosis and raises the question as to whether fluoride dosage should be reduced in towns at a high altitude.

The explanation of this effect is not known, but a possibility is suggested by the experiments of Birdsong-Whitford, Dickinson and Whitford (1986) on the effect of the haematocrit on the distribution of fluoride between plasma and cells. When the haematocrit was increased, the fluoride of the plasma rose at the expense of the fluoride in the red cells and the polycythaemia induced by residence at high altitudes would therefore tend to raise plasma fluoride.

Fluoride as a factor in repetitive strain injury

Repetitive strain injury (RSI) is a recently recognized syndrome in which patients who carry out repetitive movements with their hands (e.g. musicians and typists) suffer from pain in the wrists, forearm, hands and fingers. Smith (1985a) reported that bone samples, removed after dental extractions from the alveolar bone between the roots of molars, from 12 RSI patients in Melbourne, Australia, contained significantly higher fluoride concentrations (mean 2734 ppm) than 12 controls of similar age free from the disease (1687 ppm). It was also stated (Smith, 1985b) that 8 of the patients experienced a marked relief from symptoms when they ingested less fluoride (and more magnesium which was considered to be low in their diet). Smith (1985b) suggests that excess fluoride released from bone may affect neighbouring cells adversely, in an unknown way, and cause the symptoms. No other work along these lines appears to have been reported.

Acute fluoride poisoning

A review by Hodge and Smith (1965) of the 607 fatal cases of fluoride poisoning (mostly suicides) then known, concluded that the fatal dose of sodium fluoride was between 5 and 10 g (2.2 and 4.4 g F) for a typical adult weighing 70 kg (32–64 mg F/kg body weight). The basis for this conclusion was somewhat arbitrary, however, because neither the precise dose nor the body weight of most of the victims was known.

It would obviously be impossible for fluoridated water to cause acute fluoride poisoning, because in order to receive 1 g F one would have to consume 1000 litres of water. However, the availability of tablets, gels and mouthrinses containing potentially lethal doses of fluoride does present a problem which can be minimized by the use of child-proof containers (see pages 357–360). The plasma fluoride after the application (without the use of saliva ejectors) of a gel containing 1.23% F was studied in 8 subjects by Ekstrand *et al.* (1981). The concentration rose from a baseline value of 0.012 ppm to, in two out of the eight subjects, more than 1 ppm for over 2 h and, in the subjects least affected, reached a peak of 0.3 ppm. The highest levels probably exceed the nephrotoxic dose and may lead to diuresis. The direct irritant effect of HF formed in the stomach is probably responsible for the gastric discomfort which has occasionally been reported following the use of fluoride gels.

Three fatal cases of poisoning by such products are on record. In one, a 3-year-old boy swallowed 45 ml of a 4% SnF_2 mouthrinse (about 435 mg F) and died 3 h later (Church, 1976); in another case, death occurred 7 h after swallowing 200 fluoride tablets (Eichler *et al.*, 1982); and in the third, a 27-month-old boy died 5 days after swallowing about 100 0.5 mg F tablets – a probable dose of less than 5 mg/kg body weight (Dukes, 1980) which can therefore be regarded as the potentially lethal dose.

The most serious accidental poisoning from fluoride occurred in Oregon State Hospital where 17 lb (8 kg) of NaF (used as an insecticide) were inadvertently added, in a mistake for powdered milk, to 10 US gal (38 litres) of scrambled eggs being prepared in the hospital kitchen. As a result, 236 of the patients became ill, of whom 47 died (Lidbeck, Hill and Beeman, 1943).

The symptoms of acute fluoride poisoning are nausea, vomiting and gastrointestinal pain, followed later by muscular weakness, spasms and tetany as the fluoride combines with blood Ca ions. Emergency treatment consists of emptying the stomach by stomach pump or emetic (with precautions to avoid inhalation of the vomit) and providing Ca-containing solutions to precipitate the fluoride and to restore blood Ca (Bayliss and Tinanoff, 1985; Whitford, 1987). It is suggested that if the dose exceeds 5 mg F/kg body weight, the patient should be sent to hospital.

An important site of a toxic reaction is the stomach. When fluoride is swallowed and reacts with the HCl of the gastric juice, it is converted into the highly irritant HF. Concentrations of 10 mmol/litre (190 ppm) have been shown in dogs and rats to produce effects varying from patchy loss of the mucous membrane to erosion sufficiently severe to expose the underlying lamina propria (for references see Whitford, 1990). The threshold for changes in gastric function is between 1 and 5 mmol F/litre (19–95 ppm), concentrations that could be reached by swallowing several dental products in small amounts (e.g. 2.0 ml of APF gel).

The original studies on the toxicity of MFP suggested that it is less toxic than NaF, but this has not been confirmed by more recent work (Whitford, 1990). Although the general systemic effects of MFP and NaF are similar (because MFP is broken down to F ions in the blood), MFP is much less toxic to the stomach where it remains largely intact (see page 276) and is not itself an irritant. This may not be important in choosing a toothpaste, because very little is swallowed, but may be a major factor in treating osteoporosis which involves large and prolonged dosage.

References

Angmar-Mansson, B. and Whitford, G. A. (1982) Plasma fluoride levels and enamel fluorosis in the rat. *Caries Res.*, **16**, 334–339

Angmar-Mansson, B. and Whitford, G. M. (1984) Enamel fluorosis related to plasma F levels in the rat. *Caries Res.*, **18**, 25–32

Angmar-Mansson, B. and Whitford, G. A. (1985) Single fluoride doses and enamel fluorosis in the rat. *Caries Res.*, **19**, 145–152

Angmar-Mansson, B., Whitford, G. M., Allison, N. B., Devine, J. A. and Maher, J. T. (1984) Effects of simulated altitude on fluoride retention and enamel quality. *Caries Res.*, **18**, 165 (Abstract 36)

Baylink, D. J., Duane, P. B., Farley, S. M. and Farley, J. R. (1983) Monofluorophosphate physiology: the effects of fluoride on bone. *Caries Res.*, **17**, Suppl. 1, 56–76

Baylink, D. J., Wergedal, J., Stauffer, M. and Rich, C. (1970) Effects of fluoride on bone formation, mineralization, and resorption in the rat. In *Fluoride in Medicine* (ed. T. K. Vischer), Huber, Berne, pp. 37–69

Bayliss, J. S. and Tinanoff, N. (1985) Diagnosis and treatment of acute fluoride toxicity. *J. Am. Dent. Ass.*, **110**, 209–211

Bernstein, D. S. *et al.* (1963) The use of sodium fluoride in metabolic bone disease. *J. Clin. Invest.*, **42**, 916

Bhussry, B. R. (1959) Chemical and physical studies of enamel from human teeth, IV. Density and nitrogen content of mottled enamel. *J. Dent. Res.*, **38**, 369–373

Birdsong-Whitford, N. L., Dickinson, A. and Whitford, G. M. (1986) Effect of haematocrit on plasma F concentrations. *J. Dent. Res.*, **184** (Abstract 129)

Bowes, J. H. and Murray, M. M. (1936) A chemical study of 'mottled teeth' from Malden, Essex. *Br. Dent. J.*, **60**, 556–562

Buttner, W. (1966) In *Advances in Fluorine Research and Dental Caries Prevention* (eds P. M. C. James *et al.*), Proceedings 12th O.R.C.A. Congress, Utrecht, 1965, Vol. 4, pp. 193–200

Carbone, P. P., Zipkin, I., Sokoloff, L. *et al.* (1968) Fluoride effect on bone in plasma cell myeloma. *Arch. Intern. Med.*, **121**, 130–140

Church, L. E. (1976) Fluorides: use with caution. *Maryland Dent. Ass.*, **19**, 106

DenBesten, P. K. (1986) Effect of fluoride on protein secretion and removal during enamel development in the rat. *J. Dent. Res.*, **65**, 1272–1277

DenBesten, P. K. and Crenshaw, K. (1984) The effect of chronic high fluoride levels on forming enamel in the rat. *Arch. Oral Biol.*, **29**, 675–679

Dukes, M. N. G. (1980) Fluorides. In *Side Effects of Drugs Annual*, Vol. 4, Excerpta Medica, Oxford, p. 354

Eastoe, J. E. (1979) Enamel protein chemistry – past, present and future. *J. Dent. Res.*, **58**, 753–763

Eichler, H. G., Lenz, K., Fuhrmann, M. and Hruby, K. (1982) Accidental ingestion of NaF tablets by children: report of a poison control centre and one case. *Int. J. Clin. Pharmacol. Ther. Toxicol.*, **20**, 334–338

Ekstrand, J., Koch, G., Lindgren, L. E. and Petersson, L. G. (1981) Pharmacokinetics of fluoride gels in children and adults. *Caries Res.*, **15**, 213–220

Faccini, J. M. (1969) Fluoride and bone. *Calcif. Tissue Res.*, **3**, 1–16

Geever, E. F., Leone, N. C., Geiser, P. and Lieberman, J. E. (1958a) Pathological studies in man after prolonged ingestion of fluoride in drinking water. *Public Health Rep.*, **73**, 721–731

Geever, E. F., Leone, N. C., Geiser, P. and Lieberman, J. E. (1985b) Pathological studies in man after prolonged ingestion of fluoride in drinking water, I. Necropsy findings in a community with a water level of 2.5 ppm. *J. Am. Dent. Assoc.*, **56**, 499–507

Glas, J. E. (1962) Studies on the ultrastructure of dental enamel, VI. Crystal chemistry of shark's teeth. *Odont. Revy*, **13**, 315–326

Higgins, B. A., Nassim, J. R., Alexander, R. and Hilb, A. (1965) Effect of sodium fluoride on calcium phosphorus and nitrogen balance in patients with Paget's disease. *Br. Med. J.*, **1**, 1159–1161

Hodge, H. C. and Smith, F. A. (1965) Biological properties of inorganic fluorides. In *Fluoride Chemistry* (ed. J. H. Simons), Academic Press, New York, pp. 1–42

Jowsey, J., Riggs, B. L., Kelly, P. J. and Hoffman, D. L. (1972) Effects of combined therapy with sodium fluoride, vitamin D and calcium in osteoporosis. *Am. J. Med.*, **53**, 43–49

Kuzemko, J. A. (1970) Osteogenesis imperfecta tarda treated with sodium fluoride. *Arch. Dis. Child.*, **45**, 581–582

Kvam, T. (1950) *K. Norske Vidensk. Selskab.* (*Trondhjem*)

Largent, E. J., Bovard, P. G. and Heyroth, F. F. (1951) Roentgenographic changes and urinary fluoride excretion among workmen engaged in the manufacture of inorganic fluorides. *Am. J. Roentgenol. Radium Ther. Nucl. Med.*, **65**, 42–48

Larsen, M. J., Richards, A. and Fejerskov, O. (1985) Development of dental fluorosis according to age at start of fluoride administration. *Caries Res.*, **19**, 514–527

Leone, N. C., Shimkin, M. B., Arnold, F. A., Stevenson, C. A., Zimmerman, E. R., Geiser, P. B. and Lieberman, J. E. (1954) Medical aspects of excessive fluoride in a water supply. *Public Health Rep.*, **69**, 925–936

Lidbeck, W. L., Hill, I. B. and Beeman, J. (1943) Acute sodium fluoride poisoning. *J. Am. Med. Ass.*, **121**, 826–827

Lison, L. (1941) Sur la structure des dents poissons dipneustes. La Petrodentine. *C. R. Séanc. Soc. Biol.* (*Paris*), **135**, 431–443

Liu, C. C. and Baylink, D. J. (1977) Stimulation of bone formation and bone resorption by fluoride in thyroparathyroidectomised rats. *J. Dent. Res.*, **56**, 304–311

Morris, J. W. (1965) Skeletal fluorosis among Indians of the American South West. *Am. J. Roentgenol. Radium Ther. Nucl. Med.*, **94**, 608–615

Nordin, B. E. C. (1973) *Metabolic Bone and Stone Disease*, Churchill Livingstone, Edinburgh

Ockerse, T. (1946) *Endemic Fluorosis in South Africa. Thesis*, University of Witwatersrand. Pretoria, Government Printers

Patterson, C. M., Basford, K. E. and Kruger, B. J. (1976) The effect of fluoride on the immature enamel matrix of the rat. *Arch. Oral Biol.*, **21**, 131–132

Patterson, C. M., Kruger, B. J. and Dales, J. J. (1977) Differences in fluoride levels in the blood between sheep, rabbit and rat. *Arch. Oral Biol.*, **22,** 419–423

Pindborg, J. J. (1970) *Pathology of the Dental Hard Tissues*, Copenhagen, Munksgaard

Posner, A. S., Eanes, E. D., Harper, R. A. and Zipkin, I. (1963) X-ray diffraction analysis of the effect of fluoride on human bone apatite. *Arch. Oral Biol.*, **8,** 549–570

Raisz, L. G. and Taves, D. R. (1967) The effect of fluoride in parathyroid function and responsiveness in the rat. *Calcif. Tiss. Res.*, **1**, 219–228

Rich, C. and Ensinck, J. (1961) Effect of sodium fluoride on calcium metabolism of human beings. *Nature* (*Lond.*), **191**, 184–185

Richards, A. (1990) Nature and mechanisms of dental fluorosis in animals. *J. Dent. Res.*, **69**, 701–705

Richards, A., Kragstrup, J., Josephsen, K. and Fejerskov, O. (1986) Dental fluorosis developed in post-secretory enamel. *J. Dent. Res.*, **65**, 1406–1409

Riggs, B. L., Hodgson, S. F. and O'Fallon, W. M. (1990) Effect of fluoride treatment on the fracture rate of postmenopausal women with osteoporosis. *N. Engl. J. Med.*, **322**, 802–809

Riggs, B. L., Seeman, E., Hodgson, S. F., Taves, D. R. and O'Fallon, W. M. (1982) Effect of the fluoride/calcium regimen on vertebral fracture occurrence in postmenopausal osteoporosis: comparison with conventional therapy. *N. Engl. J. Med.*, **306**, 446–450

Roholm, K. (1937) *Fluorine Intoxication: A Clinical-hygienic Study with a Review of the Literature and Some Experimental Investigations*, London, Lewis

Russell, A. L. (1964) In *The Dentist, His Practice and His Community* (eds W. O. Young and D. F. Striffer), Saunders, Philadelphia

Schenk, R. K., Merz, W. A. and Reutter, F. W. (1970) Fluoride in osteoporosis: quantitative histological studies on bone structure and bone remodelling in serial biopsies of the iliac crest. In *Fluoride in Medicine* (ed. T. L. Vischer), Huber, Berne, pp. 153–168

Schlesinger, E. R., Overton, D. E., Chase, H. C. and Cantwell, K. T. (1956) Newburgh–Kingston caries-fluorine study, XIII. Pediatric findings after ten years. *J. Am. Dent. Ass.*, **52**, 296–306

Schmidt, W. J. and Keil, A. (1958) *Die gesunden und die erkrankten Zahngewebe des Menschen und der Wirbeltiere im Polarisationsmikroskop.* Hanser, Munich

Schour, I. and Smith, M. C. (1934) The histological changes in enamel and dentine of rat incisor in acute chronic experimental fluorosis. *Univ. Arizona Agric. Exp. Stat. Tech. Bull.*, **52**, 69–91

Singh, A., Dass, R., Hayreh, S. S. and Jolly, S. S. (1962) Skeletal changes in endemic fluorosis. *J. Bone Joint Surg.*, **44B**, 806–815

Singh, M. and Susheela, A. K. (1982) Adenyl cyclase activity and cystic AMP levels following F^- ingestion in rabbits and human subjects. *Fluoride,* **15**, 202–208

Smith, G. E. (1985a) Simple method for obtaining bone biopsy specimens for fluoride analysis and some preliminary results. *N.Z. Med. J.*, **98**, 454–455

Smith, G. E. (1985b) Repetitive strain injury (RSI) and magnesium and fluoride intake. *N.Z. Med. J.*, **98**, 556–557

Srikantia, S. G. and Siddiqui, A. H. (1965) Metabolic studies in skeletal fluorosis. *Clin. Sci.*, **28**, 477–485

Steinberg, C. L., Gardner, D. E., Smith, F. A. and Hodge, H. C. (1955) Comparison of rheumatoid (ankylosing) spondylitis and crippling fluorosis. *Ann. Rheum. Dis.*, **14**, 378–384

Stevenson, C. A. and Watson, A. R. (1957) Fluoride osteosclerosis. *Am. J. Roentgenol. Radium Ther. Nucl. Med.*, **78**, 13–18

Susheela, A. K. and Sharma, Y. D. (1982) Certain facets of F^- action on collagen protein in osseous and non-osseous tissue. *Fluoride,* **15**, 177–190

Weatherell, J. A. and Weidmann, S. M. (1959) The skeletal changes of chronic experimental fluorosis. *J. Pathol. Bacteriol.*, **78**, 233–241

Weidmann, S. M., Weatherell, J. A. and Jackson, D. (1963) The effect of fluoride on bone. *Proc. Nutr. Soc.*, **22**, 105–110

Whitford, G. M. (1987) Fluoride in dental products: safety considerations. *J. Dent. Res.*, **66**, 1056–1060

Whitford, G. M. (1990) *The Metabolism and Toxicity of Fluoride*, Monographs in Oral Science No. 13, Karger, Basel

Whitford, G. M., Allison, N. B., Devine, J. A., Maher, J. T. and Angmar-Mansson, B. (1983) Fluoride metabolism at simulated altitude. *J. Dent. Res.*, **62**, 262 (Abstract 840)

World Health Organisation (1970) *Fluorides and Human Health*, WHO Monogr. Ser. No. 59, WHO, Geneva, pp. 278–279

Yaeger, J. A. (1966) The effects of high fluoride diets on developing enamel and dentine in the incisors of rats. *Am. J. Anat.*, **118**, 665–683

Zipkin, I. and McClure, F. J. (1952) Deposition of fluoride in bone and teeth of growing rats. *J. Dent. Res.*, **31**, 494–495 (Abstract)

Zipkin, I., McClure, F. J. and Lee, W. A. (1960) Relation of the fluoride content of human bone to its chemical composition. *Arch. Oral Biol.*, **2**, 190–195

Chapter 17

Health and water fluoridation

It has been suggested over the years that many different disorders can be caused or aggravated by fluoridation. A summary of these disorders, compiled by the Royal College of Physicians (1976), is given in Table 17.1. Recently, further information on urban mortality, cancer mortality and congenital malformation in relation to fluoridation has been published and these data will be reviewed.

Urban mortality

Rogot *et al.* (1978) sampled 473 urban areas of the USA that had populations of over 25 000 in 1950. These cities had a combined population of 61 million in 1950 and 71 million in 1970, constituting 40.6% and 35%, respectively, of the total US population in those years. Numbers of deaths from all causes and from cardiovascular, renal and heart disease and cancer separately in each urban area were obtained from official vital statistics for the years 1949–50, 1959–61 and 1969–71. To allow comparison of mortality in cities whose age, race and sex compositions varied, the method of indirect adjustment was employed using the US 1960 mortality rates as standard.

For the three census years 1950, 1960 and 1970, each city's population in each of 76 age–race–sex subgroups was multiplied by the US 1960 standard rates and by the number of years in the peri-censal period to give the expected number of deaths in that city for the particular census period. The ratio of the number of deaths which occurred to the number of deaths expected was called the 'mortality ratio'. The Average Mortality Ratio (AMR) was obtained for groups of cities by summing individual mortality ratios for each city and dividing by the number of cities in the group. (This gives cities equal weight to one another. In preliminary analyses, average mortality ratios weighted by city size were also used. The results of the two sets of analyses were similar.)

Of the 473 study cities, 260 had fluoridated some time before 1970 and 213 had not. Of the fluoridated cities, 26 had discontinued fluoridation at some time before 1970, 4 had incomplete coverage and 3 had been on water with a high natural fluoride content before switching sources and fluoridating. These 33 cities were considered of uncertain fluoridation status, leaving for analysis 227 cities which originally received water with a low fluoride content, then fluoridated, and maintained complete and continuous coverage until 1970. Of the cities which never fluoridated, 187 were using water with an average fluoride content of less than 0.7 ppm and 26 had water ranging from 0.7 to 2.7 ppm F.

Table 17.1 Disorders claimed to be caused or aggravated by fluoridation (From Royal College of Physicians, 1976)

Gastrointestinal disorders:	Flatulence Nausea Abdominal pain Vomiting Haematemesis Peptic ulcer	Diarrhoea Constipation Gingivitis Stomatitis Oral ulcers
Neurological and mental disorders:	Headache Migraine Depression Paraesthesiae Painful numbness in the limbs	Mental deterioration Convulsions Personality change Deafness
Urinary tract disorders:	Urethritis Cystitis Pyelitis	Nephritis
Skin disorders:	Urticaria Rashes Dermatoses	Furunculosis Brittle nails Alopecia
Musculoskeletal disorders:	Skeletal Fluororis Backache Pain or muscular assertion of the ribs (sic)	Arthritis Renal osteodystrophy Scheuermann's disease
Dental disorders:	Mottling of the teeth	
Ocular disorders:	Optic neuritis	
Endocrine disorders:	Thyroid enlargement Diabetes mellitus	Parathyroid disorders Adrenal disorders
Cardiovascular disorders:	Heart disease Arteriosclerosis	
Congenital malformations:	Mongolism Anencephalus Spina bifida	
Non-specific disorders:	Lethargy Exhaustion after sleep Muscular weakness	

Table 17.2 Populations and Average Mortality Ratios (AMR) for 1950, 1960 and 1970 periods and average percentage change from 1950 to 1970, 1950 to 1960, and 1960 to 1970 for cities by fluoridation status: US, selected study cities (From Rogot *et al.*, 1978)

*Fluoridation group**	*Combined population (millions)*			*AMR*			*Average % change from*		
	1950	*1960*	*1970*	*1950*	*1960*	*1970*	*1950–1970*	*1950–1960*	*1960–1970*
F	37.7	39.6	40.5	1.13	1.03	0.97	−14	−8	−6
NF	17.9	20.7	22.4	1.16	1.07	0.99	−14	−7	−7
H	2.1	3.1	4.0	1.19	1.02	0.96	−19	−14	−6
U	3.6	4.2	4.4	1.15	1.02	0.97	−15	−10	−5
T	61.2	67.5	71.1	1.15	1.05	0.98	−14	−8	−6

* F, 227 cities that fluoridated in the period 1945–69; NF, 187 cities with low natural fluoride (less than 0.7 ppm), that had not fluoridated by 1970; H, 26 cities with high natural fluoride (0.7 ppm or greater); U, 33 cities of uncertain fluoridation status; T, total of 473 cities.

The findings for total deaths is given in Table 17.2. The AMR for the 227 cities which had fluoridated declined from 1.13 to 0.97 over the 20-year period; the corresponding figures for the 187 non-fluoridated cities were 1.16–0.99. For the fluoridated cities, 11 cities showed increases in their AMR; for the non-fluoridated group, 10 cities showed increases in their AMR. Overall the basic trend showed a decline in mortality over the 20 years of the study – a mean percentage drop of 13.5 in fluoridated cities compared with 13.6 in the non-fluoridated cities. The overall findings clearly showed no consistent relation between fluoridation and observed changes in mortality over the 20-year period studied.

Cancer mortality

Data purporting to show the age dependence of cancer mortality related to artificial fluoridation have been put forward by Yiamouyiannis and Burk (1977). The 10 largest fluoridated cities in the USA were taken as the experimental group. The 10 largest cities in the USA which had not fluoridated as of 1969 but had a cancer death rate greater than 155 per 100 000 per year were taken as the control group. The results show that the crude cancer death rates of both groups of cities had a strikingly similar trend between 1940 and 1950. Subsequent to fluoridation, however, a divergence could be observed that was maintained up to 1969, the last year of the study. The authors deduced from their data that 25 000 excess cancer deaths per year would be caused by fluoridation of all US water supplies (Figure 17.1).

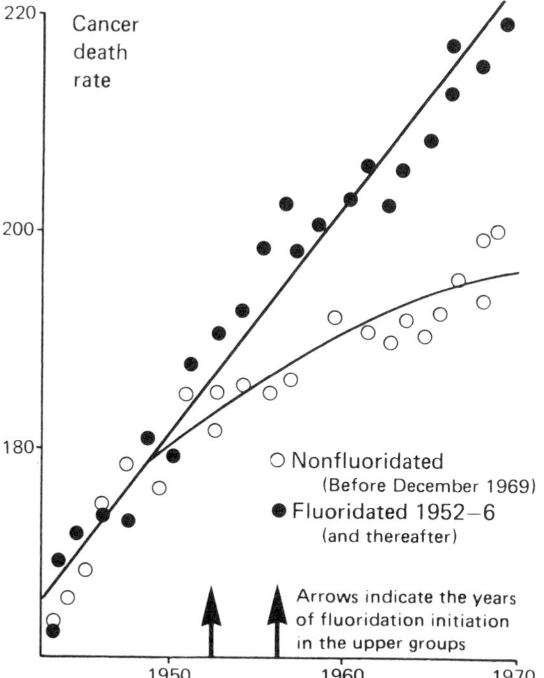

Figure 17.1 Comparison of cancer death rates in the 10 largest American cities fluoridated since 1952–56 with 10 American cities which had not fluoridated before 1969 (From Yiamouyiannis and Burk, 1977). See text for discussion of these data

The US National Cancer Institute asserted that the rise in cancer deaths could be explained by the different age–sex–race structures of the population in the two groups of cities, and this aspect was considered further by Oldham and Newell (1977), on behalf of the Royal Statistical Society (England) at the request of the Royal College of Physicians, London. They reported: 'Our analysis shows that the two groups of 10 cities differed in their age–sex–race structure in 1950. The cities which were to be fluoridated started with many fewer elderly white females, somewhat fewer elderly white males and more non-whites at all ages below 50. By 1970, the two sets of cities differed much more in their demographic structure than they had in 1950. The fluoridated cities now had many more non-whites of all ages in their populations, and many fewer whites under the age of 55. When the demographic changes are taken into account we find, in proportional terms, that the excess cancer rate increased by 1% over the 20 years in the fluoridated cities, but it also increased by 4% in the unfluoridated control cities, giving a difference of 3% to the advantage of the fluoridated cities.' This point is also made by Newbrun (1977), who showed that although Yiamouyiannis and Burk (1977) claimed that the death rate from cancer increased in San Francisco after fluoridation, their supporting data were not adjusted for age. The US Census shows a steady increase in the older population residing in San Francisco. The percentage of the population of people over 65 was 9.7% in 1950 but had risen to 14.1% by 1970; as cancer mortality rate increases dramatically with advancing age it is not surprising that San Francisco cancer mortality rates rose during the 20-year period. However, if the change in the age distribution is taken into account, there is no trend in the cancer mortality rate in San Francisco (Table 17.3).

Table 17.3 San Francisco – population and cancer mortality rates 1950–70 (From Newbrun, 1977)

Year	*Total population*	*Age 65 and over*		*Cancer mortality rates (per 100 000)*	
		No.	*% of total*	*Unadjusted*	*Age adjusted**
1950	762 082	74 050	9.7	239	239
1960	727 898	91 603	12.6	249	216
1970	706 601	99 738	14.1	266	230

* San Francisco's water supply has been fluoridated since 25 August 1952. Adjusted for age 5 and over, based on 1950 San Francisco population.

In Great Britain, the incidence of cancer has been investigated in relation to water fluoride level. By means of the national cancer registration scheme it was possible to compare cancer incidence in areas with contrasting levels of fluoride in the water.

For each local authority districts with a water fluoride level of 1 mg/litre or over ('high'), one or more nearby district of similar size with a fluoride level of 0.2 mg/litre or less ('low') was selected for comparison. For areas with a fluoride level in the range 0.5–0.99 mg/litre ('high'–'medium'), control areas were chosen with fluoride levels of 0.1 mg/litre or less ('very low'). The numbers of cancers of each anatomical site were arranged by age group, sex and water fluoride level. For each anatomical site, the numbers of cancers observed were then compared, within each age group, sex and area, with the numbers expected if the incidence of the disease had been uniform throughout the four areas (Royal College of Physicians, 1976). Table 17.4 shows, for cancers of the thyroid, kidney, stomach, oesophagus, colon, rectum, bladder, bone and breast, the numbers observed in each of the four sets of districts grouped by water fluoride level, together with the ratios of observed to expected numbers. It will be seen that there is no tendency for the ratio for any cancer to be greater in the high-fluoride areas than in the low-fluoride areas.

Table 17.4 Ratios of observed to expected numbers of cancers in certain organs in areas with different levels of fluoride in water in Great Britain (From Royal College of Physicians, 1976)

Site of cancer	*High F (1 ppm)*	*High–medium F (0.5–0.99 ppm)*	*Low F (0.2 ppm)*	*Very low F (0.1 ppm)*
Thyroid	1.05 (45)*	0.79 (54)	1.27 (57)	1.02 (84)
Kidney	1.01 (129)	1.00 (198)	1.02 (131)	0.98 (233)
Stomach	0.88 (375)	1.15 (733)	0.90 (327)	1.05 (815)
Oesophagus	0.87 (73)	1.02 (131)	0.87 (73)	1.13 (177)
Colon	0.96 (386)	1.03 (618)	0.99 (385)	1.00 (719)
Rectum	0.93 (273)	1.11 (486)	0.94 (264)	0.99 (519)
Bladder	1.00 (430)	0.96 (632)	1.06 (444)	1.00 (786)
Bone	1.00 (18)	1.06 (30)	1.02 (19)	0.94 (31)
Breast	0.92 (567)	1.06 (999)	1.08 (650)	0.97 (1105)
Total population	482 398	779 054	510 045	896 625

* The total numbers of cancers observed are given in parentheses.

Since the report by the Committee of the Royal College of Physicians, the results of a number of new epidemiological investigations have become available and the authors of some of the studies claimed that increased cancer rates are associated with fluoridation. The Department of Health and Social Security set up a Working Party with the following terms of reference: 'To appraise the published and otherwise available data and conclusions on cancer incidence and mortality amongst populations whose drinking water is either artificially fluoridated or contains high levels of fluoride from natural sources.'

The report, referred to as the Knox Report after the Chairman, Professor E. G. Knox, was published in 1985 (Knox, 1985). The Working Party considered the claims by Yiamouyiannis and Burk and concluded that 'each of these analyses by Yiamouyiannis and Burk were defective. None justifies their conclusion that fluoridation affects cancer mortality'. With regard to studies in the UK, they reported that 'no subsequent studies revealed any association in the United Kingdom between fluoride concentrations and cancer of any part of the body'. The report concluded:

(i) We have found nothing in any of the major classes of epidemiological evidence which could lead us to conclude that either fluoride occurring naturally in water, or fluoride added to water supplies, is capable of inducing cancer, or of increasing the mortality from cancer. This statement applies both to cancer as a whole, and to cancer at a large number of specific sites. In this we concur with the great majority of scientific investigators and commentators in this field. The only contrary conclusions are in our view attributable to errors in data, errors in analytical technique, and errors in scientific logic.

(ii) The evidence permits us to comment positively on the safety of fluoridated water in this respect. The absence of demonstrable effects on cancer rates in the face of long-term exposures to naturally elevated levels of fluoride in water: the absence of any demonstrable effect on cancer rates following the artificial fluoridation of water supplies: the large human populations observed: the consistency of the findings from many different sources of data in many different countries: lead us to conclude that in this respect the fluoridation of drinking water is safe.

(iii) The routine monitoring of public health has been an important feature of many fluoridation programmes, and has contributed to the confidence with which we can assert the safety of fluoridation with respect to cancer. We recommend that such monitoring should continue.

Congenital anomalies

The suggestion that fluoride is a cause of mongolism (Down's syndrome) derives from two studies by Rapaport (1959, 1963) in the USA. His results are summarized in Table 17.5, and at first sight the correlation between the incidence of mongolism and the fluoride content of the water is impressive. But, as the report by the Royal

Table 17.5 Incidence of mongolism in Illinois (After Rapaport, 1959, 1963) (From Royal College of Physicians, 1976)

Size of towns	*No. towns*	*Fluoride in water* (mg/litre)	*Down's syndrome*	
			No. cases	*Frequency per 1000 births*
10 000–100 000 inhabitants	15	0.0	15	0.24
	24	0.1–0.2	52	0.39
	17	0.3–0.7	33	0.47
	12	1.0–2.6	48	0.72
5000–10 000 inhabitants	–	0.0–0.2	10	0.40
	–	0.3–2.6	19	0.78

College of Physicians (1976) shows, the highest rates found by Rapaport are only about half those that are normally reported after intensive case finding, while the lowest rates are only about one-sixth as high. Intensive investigation has shown that the incidence of mongolism is remarkably constant, the rate ranging from 1.15 to 1.92 per 1000 births (median value of 1.5 per 1000) in Denmark, Great Britain, Switzerland and the USA. Rates at this level are universally accepted by paediatricians as compatible with complete ascertainment. To obtain such a level of ascertainment, however, it is usually necessary to utilize, in addition to the sources used by Rapaport (1959, 1963), a range of further information, including the records of community physicians, school doctors, midwives, health visitors, social workers and others concerned with the welfare of mongols. It is difficult to attach any meaning to Rapaport's limited enquiry, missing, as it would, most surviving children with mongolism who were cared for at home.

Berry (1958) undertook a similar study in nine English towns, making the sort of intensive enquiries that are needed for complete ascertainment. His results are summarized in Table 17.6 along with those obtained by other British investigators (see R.C.P. Report, 1976). These data provide no evidence that the incidence of mongolism bears any relationship to the fluoride content of the drinking water. The absence of any relationship is, moreover, confirmed by the experience in Birmingham where fluoridation has been practised since 1964.

Table 17.6 Incidence of mongolism in England (After Berry, 1958, 1962) (From Royal College of Physicians, 1976)

Place	*Fluoride in water* (ppm)	*Down's syndrome*	
		No. cases	*Frequency per 1000 live births*
High Wycombe	Less than 0.2	9	1.31
Reading		30	1.53
Tynemouth		24	1.90
Carlisle		19	1.64
Gateshead		37	1.65
Stockton		16	1.08
Slough	0.9	13	1.37
South Shields	0.7–1.1	33	1.59
W. Hartlepool	1.9–2.0	16	1.23
6 towns	Less than 0.2	135	1.53
3 towns	More than 0.7	64	1.42
Liverpool	–	18	1.29*
UK	–	7	1.69
London	–	107	1.50*
Rural Northants	–	86	1.63*

* Live and still births.

Further evidence that mongolism (Down's syndrome) and other selected congenital malformations are not associated with water fluoridation is given by Erickson *et al.* (1976) in a very large study of 1 387 027 births using two sources: the Metropolitan Atlanta Congenital Malformation Surveillance Program and the National Cleft Lip and Palate Intelligence Service. Their results are given in Table 17.7 and show no association between water fluoridation and the incidence of congenital malformations.

Aluminium–fluoride interactions

The early work on the interaction of dietary Al and fluoride was concerned with the possibility that the Al in some waters (largely from the alum used in water purification) might form complexes with the fluoride and reduce its absorption and effectiveness as a cariostatic agent. The addition of 0.2 ppm Al to a solution of 1 ppm F reduces the ionic fluoride by 25–30% (Brudevold, Moreno and Bakhos, 1973). Weddle and Muhler (1957) fed 24 mg F daily to rats with or without a range of doses of Al and found that 0.1% in the water reduced the skeletal retention of fluoride from 43% in the control (no Al) to 30%, clearly showing that the Al–F complex, probably AlF_6^{-3}, was not readily absorbed.

Table 17.7 Incidence of selected common congenital malformations in areas with and without fluoridated water (From Erikson *et al.*, 1976)

Malformation	*Metropolitan Atlanta 1967–73*					*NIS surveillance areas, 1961–66*				
	Fluoride (95 254 total births)		*Non-fluoride (25 373 total births)*		χ^2	*Fluoride (234 300 total births)*		*Non-fluoride (1 032 100 total births)*		χ^2
	No. cases	*Rate/10 000 white births*	*No. cases*	*Rate/10 000 white births*		*No. cases*	*Rate/10 000 white births*	*No. cases*	*Rate/10 000 white births*	
Anencephaly	101	10.6	33	13.0	0.83	70	3.0	275	2.7	0.62
Cardiac and other circulatory system defects	379	39.8	78	30.7	4.11	120	5.1	456	4.4	1.93
Cleft lip with/without cleft palate	107	11.2	35	13.8	0.91	185	7.9	784	7.6	0.19
Cleft palate	50	5.2	20	7.9	1.96	94	4.0	331	3.2	3.45
Clubfoot	414	43.5	96	37.8	1.38	303	12.9	1 642	15.9	10.84
Down's syndrome	166	9.9	86	8.5	1.41	115	4.9	524	5.1	0.08
Hydrocephalus	77	8.1	34	13.4	5.59	70	3.0	299	2.9	0.03
Hypospadias	237	24.9	47	18.5	3.18	198	8.5	736	7.1	4.33
Reduction deformities	82	8.6	14	5.5	2.03	79	3.4	358	3.5	0.03
Spina bifida	149	15.6	37	14.6	0.09	146	6.2	535	5.2	3.71
All malformation cases	2787	292.6	685	270.0	3.58	2264	96.6	10 526	102.0	5.43

Degree of freedom corrected for continuity; $P0.05 = 3.84$.
Data given here refer to a 1% sample of NIS records.

Interest in the Al–F relationship has been renewed in recent years because of the possibility that excessive intake of Al might be a factor in promoting Alzheimer's disease, in view of the high levels of Al in the brains of patients with this disease. Fluoride became linked with Al intake after it was stated that when water acidified with citric acid or certain acid foods (crushed tomatoes) was boiled in an aluminium pan, the leaching of Al by the acid was increased a thousandfold if the water contained 1 ppm F (Tennakone and Wickramanayake, 1987a). These experiments were repeated by Savory, Nicholson and Willis (1987) with deionized water, citric acid and crushed tomatoes in 15 different aluminium pans (some old, some new), but they found only a 15% increased leaching with fluoride and citric acid and a marked *decrease* with crushed tomatoes. Later, Tennakone and Wickramanayake (1987b) withdrew their original statement as they had found an analytical error in their Al estimations, but maintained that 10 ppm F did have a significant effect on leaching. This was confirmed by Moody, Southam and Buchan (1990) who found a negligible effect in water alone but a marked effect if the water contained citric acid (a common constituent of food additives, fruits and soft drinks) which was proportional to the concentration of fluoride up to a ceiling of 50 ppm. For example, the Al leached in citric acid increased from 16 ppm without fluoride to 35.4 ppm with 5 ppm F. Concentrations of around 5 ppm F could conceivably be reached in a domestic situation if fluoridated water was frequently boiled in a kettle, some water poured off and the kettle refilled without the residue ever being poured away completely. However, the evidence as a whole suggests that only a most unusual combination of circumstances (fluoridated water boiled to small bulk in an aluminium vessel in the presence of citric acid) would lead to undesirably high levels of Al. Only a small proportion of Al salts are normally absorbed from the gut, so even if an Al–F complex did form, it would be most unlikely to be absorbed.

Conclusions

Schemes for the fluoridation of public water supplies have now been operated for over 40 years, although in the past few years the progress of water fluoridation has been slow, especially in Western Europe. The main obstacles to further implementation seem to be sociopsychological and political factors which are determining attitudes, rather than technical or economic problems. The results of our review of 113 community water fluoridation schemes show, beyond reasonable doubt, that artificial fluoridation is effective in reducing caries experience by approximately 50%, regardless of climate, race or social conditions (see page 86). The effect of water fluoridation on general health has been thoroughly investigated in a series of population studies. There is no evidence that the consumption of water containing approximately 1 ppm F (in a temperate climate) is associated with any harmful effect.

References

Berry, W. T. C. (1958) Study of incidence of mongolism in relation to fluoride content of water. *Am. J. Ment. Defic.*, **62**, 623–636

Brudevold, F., Moreno, E. and Bakhos, Y. (1973) Fluoride complexes in drinking water. *Arch. Oral Biol.*, **17**, 1155–1164

Erickson, J. D., Oakley, G. P., Flynt, J. W. and Hay, S. (1976) Water fluoridation and congenital malformations: no associations. *J. Am. Dent. Ass.*, **93**, 981–984

Knox, E. G. (1985) *Fluoridation of Water and Cancer: A Review of the Epidemiological Evidence*, Report of the DHSS Working Party, HMSO, London

Moody, G. H., Southam, J. C. and Buchan, S. A. (1990) Aluminium leaching and fluoride. *Br. Dent. J.*, **169**, 47–50

Newbrun, E. (1977) The safety of water fluoridation. *J. Am. Dent. Ass.*, **94**, 301–304

Oldham, P. D. and Newell, D. J. (1977) Fluoridation of water supplies and cancer – a possible association. *J. R. Statist. Soc. Ser. C (Appl. Statist.)*, **26**, 125–135

Rapaport, I. (1959) Nouvelles recherches sur le mongolisme à propos du rôle pathogénique du fluor. *Bull. Acad. Nat. Med. (Paris)*, **143**, 367–370

Rapaport, I. (1963) Oligophrénie mongolienne et caries dentaires. *Rev. Stomatol. (Paris)*, **46**, 207–218

Rogot, E., Sharrett, A. R., Feinleib, M. and Fabsitz, R. R. (1978) Trends in urban mortality in relation to fluoridation status. *Am. J. Epidemiol.*, **107**, 104–112

Royal College of Physicians (1976) *Fluoride Teeth and Health*, Royal College of Physicians, London

Savory, J., Nicholson, J. R. and Wills, M. R. (1987) Is aluminium leaching enhanced by fluoride? *Nature,* **327**, 107–108

Tennakone, K. and Wickramanayake, S. (1987a) Aluminium leaching from cooking utensils. *Nature,* **325**, 202

Tennakone, K. and Wickramanayake, S. (1987b) Aluminium and cooking. *Nature,* **329**, 398

Weddle, D. A. and Muhler, J. C. (1957) The effect of inorganic salts on fluorine storage in the rat. *J. Nutr.*, **54**, 437–442

Yiamouyiannis, J. and Burk, D. (1977) *Fluoridation and cancer: age dependence of cancer mortality related to artificial fluoridation.* Presented at the 8th International Society for Fluoride Research Conference, Oxford, England, May 29–31

Chapter 18

Fluoridation and the law

In Chapter 2, reference was made to judgements in the Irish High Court and the Court of Session in Edinburgh. Roemer (1983) reviewed the question of legislation on fluorides and dental health. In order to provide for fluoridation of public water supplies, legislation is of two kinds. It may be mandatory, requiring the health ministry or communities of a certain size to fluoridate public water supplies, or it may be of the enabling type, empowering but not requiring authorities to introduce fluoridation.

Mandatory legislation

Legislation making fluoridation of public water supplies compulsory has been enacted under at least the following jurisdictions: Argentina, Bulgaria, Greece, Ireland, one Canadian province, five states of the USA and one constituent Republic of Yugoslavia.

The earliest national statute is the Health (Fluoridation of Water Supplies) Act 1960 of Ireland, requiring the health authority to make all arrangements necessary for the fluoridation of piped water supplied to the public by the health authorities. A lawsuit filed by a member of the public claimed that the Act was unconstitutional in infringing the right of parents to educate their children as they saw fit, the guarantee of protection of the family as an entity, and the personal rights of the citizen, which included the right to bodily integrity. In July 1964, following an exhaustive legal review of the scientific evidence on fluoridation, the Supreme Court rejected all these arguments and held the Act to be constitutional.

In Greece, Regulations issued in 1974 provide for the compulsory fluoridation of water-supply systems serving more than 10 000 persons, and prescribe that fluoridation may be required for other systems on public health grounds where this measure can be safely and successfully implemented (the prescribed concentration of fluorine compounds is 0.8 mg/litre, with variations permitted between 0.7 and 1.0 mg/litre). The Regulations further provide for the adoption of control and safety measures, and make the agency in charge of the water supply system liable in the event of the occurrence of any excess concentration of fluorine that may jeopardize public health.

In New Zealand, local government councils are empowered by the Local Government Act 1974 to provide waterworks, and are further required under the Health Act 1956 to ensure that only wholesome water enters public supply systems (as a measure of wholesomeness, New Zealand has adopted, *inter alia*, a fluoride concentration of 1 mg/litre ± 0.1 mg/litre).

In the USA, the first compulsory fluoridation was introduced by municipal ordinance in various large or medium-sized cities, currently including Baltimore, Chicago, Denver, Detroit, Miami, New York, San Francisco, St Louis and Washington DC. Some of these cities have been fluoridating their water supplies for 25 or 30 years, and dramatic improvements in the dental health of their populations have occurred over that period. A number of these municipal ordinances have been challenged as an unconstitutional invasion of personal liberty, as invalid 'class legislation' that benefits only children, and as a violation of the constitutional guarantee of religious liberty; however, the courts have systematically rejected all such arguments.

While the constitutionality of community water fluoridation is clearly established in the USA, its legality in the UK has been subject to question. In 1976, the Medical Adviser to the Thames Water Authority, Dr P. S. Fuller, stated that the Authority had no duty to comply with a request from an area health authority to add fluorides to the water supply, that he in fact doubted whether the Authority had the power to do so as a supplier and distributor of water, and that the Authority would thus incur no legal liability for refusing to comply with such a request. Commenting on this statement, an editorial in the journal *Dental Update* called on the Secretary of State for Social Services (whose Department, it said, 'has consistently endorsed fluoridation for many years') to take steps to introduce the necessary legislation to enable water authorities in the UK to fluoridate their water supplies with clear legal authority (Editorial, 1976).

Enabling legislation

Enabling legislation authorizes national health authorities or local governments to institute community water fluoridation. While such legislation does not automatically lead to fluoridation of water supplies, it opens the way for national or local health officials to act on the matter. Examples of countries with enabling legislation are several states of the USA, Australia, German Democratic Republic, Israel, New Zealand, Canada and the United Kingdom. Roemer (1983) concluded:

> Members of the public may well ask: 'If water fluoridation is so beneficial, why doesn't the Government do something about it?' Such a question highlights the importance of legislation in this area. While in some jurisdictions fluoridation can be introduced under existing public health legislation, the controversy that has surrounded this in the past makes it imperative for governments to pass legislation expressly setting forth official endorsement of fluoridation. Such legislation can also set standards for a safe, wholesome, and high-quality water supply, authorize action by health officials and operators of waterworks, and remove any lingering doubts and ambiguities about the propriety and legality of community water fluoridation and other fluoride programmes. Legislation is a reflection of official policy.

The Strathclyde fluoridation case

The issues raised by Roemer are relevant to a consideration of the Court Case in Edinburgh involving Strathclyde Regional Council.

Background
In 1978, Strathclyde Regional Council, as a statutory water authority in Scotland, agreed to co-operate with local Health Boards by fluoridating water supplies for which they were responsible. Mrs Catherine McColl, a Glasgow citizen, applied for an interdict to restrain Strathclyde Regional Council from implementing its decision. The interdict was based on four main grounds:

1. Fluoridation would be *ultra vires*, i.e. beyond the legal powers of the Regional Council.
2. It would be a nuisance and being a toxic substance, harmful to consumers, particularly in relation to cancer.
3. It would be a breach of the Water Act in that the Council would be failing in their duty to provide a supply of wholesome water.
4. It would be unlawful in that the Council would be providing a medicinal product for a medicinal purpose without having a product licence.

The hearings, held in the Court of Session, Edinburgh, commenced on 23 September 1980 and continued (after a few breaks) until 26 July 1982. The court sat on 201 days, making it the longest and costliest case in Scottish legal history. The judge, Lord Jauncey, took almost 12 months to consider the massive evidence and gave his verdict on 29 June 1983 (Jauncey, 1983). His judgement was contained in a 400-page document. He summarized his conclusions, in relation to the general topics which were canvassed in evidence, as follows:

> *Summary*
> Before turning to consider the law it may be convenient to summarize my conclusions in relation to the general topics which were canvassed in evidence:
>
> 1. Fluoride at a concentration of 1 ppm is not mutagenic.
> 2. No biochemical mechanism has been demonstrated whereby fluoride at a concentration of 1 ppm is likely to cause cancer or accelerate existing cancerous growth.
> 3. No association between fluoridation of water supplies and increased CDRs (crude death rates) in the consumers has been demonstrated.
> 4. There is no reason to anticipate that fluoride at a concentration of 1 ppm is likely to have an adverse effect upon the migration of leucocytes in the consumer.
> 5. There is no reasonable likelihood that CRF (chronic renal failure) patients drinking water fluoridated to 1 ppm will suffer harm.
> 6. Fluoridation of water supplies in Strathclyde would be likely to reduce considerably the incidence of caries.
> 7. Such fluoridation would be likely to produce a very small increase in the prevalence of dental mottling which would only be noticeable at very close quarters and would be very unlikely to create any aesthetic problems.
> 8. The present low levels of fluoride in the water supplies in Strathclyde do not cause caries.
>
> I am not therefore prepared to make a finding that the present concentration of fluoride in the water in Strathclyde causes caries. However, I have no doubt that increasing the present concentrations to 1 ppm would considerably reduce the incidence of that disease. [Opinion of Lord Jauncey, pp. 326–63.]

He then dealt with the four questions of Law. Namely, (1) *ultra vires*; (2)

nuisance; (3) breach of the Water (Scotland) Act 1980; and (4) breach of the Medicines Act 1968. He repelled the last three legal arguments but upheld that part of her case which claimed that water fluoridation was *ultra vires*.

The judge's opinion on the legal point of *ultra vires* centred around the meaning of the word 'wholesome'. The relevant section of the Act provided 'it shall be the duty of every local authority to provide a supply of wholesome water in pipes to every part of their district where a supply of water is required for domestic purposes and can be provided at reasonable cost'.

The judge considered in detail the judgement in the Lower Hutt Case in New Zealand, which had ruled in favour of fluoridation. He decided that

> the question is a narrow and difficult one but I consider that there are material differences between the circumstances in the Lower Hutt case and the present. . . . In my view the word 'wholesome' falls properly to be constructed in the more restricted sense advocated by the petitioner as relating to water which was free from contamination and pleasant to drink. It follows that fluoridation which in no way facilitates nor is incidental to the supply of such water is out with the powers of the respondents. The petitioner therefore succeeds on this branch of her case.

The UK Government's response

The Government's response was given by the Secretary of State for Social Services.

> Fluoridation has been supported by successive Governments as a safe and effective public health measure and we consider that Lord Jauncey's opinion amply demonstrates that the Government should continue to support fluoridation as a positive means to promote good dental health. It is therefore the Government's intention, when the Parliamentary timetable permits, to bring forward legislation which will clarify the power of water authorities in Scotland to add fluoride to the water supply on the recommendation of the appropriate Health Boards.

The Fluoridation Bill was laid before Parliament in February 1985. It passed through its last stage on 30 October 1985, supported by the leaders of all the main political parties, and received the Royal Assent (the Bill is reproduced at the end of the chapter). This legislation enables a health authority to make arrangements with a 'statutory water undertaker' to add fluoride to the water supply. The Bill requires the health authority, before implementing their proposal, to inform the public by publishing details in a newspaper and informing every local authority whose area falls wholly or partly within the area affected by the proposal.

Thus the UK has improved its 'enabling legislation' and introduced a clause whereby the public must be informed before any decision is taken on the subject. The reality is that fluoridation schemes in Scotland that had to be stopped as a result of Lord Jauncey's judgement in 1983 have not been restarted and no new major scheme has been implemented in England and Wales.

References

Editorial (1976) Water fluoridation – an illegal procedure? *Dental Update*, Nov.–Dec., pp. 269–279

Jauncey, Lord (1983) Opinion of Lord Jauncey in causa Mrs Catherine McColl against Strathclyde Regional Council. The Court of Session, Edinburgh

Roemer, R. (1983) Legislation on fluorides and dental health. *Int. Digest Hlth Legis.*, **34**(1), 3–31

Water (Fluoridation) Act 1985

1985 CHAPTER 63

An Act to make provision with respect to the fluoridation of water supplies. [30th October 1985]

BE IT ENACTED by the Queen's most Excellent Majesty, by and with the advice and consent of the Lords Spiritual and Temporal, and Commons, in this present Parliament assembled, and by the authority of the same, as follows:—

Fluoridation of water supplies at request of health authorities.

1.—(1) Where a health authority have applied in writing to a statutory water undertaker for the water supplied within an area specified in the application to be fluoridated, that undertaker may, while the application remains in force, increase the fluoride content of the water supplied by them within that area.

(2) For the purposes of subsection (1) above, an application shall remain in force until the health authority, after giving reasonable notice to the statutory water undertaker in writing, withdraw it.

(3) The area specified in an application may be the whole, or any part, of the area or district of the authority making the application.

(4) Where, in exercise of the power conferred by this section, the fluoride content of any water is increased, the increase may be effected only by the addition of one or more of the following compounds of fluorine—

hexafluorosilicic acid (H_2SiF_6);

disodium hexafluorosilicate (Na_2SiF_6).

(5) Any health authority making arrangements with a statutory water undertaker in pursuance of an application shall ensure that those arrangements include provisions designed to secure that

the concentration of fluoride in the water supplied to consumers in the area in question is, so far as is reasonably practicable, maintained at one milligram per litre.

(6) Water to which fluoride has been added by a statutory water undertaker in exercise of the power conferred by this section (with a view to its supply in any area) may be supplied by that or any other statutory water undertaker to consumers in any other area if the undertaker or undertakers concerned consider that it is necessary to do so—

(*a*) for the purpose of dealing with an emergency, or

(*b*) in connection with the carrying out of any works (including cleaning and maintenance) by any of them.

Power to vary permitted fluoridation agents.

2.—(1) The Secretary of State may by order amend section 1(4) of this Act by—

(*a*) adding a reference to another compound of fluorine ; or

(*b*) removing any reference to a compound of fluorine.

(2) The power to make orders under this section shall be exercisable by statutory instrument subject to annulment in pursuance of a resolution of either House of Parliament.

Continuity of existing fluoridation schemes.

3.—(1) Where, in pursuance of arrangements entered into by a statutory water undertaker before 20th December 1984—

(*a*) a scheme for increasing the fluoride content of water supplied by the undertaker in any part of England and Wales was in operation immediately before that date ; or

(*b*) work had been begun by the undertaker, before that date, for the purpose of enabling such a scheme to be brought into operation ;

the undertaker may, while the conditions mentioned in subsection (2) below are satisfied, operate the scheme.

(2) The conditions are that the arrangements under which the scheme operates require—

(*a*) fluoridation to be effected only by the addition of one or more of the compounds of fluorine mentioned in section 1(4) of this Act ; and

(*b*) the concentration of fluoride in the water supplied to consumers to be maintained, so far as is reasonably practicable, at one milligram per litre.

(3) Where a statutory water undertaker is operating a fluoridation scheme by virtue of this section—

(*a*) subsection (6) of section 1 of this Act shall apply in relation to the scheme as it applies in relation to any scheme operated in exercise of the power conferred by that section;

(*b*) the scheme shall cease to have effect upon the appropriate authority giving to the undertaker reasonable notice of the authority's desire to terminate it; and

(*c*) the arrangements under which the scheme is operated may be varied to take account of any amendment of section 1(4) of this Act made under section 2.

4.—(1) This section applies where a health authority propose— Publicity and consultation.

(*a*) to make or withdraw an application; or

(*b*) to terminate a scheme which may be operated by virtue of section 3 of this Act (" a preserved scheme ").

(2) At least three months before implementing their proposal, the health authority shall—

(*a*) publish details of the proposal in one or more newspapers circulating within the area affected by the proposal; and

(*b*) in the case of an authority in England and Wales, give notice of the proposal to every local authority whose area falls wholly or partly within the area affected by the proposal.

(3) Before implementing the proposal the health authority shall consult each of the local authorities (if any) to whom they are required by subsection (2)(*b*) above to give notice of the proposal.

(4) The health authority shall, not earlier than seven days after publishing details of the proposal in the manner required by subsection (2)(*a*) above, republish them in that manner.

(5) Where a health authority have complied with this section in relation to the proposal they shall, in determining whether or not to proceed, have such regard as they consider appropriate—

(*a*) to any representations which have been made to them with respect to it; and

(*b*) to any consultations held under subsection (3) above.

(6) The Secretary of State may direct that this section shall not apply in relation to any proposal of a health authority to withdraw an application or to terminate a preserved scheme.

(7) Where, at any meeting of a health authority, consideration is given to the question whether the authority should make or withdraw an application or terminate a preserved scheme, section 1(2) of the Public Bodies (Admission to Meetings) Act 1960 (which would have allowed the authority to exclude the public from the meeting in certain circumstances) shall not apply to any proceedings on that question. 1960 c. 67.

Interpretation, etc.

5.—(1) In this Act—

"application" means an application under section 1(1);

"appropriate authority", in relation to a fluoridation scheme which is operated by virtue of section 3, means the Regional or District Health Authority to whom the statutory water undertaker concerned are answerable in accordance with the arrangements under which the scheme is operated;

"emergency" means an existing or threatened serious deficiency in the supply of water (whether in quantity or quality) caused by an exceptional lack of rain or by any accident or unforeseen circumstances;

"health authority" means—

(a) in relation to England and Wales, any District Health Authority (within the meaning of the National Health Service Act 1977); and

1977 c. 49.

(b) in relation to Scotland, any Health Board (within the meaning of the National Health Service (Scotland) Act 1978);

1978 c. 29.

local authority" means the council of a county or district, the council of a London borough or the Common Council of the City of London; and

"statutory water undertaker" means—

(a) in relation to England and Wales, any water authority or statutory water company within the meaning of the Water Act 1973; and

1973 c. 37.

(b) in relation to Scotland, any water authority within the meaning of the Water (Scotland) Act 1980.

1980 c. 45.

(2) The provisions of this Act apply to the Isles of Scilly as if the Council of the Isles of Scilly were a water authority and as if the Isles were the area of that water authority.

Short title, commencement and extent.

6.—(1) This Act may be cited as the Water (Fluoridation) Act 1985.

(2) This Act does not extend to Northern Ireland.

PRINTED IN ENGLAND BY W. J. SHARP, CB
Controller and Chief Executive of Her Majesty's Stationery Office and
Queen's Printer of Acts of Parliament

LONDON: PUBLISHED BY HER MAJESTY'S STATIONERY OFFICE

(546351) 80p net

ISBN 0 10 546385 X

Chapter 19

Fluoride therapy planning for the individual and the community

Previous chapters have described the types of fluoride therapy that are available. Each type has been considered individually with particular regard to efficacy, and enamel opacities, toxicity and the modes of action of fluoride were described in separate chapters. The choice between the various methods and their place in the total treatment plan of an individual patient has not been fully discussed, and planners of dental services may wish to compare the merits of the various methods of fluoride therapy in relation to levels of caries experience and resources available in their community. The use of various materials has evolved in different areas of the world because of different needs, demands and resources. The purpose of this chapter is to describe the extent to which fluoride therapies are used throughout the world, and to discuss issues relevant to their use in the care of an individual patient and on a community scale.

Use of fluorides throughout the world

A very tentative estimate of the number of people using various types of fluoride therapy is given in Table 19.1. Accurate figures would be almost impossible to obtain, and the data given are likely to be very approximate only. Nevertheless, the conclusion to be drawn from the table – that water and toothpaste are by far the most widely available vehicles for fluoride – is almost certainly true. The worldwide use of the other methods is small, relative to the availability of fluoride-containing

Table 19.1 Estimate of number of people throughout the world using various types of fluoride therapy*

Type of therapy	*People* (million)
Water fluoridation (artificial)	210
School fluoridation	0.2
Fluoridated salt	4
Drops/tablets	20
Mouthrinses	20
Clinical topicals	20
Fluoride toothpastes	450

* Figures are based on population statistics and published data on the use of fluorides; likely to be very approximate.

water and toothpaste, but each of them has had, and probably will continue to have, an important role in caries prevention under particular circumstances.

Water fluoridation is a community preventive measure 'par excellence'. It is also reasonable to label the widespread use of fluoride toothpastes as community prevention since, although individuals can be encouraged to use them, their use in many developed countries is now so well established that other therapies have to take this background exposure to fluoride toothpastes into account.

School water fluoridation is used in the USA in some areas where fluoridation of public water supplies is not feasible. Salt fluoridation has many advantages as a community measure and its use is spreading. Milk fluoridation has not progressed on a community scale because of perceived logistical problems. Fluoride mouthrinses are used in many countries in school-based community programmes and also prescribed for individual patients. Clinical topical applications of fluoride are given, almost exclusively, as part of the care of individual patients. The use of fluorides in community programmes and factors to consider when planning these programmes will be considered after fluoride therapy for the individual.

Fluoride therapy for the individual

The dental practitioner is faced with a large number of methods for administering fluoride, often capable of being used at different concentrations and amounts and frequencies. In the first place it is helpful to divide these into those methods primarily aimed at systemic administration and those formulated for topical oral use only (Table 19.2). In general, methods of systemic fluoride administration will

Table 19.2 Methods of fluoride administration

Systemic	*Topical*
Public water fluoridation	Clinical topical application
School water fluoridation	Fluoride mouthrinse
Fluoridized salt	Fluoride toothpaste
Fluoridized milk	
Fluoride drops/tablets	

provide fluoride at an optimal dosage level. If the dosage is optimal, then only one method of systemic fluoride therapy should be given to any one individual. For example, if a child lives in an area of England supplied with drinking water containing about 1 ppm F, this will provide the child with a sufficient amount of ingested fluoride and no other systemic fluoride (e.g. drops or tablets) should be prescribed. If a young child did ingest both fluoride tablets and adequately fluoridated water, there would be a risk of fluorosis in developing enamel (see Chapter 13). Very occasionally this rule of 'only one method of systemic administration' might be broken, if prevention of caries is more important than aesthetics: this might be so in the case of severely medically handicapped children in whom a carious tooth might be a threat to life or the severely mentally handicapped in whom topical fluoride therapy and treatment may be very difficult.

Systemic fluoride administration is usually considered desirable only when enamel is forming before the teeth erupt, and considered no longer beneficial in adults. While the possibility that the slightly raised fluoride level in saliva and gingival fluid after fluoride ingestion may have a caries-preventive effect should be investigated, it is likely that this action is much less important than the local effect of fluoride in the mouth, So, although there would appear to be no harm in continuing with systemic administration of fluoride (such as tablets) in adulthood, the caries-preventive effect is likely to be limited to the local action in the mouth. In practical terms, the only method of systemic fluoride therapy under the control of the dental practitioner is the prescription of fluoride drops or tablets, since there are no UK school fluoridation schemes and fluoridized salt and milk are not on sale in the UK.

Four aspects of fluoride therapy in treatment planning for the individual will be considered: safety, cooperation, age of the child, and caries prediction.

Safety of fluoride in the care of the individual patient

Although a patient should receive only one source of systemic fluoride, this restriction does not apply to those methods aimed solely at a topical effect. If no fluoride is ingested there is no toxicological reason why all three of the topical methods (see Table 19.2) should not be given in combination. However, some mouthrinse, toothpaste and topical fluoride solutions, gel or varnish is swallowed and the effect of this has been investigated from the points of view of acute and chronic toxicity.

Broader aspects of fluoride toxicity have been considered in Chapter 16, and the relative importance of various fluoride vehicles as causes of dental fluorosis was discussed in Chapter 13.

It is generally agreed that fluoride mouthrinsing should not be commenced before the age of 6 years (Health Education Authority, 1989) because children under this age are likely to ingest a high proportion of the rinse (see Chapter 10 for a discussion of the relevant literature).

One of the conclusions from a survey of the literature concerning causes of enamel fluorosis in Chapter 13 was that increased levels of fluorosis were associated with early introduction of the young child to fluoride toothpastes. It should again be emphasized that the levels of fluorosis observed were very mild. Nevertheless, some advice to parents of young children is necessary. There are basically two choices: first, to advise that only a small amount of toothpaste is used, or, secondly, to advise the use of a toothpaste with a lower fluoride content. The British Association for the Study of Community Dentistry (1988) and the Health Education Authority (1989) agree that parents should supervise their child's toothbrushing, the amount of paste placed on the child's brush by the parent should be limited to the size of a small pea (or a 'smear of toothpaste') and that children should be encouraged to spit the toothpaste out after brushing. Several manufacturers conscientiously put this advice on their products which are likely to be used by young children.

The second approach is to advise parents to use a toothpaste which contains less fluoride. Several 'Junior' brands now contain about 500 ppm F, which is one-half to one-third of the concentration of fluoride in most toothpastes. However, it is worth recalling (see Chapter 9) that the caries-inhibiting effect of toothpastes was, overall, directly related to the fluoride content of the paste. It is thus likely that toothpastes with a fluoride content of about 500 ppm will be slightly less effective than those with 1000 or 1450 ppm F. The dental practitioner and mother of the young patient should be aware of the balance between the slight risk of fluorosis from the swallowing of high-concentration fluoride toothpastes and the slightly reduced effectiveness of a toothpaste with a lower fluoride content. Some children enjoy eating toothpaste and in these cases it would be wise to recommend that a fluoride-free toothpaste is available.

Clinical topical applications of fluoride are given in the dental surgery and are thus under the control of the dentist. The amount of fluoride ingested during and immediately after a clinical topical application of fluoride should be low if the technique is good. Applications tend to be infrequent, lessening the risk of chronic fluoride ingestion and possible enamel fluorosis. Risks are therefore of acute toxicity.

Ekstrand *et al.* (1981) reported that the average quantity of fluoride ingested, in 8 children, was 31.2 mg F after a mean of 3.33 g of gel (1.23% F) was applied in a pair of custom-fitted trays. This indicates that 78% of the gel was swallowed and only 22% removed with the tray or spat out. The 1-hour plasma fluoride level ranged from 300 to 1443 ng/ml (0.3–1.4 ppm F in plasma) in these children. In adults, who received 5 g gel in commercially available disposable trays, plasma levels ranged from 300 to 980 ng/ml, but levels were reduced to a maximum of 230 ng/ml in these adults when custom-fitted trays were used. The authors point out that plasma fluoride levels in excess of 950 ng/ml are likely to be nephrotoxic and warn against the frequent use at home of gels containing fluoride concentrations as high as 1.23%.

Saliva ejectors do not appear to have been used in the study of Ekstrand and colleagues, and the results highlight the need for some salivary removal system during application (especially since highly flavoured acid gels induce high salivary flow) and the use of accurately fitting trays.

Tyler and Andlaw (1987) investigated the amount of fluoride dispensed during application of fluoride gel in trays in 13 children aged 5–13 years, in England. Suction was used during applications. The gel contained 1.23% F or 12 300 ppm F. The mean amount of gel dispensed per tray was 2.5 g, which contained 30 mg F. They found that 46% of the fluoride dispensed was recovered with the paper liner, 18% by suction and 7% by a gauze wipe. Only 19% (5.6 mg F) of the gel dispensed remained in the mouth. If both maxillary and mandibular dentitions were treated, fluoride retention would double to 11.3 mg F, but this is considerably lower than the 31.2 mg F reported by Ekstrand *et al.* (1981) and the 23.3 mg F reported by McCall *et al.* (1983). The results of Tyler and Andlaw (1987) agree with those of LeCompte and Doyle (1985), in the USA, and highlight the importance of controlling the amount of gel dispensed into the tray as well as careful removal of excess gel after removing the trays. In this latter respect, LeCompte and Doyle (1985) used suction to remove excess gel rather than a gauze wipe. Guidelines for the technique of tray and gel application have been published in the USA (Table 19.3).

The effectiveness of fluoride varnishes was discussed in Chapter 11. They are very suitable for use in young children, since application is quicker and easier compared with gel and tray. Roberts and Longhurst (1987) investigated the amount of varnish applied and retained in a study on 111 children aged 2–14 years. One ml of the varnish weighed 1.0 g and contained 50 mg NaF (22.6 mg F). The mean amount of fluoride applied per patient was 5 mg F, and this varied only slightly with age. It can be assumed that virtually all of this fluoride would be ingested, but the amount of fluoride ingested after varnish application is less than that during or after gel application.

Table 19.3 Recommended guidelines for professional application of high-fluoride concentration products (From LeCompte, 1987)

1. Apply not more than 2 g of gel per tray (approximately 40% of tray capacity)
2. Use a saliva ejector during the 4 min application procedure and have the patient tilt his head forward during the fluoride application
3. Instruct patients to expectorate thoroughly for from 30 s to 1 min immediately following the application procedure
4. When one is utilizing custom-made trays, only from 5 to 10 drops of product should be dispensed per tray

From the discussions in the present chapter, fluoride products are generally very safe. As described in Chapter 16, accidents have occurred but these very rare events have followed only gross accidental over-dosage. However, as with all materials, caution is needed to avoid untoward side-effects and, as a warning, it is relevant to recall that a 3-year-old child died a few years ago as the result of fluoride treatment in the dental surgery. Undoubtedly, the materials were misused. A prophylaxis was given with a mixture of pumice and 4% SnF_2 applied to the teeth with a cotton swab. The excess pumice was removed with a swab dipped in 4% SnF_2 solution, and the child then instructed to rinse his mouth with 4% SnF_2. He died about three hours later. It was estimated that he swallowed about 45 ml of the solution and ingested about 435 mg F from the rinse alone (Horowitz, 1977). As Horowitz says, this is not an indictment against stannous fluoride, for the results might have occurred with any fluoride compound, but it is a warning that all agents should be handled with care and intelligence.

About 50 children die a year in this country from consuming household poisons; fluoride is exceedingly rarely involved. The certainly lethal dose (CLD) for an adult is 5–10 g NaF, or 32–64 mg F/kg body weight. The safely tolerated dose (STD) is 8–16 mg F/kg body weight. To assist calculating amounts in terms of body weight, children aged 1–2 years weigh about 10 kg; 2–4 years, 15 kg; 4–6 years, 20 kg, and 6–8 years, 23 kg.

A first step in any case of suspected fluoride poisoning is to obtain a history in order to estimate the amount swallowed. If the amount of ingested fluoride is estimated to be less than 5 mg F/kg transfer to hospital is unnecessary, but milk can be given in order to slow the absorption of fluoride which usually occurs very rapidly in the stomach. If the amount of fluoride swallowed is estimated to be 5–15 mg F/kg, the stomach should be emptied. This should not be attempted if there is a possibility that any other poison had been swallowed. Ipecacuanha emetic mixture, Paediatric BP (Ipecac syrup), is widely recommended, at a dosage of 10 ml for children aged 6–18 months, 15 ml for older children and 30 ml for adults. Milk, Epsom salts or aluminium hydroxide antacid mixture will help to slow the absorption of any remaining fluoride. If the amount swallowed is estimated to be greater than 15 mg F/kg body weight, immediate transfer to hospital is necessary. The effect of fluoride over-dosage is nausea, vomiting, hypersalivation, abdominal pain (from production of HF) and diarrhoea. Subsequently, depression of plasma calcium levels resulted in convulsions, and cardiac and respiratory failure.

In order to put these figures into perspective, let us consider the case of a 2-year-old child. The CLD would be about 320 mg F and the STD 80 mg F. Toothpaste (at 1000 ppm) contains 1 mg F/g of paste – about 1 in (25 mm). Tube sizes commonly range from 25 g to 140 g, and contain well below the CLD for a 2-year-old who would certainly be sick before finishing a large tube of toothpaste.

Fluoride mouthrinses (0.05% NaF) are usually sold in 500 ml bottles which thus contain 115 mg F. Again, if a 2-year-old child managed to consume a full bottle, the amount of fluoride ingested would only be slightly over the STD. Containers of fluoride tablets hold 120–200 tablets. At 1 mg F per tablet, 200 mg F is the maximum in a container, again well below the CLD for a 2-year-old child. Child-resistant lids are fitting to bottles of fluoride rinse and containers of fluoride tablets, and it is important that parents replace these lids after use. It can be seen that the chance of acute fluoride poisoning from reasonable use of fluoride products in the home is exceedingly small.

For further information on safety consideration of fluoride therapy for patients, see Heifetz and Horowitz (1984).

Level of cooperation

The daily use of fluoride drops, tablets or mouthrinse at home requires considerable effort and a high level of motivation. The daily use of a toothpaste is an established practice but, as long as the patient attends the surgery, only minimum cooperation is required for clinical topical fluoride application. Therefore, if cooperation is in doubt, topical application in the surgery may be first choice.

Age of the patient and planning other treatment

The third consideration is the age of the patient. We have already said that there appears to be little point in recommending systemic fluorides after about 18 years of age; the younger end of the age range is more important in order to obtain a pre-eruptive effect. Fluoride tablet dosage at various ages has been discussed in Chapter 8. There would appear to be no lower age limit on clinical topical application of fluoride, although it is usually limited by lack of cooperation for such a lengthy procedure. It has already been noted that limiting the amount of varnish or gel applied and adequate removal of excess gel are essential. The use of mouthrinses should not be recommended below about 6 years, and parental supervision of the amount of fluoride toothpaste used (so that it does not exceed the size of a small pea) would also be prudent below this age.

It is usually recommended that a prophylaxis be carried out to clean the teeth before topical application in the surgery. Recent data suggest that the efficacy of the application is unaltered by the omission of plaque removal, although this may only be relevant to application of solution, and plaque may reduce the efficacy of gel application (Horowitz *et al.*, 1974). However, plaque removal is so important as far as gingival health is concerned that it may be necessary to include it, for this reason, in the treatment plan.

The point at which various fluoride therapies occur in a treatment plan should be considered. As mentioned earlier, the home use of tablets and mouthrinses requires considerable cooperation and it may be sensible to delay recommending these until the degree of cooperation expected is assessed. If it is planned to fissure-seal teeth, topical fluoride application should be delayed until after this has been completed, since, in theory, the raised enamel fluoride level resulting from the topical fluoride application might lessen the effectiveness of enamel etching prior to sealing. This precaution might not be completely necessary, as it is known that the retention of fissure sealants is as good in fluoridated as in fluoride-low areas.

Caries prediction

The last aspect to consider is the most difficult – determining the cost–benefit ratio of the proposed treatment plan. This involves predicting how much caries the patient is likely to develop over the next few years. If the patient is expected to develop many carious lesions, it would be justified to recommend a high level of fluoride therapy to try to prevent the carious lesions developing. But if little or no caries development is expected, it would not be justified in recommending extensive fluoride therapy for so little gain. It is important that adequate information is given about the likely benefit from the therapy.

Methods of predicting future caries increments have been the subject of many studies, particularly in the past 10–15 years – since the decline in caries has become a reality. The profile of dental caries in children in many developed countries has changed so that now quite a proportion of children develop little or no caries and, at the other end of the distribution, there are children who develop much caries. The problem is to identify this latter group. A full discussion of caries prediction is outside the scope of this book (see Krasse, 1985; De Liefde, 1989; Russell *et al.*, 1990; Demers *et al.*, 1990), but methods studied most thoroughly include examination of saliva (e.g. for *S. mutans* and lactobacillus levels, flow rate or buffering capacity), and teeth (e.g. past caries experience, at risk sites), although plaque quality and dietary factors have also been considered. Overall, past caries experience and microbiological counts alone or in combination seem to be the best predictors, although not outstandingly so. Disney *et al.* (1990b) reported that 'dentist intuition' was as good as any of the more material predictors.

In a study of New Zealand children, De Liefde (1989) divided children into low risk or high risk on the basis of the presence of 3 dmft at the age of 5 years, or one or more first permanent molars becoming carious within 2 years of eruption. These criteria proved to be good predictors of future caries experience and easily applicable to dental practice. It would, of course, be more useful to predict persons at risk before any caries developed, but this is much more difficult. It may be that, at the present time, dentist intuition, which takes into consideration family history and socioeconomic factors, is the best available.

Almost all of the studies concerned with identifying predictors of dental caries have involved children. At the present time there are no adequate predictors of root caries in adults. The ability of fluoride to prevent root caries was discussed in Chapters 4 and 11.

Some patients are more easily identified as being at risk of developing caries. Hyposalivation or xerostomia (dry mouth) is clearly a risk factor, since extensive caries develops in people whose salivary flow is restricted (Kidd and Joyston-Bechal, 1987). Intense fluoride therapy is advocated for these patients, involving daily topical application of fluoride gels and fluoride mouthrinses, with or without the concurrent use of chlorhexidine (see Chapter 11).

Many orthodontists feel that they wish to do all they can to prevent caries occurring in patients wearing fixed or removable orthodontic appliances. Certainly, caries does occur around brackets or beneath loose bands or wires (Gorelick, Geiger and Gwinnett, 1982; Artun and Brobakken, 1986) and areas of decalcification can persist many years after orthodontic treatment (Ogaard, 1989). Daily rinsing and topical applications of fluoride have been shown to reduce the prevalence and severity of those lesions (Ogaard *et al.*, 1988).

Stephen and MacFadyen (1977) described a very effective caries-preventive scheme for children with cleft palate, which involved frequent applications of fluoride gel in special trays in addition to the use of fluoride dietary supplements. Children or adults with overlay dentures can also be considered to be at special risk of dental caries.

So, for a cooperative child, over about 8 years, living in an area with a fluoride-low water supply and considered to be at high caries risk, one could recommend the daily ingestion of fluoride tablets, the use of a fluoride mouthrinse and toothpaste at home and clinical topical applications in the surgery – the greater the caries risk, the more frequent could be the clinical applications of fluoride as long as precautions are taken to reduce ingestion of the fluoride solution or gel.

Summary

It is possible to construct tables giving possible fluoride regimens for patients at differing risk of caries. Ripa (1984) published one such guide, identifying three variables – age, concentration of water-borne fluoride, and caries status. The tables in his report were based on those recommended by the US National Foundation of Dentistry for the Handicapped. There are three tables, depending on the level of water-borne fluoride (less than 0.3 ppm; 0.3–0.7 ppm; greater than 0.7 ppm). Use of fluoride dentifrice was recommended for all groups, and fluoride dietary supplements were prescribed if the water-borne fluoride concentration was less than 0.7 ppm. The use of self-applied topical fluoride (gel in tray, or fluoride mouthrinse) and the professional application of fluoride (gels or varnishes) depended upon three variables: water F level, age, and caries status. This scheme is useful, although self-applied topical fluoride (gels or mouthrinses) would not normally be recommended in the UK for children as young as 3 years.

The dental practitioner can benefit greatly the dental health of patients by judicious use of fluorides. The types of fluoride therapy he may wish to use will depend upon the factors listed above. Fluoride therapy should become part of the overall treatment plan for the patient which will involve other preventive methods such as plaque control instruction, dietary advice and fissure sealing, as well as any restorative procedures necessary. Many types of fluoride therapy, especially those designed for home use, require constant monitoring, encouragement of the patient and reassessment. When this is done, the occurrence of caries can be reduced to almost negligible levels.

Fluoride therapy in the community

Treatment of an individual patient involves explanation by the dental practitioner of the alternatives available and agreement between the two parties on the proposed treatment plan. In some cases, a patient may be prepared to pay more for receiving caries-preventive therapy than he would need to pay to have restored the teeth which would have become carious without the preventive therapy. This is perfectly ethical as long as the patient is fully informed. But decisions in public health about different health-care strategies are usually made solely on a monetary basis. The community will demand that the health planner provides the best possible health services for their money. Since the planner will have to decide between various strategies he will have to be able to estimate (a) the cost of the proposed measure and (b) the benefit likely to accrue from that measure – both in monetary terms. This is called cost–benefit analysis and is a well-recognized procedure in public health planning.

Before discussing the limited amount of information available on the cost and cost–benefit of various fluoride procedures, two related topics will be briefly reviewed: first, the role of fluoride in the decline in dental caries seen in many developed countries and, secondly, fluoride-based community preventive schemes which have operated in various countries for many years. An overview of the appropriate use of fluorides has been published by WHO (Murray, 1986).

Decline in caries in many developed countries

A few countries have carried out national surveys of the dental health of children and adults for many years, e.g. Japan and the UK. Other countries have regularly monitored the dental health of children, e.g. Denmark. But, on a worldwide scale, the creation of the WHO Global Data Bank on Oral Health in 1969 has enabled trends in dental health to be recognized. These trends have been described by Murray (1986). The first clear trend affecting large numbers of countries, recorded in 1974, was an increase in caries prevalence in developing countries, particularly in urban areas. The widespread trend of decreasing national caries levels in highly industrialized countries did not become clear from the WHO Global Data Bank until 1978. In the UK, the first signs of improving dental health of children became evident in the late 1970s (Palmer, 1980; Anderson, 1981).

In the early 1980s, two groups decided to investigate the reasons for the decline in caries observed in many countries. The report of the first conference (Glass, 1982) held in Boston USA in 1982, included the following summary: 'All 16 speakers agreed that the prevalence of dental caries has declined substantially in several countries represented in areas both with and without organized preventive programmes or fluoridation. Most agreed that fluoride in toothpastes, rinses and community water supplies provides the best single association and that there were many other factors, including unknowns, which might be involved.'

The second publication (WHO/FDI, 1985) concluded that 'the most probable reasons for the decrease in dental caries in children in the developed countries were considered to be associated with: (1) the widespread exposure to fluoridated water and/or fluoride supplements, especially the regular use of fluoride toothpaste. . . . The factors common to all countries with a substantial reduction in caries was fluoride, either as fluoridated water or toothpaste'. This last point is in line with the widespread use of these two vehicles, indicated in Table 19.1 (page 355). Further discussion of the data collected from the 20 selected developed and developing countries considered by the WHO/FDI Working Group has been given by Renson (1986, 1989).

A small minority of people have questioned the role of fluoride, and particularly fluoridation, in the decline in caries (Diesendorf, 1986; Colquhoun and Mann, 1986). These assertions have been effectively answered (Murray and Rugg-Gunn, 1987; Brown, 1988; Rugg-Gunn, 1990). In simple terms, while sugar consumption has been responsible for the increase in caries prevalence, fluoride has been responsible for its decline (Renson, 1986, 1989).

Community prevention in Sweden, Norway, Finland and Denmark

Fluoridation of public water supplies does not exist in Sweden, Norway or Denmark, and involves only one major community in Finland (Chapter 5). Caries experience has been extremely high in these countries (Murray, 1986), and it is due to high expenditure on dental services and a commitment to school-based preventive programmes that caries experience has decreased dramatically in these countries. It is worth considering how these improvements have been achieved.

Sweden can be considered the birthplace of school-based caries-preventive programmes, with virtually all Swedish schoolchildren participating in some fluoride programme.

While in and around Stockholm children brushed with fluoride solutions 4 times per year (Berggren and Welander, 1960), most children in the rest of Sweden rinsed with 0.2% NaF either weekly or fortnightly. Supervised fortnightly fluoride mouthrinsing began in Göteborg in 1960 and by 1963 all schoolchildren in the city were involved. Because dental services in Göteborg are so comprehensive, the record of the number of fillings inserted per child per year provided an excellent estimate of the effectiveness of the caries-preventive programme. The number of fillings inserted fell from nearly 5/child/year in 1960 to 2/child/year in 1973 (Figure 19.1). During the same period, the number of extractions per 100 children/year fell

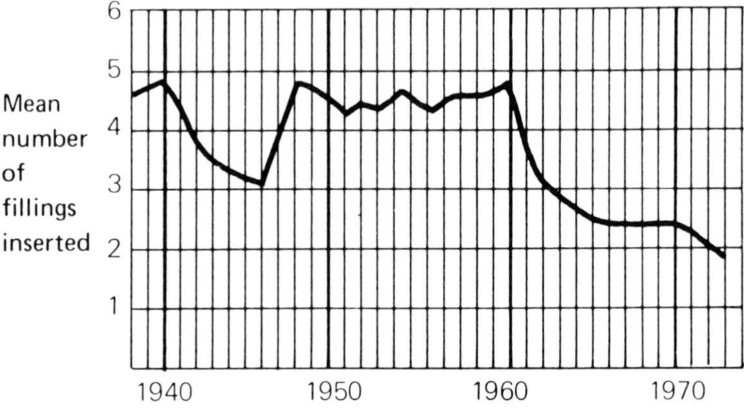

Figure 19.1 Mean number of fillings inserted for each child, 6–15 years of age, by the Public Dental Service of Göteborg, Sweden between 1938 and 1973 (about 40 000 children) (From Torell and Ericsson, 1974; reproduced by courtesy of the authors)

from 13 to 4, and the number of endodontic treatments fell from 4 to 1 per 100 children/year (Torell and Ericsson, 1974). Torell and Ericsson (1974) also showed that the cost–benefit ratios for the fluoride rinse schemes were favourable in four Swedish communities (Table 19.4).

Fluoride dentifrices were introduced into Sweden during the 1970s, and by 1982 80% of toothpaste sold contained fluoride (Renson, 1986). When reviewing the reasons for decline in caries in Sweden, Koch (1982) suggested that the extensive use of fluoride rinses and dentifrices, plus the possible decrease in frequency of sugar intake in Swedish children, were the most likely reasons for the greatly improved dental health. More recently, the necessity for continuing the school fluoride programmes for all children has been questioned. Widenheim *et al.* (1989) have pointed out that several trials have indicated that combining the use of fluoride rinses and fluoride dentifrices leads to little or no advantage over the use of one method alone. However, in some of these trials rinsing was done straight after

Table 19.4 Cost–benefit analysis of supervised school-based fluoride mouthrinsing in Sweden (From Torell and Ericsson, 1974)

Community	*No. children involved in 1971*	*Cost: benefit ratio**
Fortnightly rinsing		
Göteborg	40 000	1:6
Weekly rinsing		
Halland County	59 000	1:8
Norrbotten	39 000	1:2.7
Kronberg County	20 000	1:3.5

* The ratio of the cost of the fluoride mouthrinsing scheme to the estimated cost of dental treatment prevented.

the brushing, therefore not increasing the frequency of exposure to fluoride. Widenheim *et al.* (1989) investigated the effect of discontinuing fluoride mouthrinsing in school between the ages of 13 and 16 and concluded that there was a small increase in the incidence of approximal caries compared with children of the same age who had participated continuously in the programme (from age 6 years). The possibility that school fluoride programmes should be selective was discussed by Bawden *et al.* (1980), since fluoride mouthrinses were more effective in Swedish children with high caries experience. The effect of any discontinuation of school-based fluoride programmes in Sweden will be of considerable interest.

Like Sweden, in the absence of water fluoridation, Norway has developed alternative fluoride schemes. Fluoride rinsing and brushing programmes have expanded continuously since 1960 to cover more than 90% of the schoolchildren by the early 1980s (Von der Fehr, 1982). By 1983, fluoride toothpastes occupied 70% of the market (Renson, 1986). Fluoride tablets were introduced systemically through 'well baby' clinics, so that the proportion of young children taking fluoride tablets increased from less than 1% in 1971 to 50% in 1976 (Lokken and Birkeland, 1978). Since 1977, sales have declined (Von der Fehr, 1982; Renson, 1986). In addition to the organized fluoride rinsing and brushing programmes which have taken place in many Norwegian schools for 20 years and reached 90% of children by 1977 (Rise and Haugejorden, 1980), topical application of fluoride varnishes is now widespread (Rolla and Ogaard, 1987).

The Scandinavian countries have comprehensive school dental services and the number of restorations placed is a good indicator of dental health. Figure 19.2 shows that the improvement between 1971 and 1975 affected all ages, but especially those aged 14 to 16 years, while Figure 19.3 highlights the dramatic improvement in the dental health of Norwegian children, albeit from the very high level of the 1960s. There has been concern that the cariostatic effect of school-based topical fluoride programmes might be lost after the person leaves school. Haugejorden, Lervick and Riordan (1985) showed that the benefits of fluoride rinsing or fluoride brushing was still substantial at the age of 21 years, 6–7 years after discontinuation of the school-based programme, at a time when most toothpastes used contained fluoride.

The only town in Finland to receive artificially fluoridated water is Kuopio (Chapter 5). Fluoride rinsing programmes were introduced into some primary

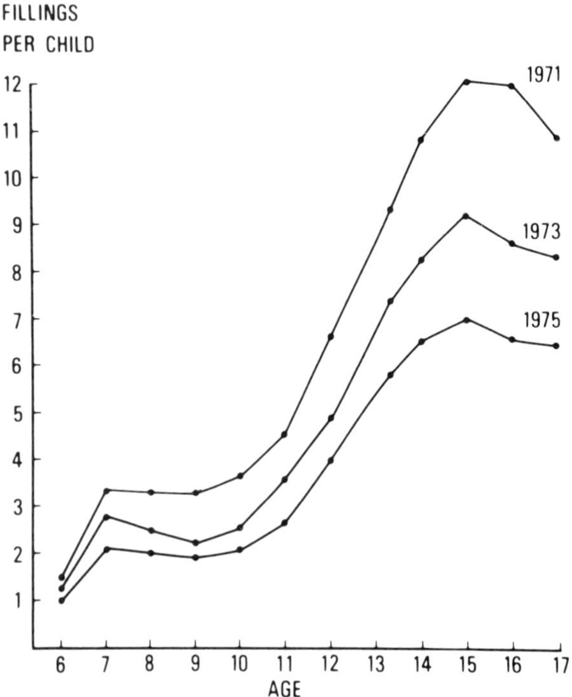

Figure 19.2 Mean number of fillings (filled surfaces) inserted in Norwegian children in 1971, 1973 and 1975, by age (6–17 years) (From Lokken and Birkeland, 1978; reproduced by courtesy of the Editor, *Community Dent. Oral Epidemiol.*)

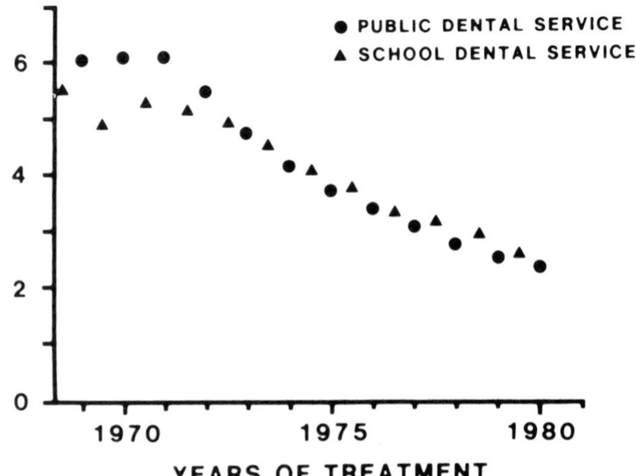

Figure 19.3 Mean number of fillings per child per year provided when treating about 250 000 children in the School Dental Service and 150 000–400 000 in the Public Dental Service in Norway (From Von der Fehr, 1982, with kind permission of the Editor, *Journal of Dental Research*)

schools in the early 1960s, and by 1972 most schoolchildren rinsed fortnightly. The use of dentifrices has increased very greatly from about 33 ml/person in 1962 to 150 ml/person in 1984 (Tala, 1987), with the proportion containing fluoride now over 95%. Fluoride tablets were introduced in 1968 but, although recommended by the National Board of Health, tablet programmes have been very vulnerable to anti-fluoride controversy, as in Norway. Their use is declining, and never reached more than 10% of eligible children (Tala, 1987). Honkala, Nyyssonen and Rimpela (1984) reported that only a modest proportion of Finnish schoolchildren received fluoride other than home use of fluoride toothpaste and concluded that the 'use of fluoride tablets and topical fluorides do not seem to be a practical alternative to drinking-water fluoridation'.

Like Sweden and Norway, Denmark has comprehensive dental services for children. The first children's dental clinics were opened in 1910. Now, virtually all children aged 0–16 years are cared for by this service which is seen as responsible for the very great improvement in the dental health of Danish children (Schwarz, 1987). This is seen clearly in Figures 19.4 and 19.5 which are taken from records collected at Hillerod, 40 km north of Copenhagen. In this community, the school dental service began in 1957; school-based fortnightly rinsing with 0.2% NaF began in 1962 and varnish or solution has been applied to the teeth of children with high caries activity since 1960 (Helm and Helm, 1990). Fluoride dentifrices were introduced into Denmark in 1964 and their share of the market had reached 95% by 1982 (Renson, 1986). Fissure sealants have been used fairly extensively since 1978 and some of the improvement evident in Figures 19.4 and 19.5 is likely to be due to their use.

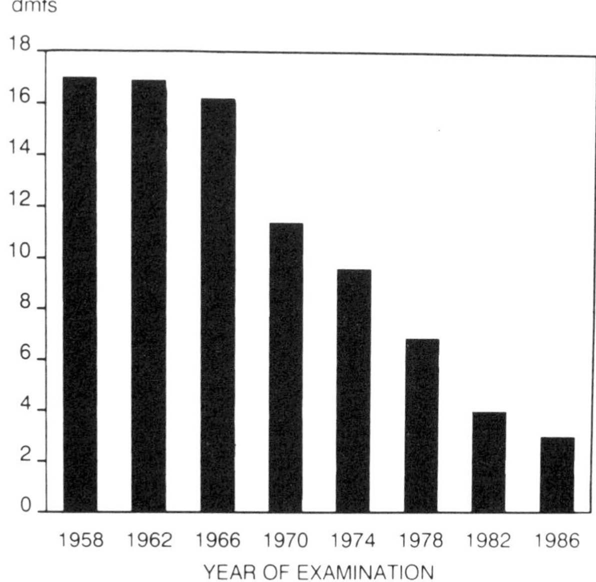

Figure 19.4 Mean dmfs in 8-year-olds living in Hillerod, Denmark, from 1958 to 1986 (From Helm and Helm, 1990, with kind permission of the Editor, *Community Dent. Oral Epidemiol.*)

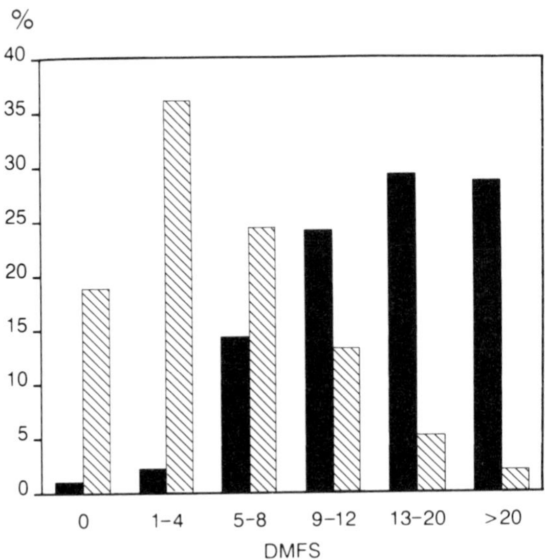

Figure 19.5 Percentage distribution of 16-year-old children living in Hillerod, Denmark, according to DMFS scores. Data for 1966 shown as dark bars (left column) and 1986 as hatched bars (From Helm and Helm, 1990, with kind permission of the Editor, *Community Dent. Oral Epidemiol.*)

Community prevention in Switzerland and mainland Europe

Switzerland is the home of salt fluoridation, which was discussed fairly fully in Chapter 7. In addition to the introduction of salt fluoridation, other fluoride-based community preventive measures have been introduced. One of the interesting features of community fluoride prevention in Switzerland has been the use of both systemic and topical methods. Two of the best reviews of caries prevention in Switzerland are by Marthaler (1987) and Tremp (1987) – Marthaler has led caries prevention in Switzerland for over 30 years. One major city – Basel (population 230 000) – fluoridated in 1962 and the subsequent trend in caries in Basel schoolchildren has been reported at intervals (Chapter 5). At about the same time, school-based preventive programmes were introduced in the Cantons of Zurich and St. Gall, and DMFT averages per child were reduced by 60–72% during the period 1963–64 to 1983–84. The preventive programmes involved supervised tooth-brushing with fluoride solutions or with fluoride tablets. These were supervised three times a year by especially trained chairside assistants who also discussed diet and plaque control. Teachers were supposed to supervise fluoride brushing a further three times a year, but the actual number of brushings per child per year was between 4 and 6. Fluoride rinsing has never been used in Switzerland.

In the Canton of Glarus, caries prevalence declined substantially during the first 8 years after the introduction of universal salt fluoridation in 1975–76. Perhaps the oldest school-based fluoride programmes in Switzerland were the distribution of fluoride tablets, which began in the Canton of Vaud in 1953. However, the use of tablets has been withdrawn as salt fluoridation has spread. In 1955, production of salt containing 90 mg F/kg started at the United Swiss Salt Works. In 1983, the fluoride level was increased to 250 mg/F kg, and by 1985 the market share of fluoridated domestic salt was 72%. As Marthaler (1987) says: 'It is evident that 5.3 million Swiss inhabitants (83% of population) are profiting from an optimal or nearly optimal fluoride ingestion. Of the remaining 1.1 million, an unknown small fraction may use fluoride tablets for preventing decay in their children. Further reductions in caries are expected in Switzerland as the optimum level of fluoride in salt was only reached in 1983.'

Information concerning community fluoride schemes in the rest of mainland Europe is limited. In the Netherlands, caries has declined dramatically, but this has not been associated with any particular community programme (Konig, 1987). In France, salt fluoridation (with KF, at 250 mg F/kg) has been authorized (Rey, 1987), but it is too early to judge the efficiency of this measure (Frank and Cahan, 1987). An analysis of the laws and regulations governing the use of fluorides in Europe has been made by Pinet (1987).

Community prevention in the UK and Eire

The backbone of the British national caries-preventive strategy has been fluoridation of public water supplies. Fluoridation began in 1955 and its effectiveness has been monitored extensively (see Chapters 2–5). Despite its effectiveness, less than 10% (about 5 million people) of the UK population receive fluoridated water. The most widely used fluoride agent is toothpaste, and fluoride toothpastes have exceeded 95% of toothpaste sales since 1979. Moreover, toothpaste sales increased by 20% between 1977 and 1986, with an equivalent of one standard tube being purchased by an average household each fortnight (Downer, 1987). The increasing use of fluoride toothpastes is by far the most likely reason for the decline in caries observed in the UK: between 1973 and 1983 caries experience fell by 50% in 5-year-olds and 40% in 12-year-olds (Todd and Dodd, 1985). The use of fluoride dietary supplements is not extensive (about 50 million tablets per year; enough to supply 1–2% of eligible children) and the use of fluoride rinses, gels and varnishes is spasmodic.

The main alternative in the UK to water fluoridation has been fluoride tablets. Some authorities have attempted to encourage their wider use. Many years ago, Smyth and Withnell (1974) reported a scheme where parents of 3500 pre-school children in Gloucestershire were asked to give their children fluoride tablets. Only 759 (22%) entered the scheme and only 70 (2%) were still giving tablets at the end of 9 months despite the wide publicity and subsidy of the cost of the tablets. More recently, Holt *et al.* (1983, 1985, 1989) reported a dental health education programme in Hillingdon, London, in which mothers were offered a free supply of fluoride drops for their very young children. The message was conveyed by health visitors who visited the homes 3 times a year. All the 438 mothers accepted the drops, 65% were still using them after 14–16 months and 25% after 5 years.

Three school-based fluoride tablet programmes have been reported in the UK (Stephen and Campbell, 1978; Allmark *et al.*, 1982; O'Rourke, Attrill and Holloway, 1988). They all reported substantial reductions in dental caries (about 50% or more). The Portsmouth study (Allmark *et al.*, 1982) and the Manchester study (O'Rourke, Attrill and Holloway, 1988) were of marginal cost–benefit advantage. As O'Rourke and colleagues commented, the unfavourable ratio of cost to benefit observed in their trial in Manchester could have been reversed if the scale of tablet distribution had been larger. The study by Stephen and Campbell (1978) in social classes IV and V children in Glasgow showed an 81% caries reduction equivalent to an estimated monetary saving of about £3 per child over 3 years.

Bennie *et al.* (1978) reported results of a programme (largely fortnightly fluoride rinsing) in the county of Sutherland, Scotland. Substantial reductions in caries were observed after 5 years. Children in Edinburgh participated in fluoride rinsing programmes in school for many years, but few data have been published.

In contrast to the UK, over 65% of the population of Eire reside in communities served with fluoridated water supplies (see Chapter 5). School-based fluoride mouthrinsing programmes in non-fluoridated areas have been in operation since the early 1970s (O'Mullane, 1987). Fluoride toothpastes were first introduced to Eire in the early 1970s and by 1985 constituted 95% of sales. Sales of toothpaste increased by 27% between 1971 and 1981.

One study of the effectiveness of a fortnightly fluoride rinsing programme was reported by Holland, O'Leary and Mullane (1987). The children began rinsing at the age of 6 years and substantial benefits were observed at the age of 12 years (after 6 years of continuous rinsing in school). Results from the survey on Children's Dental Health in Ireland (O'Mullane *et al.*, 1986) recorded that the mean DMFT for 12-year-olds who had been lifetime residents in fluoridated communities nationally was 2.6, whereas the mean DMFT for 12-year-olds who had participated in school fluoride rinsing programmes nationally was 2.5. However, the authors warn against direct comparisons and suggest that further long-term studies are needed. Holland, O'Leary and Mullane (1987) remarked that the per capita operating costs of the mouthrinsing programme were considerably in excess of operating costs for fluoridation programmes. Recent information on the cost of fortnightly rinsing in Eire indicated that the annual cost, for a programme involving 6300 children in western Eire, was IR£1.60 per participant. The cost of water fluoridation is quoted as IR£0.37 per participant (O'Mullane, 1990). Despite widespread use of fluoride rinsing in some areas of Europe, this is the only time that direct cost comparisons between fluoridation and rinsing has been made in Europe.

Community prevention in the USA

Assessment of any community preventive programme must be made in the light of the cost of disease. To quote Newbrun (1989): 'Americans spent almost 30 billion dollars in 1986 to treat all their dental and oral woes. A major proportion of this amount was for the treatment of decayed teeth or the sequelae of caries'. Water fluoridation has always been the most important community measure for caries prevention in the USA (see Chapter 5), and Newbrun (1989) reassessed its value in the late 1980s. He concluded that 'communal water fluoridation is the cornerstone of caries prevention; it is safe, inexpensive, and non-discriminatory'. Percentage and absolute caries reductions due to water fluoridation are less than they were 20–30 years ago, but they are still very important. He also warned that 'clearly, abandoning water fluoridation and relying only on topical forms of fluoride therapy is a mistake and is not justified by the available evidence'.

Brunelle and Carlos (1990) reviewed the interaction between fluoridation and the decline in caries in the USA. Using data from the 1987 national survey of children's dental health, they reported that children who had always been exposed to community water fluoridation had a mean DMFS about 18% lower than those children who had never lived in fluoridated communities. When some of the 'background' effect of topical fluoride was controlled, this difference increased to 25%. They concluded 'that water fluoridation has played a dominant role in the decline in caries and must continue to be a major prevention methodology'. In addition to widespread water fluoridation, over 80% of toothpaste sales in the USA have been fluoride containing for many years (Renson, 1986).

Eichenbaum, Dunn and Tinanoff (1981) and Grembowski (1984) have investigated the impact of fluoridation upon dental practice in the USA. The type of treatment provided had changed dramatically between 1948 and 1979, especially in the prevalence of dental pulp pathologies.

Although school water fluoridation has been studied extensively, it has never been widely implemented. At its height, only slightly more than 200 000 schoolchildren attending about 500 schools were included in such schemes (Horowitz, 1990). The possibility of accidents with these small plants, as reported by Hoffman *et al.* (1980), must be considered. School-based fluoride tablet programmes are rare in the USA, but they are prescribed fairly widely by general medical and dental practitioners. Using data from the 1987 national children's survey, Brunelle and Carlos (1990) reported that 54% of children in non-fluoridated areas had been given fluoride drops or tablets and, surprisingly, 15% of children with lifelong exposure to fluoridated water had been given fluoride drops or tablets. In addition, about 50% of American children had received topical fluoride applications in a dentist's office (surgery) (Brunelle and Carlos, 1990). Siegel and Gutgesell (1982) reported that inadequate knowledge by physicians in Texas concerning fluoride tablet supplementation, and ways to improve knowledge and awareness, were discussed by Horowitz (1985).

School-based fluoride mouthrinsing is the second most prevalent method of community caries prevention in the USA, after water fluoridation. In 1975, about 2 million American children participated in school-based fluoride mouthrinsing (FMR) programmes, and this had risen to about 12 million by 1983 (Miller and Brunelle, 1983; Ripa, 1987). The recommended programme is rinsing once a week with 10 ml (5 ml for kindergarten children) of 0.2% NaF for 60 s. This is based, to some extent, on the trial of Heifetz, Meyers and Kingman (1982) which compared the daily rinsing (in school) with 0.05% NaF and weekly rinsing with 0.2% NaF. The results were in line with those described in Chapter 10 which indicated that daily rinsing was more effective – Heifetz and colleagues reported a 34% reduction with daily rinsing and 24% reduction with weekly rinsing. But because costs of daily rinsing was four times that for weekly rinsing and compliance was more difficult with daily rinsing, weekly rinsing was recommended.

Despite its widespread use in the USA in the early 1980s, its value as a community measure is being reassessed. There are two studies of great significance in this debate: first, the Community Caries Prevention Demonstration Programme (CCPDP) conducted between 1975 and 1980 and, secondly, the National Preventive Dentistry Demonstration Programme (NPDDP) which ran between 1977 and 1982. Both of these studies were very large and the findings have been well and extensively reported. They are of considerable interest to community dental health workers outside as well as inside the USA. The CCPDP investigated fluoride mouthrinsing only, while the NPDDP studied several methods of caries prevention (fissure sealants, classroom education, fluoride gels, fluoride tablets and fluoride rinses).

The CCPDP was funded and organized by the National Caries Program, part of the federal-funded National Institute of Dental Research, Washington DC. The aim was to 'demonstrate the community acceptance and cost-effectiveness of this school-based rinse procedure' (Miller and Brunelle, 1983). Seventeen sites were involved, across America, in parallel. Approximately 75 000 children in more than 3500 classrooms, in classes kindergarten to grade 6 or 8 (ages 6 to 12/14 years), volunteered to participate. The rate of participation for all sites for the 4-year programme was 83% of the eligible children. Although participation varied from 62% to 95% between the 17 sites, it did not diminish during the 4 years and, on the whole, teachers were enthusiastic. The cost of equipment and supplies was low – $0.28–$1.09 per child per year. The major cost variant was personnel, which ranged from $0.41 to $8.63. Almost all sites used parent, student or other community volunteers to supplement the paid programme personnel. The total cost therefore ranged from $0.71 to $9.27 (Miller and Brunelle, 1983). Only part of the purpose of the study was to evaluate the caries-preventive effectiveness of the programme. A sub-sample of children were examined at baseline, during and at the end of the 4-year study. Caries inhibition ranged from 11% to 54% (in DMFS) across the 17 sites. It is important to realize, however, that these calculations used retrospective control data and that there was no parallel control group.

The study was seen as a success. Miller and Brunelle (1983) reported that 'The increased number of children using fluoride rinses is assumed to be an important contributing factor to the recently reported decline of dental caries throughout the United States. Rinse programs implemented in areas with optimally fluoridated water supplies have also provided significant added protection against dental caries. Within this decade, it is hoped that self-applied fluoride rinse programs will be available to all US children in fluoridated and non-fluoridated areas'. There were several reports in dental journals of the success of locally organized mouthrinse programmes (e.g. Dismer, 1982; Osterbrock, 1985). In the late 1970s and early 1980s, the National Caries Program initiated nationwide promotion of fluoride mouthrinsing. These included development of guidebooks, films, extensive mailings and presentations at national and local meetings. Twelve million American children rinsing by the mid-1980s is a tribute to the success of this effort. The attitude of teachers and parents, and the processes of adoption and implementation, have been investigated (e.g. Scheetz, Suddick and Fields, 1984; Scheirer, Allen and Rausch, 1987) and generally the reports are favourable.

However, the results and the interpretation of the results of the CCPDP, as well as the continuing promotion of FMR, has been severely criticized by Stamm *et al.* (1984). The aim of their critique was to answer the question: 'Is this procedure worth doing compared to other things that could be done with these same resources?' In their review of the literature on the efficacy of weekly fluoride mouthrinses, they separate trials into randomized clinical trials which had a parallel control group, and studies using retrospective, or historical control comparisons. Historical controls were acceptable in the days when background caries prevalence in the population was not changing. The CCPDP was planned about 1974 (it began in 1975) when there was no sign of any decline in caries. In the event, the national decline in caries became apparent as the CCPDP was in progress and, as Stamm *et al.* (1984) point out, this makes estimation of efficacy from this important study very difficult. Commenting on the figure of 0.33 DMFS increment saved per child per year (Miller and Brunelle, 1983), Stamm *et al.* (1984) say: 'This over-estimation arises because the historical comparison design cannot separate the unique contribution of FMR from the impact of the secular caries decline with respect to the overall reduction in caries increment in children'. They also suggest that the total costs of FMR have been underestimated and that a realistic figure, at 1981 prices, might be $50 000 per year for 10 000 children. Their calculations on cost-effectiveness of weekly FMR led them to conclude that 'unless a weekly fluoride mouthrinsing program can reduce the target population's mean caries increment by approximately 0.25 surfaces a year or more, the efficiency of the FMR program may be sufficiently low as to cast doubt on its economic viability'. Annual savings were often less than 0.25 surfaces per child. Finally, they also concluded that 'the problems with longer term compliance are generally disregarded'.

The second important study in community prevention of dental caries was the NPDDP. The study was conceived in the mid-1970s and the design was based on a number of assumptions, two of which were that caries levels would remain high in American children, and that combinations of methods might reduce caries by as much as 90% (Bohannan *et al.*, 1985a). The study ran for 4 years between 1977 and 1982, at 10 sites (5 fluoridated and 5 fluoride-deficient) across America. Twenty-five thousand children in grades 1–8 (ages 6–13 years) participated. Twenty thousand children in grades 1, 2 and 5 formed the longitudinal cohorts, while the remaining 5000 children in grades 3, 4, 6, 7 and 8 constituted control groups for cross-sectional comparisons. At each site, schools were assigned to one of 6 regimens (Table 19.5). One regimen included only clinical procedures, two

Table 19.5 Types of treatment procedures undertaken for the 6 regimens in the NPDDP* (From Disney *et al.*, 1990a)

Regimen	*Fluoride-deficient*		*Fluoridated sites*	
	Clinic	*Classroom*	*Clinic*	*Classroom*
1. Comprehensive	Sealants Prophy/gel	Rinse/tablet Education	Sealants Prophy/gel	Rinse Education
2. Modified comprehensive	Prophy/gel	Rinse/tablet Education	Sealants	Rinse Education
3. Clinic	Sealants Prophy/gel		Sealants Prophy/gel	
4. Classroom		Rinse/tablet Education		Rinse Education
5. Education		Education		Education
6. Longitudinal comparison				

* Of the 10 sites in total, 5 were in fluoridated areas and 5 were in fluoride-deficient areas. Some of the procedures were performed in clinics and some in classrooms. Regimen 6 was a longitudinal control group.

were limited to classroom procedures, and two contained both clinical and classroom procedures. Children in regimen 6 served as a longitudinal control and received only annual examinations. Whereas in the fluoride-deficient areas, weekly fluoride rinsing was given as well as daily administration of fluoride tablets, in the fluoridated area, weekly rinsing only was performed and no tablets were given. All children received annual clinical and radiological examinations each year for 4 years: this was limited to permanent teeth. There were 31 examiners.

Baseline scores were lower in fluoridated sites than in fluoride-deficient sites, although the differences were in the range 20–35% rather than the usually quoted 40–60% (see Chapter 5). The mean DMFS increments are given in Table 19.6, for the 9566 continuous participants (about 50% of the original sample). Data were adjusted by covariance analysis for baseline imbalance between groups.

Table 19.6 Mean 4-year DMFS increments observed in the NPDDP (From Disney *et al.*, 1990a)

Regimen	*Fluoride-deficient*		*Fluoridated*	
	Grades 1+2 (6/7 yr)*	*Grade† 5 (10 yr)*	*Grades* 1+2 (6/7 yr)*	*Grade† 5 (10 yr)*
1. Comprehensive	1.23‡	2.84‡	0.90‡	1.05‡
2. Modified comprehensive	2.45‡	4.10	1.19‡	1.45‡
3. Clinic	1.45‡	2.92‡	0.95‡	1.33‡
4. Classroom	2.46‡	5.30	2.15	3.68
5. Education	3.01	5.35	2.44	3.49
6. Control	3.13	4.75	2.19	3.07

* Children who were initially in grades 1 and 2 were combined a single cohort (aged 6/7 years).
† Children who were initially in grade 5 (aged 10 years).
‡ Differs from the control regimen at the 0.001 level.

The results show that the most comprehensive procedure (regimen 1) prevented 40–66% of DMFS increment. However, because of the (unexpectedly) low incidence of decay, this represents a saving of between one and two DMFS over the 4 years. Virtually all the treatment effect resulted from the clinical procedures (Table 19.7). Only in one regimen did the combination of fluoride mouthrinse and

Table 19.7 Reductions in 4-year DMFS increments, recorded in the NPDDP, calculated for each procedure* (From Disney *et al.*, 1990a)

Procedure	*Fluoride-deficient*		*Fluoridated*	
	Grades 1+2 (6/7 yr)	*Grade 5 (10 yr)*	*Grades 1+2 (6/7 yr)*	*Grade 5 (10 yr)*
Clinic				
Sealants	1.33†	1.11‡	0.96†	2.00†
Prophy/gel	0.12	1.04	0.29	0.18
Total clinic	1.46†	2.15†	1.25†	2.18†
Classroom				
Mouthrinse/tablets**	0.44‡	0.21	0.29	0.03
Health lessons††	0.01	–0.44	–0.24	–0.20
Total classroom	0.45†	–0.24	0.05	–0.16

* The analysis of a procedure's effect involved children from several regimens; e.g., only regimen 2's data were excluded from the measurement of the mouthrinse effect.
† Differs significantly from zero at 0.001 level.
‡ Differs significantly from zero at 0.05 level.
** Fluoride tablets were offered only at non-fluoridated sites.
†† Includes bi-weekly brushing and flossing plus home supply of fluoride dentifrice.

fluoride tablets achieve a statistically significant effect, and even this amounted to only 0.44 surfaces per child over 4 years. Health lessons in the classroom were ineffective.

Further analyses of the data by Disney *et al.* (1989) showed that while FMR had little effect overall (0.65 surfaces saved over 4 years in the non-fluoridated area, and 0.25 surfaces saved in the fluoridated area over 4 years), the number of surfaces saved was greater for children retrospectively classed as high caries formers.

The costs, in 1981 US dollars, are given in Table 19.8. They include direct costs only (labour, materials and capital costs) and not indirect costs or overheads such as the time spent by volunteers: calculations revealed that the indirect costs about equalled the direct costs. It can be estimated from these figures that the cost of

Table 19.8 Average direct costs per child per year (in 1981 US dollars) (From Disney *et al.*, 1990a)

Regimen procedures	*Labour*	*Materials*	*Capital*	*Total*
1. Sealants Prophy/gel Fluoride mouthrinse Plaque control Education	39.92	10.89	4.11	54.92
2. Sealants or prophy/gel Fluoride mouthrinse Plaque control Education	26.69	8.92	2.35	37.97
3. Sealants Prophy/gel	31.80	3.95	4.26	40.02
4. Fluoride mouthrinse Plaque control Education	8.21	6.94	–	15.15
5. Plaque control Education	7.36	4.38	–	11.74

adding FMR to an existing dental education programme would be $3.41 per child per year, or adding FMR plus educational programme to the clinical programme would be $14.90.

The report of this very large study is important and has aroused much controversy in the USA (Bohannan *et al.*, 1985b, 1985c; Disney *et al.*, 1989, 1990a). The most controversial aspect concerns the place of weekly fluoride mouthrinsing, since this was shown to be of very marginal benefit in the fluoride-deficient areas and of no benefit in the fluoridated areas. One relevant point is that the NPDDP was conceived and managed by the American Fund for Dental Health (AFDH), funded by the Robert Wood Johnson (RWJ) Foundation and analysed by the Rand Corporation. It was therefore independent of NIDR. The findings on the value of FMR ran contrary to the views of NIDR which at that time was actively promoting the use of FMR in schools. These aspects and the lessons to be learned are well discussed by Disney *et al.* (1990a). The future use of fluoride rinsing as a school-based community measure in the USA will be watched with interest by dental public health workers in many countries, who are grateful that the USA has been able to undertake, report and discuss these studies in such an informative way.

Community prevention in Australia

Fluoridation is widespread in Australia, and its effectiveness in terms of reduction in caries experience has been discussed in Chapter 5. In addition, there have been some estimates of the effect of fluoridation on the cost of treating caries. Carr, Dooland and Roder (1980) compared the costs of dental treatment in the South Australian Dental Service in 1977 with the cost of fluoridation, which began in 1971. Costs and savings were adjusted to constant denominators by processes of deflation and application of discount rates, and they concluded that 'Water fluoridation in South Australia is presenting highly desirable cost-benefit characteristics'. Using a similar database, Roder and Sundram (1980) reported a 40% reduction in the number of restorations placed and a 38% reduction in the time required for dental care.

Fluoride drops and tablets have been widely recommended in areas without fluoridation and many authors have reported the extent of their use. Medcalf and O'Grady (1983) reported that 63% of parents of children born in the city of Bunbury, Western Australia, began daily administration of fluoride supplements, but only 11% had maintained it to the age of 8 years and 9% to the age of 15 years. Smyth (1984) found that 27% of children aged 4–12 years were taking fluoride tablets daily, while a further 28% did so occasionally. He reported better dental health and more regular dental attendance in the tablet-takers, in agreement with findings of Fanning and Somerville (1974) in South Australia. More recently, Seow, Humphrys and Powell (1987) reported a fall in the use of fluoride tablets in Brisbane (the only non-fluoridated capital city in Australia). While McEniery and Davies (1979) reported that about 50% of Brisbane children were taking fluoride supplements in 1977, the percentage had fallen to 15% in 1985. The proportion of toothpastes in Australia that contain fluoride rose from 26% in 1971, to 62% in 1976, to 94% in 1982 (Renson, 1986).

Interesting analyses of the association between three fluoride vehicles and caries experience of Australian adolescents were made by Spencer (1986a). The three vehicles were water, dietary supplements and toothpaste. The years of study were 1965–78 and the caries data came from 21 Australian surveys. All three fluoride vehicles were significantly and negatively associated with caries experience. The magnitude of regression coefficients indicated that the most important association was with fluoridated water supplies, followed by fluoride supplements, followed by fluoride-containing dentifrices. Spencer (1986b) predicted trends in caries experience in Australian adolescents between 1978 and 1990. Caries experience was expected to fall further and the three fluoride vehicles responsible for this were (in order of magnitude of effect): water fluoridation, fluoride dentifrices and fluoride tablets. There was, thus, a decline in the relative importance of fluoride tablets, on a national scale.

Cost–benefit analysis

Horowitz and Heifetz (1979) have pointed out that cost–benefit analysis is of value in deciding between alternative public health programmes where the primary objective differs (e.g. comparing a day-stay unit for dental procedures with an orthodontic screening service in schools). Here, both the cost of the benefits and the cost of implementation have to be calculated. In caries prevention it is frequently necessary to decide between alternative ways of achieving the same primary objective of caries prevention. It then becomes unnecessary to calculate the benefit in monetary terms and this can then be expressed in terms of the number of carious teeth or surfaces prevented. This is cost-effectiveness analysis, which enables the planner to determine the least expensive of several alternatives of achieving a stated objective.

It is not intended that this book should contain a full discussion of cost–benefit and cost-effectiveness analysis and the reader is referred to the Technical Report No. 13 of the Fédération Dentaire Internationale (1981) which contains an outline of methods with references.

It must be recognized that all such calculations are imperfect and serve only as the best available information for the planner. Of particular relevance is our lack of long-term knowledge of the caries-preventive effect of various fluoride procedures. Many procedures are school based and the benefits may be lost after the participants leave school. Public water fluoridation is the only fluoride therapy for which there is information on its lifelong effectiveness. Almost all the studies reported in the previous chapters have been short-term clinical trials, or what O'Mullane (1976) has classed as 'experimental clinical trials', where the agent or procedure is given the greatest chance of showing its effectiveness. The effectiveness of a preventive regimen may differ when implemented on a community basis from that observed in an experimental clinical trial, although the limited amount of data available, given in this chapter, seems to indicate that percentage reductions in community preventive schemes and experimental clinical trials are fairly similar.

Examples of cost–benefit analysis in caries prevention have increased over recent years and, in addition to examples already mentioned in this chapter, two other aspects of analysis are worth discussing. The first is analysis of data with respect to water fluoridation, whereas the second concerns fluoride rinsing.

One of the first investigations of the economics of fluoridation in the UK was by Dowell (1976). He highlighted the economies of scale and the necessity for discounting costs in analyses of water fluoridation. More recently, Birch (1990) presented data on the cost-effectiveness of water fluoridation using data collected in England between 1973 and 1985. Using the traditional model of economic evaluation, he showed that one of the most important variables was the existing level of caries experience, but economics of scale were also very relevant. He gave the example that the cost per unit benefit from fluoridating water for a small population with high caries experience was roughly the same as fluoridating water for a population 10 times as large but with low caries experience.

The economic costs and benefits of water fluoridation in Townsville, Australia, has been quantified by Doessel (1985). After using systematic disaggregation and valuation of demographic, dental and economic data, he concluded that significant economic benefits accrue to the Townsville community through water fluoridation.

Analyses of the economic costs incurred in school-based fluoride mouthrinsing programmes have been presented by Doherty *et al.* (1984), Doherty and Martie (1988) and Doherty (1990). The Community Caries Prevention Demonstration Program (Miller and Brunelle, 1983) was the database used. Costs were divided into explicit costs (direct expenditures for providing FMR) and implicit costs (the opportunity costs of resources donated or otherwise provided at no charge to the programme). Explicit costs were 68% of the total cost, and labour accounted for about four-fifths of the total costs. Explicit costs were found to increase as the number of participants in a program increased (Table 19.9), contrary to what might be expected. This has been termed a diseconomy of scale: it should be remembered that water fluoridation shows a strong economy of scale (unit cost decreases as number of participants increases). With each 1% increase in the FMR programme size, there was a 0.33% increase in per subject cost (Doherty and Martie, 1988). These findings illustrate the need to determine the optimum economic size for preventive programmes (Doherty, 1990).

Table 19.9 Estimated average explicit costs per participant in the US FMR Demonstration Program. Values given as US dollars, 1978 (From Doherty *et al.*, 1984)

No. participants ('000)	*Cost ($)*	
	Year 1	*Year 2*
1	1.37	2.17
2	2.31	2.58
3	3.25	2.99
4	4.19	3.30
5	5.03	3.81

There have been a number of attempts to review the cost-effectiveness of several methods for preventing dental caries – most of the methods being fluoride based. One of the most thorough reviews was achieved at a conference in Ann Arbor, Michigan, in 1978 (Burt, 1978). Table 19.10 is taken from this publication and provides a guide to the order of efficiency of fluoride programmes. The table is

Table 19.10 Ranking of alternative fluoride therapies according to estimated cost-effectiveness (From Newbrun, 1978 and Heifetz, 1978)

Procedure	*Estimated percentage caries reduction*	*Annual cost per capita ($)*	*Cost per 1 DMFS saved ($)*	*Rank*
Systemic				
Public water fluoridation	50	0.20	0.20	1
Fluoride tablet distribution	35	0.40	0.57	3
School water fluoridation	40	1.50	1.88	3
Topical				
Weekly mouthrinse (0.2% NaF)	25	0.50	1.00	1
Clinical application (multiple chair) (2% NaF)	40	2.06	2.60	2
Clinical application (annual) (1.23% F APF gel in tray)	40	3.50	4.40	3
Toothbrushing in school (5 × /yr) (0.6% F solution)	20	2.23	5.60	4
Toothbrushing at home (0.1% F toothpaste)	20	4.00	10.00	5
Daily self-application by tray (0.5% F APF gel)	80	34.09	21.30	6

compiled with the assumption of a caries increment of 2 DMFS per child per year in a low-fluoride area, and the costing is given in US dollars as calculations were made on US wages and material costs. For further details of how the costs were calculated, the reader is referred to the workshop report (Burt, 1978). These data are also reproduced (with very minor modifications) in the report of the Fédération Dentaire Internationale (1981). To emphasize how difficult it is to calculate the cost–benefit and cost-effectiveness of community programmes, Table 19.11 lists factors which may be excluded from analyses. For example, the estimation of the cost of weekly fluoride mouthrinsing (Table 19.10) excluded the cost of the teachers' time, which may have to be included in some communities. It is probable that in many estimates both the cost and the benefit are underestimated, although benefits are more likely to be underestimated than costs (Burt, 1978). Because

Table 19.11 Factors which are frequently excluded from cost–benefit analysis

Cost	*Benefit*
1. Teachers' time supervising preventive measure	1. Repeat treatment (e.g. fillings) of teeth not included in DMF index
2. Subjects' time doing preventive measure	2. Subjects' (and parents') time and cost of attending surgery for treatment
3. Discounting of costs (benefits accrue later)	3. Freedom from pain, infection, etc.
	4. Post-treatment benefit
	5. Benefit to deciduous teeth
	6. Effect on gingival health of a complete dentition and unrestored teeth

disease levels and resources will vary from community to community, a public health planner must estimate cost-effectiveness ratios based as much as possible on local information.

As mentioned earlier, lack of information on the effectiveness of school-based fluoride schemes after the child leaves school (post-treatment effect) is a serious gap.

Another attempt at calculating benefit–cost and cost-effective ratios has been published by Niessen and Douglass (1984). They evaluated four preventive programmes in a hypothetical community using established economic methods, both for a 'steady-state year' (one-year costs and benefits assuming maximum caries reduction in that year) and then over a 20-year period (which requires application of discounting) (Table 19.12). Community water fluoridation yielded the greatest net benefits and the most favourable B-C and C-E ratios. For example, looking at the top of the first data column, the data show that for every dollar spent on water fluoridation, benefits would be worth \$11.6. If the full benefits were realized only after 20 years, the benefits were reduced to \$8.2 (top of second data column). All these analyses are based on a wide range of assumptions; it is important that the reader is aware of these and does not take these figures at face value. They are, however, a most helpful guide to methods used in cost–benefit and cost-effectiveness calculations.

Using data from Canada and the USA, Clark and Trahan (1985) estimated the cost-effectiveness of four fluoride-based community programmes: water fluoridation, school water fluoridation, fluoride tablet programmes, and fluoride mouthrinse programmes. The same trend was seen of public water fluoridation

Table 19.12 Benefit-cost (B-C) ratios and cost-effectiveness (C-E) ratios calculated for four community preventive measures* (From Niessen and Douglass, 1984)

Programme	*Ratios*			
	B-C		*C-E*	
	Steady-state	*20-yr*	*Steady-state*	*20-yr*
Community water fluoridation	11.6	8.2	0.9	1.2
School water fluoridation	7.2	5.1	1.4	2.0
School-based FMR (incl. teachers' time)	1.8	1.6	5.4	6.3
School-based FMR (excl. teachers' time)	7.0	6.1	1.4	1.7
School-based sealant programme	0.9	0.9	11.3	11.8

* Data calculated for 'steady-state year' (assume maximum caries reduction in that year) and 20-year costs and benefits at present values (obtained by discounting).

being the most cost-effective, whereas mouthrinsing programmes were seen as slightly less favourable than fluoride tablet programmes, and possibly not a cost-effective approach in Canada.

Cost–benefit analysis is important to those involved in dental public health, and further developments in this area will undoubtedly occur.

Conclusions

The inspired observations by McKay in Colorado Springs at the very beginning of this century, followed by his persistent search for the cause of enamel mottling and caries inhibition, led eventually to the discovery of fluoride in drinking water. McKay's work was continued by H. Trendley Dean and other researchers, who showed that the adjustment of water fluoride levels could reduce dental caries, and the effectiveness of water fluoridation has now been documented throughout the world. The study of the systemic and topical effects of fluoride has produced a tremendous outpouring of research, particularly over the past 60 years, and our knowledge of dental epidemiology, clinical trials, dental public health, dental plaque, physiology, biochemistry, toxicity and aspects of general health has increased enormously as a result. Dental health of children has improved dramatically in some countries due to the wider use of fluorides. Fluorides have a vital role in reversing the trend of increasing caries experience in some developing countries. Our aim has been to review the development of these various strands and to try to draw them together in order to give the reader a perspective of the vital part that fluorides can play in caries prevention.

References

Allmark, C., Green, H. P., Linney, A. D., Wills, D. J. and Picton, D. C. A. (1982) A community study of fluoride tablets for schoolchildren in Portsmouth. *Br. Dent. J.*, **153,** 426–430

Anderson, R. J. (1981) The changes in the dental health of 12-year-old schoolchildren in two Somerset schools; a review after an interval of 15 years. *Br. Dent. J.*, **150**, 218–221

Artun, J. and Brobakken, B. O. (1986) Prevalence of carious white spots after orthodontic treatment with multibonded appliances. *Eur. J. Orthodont.*, **8**, 229–234

Bawden, J. W., Granath, L., Holst, K., Koch, G., Krasse, P. and Rootzen, H. (1980) Effect of mouthrinsing with a sodium fluoride solution in children with different caries experience. *Swed. Dent. J.*, **4**, 111–117

Bennie, A. M., Tullis, J. I., Stephen, K. W. and MacFadyen, E. E. (1978) Five years of community preventive dentistry and health education in the County of Sutherland, Scotland. *Community Dent. Oral Epidemiol.*, **6**, 1–5

Berggren, H. and Welander, E. (1960) Supervised toothbrushing with a sodium fluoride solution in 5000 Swedish schoolchildren. *Acta Odontol. Scand.*, **18**, 209–234

Birch, S. (1990) The relative cost effectiveness of water fluoridation across communities; analysis of variations according to underlying caries levels. *Community Dent. Hlth*, **7**, 3–10

Bohannan, H. M., Graves, R. C., Disney, J. A., Stamm, J. W., Abernathy, J. B. and Bader, J. D. (1985b) Effect of secular decline in caries on the evaluation of preventive dentistry demonstrations. *J. Publ. Hlth Dent.*, **45**, 83–89

Bohannan, H. M., Klein, S. P., Disney, J. A., Bell, R. M., Graves, R. C. and Foch, C. B. (1985a) A summary of the results of the national preventive dentistry demonstration program. *J. Can. Dent. Ass.*, **51**, 435–441

Bohannan, H. M., Stamm, J. W., Graves, R. C., Disney, J. A. and Bader, J. D. (1985c) Fluoride mouthrinse programmes in fluoridated communities. *J. Am. Dent. Ass.*, **111**, 783–789

British Association for the Study of Community Dentistry (1988) *The Home Use of Fluorides for Pre-school Children. A Policy Document.* B.A.S.C.D., Cardiff

Brown, R. H. (1988) Fluoride and the prevention of dental caries; part 1; the role of fluoride in the decline of caries. *N.Z. Dent. J.*, **84**, 103–108

Brunelle, J. A. and Carlos, J. P. (1990) Recent trends in dental caries in US children and the effect of water fluoridation. *J. Dent. Res.*, **69** (spec. issue), 723–727

Burt, B. A. (1978) *The Relative Efficiency of Methods of Caries Prevention in Dental Public Health*, Proceedings of a Workshop at the University of Michigan, June 5–8, 1978, University of Michigan, Ann Arbor

Carr, S. M., Dooland, M. B. and Roder, D. M. (1980) Fluoridation, II; an interim economic analysis. *Austral. Dent. J.*, **25**, 343–348

Clark, D. C. and Trahan, L. (1985) Fluorides for community programs. *J. Can. Dent. Ass.*, **51**, 773–777

Colquhoun, J. and Mann, R. (1986) The Hastings fluoridation experiment; science or swindle? *The Ecologist*, **16**, 243–248

De Liefde, B. (1989) Identification and preventive care of high caries-risk children; a longitudinal study. *N.Z. Dent. J.*, **85**, 112–116

Demers, M., Brodeur, J.-M., Simard, P. L., Mouton, C., Veilleux, G. and Frechette, S. (1990) Caries predictors suitable for mass-screenings in children; a literature review. *Community Dent. Hlth*, **7**, 11–21

Diesendorf, M. (1986) The mystery of declining tooth decay. *Nature*, **322**, 125–129

Dismer, G. A. (1982) Sodium fluoride mouthrinse; three year study. *Illinois Dent. J.*, **51**, 158–160

Disney, J. A., Bohannan, H. M., Klein, S. P. and Bell, R. M. (1990a) A case study in contesting the conventional wisdom; school-based fluoride mouthrinse programmes in the USA. *Community Dent. Oral Epidemiol.*, **18**, 46–56

Disney, J. A., Graves, R. C., Stamm, J. W., Bohannan, H. M. and Abernathy, J. R. (1989) Comparative effects of a four-year fluoride mouthrinse program on high and low caries forming grade 1 children. *Community Dent. Oral Epidemiol.*, **17**, 139–143

Disney, J. A., Stamm, J. W., Graves, R. C., Abernathy, J. R. *et al.* (1990b) Description and preliminary results of a caries risk assessment model. In *Risk Assessment in Dentistry* (ed. J. D. Bader), University of North Carolina, Chapel Hill, pp. 204–214

Doessel, D. P. (1985) Cost-benefit analysis of water fluoridation in Townsville, Australia. *Community Dent. Oral Epidemiol.*, **13**, 19–22

Doherty, N. J. G. (1990) Resource productivity and returns to scale in school-based mouthrinsing programs. *Community Dent. Oral Epidemiol.*, **18**, 57–60

Doherty, N. J. G., Brunelle, J. A., Miller, A. J. and Li, S. H. (1984) Costs of school-based mouthrinsing in 14 demonstration programmes in USA. *Community Dent. Oral Epidemiol.*, **12**, 35–38

Doherty, N. J. G. and Martie, C. W. (1988) Effects of wages and scale on the costs of school-based mouthrinsing programs in the USA. *Community Dent. Oral Epidemiol.*, **16**, 27–29

Dowell, T. B. (1976) The economics of fluoridation. *Br. Dent. J.*, **140,** 103–106

Downer, M. C. (1987) Dental caries prevention in the United Kingdom and its statutory basis. In *Strategy for Dental Caries Prevention in European Countries According to their Laws and Regulations* (eds R. M. Frank and S. O'Hickey), IRL Press, Oxford, pp. 37–39

Eichenbaum, I. W., Dunn, N. A. and Tinanoff, N. (1981) Impact of fluoridation in a private pedodontic practice; thirty years later. *J. Dent. Child.*, **48**, 211–214

Ekstrand, J., Koch, G., Lindgren, L. E. and Petersson, L. G. (1981) Pharmacokinetics of fluoride gels in children and adults. *Caries Res.*, **15**, 213–220

Fanning, E. A. and Somerville, C. M. (1974) South Australian kindergarten children; dental health factors in urban and country families. *Austral. Dent. J.*, **19,** 35–38

Fédération Dentaire Internationale (1981) Cost effectiveness of community fluoride programmes for caries prevention. *FDI Technical Report 13*, FDI, London

Frank, R. M. and Cahan, P. M. (1987) Dental caries in France; epidemiology and prevention studies. In *Strategy for Dental Caries Prevention in European Countries According to their Laws and Regulations* (eds R. M. Frank and S. O'Hickey), IRL Press, Oxford, pp. 145–154

Glass, R. L. (1982) The first international conference on the declining prevalence of dental caries. *J. Dent. Res.*, **61** (special issue), 1301–1383

Gorelick, L., Geiger, A. M. and Gwinnett, A. J. (1982) Incidence of white spot formation after bonding and banding. *Am. J. Orthodont.*, **81**, 93–98

Grembowski, D. (1984) The effects of fluoridation on dental care demand. *Compend. Contin. Educ.*, **5**, 689–695

Haugejorden, O., Lervick, T. and Riordan, P. J. (1985) Comparison of caries prevalence 7 years after discontinuation of school-based fluoride rinsing or toothbrushing in Norway. *Community Dent. Oral Epidemiol.*, **13**, 2–6

Health Education Authority (1989) *The Scientific Basis of Dental Health Education. A Policy Document*, 3rd edn, H.E.A., London

Heifetz, S. B. (1978) Cost-effectiveness of topically applied fluorides. In *The Relative Efficiency of Methods of Caries Prevention in Dental Public Health* (ed. B. A. Burt), University of Michigan, Ann Arbor, pp. 69–104

Heifetz, S. B. and Horowitz, H. S. (1984) The amounts of fluoride in current fluoride therapies; safety considerations for children. *J. Dent. Child.*, **51,** 257–269

Heifetz, S. B., Meyers, R. J. and Kingman, A. (1982) A comparison of the anti-caries effectiveness of daily and weekly rinsing with sodium fluoride solutions; final results after three years. *Pediat. Dent.*, **4**, 300–303

Helm, S. and Helm, T. (1990) Caries among Danish schoolchildren in birth-cohorts 1950–78. *Community Dent. Oral Epidemiol.*, **18,** 66–69

Hoffman, R., Mann, J., Calderone, J., Trumbull, J. and Burkhart, M. (1980) Acute fluoride poisoning in a New Mexico elementary school. *Pediatrics*, **65**, 897–900

Holland, T., O'Leary, K. and O'Mullane, D. (1987) The effectiveness of a fortnightly mouthrinsing programme in the prevention of dental caries in schoolchildren. *J. Irish Dent. Ass.*, **33**, 24–27

Holt, R. D., Winter, G. B., Fox, B. and Askew, R. (1985) Effects of dental health education for mothers with young children in London. *Community Dent. Oral Epidemiol.*, **13**, 148–151

Holt, R. D., Winter, G. B., Fox, B. and Askew, R. (1989) Second assessment of London children involved in a scheme of dental health education in infancy. *Community Dent. Oral Epidemiol.*, **17**, 180–182

Holt, R. D., Winter, G. B., Fox, B., Askew, R. and Lo, G. L. (1983) Dental health education through home visits to mothers with young children. *Community Dent. Oral Epidemiol.*, **11**, 98–101

Honkala, E., Nyyssonen, V. and Rimpela, A. (1984) Use of fluorides by Finnish adolescents. *Scand. J. Dent. Res.*, **92**, 517–523

Horowitz, A. M. (1985) Ways to improve/increase appropriate use of dietary fluorides. *J. Dent. Child.*, **52**, 269–274

Horowitz, H. S. (1977) Abusive use of fluoride. Editorial. *J. Public Hlth Dent.*, **37**, 106–107

Horowitz, H. S. (1990) The future of water fluoridation and other systemic fluorides. *J. Dent. Res.*, **69** (special issue), 760–764

Horowitz, H. S. and Heifetz, S. B. (1979) Methods for assessing the cost-effectiveness of caries preventive agents and procedures. *Int. Dent. J.*, **29**, 106–117

Horowitz, H. S., Heifetz, S. B., McClendon, J., Viegas, A. R., Guimaraes, L. O. C. and Lopes, E. S. (1974) Evaluation of self-administered prophylaxis and supervised toothbrushing with acidulated phosphate fluoride. *Caries Res.*, **8**, 39–51

Kidd, E. A. M. and Joyston-Bechal, S. (1987) *Essentials of Dental Caries*, Wright, Bristol

Koch, G. (1982) Evidence for declining caries prevalence in Sweden. *J. Dent. Res.*, **61** (special issue), 1340–1345

Konig, K. G. (1987) Results obtained and methods used in caries prevention in the Netherlands. In *Strategy for Dental Caries Prevention in European Countries According to their Laws and Regulations* (eds R. M. Frank and S. O'Hickey), IRL Press, Oxford, pp. 61–73

Krasse, B. (1985) *Caries Risk*, Quintessence, Chicago

LeCompte, E. J. (1987) Clinical aspects of topical fluoride products – risks, benefits and recommendations. *J. Dent. Res.*, **66**, 1066–1071

LeCompte, E. J. and Doyle, T. E. (1985) Effects of suctioning devices on oral fluoride retention. *J. Am. Dent. Ass.*, **110**, 357–360

Lokken, P. and Birkeland, J. M. (1978) Acceptance, caries reduction and reported adverse effects of fluoride prophylaxis in Norway. *Community Dent. Oral Epidemiol.*, **6**, 110–116

McCall, D. R., Watkins, T. R., Stephen, K. W., Collins, W. J. N. and Smalls, M. J. (1983) Fluoride ingestion following APF gel application. *Br. Dent. J.*, **155**, 333–336

McEniery, M. and Davies, G. N. (1979) Brisbane dental survey 1977: a comparative study of caries experience of children in Brisbane, Australia over a 20 year period. *Community Dent. Oral Epidemiol.*, **7**, 42–50

Marthaler, T. M. (1987) Results obtained and methods used in caries prevention in Switzerland. In *Strategy for Dental Caries Prevention in European Countries According to their Laws and Regulations* (eds R. M. Frank and S. O'Hickey), IRL Press, Oxford, pp. 159–172

Medcalf, G. W. and O'Grady, M. J. (1983) The dental health of children eight and fifteen years of age living in Bunbury, Western Australia. *Austral. Dent. J.*, **28**, 162–165

Miller, A. J. and Brunelle, J. A. (1983) A summary of the NIDR community caries prevention demonstration program. *J. Am. Dent. Ass.*, **107**, 265–269

Murray, J. J. (1986) *Appropriate Use of Fluorides for Human Health*, World Health Organisation, Geneva

Murray, J. J. and Rugg-Gunn, A. J. (1987) *Fluoridation and Declining Decay; a Reply to Diesendorf*, British Fluoridation Society, London

Newbrun, E. (1978) Cost-effectiveness and practicality features in the systemic use of fluorides. In *The Relative Efficiency of Methods of Caries Prevention in Dental Public Health* (ed. B. A. Burt), University of Michigan, Ann Arbor, pp. 27–48

Newbrun, E. (1989) Effectiveness of water fluoridation. *J. Publ. Hlth Dent.*, **49**, 279–289

Niessen, L. C. and Douglass, C. W. (1984) Theoretical considerations in applying benefit-cost and cost-effectiveness analyses to preventive dental programmes. *J. Publ. Hlth Dent.*, **44**, 156–167

Ogaard, B. (1989) Prevalence of white spot lesions in 19-year-olds: a study on untreated and orthodontically treated persons 5 years after treatment. *Am. J. Orthodont. Dentofacial Orthopaedics*, **96**, 423–427

Ogaard, B., Rolla, G., Arends, J. and ten Cate, J. M. (1988) Orthodontic appliances and enamel demineralization. Part 2: Prevention and treatment of lesions. *Am. J. Orthodont. Dentofacial Orthopaedics*, **94**, 123–128

O'Mullane, D. M. (1976) Efficiency in clinical trials of caries preventive agents and methods. *Community Dent. Oral Epidemiol.*, **4**, 190–194

O'Mullane, D. M. (1987) Changes in the prevalence of dental caries in Irish schoolchildren between 1961 and 1984. In *Strategy for Dental Caries Prevention in European Countries According to their Laws and Regulations* (eds R. M. Frank and S. O'Hickey), IRL Press, Oxford, pp. 197–206

O'Mullane, D. M. (1990) The future of water fluoridation. *J. Dent. Res.*, **69** (special issue), 756–759

O'Mullane, D. M., Clarkson, J., Holland, T., O'Hickey, S. and Whelton, H. (1986) *Children's Dental Health in Ireland*, Stationery Office, Dublin

O'Rourke, C. A., Attrill, M. and Holloway, P. J. (1988) Cost appraisal of a fluoride tablet programme to Manchester primary schoolchildren. *Community Dent. Oral Epidemiol.*, **16**, 341–344

Osterbrock, N. L. (1985) Fluoride mouthrinsing in Cincinnati elementary schools. *Bull. Cinci. Dent. Soc.*, **54**, 17–18

Palmer, J. D. (1980) Dental health in children – an improving picture? *Br. Dent. J.*, **149**, 48–50

Pinet, G. L. (1987) Analysis of laws and regulations related to caries prevention in Europe; a synthesis. In *Strategy for Dental Caries Prevention in European Countries According to their Laws and Regulations* (eds R. M. Frank and S. O'Hickey), IRL Press, Oxford, pp. 243–262

Renson, C. E. (1986) Changing patterns of dental caries; a survey of 20 countries. *Ann. Acad. Med. Singapore,* **15**, 284–298

Renson, C. E. (1989) Global changes in caries prevalence and dental manpower requirements: 2. The reasons underlying the changes in prevalence. *Dental Update,* **16**, 345–351

Rey, J. (1987) Legal aspects related to caries prevention in France. In *Strategy for Dental Caries Prevention in European Countries According to their Laws and Regulations* (eds R. M. Frank and S. O'Hickey), IRL Press, Oxford, pp. 155–157

Ripa, L. W. (1984) A personalized regimen of multiple fluoride therapy for child patients. *N.Y. State Dent. J.*, **54**, 59–64

Ripa, L. W. (1987) Caries prevention in children; the use of fluoride mouthrinses and pit and fissure sealants. *N.Y. State Dent. J.*, **53**, 16–20

Rise, J. and Haugejorden, O. (1980) Monitoring and evaluation of results of community fluoride programs in Norway during the 1960s and 1970s. *Community Dent. Oral Epidemiol.*, **8**, 79–83

Roberts, J. F. and Longhurst, P. (1987) A clinical estimation of the fluoride used during application of a fluoride varnish. *Br. Dent. J.*, **162**, 463–466

Roder, D. M. and Sundram, P. S. (1980) Fluoridation, 1; effects on children's caries rates and professionally defined requirements for dental care. *Austral. Dent. J.*, **25**, 76–80

Rolla, G. and Ogaard, B. (1987) Reduction in caries incidence in Norway from 1970 to 1984 and some considerations concerning the reasons for this phenomenon. In *Strategy for Dental Caries Prevention in European Countries According to their Laws and Regulations* (eds R. M. Frank and S. O'Hickey), IRL Press, Oxford, pp. 223–229

Rugg-Gunn, A. J. (1990) *A Critique of the Publications of John Colquhoun Concerning the Benefits and Risks of Fluoridation*, British Fluoridation Society, London

Russell, J. I., MacFarlane, T. W., Aitchison, T. C., Stephen, K. W. and Burchell, C. K. (1990) Caries prevalence and microbiological and salivary caries activity tests in Scottish adolescents. *Community Dent. Oral Epidemiol.*, **18**, 120–125

Scheetz, J. P., Suddick, R. P. and Fields, W. T. (1984) Attitudes of school personnel and parents towards a school-based fluoride mouthrinse program. *Community Dent. Oral Epidemiol.*, **12**, 82–88

Scheirer, M. A., Allen, B. F. and Rauch, H. J. (1987) The adoption and implementation of the fluoride mouthrinse program; descriptive results from school districts. *J. Publ. Hlth Dent.*, **47**, 98–107

Schwarz, E. (1987) Dental caries prevention and legislation in Denmark. In *Strategy for Dental Caries Prevention in European Countries According to their Laws and Regulations* (eds R. M. Frank and S. O'Hickey), IRL Press, Oxford, pp. 89–102

Seow, W. K., Humphrys, C. and Powell, R. N. (1987) The use of fluoride supplementation in a non-fluoridated city in Australia in 1985. *Community Dent. Hlth,* **4**, 97–105

Siegel, C. and Gutgesell, M. E. (1982) Fluoride supplementation in Harris County, Texas. *Am. J. Dis. Child.*, **136**, 61–63

Smyth, J. S. (1984) Fluoride tablets and dental health. *Austral. Dent. J.*, **29**, 296–299

Smyth, J. F. A. and Withnell, A. (1974) Daily fluoride tablets. *Hlth Soc. Sci. J.*, **84**, 419–423

Spencer, A. J. (1986a) Past association of fluoride vehicles with caries severity in Australian adolescents. *Community Dent. Oral Epidemiol.*, **14**, 233–237

Spencer, A. J. (1986b) Contribution of fluoride vehicles to change in caries severity in Australian adolescents. *Community Dent. Oral Epidemiol.*, **14**, 238–241

Stamm, J. W., Bohannan, H. M., Graves, R. C. and Disney, J. A. (1984) The efficiency of caries prevention with weekly fluoride mouthrinses. *J. Dent. Educ.*, **48**, 617–624

Stephen, K. W. and Campbell, D. (1978) Caries reduction and cost benefit after three years of sucking fluoride tablets daily at school. *Br. Dent. J.*, **144,** 202–208

Stephen, K. W. and MacFadyen, E. E. (1977) Three years of clinical caries prevention for cleft palate children. *Br. Dent. J.*, **143**, 111–113

Tala, H. (1987) Strategy of dental caries prevention in Finland according to the health legislation and other legal regulations. In *Strategy for Dental Caries Prevention in European Countries According to their Laws and Regulations* (eds R. M. Frank and S. O'Hickey), IRL Press, Oxford, pp. 103–117

Todd, J. E. and Dodd, T. (1985) *Children's Dental Health in the United Kingdom 1983*, HMSO, London

Torell, P. and Ericsson, Y. (1974) The potential benefits to be derived from fluoride mouthrinses. In *International Workshop on Fluorides and Dental Caries Reductions* (eds D. J. Forrester and E. M. Schulz), University of Maryland, Baltimore, pp. 113–176

Tremp, E. (1987) Dental caries prevention, laws and regulations in Switzerland. In *Strategy for Dental Caries Prevention in European Countries According to their Laws and Regulations* (eds R. M. Frank and S. O'Hickey), IRL Press, Oxford, pp. 173–179

Tyler, J. E. and Andlaw, R. J. (1987) Oral retention of fluoride after application of acidulated phosphate fluoride gel in air-cushion trays. *Br. Dent. J.*, **162,** 422–425

Von der Fehr, F. R. (1982) Evidence of decreasing caries prevalence in Norway. *J. Dent. Res.*, **61** (special issue), 1331–1335

WHO/FDI (1985) Report of a Working Group convened jointly by the FDI and the WHO: changing patterns of oral health and implications for oral health manpower, part 1. *Int. Dent. J.*, **35**, 235–251

Widenheim, J., Birkhed, D., Hase, J. C. and Olavi, G. (1989) Effect on approximal caries in teenagers of interrupting a school-based weekly NaF mouthrinse program for 3 years. *Community Dent. Oral Epidemiol.*, **17**, 83–86

Index